Vaccine
**Religious Exemption
Essentials**

"O Timothy, keep that which is committed to thy trust, avoiding profane and vain babblings, and oppositions of science falsely so called." (1 Timothy 6:20)

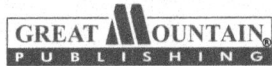

Copyright © 2025 by Edward Hendrie
All Rights Reserved
ISBN: 978-1-943056-20-0
Other books from Great Mountain Publishing®

- Hoax of Biblical Proportions
- Yahweh Is NOT the LORD JEHOVAH
- 9/11-Enemies Foreign and Domestic
- Solving the Mystery of BABYLON THE GREAT
- The Anti-Gospel
- Bloody Zion
- What Shall I Do to Inherit Eternal Life?
- Murder, Rape, and Torture in a Catholic Nunnery
- Antichrist: The Beast Revealed
- The Greatest Lie on Earth
- The Greatest Lie on Earth (Expanded Edition)
- Rome's Responsibility for the Assassination of Abraham Lincoln
- The Damnable Heresy of Salvation by Dead Faith (Expanded Edition)
- The Sphere of Influence
- Vaccine Danger: Quackery and Sin

Available at:
https://greatmountainpublishing.com
https://play.google.com
www.barnesandnoble.com
www.amazon.com

Edward Hendrie rests on the authority of the Holy Bible alone for doctrine. He considers the Holy Bible to be the inspired and inerrant word of God. Favorable citation by Edward Hendrie to an authority outside the Holy Bible on a particular issue should not be interpreted to mean that he agrees with all of the doctrines and beliefs of the cited authority. All Scripture references are to the Authorized (King James) Version of the Holy Bible, unless otherwise indicated.

Table of Contents

Introduction 1

1	Vaccination: A Superstitious Religious Practice.	8
2	Heresy to Do Evil That Good May Come	34
3	The Ends Do Not Justify the Means	44
4	The Sacrament of Vaccination.	55
5	The Truth about the Polio Vaccine	66
6	Proof That the Measles Virus Does Not Exist.	77
7	The Emperor Has No Virus.	83
8	The Spanish Flu of 1918	87
9	SARS-CoV-2 Virus Has Never Been Isolated.	95
10	The Lie of Asymptomatic Virus Spread	104
11	Exosomes.	108
12	Injecting Disease	113
13	Poisonous Magic Potions.	116
14	Unsafe and Ineffective Flu Vaccines.	125
15	COVID-19 Vaccine Scam	138
16	COVID-19 Vaccines are Ineffective	170
17	COVID-19 Vaccines Are Dangerous.	213

18	CDC Changes the Definition of Vaccine	238
19	Increased All-Cause Mortality	246
20	Prion Disease	262
21	Myocarditis	265
22	Killing Children to Save Them	283
23	Sudden Adult Death Syndrome	287
24	How the Vaccine Makers Scammed the Public	289
25	Food Allergies	311
26	Toxic Excipients	315
27	Vaccines Are Dangerous Medical Quackery	337
28	Vaccines Cause Autism	377
29	Dangerous Placebos	390
30	Pediatricians Are Paid Bounties	403
31	Buying Influence to Injure and Kill	418
32	Jacobson v. Massachusetts	425
33	First Amendment Free Exercise Clause	435
34	The Religious Freedom Restoration Act	440
35	Title VII of the Civil Rights Act of 1964	443
36	Unconstitutional Accommodations	448

37	First Amendment Establishment Clause	451
38	Inflating COVID-19 Death Statistics	489
39	5G Radiation Sickness	534
40	The Disappearing Flu	542
41	State Action by Hospitals	550
42	Courts Cannot Question Religious Beliefs	557
43	Avoid The Sectarian Trap	562
44	The Military Vaccine Complex	572
45	Unlawful COVID-19 Mandates	594
46	Moral Hazard	622
Endnotes		633

Introduction

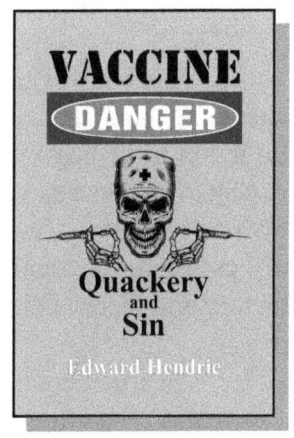

This book is largely excerpted from the 1,200 page book, *Vaccine Danger: Quackery and Sin.*[1] That book addresses many issues beyond the scope of obtaining a religious exemption from vaccination. This book has an expanded discussion of the legal standard for religious exemptions. *Vaccine Danger*, at 1200 pages, could not be expanded with additional legal analysis. Rather than having to purchase *Vaccine Danger* to obtain the vital information about the history, ineffectiveness, and dangers of vaccines that underlie an effective religious exemption claim, I incorporated those parts of *Vaccine Danger* germane to a vaccine exemption claim into this book. The concept behind this book is to provide a person with the necessary information to argue authoritatively against vaccination for his child or himself.

There are many arguments people have not made when seeking a religious exemption. Often, a person seeking a religious exemption is bulldozed by a government agency or private employer with improper inquiries into the details of a person's religious beliefs and the scope of their objection to vaccination.

This book is intended to level the playing field. Indeed, it is this author's view that there is no basis for any entity ever to deny a person's exemption based on his sincerely held religious objection to a vaccine. Once you read this book, you will have sufficient knowledge to go toe-to-toe with the administration of any organization and dismantle their arguments against your religious exemption. You will be able to see through the trickery and dishonesty that permeates the denials of religious exemptions.

This book begins by explaining the history and premise of vaccines. After that, it explains the different legal standards in litigation regarding religious exemptions. Ordinarily, one would expect to have the standard for review laid out first. Indeed, it was my first impulse to do just that. However, I realized that a detailed discussion of the legal standard requires an understanding of the history and theory behind vaccines.

An argument that litigants are not presently making is that vaccination is a religious ritual that governments impose on their citizens in violation of the Establishment Clause of the First Amendment. To understand the legal standard for that argument, it is necessary first to understand the superstitious religious origins of vaccines. It would be most beneficial for the reader to understand the history and nature of vaccines to most effectively apply the legal standards. By doing it that way, it was not necessary to repeat concepts that had already been explained in detail earlier in the book.

This book will reveal that vaccination is not a medical treatment; it is a superstitious religious ritual. You will understand that you are not seeking a religious exemption from a medical treatment but rather a religious exemption from an unsafe and ineffective religious custom. All governments that mandate vaccination violate the Establishment Clause of the First Amendment by requiring participation in a religious ritual. Unfortunately, litigants arguing for a religious exemption from vaccines are not making that claim. Typically, they limit their argument to a Freedom of Religion claim, arguing for a religious exemption from a medical treatment. Consequently, they come to court with two strikes against them.

To make a successful Establishment Clause argument, it is necessary first to understand the superstitious religious origins of vaccines, their dangers, and inefficacy. The dangers and ineffectiveness of vaccines are outgrowths of the unscientific, superstitious origins of vaccines. Indeed, it can properly be said that ineffectiveness and hazards are features of vaccines. Once a litigant raises an Establishment of Religion issue, the vaccine dangers and ineffectiveness become germane. But most people do not know that vaccination is a religious ritual. And thus, they do not know how to raise an Establishment Clause argument.

The book delves into the dangers and ineffectiveness of vaccines in great detail. That is essential information. You can use that information to support your request for a religious exemption. Entities seeking to deny a request for a religious exemption will often try to head off any discussion of the efficacy or safety of vaccines. They will disallow you from raising the issue. They will claim that such a discussion is irrelevant. But you can rebut that argument by simply citing a single Bible passage found at Romans 3:8, which admonishes Christians in the most strident language not to do evil that good may come.

The theory of vaccines is to inject poison into a healthy person (which is an evil act) so that later the person will develop an immunity to the antigen (the expected good outcome). Vaccination is premised on the heresy that it is okay to do evil so that good may come about from it. In Romans 3:8, God calls that ethic "damnable." Vaccination is a sin. No Christian should ever participate in the practice. Romans 3:8 can be the basis for both Establishment Clause and Freedom of Religion claims.

Vaccines are given to people who are well. It is against the Christian faith to be injected with a vaccine when the person is not ill. That is doing evil that good may come about. To do so is to take on a spirit of fear and reliance on man rather than God.

> But when Jesus heard that, he said unto them, They that be whole need not a physician, but they that are sick. (Matthew 9:12)
>
> For God has not given us a spirit of fear, but of power and of love and of a sound mind (2 Timothy 1:7).

Christians are bound to care for their bodies as it is the temple of the Holy Spirit.

> Know ye not that ye are the temple of God, and that the Spirit of God dwelleth in you? If any man defile the temple of God, him shall God destroy; for the temple of God is holy, which temple ye are. (1 Corinthians 3:16-17)
>
> What? know ye not that your body is the temple of the Holy Ghost which is in you, which ye have of God, and ye are not your own? For ye are bought with a price: therefore glorify God in your body, and in your spirit, which are God's. (1 Corinthians 6:19-20)

It is the wish of God that we prosper in our physical health. "Beloved, I wish above all things that thou mayest prosper and be in health, even as thy soul prospereth." 3 John 1:2. Christians sincerely believe that vaccines are detrimental to their health, and thus, it would violate a Christian's sincerely held religious beliefs to harm their body by being vaccinated.

To support the argument that vaccination is a sin that violates Romans 3:8, the Christian must be able to bring evidence proving that vaccination is evil. That evil is most clearly seen by the death and injury vaccines cause. Furthermore, it is also necessary for the Christian to set forth proof that vaccination is ineffective. Indeed, the ineffectiveness of vaccination is part and parcel of it being based on the germ theory, which has never been proven. The germ theory is actually founded on a religious superstition.

To take part in an ineffective and harmful religious practice is to approve fraud and authorize evil. Christians are to "abstain from all appearance of evil." 1 Thessalonians 5:22. Indeed, we are to reprove evil. "And have no fellowship with the unfruitful works of darkness, but rather reprove them." (Ephesians 5:11) Christians must speak out against vaccination, not take part in the evil practice. It is a sin for a Christian to get vaccinated, i.e., to go along to get along.

The gospel message is that those who have saving faith and are thus justified will live by that faith. Their faith is a living faith, not a dead faith. "For therein is the righteousness of God revealed from faith to faith: as it is written, The just shall live by faith." Romans 1:17. See also Galatians 3:11. Indeed, God has a warning for those who purport to believe but who do not live by faith. "Now the just shall live by faith: but if any man draw back, my soul shall have no pleasure in him." (Hebrews 10:38) "Not every one that saith unto me, Lord, Lord, shall enter into the kingdom of heaven; but he that doeth the will of my Father which is in heaven." (Matthew 7:21) Faith brings obedience. It is special obedience wrought by God through faith that God imparts in the believer. "But now is made manifest, and by the scriptures of the prophets, according to the commandment of the everlasting God, made known to all nations for the obedience of faith." (Romans 16:26)

There is a malevolent spirit behind vaccines. The practice of vaccination is part of a conspiracy against God and man. While most doctors are unwitting, some are willing minions of that old serpent, called the Devil, and Satan, who are quite happy to kill people for profit. Jesus describes such men:

> Ye are of your father the devil, and the lusts of your father ye will do. He was a murderer from the beginning, and abode not in the truth, because there is no truth in him. When he speaketh a lie, he speaketh of his own: for he is a liar, and the father of it. John 8:44.

All medical care and advice should be customized to the unique needs and characteristics of the patient. The author of this book is not a medical professional, and this book creates no physician-patient or lawyer-client relationship. This book is for informational and educational purposes and does not constitute medical or legal advice or professional services. The information provided in this book should not be used for diagnosing or treating a health problem or disease. That should only be done by a medical professional who knows your unique medical history and condition. If you believe your rights have been infringed, seek legal counsel.

When seeking medical advice, you should find a medical professional who is not a quack. Seek a doctor who will not blindly follow the sometimes unsafe and ineffective edicts of incompetent government bureaucrats. Do your due diligence and take charge of your medical care by being informed and asking questions. When remedying a disease, a doctor should try to find the cause of that disease rather than treat only the symptoms. If you believe a vaccine or a pharmaceutical drug has injured you, find a doctor who will at least acknowledge that possibility and thus be able to treat the cause of your illness.

Edward Hendrie
July 22, 2025

1 Vaccination: A Superstitious Religious Practice

The first mistake most people make when seeking a religious exemption from vaccination is assuming vaccination is a medical treatment. This assumption puts individuals seeking a religious exemption at a disadvantage. He comes to the plate with two strikes against him. The person seeking an exemption should frame the issue properly. The petitioner should not argue against being forced to participate in a medical treatment but rather against being forced to participate in a superstitious religious practice. To make that argument, the petitioner must educate the institution from which he seeks the exemption about the little-known history and foundational principles of vaccination.

Many attribute the practice of vaccination to the quack doctor Edward Jenner (1749-1823).[2] The very word vaccine is from the Latin word for cow. Jenner pulled a trick. He renamed cowpox *variolae vaccinae,* from which we get the word vaccine. Jenner called the cowpox that he injected into humans *variolae vaccinae*. Jenner's theory was that it would make them immune from smallpox. While Jenner is often credited with the cowpox/smallpox hypothesis, it can be traced past Jenner's first experiments in 1796 to a farmer, Benjamin Jesty (1736-1816), who first used cowpox to innoculate against smallpox in 1774.[3] Cowpox is a disease of cows' udders and has no relation to smallpox, except they both have the suffix "pox" in their names. Indeed, *variolae vaccinae*, which means smallpox of the cow, is a made-up disease. There is a disease called cowpox and a disease called smallpox, but there is no such disease as smallpox of the cow.[4] Jenner was running a medical scam.

The esteemed Dr. Charles Creighton, writing in the Ninth Edition of the Encyclopedia Britannica, described Jenner's representation of cowpox as "smallpox of the cow" as "arbitrary and untenable."[5] He explained that cowpox and smallpox are infections that are quite unlike one another. Dr. Creighton further explained the dangers of Jenner's cowpox vaccination. He listed five diseases caused by vaccination: "1) erysipelas, (2) jaundice, (3) skin eruptions, (4) vaccinal ulcers, and (5) so-called vaccinal syphilis."[6] Dr. Creighton noted a 50% increase in infant deaths from syphilis after compulsory vaccination was instituted in England in 1853. Dr. Creighton opined that vaccination may predispose infants to be beset by illnesses because the vaccines "produce a considerable constitutional disturbance,"[7] rendering the infant's immature immune system unable to resist diseases. Tragically, this often caused the premature death of children or, if they survived, lifelong illness and frailty.

The practice of inoculation also involved using *variolae* (i.e., smallpox) as the inoculating antigen. But that practice was no more successful than using cowpox. Jenner was intimately aware of the ineffectiveness of both cowpox and smallpox vaccines. Thomas Morgan writes in his book, *Medical Delusions*, that "Jenner soon discovered that vaccination did not give immunity from smallpox, including some who had been vaccinated by himself and had died from it."[8] Eleanor McBean explains that "[i]t was not long ... before Jenner's cowpox vaccinations were followed by death and disease, and that practice was also branded as dangerous and deadly."[9] But Jenner convinced the world his cowpox vaccine worked because he lied about its efficacy and safety. Jenner's unceasing promotion of the practice and subsequent government funding of his research led to compulsory vaccination in England in 1853, unsurprisingly bringing death and disease to the population.[10] The smallpox vaccine was proven to be unsafe and ineffective. Morgan summarizes the fraudulent foundations of vaccines.

> From its inception until the present day, the vaccination scheme has been an endless record of lies, deception, fraud, juggling statistics, and falsifying death certificates in order to preserve vaccination from reproach and to secure its continuation. . . and all this after more than a century of terrible experience, which has demonstrated that vaccination has killed more than smallpox, besides crippling and disfiguring millions more.[11]

But those inconvenient historical details are ignored today. While "routine vaccination against smallpox among the general public was stopped ... the U.S. government has stockpiled enough smallpox vaccine to vaccinate everyone who would need it if a smallpox outbreak were to occur."[12] And the smallpox vaccine is still being administered on a case-by-case basis today. The Mayo Clinic reveals some of the risks of the smallpox vaccine and states that "the risks of the vaccine outweigh the benefits for most people."[13]

> The ACAM2000 vaccine uses a live virus that's like smallpox, but less harmful. It can sometimes cause serious side effects, such as infections in the heart or brain. That's why the vaccine is not given to everyone. Unless there is a smallpox outbreak, **the risks of the vaccine outweigh the benefits for most people**.[14]

The term vaccination did not exist until Edward Jenner (1749-1823). Before Edward Jenner, the method of gaining immunity from smallpox was called variolation, a name drawn from variola, the scientific name for smallpox.[15] The Chinese of the 15th century practiced a form of variolation where a practitioner would use nasal insufflation, where the recipient would suck powdered smallpox scabs into his lungs. The more common method was for the practitioner to dip a swab or other implement into a smallpox pustule and then introduce that smallpox material into a cut or poke a needle containing the material into the recipient's skin. This process was thought to give the recipient a mild case of smallpox but lifelong immunity from smallpox thereafter. This process of implanting a disease agent in a person is also called inoculation.

Although inoculation is based on the germ theory, it predates the alleged discoveries of Louis Pasteur (1849–1895) by hundreds of years. Indeed, both inoculation and the germ theory began their existence not as scientific discoveries but as religious superstitions. The Hindu superstition was transformed into "science" by Louis Pasteur through plagiarism and fraud.[16] Pasteur falsely took credit for the discoveries of Antoine Bechamp. He then twisted the science of Bechamp through fraud to conjure the myth of his germ theory as the cause of illness. Pasteur's germ theory for the cause of disease is the basis for the quackery and sin of the modern practice of vaccination. Bechamp's legitimate science-backed terrain theory for the cause of illness did not serve Satan's interest in killing, injuring, and enslaving mankind. And so Pastuer was promoted, and Bechamp was suppressed. Christians are called on to "keep that which is committed to thy trust, avoiding profane and vain babblings, and oppositions of science falsely so called: Which some professing have erred concerning the faith." 1 Timothy 6:20.

Burroughs Wellcome Pharmaceutical Company presented

at the 17th International Congress of Medicine in London, England, in 1913, "The History of Inoculation and Vaccination for the Prevention of Disease."[17] In 2005, GlaxoSmithKline Pharmaceutical Company absorbed Burroughs Wellcome in a merger of the two companies. The 360-page International Congress of Medicine lecture memoranda from Burroughs Wellcome explain that inoculation against disease was started by Dhanwantari, the Vedic father of medicine, in 1500 B.C. In an account given in 1757 by one Howell, inoculation was practiced by itinerant Brahmins who went from house to house. Brahmin is the highest Varna in Vedic Hinduism. Brahmin came from the term Brahman, which is a magical force. The practice by the Brahmin required the recipients of the inoculation to "make a thanksgiving, Poojah, or offering to the goddess on their recovery."[18] Poojah is a Hindu word meaning worship, prayer, and offerings to a god or goddess.

The goddess to which an offering was to be made was Sitala, the goddess of smallpox, who "is the preeminent tutelary deity of villages in southwestern Bengal, and a goddess of the same name has a prominent role in Hindu pantheons throughout northern India."[19]

Pharmaceutical companies know full well that inoculation is a religious rite masquerading as a medical treatment. Below is a native drawing from India published in the Burroughs Wellcome lecture memoranda depicting a Malaba woman invoking the Hindu goddess of smallpox. The caption is as it appeared in the Wellcome Pharmaceutical Company lecture memoranda. Malabar is a region along the southwestern coast of India.

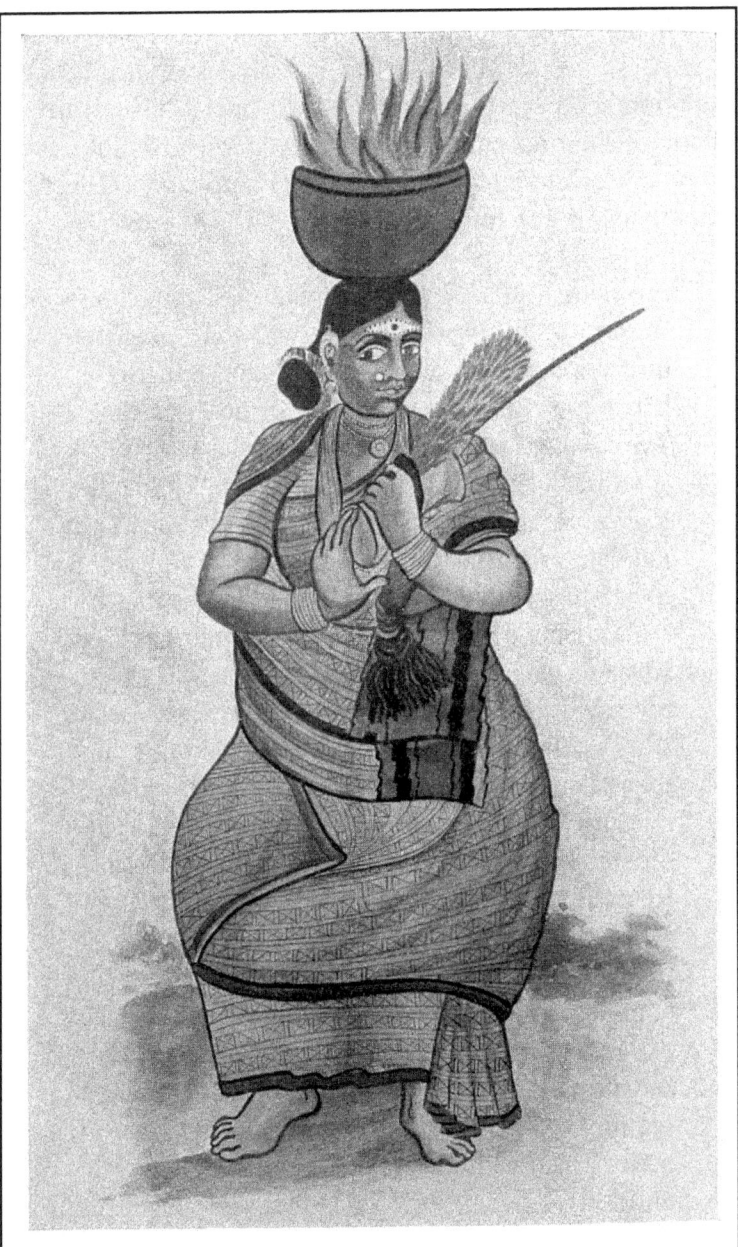

A Malaba Woman invoking the Goddess of Smallpox and carrying Fire on her Head symbolic of the disease

From a native drawing

Below is an ancient depiction of the Hindu veneration of the goddess of smallpox, which includes the practice of inoculation as part of the religious superstition. Burroughs Wellcome Pharmaceutical Company published the ancient drawing in its lecture memoranda at the International Congress of Medicine with a caption explaining:

> From an Antient Oriental Drawing. The goddess stands with two uplifted crooked daggers, threatening to strike on the right and left. Before her is a band of the executors of her vengeance. Two of them wear grinning red masks, carry black shields, and brandish naked scimitars. White lines, like, rays, issue from the bodies of the others, to indicate infection. On the left there is a group of men with spotted bodies, inflicted by the malady; bells are hung at their cinctures, and a few of them wave in their hands black feathers. They are preceded by musicians with drums, who are supplicating the pity of the furious deity. Behind the goddess, on the right, there advances a bevy of smiling young women, who are carrying gracefully on their heads baskets with thanksgiving offerings, in gratitude for their lives and their beauty having been spared. There is, besides, a little boy with a bell at his girdle, who seems to be conveying something from the right arm of the goddess. This action may probably be emblematic of inoculation. In a country where every thought, word and deed are mere repetitions of those of their progenitors, a composition like this bears the stamp of great antiquity.[20]

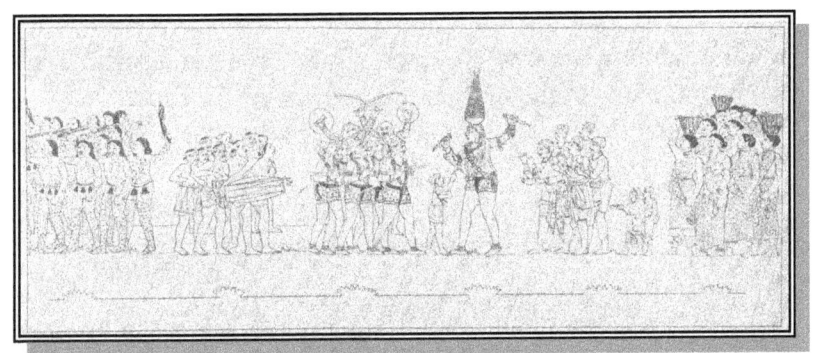

Ancient Depiction of Hindus Appeasing the Goddess of Smallpox Through the Superstitious Practice of Inoculation

Steve Halbrook confirmed that inoculation is founded on Hindu religious practices.

> James Martin Peebles, M.D., M.A., P.H.D., notes that "[s]mallpox inoculation was derived, not from scientific experimentation, but from a superstition practiced by the common people in India since the sixth century."[21] William H. York, in *Health and Wellness in Antiquity Through the Middle Ages*, elaborates:

> "Hindu mythology suggests that smallpox was likely present in India at roughly the same time as in Egypt. Religious texts make numerous allusions to the worship of Shitala, the goddess of smallpox, who was supposed to possess the body of individuals, thereby causing the disease. The Atharvaveda also describes a series of services and prayers that Brahmin priests would offer for the worship of Shitala, which included a ritual of inoculation in which people would breathe in dried scabs from smallpox lesions to induce a mild case of the disease. These unsystematic rituals likely led

to the death of many and were probably not effective enough to have thwarted large-scale outbreaks of the disease, but they offer the earliest account of inoculation measures in the world."[22]

James Martin Peebles explains that the superstitious religious practice of inoculation was not limited to India:

Mr. Porter, who was English ambassador at Constantinople in 1755, informs us, (Gentleman's Magazine, for October of that year): "It is the tradition and opinion of the inhabitants of the country that a certain angel presides over this disease. That it is to bespeak his favor and evince their confidence that the Georgians take a small portion of variolous matter, and, by means of scarification, introduce it between the thumb and the forefinger of a sound person. The operation is supposed to never miss its effect. To secure beyond all uncertainty the good will of the angel, they hang up scarlet cloths about the bed, that being the favorite colour of the Celestial inhabitants they wish to propitiate."[23]

Inoculation is a superstitious religious custom. Inoculation causes death and disease. Edward Jenner and Benjamin Jesty thought that by using cowpox puss as the antigen, they could induce an immune response to smallpox while reducing the risk of death because cowpox was much less deadly than smallpox. Today, the Jenner quackery continues on the theory that vaccination with something other than smallpox will give immunity to smallpox. The U.S. Food and Drug Administration (FDA) has licensed ACAM2000®, as a vaccine for smallpox.[24] The vaccine does not contain any smallpox (variola) virus. It contains a vaccinia virus in the genus Orthopoxvirus. While the virus is not cowpox, it is in the same genus (Orthopoxvirus) as cowpox. It is a variation of Jenner's cowpox vaccine. The consequences have proven to be the same, death and illness. The smallpox vaccine, ACAM2000®, is religious superstition masquerading as a medical treatment. It is based on the corrupt ethical judgment that the few should be sacrificed for the mythical hope that it will bring about a greater good. It justifies evil means by the hope of doing good. But the good that is hoped for is a phantom. It is quackery and sin.

The Wellcome memoranda reveal that the Hindus carried out the same process of vaccination using cowpox hundreds of years before Jenner and Jesty.[25] But Dominik Wujastyk, seeking to defend the legacy of Jenner and western medicine, disputes the claim that India was the first to use cowpox to vaccinate against smallpox.[26] Today, most use the terms vaccination and inoculation interchangeably to mean the same thing. But some, like Wujastyk, distinguish between vaccination, which Wujastyk limits to describing the use of a vaccinia (e.g., cowpox) virus and inoculation, which Wujastyk limits to describe the use of variola (smallpox) virus.

Wujastyk states that his research has uncovered that "no one disputed the fact that smallpox inoculation [using variola] was frequently practiced in India before the introduction of vaccination [using cowpox]."[27] But he claims that it was not true that the early Hindus used cowpox as the antigen for vaccination. That quibble leaves standing the fact that inoculation using variola from its beginning was based on a religious superstition complete with worship prayers and offerings to a Hindu smallpox goddess called Sitala. Modern-day vaccination finds its roots in that religious superstition and continues with the quackery of Jenner and Jesty.

Vaccination is a religious practice that has been proven to be medically ineffective and harmful.[28] In addition to the Hindus, other heathen tribes had practiced inoculation for centuries past.[29] The practice was usually abandoned once the superstitious treatment was found to be useless and harmful. But the enlightened medical doctors of today seem to be slow learners and are thus slow to abandon a practice that has been proven to be dangerous and ineffective.

The Hindu religion is a heathen religion. God commands us to have nothing to do with heathen practices. "And have no fellowship with the unfruitful works of darkness, but rather reprove them." Ephesians 5:11. We are called on to avoid such practices. "Beware lest any man spoil you through philosophy and vain deceit, after the tradition of men, after the rudiments of the world, and not after Christ." Colossians 2:8.

Christians have nothing religiously in common with Hindus. We are not to practice their heathen religion that masquerades under the guise of medicine. Christians are to separate themselves from the religious practices of heathens.

> Be ye not unequally yoked together with unbelievers: for what fellowship hath righteousness with unrighteousness? and what communion hath light with darkness? And what concord hath Christ with Belial? or what part hath he that believeth with an infidel? And what agreement hath the temple of God with idols? for ye are the temple of the living God; as God hath said, I will dwell in them, and walk in them; and I will be their God, and they shall be my people. Wherefore come out from among them, and be ye separate, saith the Lord, and touch not the unclean thing; and I will receive you, And will be a Father unto you, and ye shall be my sons and daughters, saith the Lord Almighty. (2 Corinthians 6:14-18)

It is no surprise to find that the Hindu superstition of variolation (vaccination) found its way into the doctrines of the

Roman Catholic Church. Before Benjamin Jesty or Edward Jenner initiated the vaccine quackery in the West, the Jesuits were variolating (i.e., vaccinating) the indigenous population of the Amazon against smallpox in the 1720s.[30] The practice was not based on science. Indeed, there were no Western studies or scientific literature proving the efficacy and safety of the practice at that time. Vaccination is based on the myth that disease is caused by viruses. The little-known fact is that, to this day, no disease-causing virus has ever been isolated. It is based not on science but on a religious superstition. The Jesuits were experimenting on the indigenous tribes with a superstitious religious ritual borrowed from the Hindus.

To this day, the Roman Catholic Church promotes vaccination as a moral imperative, an "act of love."[31] Pope Francis said: "Getting vaccinated is a simple yet profound way to care for one another, especially the most vulnerable."[32] It is justified on moral and religious grounds. The Vatican has dismissed any moral concern regarding the use of aborted fetal tissues in the study and manufacture of vaccines.[33] The Vatican is effectively approving of the few (the aborted children) being sacrificed for the good of the many. Indeed, it is not only the aborted children who are being sacrificed, but also the thousands killed and injured by the vaccines themselves. The Vatican has adopted the heathen superstitious ethic behind the sacrifice of children to Molech.

Herbert M. Shelton describes vaccination as not merely quackery but "a criminal operation."[34] He elaborates:

> I would not go so far as to say that vaccination has never saved a single person from smallpox. It is a matter of record that thousands of the victims of this superstitious rite have been saved by the immunizing potency of death.[35]

Dr. Charles Creighton, M.A., M.D. (1847-1927) was a

recognized authority in epidemiology. He had orthodox views of vaccination and believed them to be efficacious and safe. He was selected by the publishers of the Encyclopedia Britannica, Ninth Edition, to write the article on Vaccination. He did original and exhaustive research. His research opened his eyes to the reality that vaccines were ineffective and dangerous.[36] Dr. Creighton continued his research and wrote a book titled *Jenner and Vaccination: A Strange Chapter of Medical History*. Dr. Creighton explained that the book was written as he tried to find out **"how the medical profession in various countries could have come to fall under the enchantment of an illusion."**[37] One notable statistic that Dr. Creighton cited in his Encyclopedia Britannica article was that "in Bavaria in 1871 of 30,742 cases [of smallpox] 29,429 were in vaccinated persons, or 95.7 per cent, and 1,313 in the un-vaccinated, or 4.3 per cent."[38]

Upon reading Dr. Creighton's article in the Encyclopedia Britannica, Prof. Edgar M. Crookshank, who was the bacteriologist of King's College, did his own independent research on the efficacy and safety of vaccines in an attempt to assail the findings of Dr. Creighton. He was not able to refute Dr. Creighton's findings. He ended up writing two volumes titled, *The History and Pathology of Vaccination*, in which he presented unrefutable proof that vaccination was "uncertain, unscientific and dangerous."[39]

Herbert Spencer (1820-1903), biologist, could not understand how people could defend the "medical popery" of vaccination while condemning religious popery. Notice Dr. Creighton reported that in Bavaria, 95.7% of the persons infected with smallpox were vaccinated against smallpox. That not only proves that the vaccines do not work, it shows that the vaccines cause the persons to be more suspetible to the illness they are supposed to prevent. The vaccination compromised their immune system, causing them to be more vulnerable to disease. There is no other explanation for the high percentage of vaccinated persons with smallpox. Dr. Viera Scheibner, Ph.D. principal research scientist and author of *Vaccination: 100 Years of Orthodox Research*, explains:

> The immunological research in the last 100 years has been demonstrating that vaccines actually do not immunize ... So, even the word immunize is incorrect, because that would imply that the vaccines actually immunize; they don't, they de-immunize, they suppress the immunize system, and all they cause is a harmful immune response.[40]

Dr. John Hodge concluded:

> That vaccination is not only useless, but positively injurious; That instead of protecting its subjects from the contagion of smallpox, it actually renders them more susceptible to it by depressing the vital powers and diminishing natural resistance.[41]

Dr. James Martin Peebles writes:

> The erudite Dr. A. Wilder, of New York, physician and author, assures us that if vaccination has any influence, it is that of changing the body from a natural and normal condition to an unnatural and diseased one; in which case, repeated vaccinating can be but an endeavor to make this unnatural and diseased condition permanent. The individual is thus rendered sickly, and placed in a state of chronic aptitude to contract other diseases.[42]

Dr. William Howard Hay in a 1937 address to the Medical Freedom Society explained how previously healthy children were struck with lifelong illness upon being vaccinated:

> It is now 30 years since I have been confining myself to the treatment of chronic diseases. During those 30 years I have run against so many histories of little children who had never seen a sick day until they were vaccinated and who, in the several years that have followed, have never seen a well day since. I couldn't put my finger on the disease they have. They just weren't strong. Their resistance was gone. They were perfectly well before they were vaccinated. They have never been well since.[43]

If vaccines are so clearly ineffective and dangerous, why are they falsely propagandized as safe and effective? Because the mantra of "safe and effective" is not based on science. It has become an unassailable religious maxim. It is a religious doctrine that cannot be questioned. All doctors who question the safety and effectiveness of vaccines will find themselves defrocked and relieved of their priestly duties. The so-called "science" of vaccines is a heathen religious practice. It is born of superstition and nurtured by money. The modern doctor administering vaccines is no different from a shaman priest who scares his victim into blindly following his edicts. Brett Wilcox, in his book, *Jabbed*, explains:

> Until fairly recently, traditional religion has provided the predominant paradigm that gives comfort in and purpose to pain, suffering, injustice, and death. Religion offered protection from bad weather, malignant spirits, vile people, and poor health. As the influence of religion decreased in modern society, the influence of the religion of Scientism took its place. Germs replaced evil spirits. Doctors replaced shaman. Pharmaceuticals replaced amulets and icons. And vaccines replaced prayers, ceremonies, and rites of passage.[44]

Brett Wilcox correctly characterizes the modern practice of Vaccinology as a religious rite dressed up as science.

> Framing government, medicine and pharma in a religious context may rankle those who have abandoned the confusion and chaos of religion for the perceived certainty of science, but science—as practiced in the modern profit and power-driven paradigm—is no less of a salvation-offering religion than is Christianity, Judaism or Islam. Pure science, on the other hand, is a method for uncovering facts and their interrelationship, but hardly worthy of worship. People of business have co-opted science and turned it into Scientism, the religion for the masses. Scientific bodies have displaced religious bodies just as scientific journals have displaced holy writ. The phrases "All scientists agree" and "The science is settled" have displaced phrases such as "God says" or "The Bible says."[45]

Attorney William Wagner explains in his book, *Vaccine Epidemic,* how the government has replaced God in the minds of the people, who do not question the edicts of government bureaucrats. The commands of the government to get vaccinated are not based on objective truth but rather on public policy dogma.

> The government ... increasingly substitutes itself for God, as the source of our liberty. The paradigm shifts under this evolving legal philosophy. To evaluate state action that has an impact on parental decisions, the state replaces self-evident, unalienable standards with its own morally relative, utilitarian assessments. Thus the freedom of conscience and the sanctity behind parents directing the upbringing of their children no longer

serve as moral benchmarks against which to measure whether government vaccination laws are right or wrong, good or bad, just or unjust. Instead, parents are told that questions regarding vaccination laws are public policy matters for the government to decide. Moreover, parents should not bother asking to participate in the debate if our view of the world is informed by religious principles since we are told we must only adopt public policy informed by secular dogma—without regard to any sacred, conscientious, or moral considerations. Beware. When the government eliminates a self-evident moral element from the law, it removes any moral reference point with which to measure whether laws are right or wrong, good or bad, just or unjust.[46]

People have lost sight of the truth that "the life of the flesh is in the blood." (Leviticus 17:11) They are thus easily tricked into polluting their blood with vaccines. They do not realize that vaccination is a religious ritual wherein the blood is contaminated.

The religion of Vaccinology ever so subtlety gains converts to its sacrament of vaccination by tricking people into thinking that the belief system of Vaccinology is different, it is superior, it is "science." The deluded masses do not perceive that they are being hoodwinked into turning from reliance on Almighty God in heaven to faith in science on earth. Brett Wilcox explains:

> Many people cite religious violence, intolerance, and hypocrisy as the motivation for their exodus from religious practice. However, when leaving their former faith, many of the same individuals fall to their knees in adoration of yet another object of devotion—the religion of Scientism. Despite having so plainly seen the flaws of their former

churches, they often become blind to those of the white-coated ecclesiastics of their new secular faith. This peculiar phenomenon is never more evident than in the subsect of Scientism, The Church of Vaccinology.[47]

The disciples in this new religion of Vaccinology are kept ignorant of the cost to their bodies and souls. But the cost is real; they are being sacrificed by poisoning and, tragically, unwittingly sacrificing their children to the gods of Vaccinology. Brett Wilcox explains:

> The gods of Vaccinology are jealous, destructive, and vengeful. Their thirst for blood is not quenched with the sacrifice of a virgin or two. No, they demand the blood of virtually every human upon the planet. And the blood they crave most comes from the bodies of the faith-based community because it's harder to obtain.[48]

History testifies how heathen religions like Islam and Roman Catholicism use government force to gain converts and maintain adherents.[49] Historically, the synergy between religion and government has been close and mutually beneficial. The government-authorized heathen religion keeps the people docile and obedient to the oppressive government, while the government offers special protections to the religion. The force of government is used to eliminate religious competition. The primary target for government persecution is Christianity. That is because the kingdom of Jesus Christ is a spiritual kingdom that is not of this world. The Christian Church is outside the control of the government, and thus it is viewed as an enemy.

> Jesus answered, My kingdom is not of this world: if my kingdom were of this world, then would my servants fight, that I should not be delivered to the

Jews: but now is my kingdom not from hence. Pilate therefore said unto him, Art thou a king then? Jesus answered, Thou sayest that I am a king. To this end was I born, and for this cause came I into the world, that I should bear witness unto the truth. Every one that is of the truth heareth my voice. (John 18:36-37)

A follower of Jesus Christ is called on to be unspotted by the heathen practices of vaccination. "Pure religion and undefiled before God and the Father is this, To visit the fatherless and widows in their affliction, and to keep himself unspotted from the world." James 1:27. We are not to take part in heathen religious practices like vaccination. *See* 2 Corinthians 6:14-18.

What is the religion of "scientism" to do when people object to their vaccine ritual? Simple, it uses its government partner to coerce people to get vaccinated. Laws and regulations mandate vaccinations before children can attend public or private schools. Similar regulations mandate vaccines for healthcare workers. The Center for Medicare and Medicaid Services stated: "Strategies that Work: Make the [flu] vaccinations mandatory for employees. Consequences of non-vaccination may result in termination or suspension of employment."[50] And, as has happened recently with the COVID-19 vaccines, the laws are being expanded to the entire population. Indeed, in a presidential executive order (that was later ruled unconstitutional) the government tried to mandate experimental (COVID-19) vaccines for whole swaths of the population.

Mandatory vaccinations violate the constitutional religious rights of the people. Vaccine requirements are driven by evil greed. Basic logic proves that fact. Robert F. Kennedy, Jr., used some basic grade school arithmetic to prove the point that the meningitis vaccine mandates only make sense for those who profit from the vaccine mandates:

My opposition to new meningitis mandates for every New York State seventh and twelfth grader has nothing to do with autism and everything to do with arithmetic. .... . Meningitis is a rare disease that [affected] only 390 people nationally last year. FDA and industry testing show the meningitis vaccine to be unusually low efficacy and high risk. The manufacturers' inserts predict that 1% to 1.3% of inoculated children will suffer "serious adverse effects." CDC's Pink Book forecasts that 0.3% of these will die from the vaccine. Of the 400,000 New York school children inoculated annually, some 4,000 will become [seriously] ill and nine will die in order to prevent around four people from contracting the disease. At between $84 and $117 per shot, and with the requirement for a two-shot series, the law is an $80 million annual windfall for vaccine manufacturers at taxpayer expense. This math makes sense only to the pharmaceutical companies and the Albany politicians who have taken their money.[51]

Vaccinology is a belligerent religion. It will seek to persecute those who are of a different faith. The heathen priests of Vaccinology are of the flesh. They will persecute those who have the Spirit of Jesus Christ. The Bible informs us "that was born after the flesh persecuted him that was born after the Spirit, even so it is now." Galatians 4:29.

The fact that most states allow for religious exemptions to vaccination testifies that vaccination is a religious practice. But the pharmaceutical industry, through its wholly controlled auxiliary, the American Medical Association (AMA), has been lobbying governments to disallow religious exemptions for vaccinations.

The AMA has stated that it will try to eliminate all

religious exemptions for vaccinations. In its 2015 newsletter, the AMA said, "the AMA will seek more stringent state immunization requirements to allow exemptions only for medical reasons." The AMA bemoaned the fact that "only two states bar non-medical exemptions based on personal beliefs." The AMA states:

> New AMA policy recommends that states have in place an established decision mechanism that involves qualified public health physicians to determine which vaccines will be mandatory for admission to schools and other public venues. States should only grant exemptions to these mandated vaccines for medical reasons.[52]

The AMA has succeeded in its strategy, as evidenced by the passage of California Senate Bill 277 (SB 277) in 2015. That law removed personal or religious belief as a reason for obtaining an exemption from the vaccination requirements for entering private or public elementary or secondary schools in California. It also did not allow personal or religious belief exemptions for workers in daycare centers. That is just the beginning. That bill was followed by yet another California law (SB 792) signed by Governor Jerry Brown that requires parents who volunteer at public and private daycare and pre-schools to submit to the MMR, TDaP vaccines.[53] All who refuse are barred from volunteering at those facilities unless they have a medical exemption. Religious exemptions are not allowed, per SB 277.

The religion of Vaccinology, like all heathen religions, is founded on a myth. The sacrament of vaccination is premised on the germ theory that disease is born by contagious viruses. For example, the modern medical myth is that smallpox is a contagious virus that is spread by the inhalation of airborne *variola virus*.[54] That is wrong. Dr. A.R. Campbell was a Texas doctor who discovered that smallpox was only spread by the bite of bedbugs (cimex Lectularius). Cimex is Latin for "bug" and

Lectularius is Latin for "couch" or "bed."[55] Dr. Campbell proved that smallpox is not contagious and is not an airborne disease. In 1919 Dr. Campbell was nominated for the Nobel Prize in Medicine by the resolution of the legislature of the State of Texas for his work in eradicating mosquitoes assumed to cause malaria.[56] Dr. Campbell was the head bacteriologist for the city of San Antonio, Texas. Dr. Campbell constructed bat houses and colonized bats as you would bees. The bats would completely decimate the misquotes in the surrounding area.

Dr. Cambell regularly mingled with his smallpox patients, and he never contracted smallpox. But Dr. Campbell always found bed bugs in the homes of his patients who contracted smallpox. The medical myth is that vaccines have eradicated smallpox. Indeed, the CDC claims that "[t]hanks to the success of vaccination, the last natural outbreak of smallpox in the United States occurred in 1949."[57] The truth is that smallpox has been eradicated by modern sanitation and regular washing of bedding and clothing, which serve to eliminate bed bugs.[58]

Vaccination is justified on the same basis as sacrificing children to Molech. God calls it an abomination to sacrifice children to Molech. The heathen religious practice was to immolate the children to appease the pagan god, Molech. God states: "And thou shalt not let any of thy seed pass through the fire to Molech, neither shalt thou profane the name of thy God: I am the LORD." (Leviticus 18:21)

Parents would sacrifice their child to Molech to gain future protection against disease, famine, and war. There was tremendous pressure put on families to sacrifice their children for the greater good of the community. It was viewed as beneficial to sacrifice a few for the benefit of the many.

That is the same reasoning behind vaccination. It is understood that vaccines are inherently dangerous and will kill and injure some of those who are vaccinated. Indeed, the pharmaceutical companies and the government acknowledge that vaccines are inherently dangerous, which is the basis for the government granting pharmaceutical companies immunity from civil liability. The government thinks it is beneficial to sacrifice a few for the benefit of the many even when they know that there is no benefit to the many.

Dr. Vincient Ianelli, M.D., explained the ethic of vaccinology in *Vaxopedia*. As a vaccine advocate, he explained that vaccination from its very beginning, long before Edward Jenner entered the scene, was based on the heathen moral judgment that the few must be sacrificed for the benefit of the many.

> Variolation worked, giving the person immunity to smallpox – if they survived. Unfortunately, about 1 to 3% of people who underwent variolation died. And people who had recently undergone variolation could be contagious, leading to smallpox epidemics. So why did folks undergo variolation if they had a chance of dying from the procedure? It's simple. A natural smallpox infection was so much more deadly. Up to 30% of people who got smallpox died, and many people eventually got caught up in the regular smallpox epidemics that plagued people in the pre-vaccine era.[59]

That is the religion of Molech. The few (1-3%) must be sacrificed to death now by being variolated (i.e., vaccinated) to save the many (30%) who might die later from smallpox. Vaccination is the shedding of innocent blood. One of the abominable sins of the Jews was the shedding of innocent blood through sacrificing their children to idols. "And shed innocent blood, even the blood of their sons and of their daughters, whom they sacrificed unto the idols of Canaan: and the land was polluted with blood." (Psalms 106:38)

In the case of the COVID-19 vaccines, Dr. Toby Rogers calculated that "[f]or every one child [allegedly] saved by the shot, another 117 would be killed by the shot."[60] But the CDC, has nonetheless placed the COVID-19 vaccine on the childhood vaccine schedule, with beginning doses starting at six months of age. The vaccine schedule is applied in whole or part by school districts nationwide as a prerequisite to entering school.

The concept of mandating vaccines is based on the theory of herd immunity. Under the herd immunity theory, there is indirect protection for the community from an infectious disease when a certain threshold of the population allegedly becomes immune to the disease through infection or vaccination. The World Health Organization advocates for developing so-called herd immunity through vaccination.[61] That same ethic drove parents to sacrifice their children to Molech. For the greater good of the herd, the child must be sacrificed. In the context of COVID-19, President Biden explained:

> The second reason to get vaccinated is to protect your community, your family, your friends, and your neighbors. Vaccines can save your own life, but they can also save your grandmother's life, your coworker's life, the grocery store clerk, or the delivery person helping you and your neighbors get through the crisis.[62]

Vaccination has much in common with the religion of Molech. It is the sacrifice of the few to protect the many. Doctors know that a certain percentage of children will die and be injured by vaccines. But as with the sacrifice of children to Molech, the medical community claims that "the benefits outweigh the risks and costs for many vaccines including polio, pertussis, measles, mumps and rubella. Thus, the use of these vaccines provides a net saving to society."[63] As with the worship of Molech, the few must be sacrificed for the benefit of society. Vaccination is the perverse ethic of doing evil that good may result. God calls such an ethic a damnable heresy. *See* Romans 3:8. God condemns it. The child sacrifices to Molech were ineffectual; it was based on mythology. In like manner, vaccination is ineffectual; it is also based on mythology. Just as Molech was no threat, so also viruses pose no threat. The sacrifice of the few to Molech did nothing to protect the many. In like manner, sacrificing the few to vaccination does nothing to protect the many. For example, it has been proven that the COVID-19 vaccine does not prevent the spread of the alleged virus known as SARS-CoV-2 and thus does not offer any immunity to the herd, as was alleged under the vaccine mandates.

There is scientific proof that the more vaccines administered to infants, the higher the infant death rate.[64] But vaccination is not based on science; it is based on religion. The religion of Molech. Parents obediently march their children to the pediatrician, who, like a priest of Molech, administers deadly poison to the children. The religious mantra is that vaccines are safe and effective; only a few will die. The few must die for the benefit of the many. Among the many surviving children, there will be those who will suffer lifelong ailments. And like Molech, the protection is a myth.

The First Amendment to the U.S. Constitution prohibits the government from establishing a religion or interfering with the people's God-given right to freely exercise religion. That means that the government is prohibited from requiring its citizens to engage in a religious ritual. The government cannot legally require anybody to engage in a religious rite, especially when it is known to cause death and disease. Vaccination is a heathen religious custom born from Satan's hatred of God and man. The First Amendment protects the people from religious tyranny, even when the religion is cloaked with the false patina of science. The constitutional protection should be at its zenith when the religious rite is premised on a degenerate philosophy that evil must be done so that some good may come about. God warns us about just such so-called science that would be used to deceive us.

> [K]eep that which is committed to thy trust, avoiding profane and vain babblings, and oppositions of **science falsely so called**: Which some professing have erred concerning the faith. Grace be with thee. Amen. 1 Timothy 6:20-21.

2 Heresy to Do Evil That Good May Come

Many organizations cut off any argument about the safety and efficacy of vaccines when addressing a request for a religious exemption. But the safety and effectiveness of a vaccine are of utmost relevance when seeking a religious exemption. The argument that makes the safety and efficacy of vaccines relevant to a decision about religious exemption is the prohibition in scripture forbidding Christians from committing evil so that good may come about. Romans 3:8.

The prohibition in Romans 3:8 puts the safety of vaccines front and center in deciding the merits of a request for a religious exemption. The systemic bodily insult occasioned by vaccines is relevant in establishing that vaccination is evil and causes harm. And, as a Christian, you cannot commit the evil of vaccination to gain some future benefit of immunization. The present harm is not hypothetical; it is real. Some will even die. As with the worship of Molech, the few must be sacrificed for the benefit of society. The perverse ethic of doing evil that good may result is the doctrine of Molech.

> And thou shalt not let any of thy seed pass through the fire to Molech, neither shalt thou profane the name of thy God: I am the LORD. (Leviticus

18:21)

Furthermore, the inefficacy of the vaccines is relevant to the argument that vaccinations are not based on actual science but are founded on a religious superstition. Proof of the ineffectiveness of the vaccines is relevant in establishing that the expected good (immunization) is ephemeral, nay, a phantom. Vaccination is a heathen superstition supported by fraud and deception and producing false hope conjoined to ill-health. The studies that reveal the ineffectiveness of vaccines can be introduced to prove that vaccination cannot be justified as a medical treatment because actual science has shown them to be ineffectual.

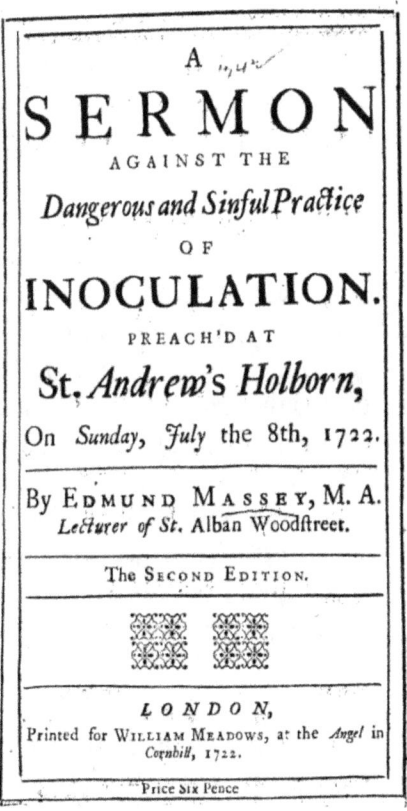

In his 1722 pamphlet, "A Sermon Against the Dangerous and Sinful Practice of Inoculation," Edmund Massey explains that vaccination is a sin. Notice that Massey's sermon was in 1722. That was 27 years before Edward Jenner was born. That is proof that the practice of administering disease into the blood of healthy persons did not start with Edward Jenner. The word vaccine had not yet been coined in the medical community when Massey gave his 1722 sermon. Massey called the practice of contaminating the blood of healthy people with disease inoculation. It was not until 1798 that Jenner published his fraudulent report and coined the term *variolae vaccinae* from which we get the word, vaccine. Massey's sermon reveals that inoculation (i.e., vaccination) is a heathen religious practice masquerading as a medical procedure.

Massey explains that the Holy Bible reveals that all diseases are under the sovereign control of God. Disease is brought upon men for one of two reasons: 1) to try our faith, and 2) to punish our sin. Indeed, God explains his sovereignty over all good and evil. "I form the light, and create darkness: I make peace, and create evil: I the LORD do all these things." (Isaiah 45:7) God uses disease and hardship to correct his elect.

> Behold, happy is the man whom God correcteth: therefore despise not thou the chastening of the Almighty: For he maketh sore, and bindeth up: he woundeth, and his hands make whole." (Job 5:17-18)

Only God can do evil so that good may come. For example, Jesus allowed himself to be crucified. Crucifixion is a torturous death; it is an evil thing. The Lord Jesus Christ did that for a good end, to atone for the sins of his elect and provide salvation to them by his grace. It is a damnable heresy for man to usurp the authority of God and do evil that good may come.

> And not rather, (as we be slanderously reported, and as some affirm that we say,) Let us do evil, that good may come? whose damnation is just. Romans 3:8.

To inject a person with poisons through vaccination causes a present offense to the body, purportedly to bring about future immunity from the injected antigen. That practice is based on a damnable religious ethic. It is doing evil that good may result.

The Bible reveals that God sometimes delegates his power to bring disease in rare occasions. For example, in Job, God permitted Satan to strike Job with a noisome disease that caused boils from head to toe. Job 2:4-7. Notice how God gave Satan permission to strike Job with disease.

> And Satan answered the LORD, and said, Skin for skin, yea, all that a man hath will he give for his life. But put forth thine hand now, and touch his bone and his flesh, and he will curse thee to thy face. And the LORD said unto Satan, Behold, he is in thine hand; but save his life. So went Satan forth from the presence of the LORD, and smote Job with sore boils from the sole of his foot unto his crown. (Job 2:4-7)

Edmund Massey opines that Job's disease was brought about by some form of infusion of a toxin similar to the practice of vaccination.

> The silence of scripture hath given interpreters occasion of guessing at the distemper, which the Devil here inflicted upon Job. But among them all, it appears not certainly what it was. I will therefore desire to give an opinion, equally I think true, with any that hath yet been taken notice of. It is this, That the Devil by some venomous Infusion into the Body of Job, might raise his blood to such a ferment, as threw out a confluence of inflammatory pustules all over him, from head to Foot. That is, his distemper might be what is now incident to most men, and perhaps conveyed to him by some such way as that of inoculation.[65]

Massey explains the motive of Satan in striking Job with the terrible disease.

The tempter's aim was still the same as before; to make his patient let go his Integrity, throw off his dependance upon Almighty God, and renounce that allegiance which is justly due to him, as creator and governor of the world.[66]

The attack on Job was unusual because God delegated his power over disease to Satan. That disease was not to punish Job for sin but to test (and prove) Job's faithfulness to God. Massey explains:

> Our Text indeed ascribes Job's distemper to the power of the Devil; but the foregoing verse shows that power to have been delegated to him, and limited by Almighty God, who alone being omnipotent, the powers that be, whether natural or Political, must all be derived from him [God]. 'Tis true, he has communicated several parts of his sovereignty to the sons of men, but still the exercise of it will ultimately be resolved into his permission. And it is as true, that there are several branches of authority, which he [God] has reserved to himself, in displaying of which, he acts upon prerogative, and without human intervention. I choose to instance in the infliction of diseases, which I will attempt to prove are utterly unlawful to be inflicted, by any who profess themselves Christians.[67]

God allowed Satan to strike Job with disease to test Job's faith. By God's grace, Job made it through the disease; God ultimately restored Job to health. Now godless and greedy men, under the auspices of Satan, are injuring people for money by the hundreds of millions. Satan's objective, as it was with Job, is to drive men to curse God. "There is no new thing under the sun." Ecclesiastes 1:9. Vaccination is an evil, devil-inspired enterprise.

The usual course is that disease is brought on directly from God. Paul offers us another example where God sent "the messenger of Satan to buffet" him by striking Paul with thorn of pain of some kind in his side. God did this to keep Paul humble. Paul explained that it was part of God's plan to make him weak in the flesh so that he would be strong in the spirit.

> And lest I should be exalted above measure through the abundance of the revelations, there was given to me a thorn in the flesh, the messenger of Satan to buffet me, lest I should be exalted above measure. For this thing I besought the Lord thrice, that it might depart from me. And he said unto me, My grace is sufficient for thee: for my strength is made perfect in weakness. Most gladly therefore will I rather glory in my infirmities, that the power of Christ may rest upon me. Therefore I take pleasure in infirmities, in reproaches, in necessities, in persecutions, in distresses for Christ's sake: for when I am weak, then am I strong. (2 Corinthians 12:7-10)

Another reason for God to bring disease is to punish a person for his sin. The malady is thought to flow from the actions of the natural laws set in place by God.

> For he that eateth and drinketh unworthily, eateth and drinketh damnation to himself, not discerning the Lord's body. **For this cause many are weak and sickly among you, and many sleep.** (1 Corinthians 11:29-30)

> And likewise also the men, leaving the natural use of the woman, burned in their lust one toward another; men with men working that which is unseemly, and **receiving in themselves that**

recompence of their error which was meet. (Romans 1:27)

Be not deceived; God is not mocked: **for whatsoever a man soweth, that shall he also reap. For he that soweth to his flesh shall of the flesh reap corruption**; but he that soweth to the Spirit shall of the Spirit reap life everlasting. Galatians 6:7-8

All elect Christians are the spiritual seed of Jesus Christ. Galatians 3:16, 29. Nonetheless, if we transgress his commandments, he will correct us. One of the means of correction is through disease. But his correction of us does not affect the eternal promise of salvation.

Also I will make him my firstborn, higher than the kings of the earth. My mercy will I keep for him for evermore, and my covenant shall stand fast with him. **His seed also will I make to endure for ever, and his throne as the days of heaven. If his children forsake my law, and walk not in my judgments; If they break my statutes, and keep not my commandments; Then will I visit their transgression with the rod, and their iniquity with stripes.** Nevertheless my lovingkindness will I not utterly take from him, nor suffer my faithfulness to fail. My covenant will I not break, nor alter the thing that is gone out of my lips. (Psalms 89:27-34)

But if we make the Lord our refuge and fortress, he will deliver us from disease. We are not to fear the pestilence by night.

I will say of the LORD, He is my refuge and my fortress: my God; in him will I trust. **Surely he**

shall deliver thee from the snare of the fowler, and from the noisome pestilence. He shall cover thee with his feathers, and under his wings shalt thou trust: his truth shall be thy shield and buckler. Thou shalt not be afraid for the terror by night; nor for the arrow that flieth by day; **Nor for the pestilence that walketh in darkness;** nor for the destruction that wasteth at noonday. (Psalms 91:2-6)

If we keep his commandments and take refuge in the Lord, no evil plague of disease will come near us.

Because thou hast made the LORD, which is my refuge, even the most High, thy habitation; **There shall no evil befall thee, neither shall any plague come nigh thy dwelling.** For he shall give his angels charge over thee, to keep thee in all thy ways. (Psalms 91:9-11)

To take a vaccine is to eschew the promises of God and put trust in man. Vaccination implicitly encourages sin by promising that there will be no consequential disease. People are beguiled by the devil's promise of immunity from future diseases. But the disease comes anyway because vaccines come with a promise that cannot be delivered. Often the disease comes from the vaccine itself. Vaccination is a sin. Those suffering from vaccine-induced disease should repent, humble themselves before God, and call on his mercy.

Massey calls vaccination a diabolical practice that promotes vice and immorality by giving people the false hope of sin without consequences by assuring them that through injection with an antigen, they will be protected from future illness. Rather than live a clean and moral life, they can now throw caution to the wind and live it up since they are immune from the consequences of their sin.

> Remembering then our text, I shall not scruple to call that a diabolical operation, which usurps an authority founded neither in the laws of nature or religion, which tends in this case to anticipate and banish providence out of the world, and promotes the increase of vice and immorality.[68]

With that in mind, it is clear that we should not purposely cause disease through vaccination. Disease is an evil that is under the control of God, and for man to usurp that power is a sin. It is a sin to do what is solely in the province of God. It is a sin to cause disease. Disease brings death, and making someone ill that could lead to his death is a violation of the commandment of God. "Thou shalt not kill." Exodus 20:13.

Jesus taught that it is a great offense to cause any harm or offense to a child. See Luke 17:1-2. Thus, injecting poisonous vaccines that cause life-long injury, such as autism, to a child is a terrible sin.

> And Jesus called a little child unto him, and set him in the midst of them, And said, Verily I say unto you, Except ye be converted, and become as little children, ye shall not enter into the kingdom of heaven. Whosoever therefore shall humble himself as this little child, the same is greatest in the kingdom of heaven. And whoso shall receive one such little child in my name receiveth me. **But whoso shall offend one of these little ones which believe in me, it were better for him that a millstone were hanged about his neck, and that he were drowned in the depth of the sea.** Woe unto the world because of offences! for it must needs be that offences come; but woe to that man

by whom the offence cometh! (Matthew 18:2-7)

Sincere Christian beliefs are founded on the Holy Bible. The Bible says:"For the life of the flesh is in the blood..." Leviticus 17:11, and "... the life of all flesh; the blood of it is for the life thereof." Leviticus 17:14. Therefore, in order to preserve the life of one's flesh, one must keep one's blood unpolluted from foreign proteins, antigens, adjuvants, and other pollutants typically found in vaccines. It is a sin to do evil that some imagined good may come. Romans 3.8.

It is a sin for a Christian to get vaccinated. It is not surprising then to find the followers of Satan, the adversary of the Lord Jesus Christ, to require his followers to commit that sin. For example, the Satanic Temple requires all attendees at their 2023 Satan Conference to be vaccinated and masked.[69] "Satancon attendees must be 18 or over and have proof of COVID vaccination. Attendees must wear an N-95, KN-95, or disposable surgical mask. Gaiters, bandanas, and cloth masks will not be allowed."[70] Satanism is founded on fear, in this case, fear of viruses. It is fear of mythical dangers that drove worshippers of Molech (i.e., Satan) to sacrifice their children. That same fear is used today to drive people to hand their children over to the priests of vaccinology. There is no fear with Jesus Christ.

> Fear thou not; for I am with thee: be not dismayed;
> for I am thy God: I will strengthen thee; yea, I will
> help thee; yea, I will uphold thee with the right
> hand of my righteousness. Isaiah 41:10.

This book sets forth the evidence establishing that vaccination is not only ineffective, but it is a dangerous and evil religious practice. Vaccination is unsupported by legitimate science. The proof is extensively supported by authority cited in endnotes so that you can bring the evidence before those who are assessing the legitimacy of your claim for a religious exemption.

3 The Ends Do Not Justify the Means

Causing disease in someone violates the great commandment that "as ye would that men should do to you, do ye also to them likewise." Luke 6:31. Edmund Massey explains:

> The Holy Scriptures give us frequent instances of God's giving power unto men to heal diseases; and by his blessing a power is still continued. But that one was ever granted to inflict diseases, will I think hardly appear; unless in the case of Moses with the Egyptians, and Elisha with his servant Gehazi. But both these cases were miraculous, and of God's own immediate appointment, to vindicate the honour of his servants the prophets, and for the punishment of sacrilege and idolatry, and cannot be drawn into precedent by any not invested with the same character and authority. Men may, and have invented racks and tortures for each other, but no man, let his Crimes be what they will, was ever yet condemned to an immediate sickness, or sentenced to lie languishing in a fever, for want of a sufficient authority, which no body but a present set of adventurous practitioners have of late

pretended to assume.[71]

It is a sin for man to kill another man. Matthew 19:18. But it is not a sin for God to kill a man. In like manner, it is a sin for a man to bring about disease in another through vaccination, but it is not sin for God to bring about disease in another.

> See now that I, even I, am he, and there is no god with me: **I kill, and I make alive; I wound, and I heal**: neither is there any that can deliver out of my hand. Deuteronomy 32:39.

Indeed, God sent disease among the Egyptians and killed the firstborn of each Egyptian household.

> He [God] made a way to his anger; he spared not their soul from death, but gave their life over to the **pestilence**; And **smote all the firstborn in Egypt**; the chief of their strength in the tabernacles of Ham. (Psalms 78:50-51)

Massey explains that disease is within the sovereign authority of God. It is not for man to usurp that authority and inject antigens to cause disease through vaccination in the hope that later the person will develop an immunity to the pathogen.

> It will easily be granted, therefore, that such a procedure, for want of a competent authority, is unlawful. That if diseases, as beforementioned, are sent unto us for the trial of our faith, or the punishment of our sins; He alone to whom our faith must approve itself, and our sins are manifest, has properly the power of inflicting them.[72]

God is sovereign. "All things were made by him; and without him was not any thing made that was made." John 1:3

"And he is before all things, and by him all things consist." (Colossians 1:17) Indeed, God knows the end from the beginning.

> According as he hath chosen us in him before the foundation of the world, that we should be holy and without blame before him in love: Having predestinated us unto the adoption of children by Jesus Christ to himself, according to the good pleasure of his will. (Ephesians 1:4-5)

Indeed, God can use evil for good ends. But don't get it twisted. What is permissible for God is not permissible for man. God is omnipotent; he knows the end from the beginning. Man is not omnipotent; man has no way of being sure that a good end will result from his evil means. While with God, good ends justify evil means, with man, good ends can never justify evil means. Man cannot commit the evil sin of injecting a vaccine containing harmful antigens, toxic adjuvants, and noxious contaminants to infect a person with a disease to accomplish the supposed good end of creating a theoretical future immunity from that disease. Indeed, the death and disease from vaccines testify to the error of man working to have the ends justify the means.

The example of Asa, King of Judah, reveals how God is displeased with evil means to accomplish good ends. In the case of Asa, he used greed and deception to trick the King of Syria into attacking Asa's enemy, the King of Israel. This displeased God because Asa relied on his own evil means to conquer his enemy, Israel. God wanted Asa to depend on him and not on his own evil devices.

> And at that time Hanani the seer came to Asa king of Judah, and said unto him, **Because thou hast relied on the king of Syria, and not relied on the LORD thy God, therefore is the host of the king of Syria escaped out of thine hand.** Were not the

> Ethiopians and the Lubims a huge host, with very many chariots and horsemen? yet, because thou didst rely on the LORD, he delivered them into thine hand. For the eyes of the LORD run to and fro throughout the whole earth, to shew himself strong in the behalf of them whose heart is perfect toward him. Herein thou hast done foolishly: therefore from henceforth thou shalt have wars. (2 Chronicles 16:7-9)

Asa started his reign as king by relying on God, but as God gave him success, he ended up relying on himself and not trusting God. As his health failed and he was struck with a disease, he acted on fear and turned to his physicians instead of turning to God. Consequently, he died of the illness. Fear is the opposite of faith.

> And Asa in the thirty and ninth year of his reign was diseased in his feet, until his disease was exceeding great: yet in his disease **he sought not to the LORD, but to the physicians.** And Asa slept with his fathers, and died in the one and fortieth year of his reign." (2 Chronicles 16:12-13)

Nationally renowned Dr. Paul Offit, M.D. condones the concept of the means justifying the ends. "Paul Offit, is a pediatrician specializing in infectious diseases and an expert on vaccines, immunology, and virology. He is the co-inventor of a rotavirus vaccine that has been credited with saving hundreds of lives every day. Offit is the Maurice R. Hilleman professor of vaccinology, professor of pediatrics at the Perelman School of Medicine at the University of Pennsylvania and director of The Vaccine Education Center at Children's Hospital of Philadelphia (CHOP). Offit is currently a member of National Institutes of Health (NIH) working group on vaccines, a subgroup of the 'Accelerating COVID-19 Therapeutic Interventions and Vaccines'

(ACTIV) comprised of experts to combat COVID-19. He is also a member of the FDA's Vaccines and Related Biological Products Advisory Committee (VRBPAC). Previously, he was a member of the Centers for Disease Control and Prevention's (CDC) Advisory Committee on Immunization Practices."[73] Dr. Offit invokes the authority of the Pope of the Roman Catholic Church as he tries to advocate for the use of evil means of using aborted fetal tissue to justify the alleged good ends of preventing disease by vaccination.

> Now, the Catholic Church, through the Pontifical Academy of Life have weighed in on this issue because obviously for the Catholic Church, abortion is a sin, a sin worthy of excommunication, a sin that causes one to lose, frankly, the ability to participate in the sacraments of the church or Catholic life. So, I think Catholics have reasonably asked the question, "Can we get these vaccines?" And the Pontifical Academy of Life, at the time headed by Joseph Ratzinger who became Pope Benedict XVI, has ruled that "yes" it is OK to get it. In fact it's important to get these vaccines because vaccines save lives; vaccines prevent suffering; vaccines prevent hospitalization and occasionally death. And the Catholic Church, like any major religion, cares deeply about the health and well-being of children.[74]

The Roman Catholic Church is the classic religious cult that justifies compromising religious principles to conform with the ways of the world. Indeed, the Roman Catholic Church is a Machievlian organization whose evil aims are hidden behind pomp and circumstance of elaborate liturgical ceremony and costumes. The Vatican is truly the habitation of seducing spirits "speaking lies in hypocrisy." See 1 Timothy 4:1-3.

The papacy presents a public facade of righteousness. That

pubic facade, however, is a smokescreen that conceals an anti-Christian agenda. The papacy is the progeny of the hypocritical scribes and Pharisees, condemned by Jesus. Matthew 23:13-15. The Roman Catholic Church funds organizations that work to undermine biblical standards, all the while claiming to uphold those very standards.

For example, the Catholic Campaign for Human Development (CCHD) gives millions of dollars in grants to numerous radical left organizations. CCHD was founded in 1970 as the Catholic bishops' anti-poverty program. In 1997 CCHD funded the following organizations, all of which endorsed the National Organization for Women's (NOW) 1996 "Fight for the Right" [to abortion] march in San Francisco: Association of Community Organizations for Reform Now (ACORN) ($310,000 grant from CCHD), Asian Immigrant Women Advocates ($20,000 grant from CCHD), the Center for Third World Organizing (CTWO) ($25,000 grant from CCHD), the Chinese Progressive Association ($30,000 grant from CCHD), and the Santa Clara Center for Occupational Safety and Health ($30,000 grant from CCHD).[75] ACORN was a co-sponsor of the February 1996 conference of the Feminist Majority Foundation which advocates abortion rights. The CTWO advocates homosexual marriage laws. CTWO in turn sponsors WAGE (Winning Action for Gender Equality), which is harshly critical of those such as Christians who support the traditional nuclear family and Christian values.

CCHD funds many radical left and communist front organizations indirectly by funding coalitions of allegedly charitable groups.[76] For example, in 1997 CCHD awarded a grant to Greater Birmingham Ministries, which in turn sponsored another coalition, Alabama Arise. Members of Alabama Arise included the AFL-CIO and the American Civil Liberties Union (ACLU).[77] CCHD also awarded a grant to the Philadelphia Unemployment Project Coalition for JOBS; that coalition included AFSCME locals, the Pennsylvania AFL-CIO, the state chapter of

NOW, and the Woman's Law Project (WLP).[78] NOW is an aggressive proponent of abortion and special sodomite rights. NOW supports partial birth abortions and opposes any restriction on abortion, including parental notification. The WLP is a legal services provider in Philadelphia that advocates lesbian and homosexual parenting rights and abortion rights. AFSME and the AFL-CIO both contribute to groups that advocate abortion rights and homosexual "marriage." The ACLU is the leading opponent of religious freedom in schools and opposes restrictions on abortions.

Some might argue that the Catholic bishops just made some errors. The evidence, however, suggests that the leftist anti-American slant to the CCHD grants is knowing and purposeful. For the past ten years the Capital Research Center has publicized to all who would listen the radical left slant to the CCHD grants, but the CCHD has done little to nothing to curtail the support of the radical anti-Christian left.[79]

The CCHD responded in 1998 to criticism by proposing changes to its guidelines. The new guidelines were adopted, and they specifically forbade the CCHD from awarding grants to organizations which "promote or support abortion, euthanasia, the death penalty, or any other affront to human life and dignity."[80] Apparently the new guidelines were merely lip service, designed to appease conservative Catholics. There, in fact, has been no significant change in the grants by the CCHD. The CCHD is still funneling money to radical left, communist, and pro abortion organizations.

For Example, not only did the CCHD not cut off its funding of ACORN in 1999-2000, they increased the funding for 17 state and local chapters of ACORN by 18%, to a total of $517,000.[81] The CCHD also continued to fund the Philadelphia Unemployment Project during 1999-2000. The project's "Jobs Campaign" coalition includes a branch of ACORN, AFSCME locals, the Pennsylvania and Philadelphia AFL-CIO, the state chapter of NOW, and the Women's Law Project, all of which support abortion rights.[82] In addition, the CCHD continues its perennial financial support to affiliates of the Industrial Areas Foundation (IAF). IAF was founded by Saul Alinsky, who was author of *Rules for Radicals*, which is a bible for left-wing political protest groups.[83] The CCHD is carrying out the official, but covert, un-American and anti-Christian policies of the Roman Catholic Church. Suzanne Belongia, CCHD director in Winona, Minnesota, in an attempt to defend CCHD pointed out that Pope John Paul II, officially endorsed CCHD when he visited Washington, D.C., early in his pontificate.[84]

The information about the CCHD grants gives us a little peak at the wolf under the sheep's clothing. Politician Huey Long once said, "if you have a reputation as an early riser, you can sleep until noon."[85] Publicly the Catholic Church is against abortion and for traditional family values; while behind the scenes the Roman church is financially supporting pro abortion and anti-Christian groups. The CCHD reveals the Roman Catholic Church as the consummate Machiavellian political organization.

A hypocrite is a person who pretends to have religious beliefs or morals that are the opposite of his behavior. The Roman Catholic hierarchy are the same as the hypocrites that Jesus criticized.

> Ye hypocrites, well did Esaias prophesy of you, saying, This people draweth nigh unto me with their mouth, and honoureth me with their lips; but their heart is far from me. But in vain they do worship me, teaching for doctrines the commandments of men. (Matthew 15:7-9)

But God is not like man. God's crucifixion of Jesus Christ illustrates how, with God, the ends justify the means. God used evil means for good ends. The crucifixion of Jesus Christ was a torturous death, but God used that evil for good; it is the means through which Jesus Christ atoned for the sins of his elect. And it was all orchestrated by God.

    Judas betrayed Jesus as prophesied by God hundreds of years earlier. Jesus stated, while praying to God the Father: "While I was with them in the world, I kept them in thy name: those that thou gavest me I have kept, and **none of them is lost, but the son of perdition; that the scripture might be fulfilled.**" (John 17:12)

    The betrayal of Jesus by Judas was planned by God. In Jeremiah we read a prophecy written approximately 600 years before the betrayal of Jesus by Judas: "Yea, mine own familiar friend, in whom I trusted, which did eat of my bread, hath lifted up his heel against me." (Psalms 41:9 AV) Jesus, referring to the prophecy in Jeremiah, told the apostles: "I speak not of you all: I know whom I have chosen: but that the scripture may be fulfilled, He that eateth bread with me hath lifted up his heel against me." (John 13:18)

    Jesus knew Judas would betray him: "For he knew who should betray him; therefore said he, Ye are not all clean." (John 13:11) Judas had no more a free will in the matter than a pencil has a free will to write. Judas, like the pencil, was an instrument completely under God's control.

    God did not leave our salvation to the chance that Judas might not betray Jesus. God is love. 1 John 4:8. It would be the very antithesis of love to leave our salvation to chance. God is not a gambler.

    Judas was preordained by God to betray Jesus. Judas had no choice in the matter. God predicted what Judas would do hundreds of years before he did it and then predicted it to his apostles moments before it happened. Jesus then personally gave Judas orders to hurry up and betray him. Judas could not resist the will of God.

> Jesus answered, He it is, to whom I shall give a sop, when I have dipped it. And when he had dipped the sop, he gave *it* to Judas Iscariot, the son of Simon. And after the sop Satan entered into him. Then said Jesus unto him, That thou doest, do quickly. (John 13:26-27)

Not only did Judas not have a free will to choose whether to betray Jesus, but every single act of Herod, Pontius Pilate, the Jews, and the Romans was preordained and orchestrated by the sovereign God of Heaven. "For of a truth against thy holy child Jesus, whom thou hast anointed, both Herod, and Pontius Pilate, with the Gentiles, and the people of Israel, were gathered together, **For to do whatsoever thy hand and thy counsel determined before to be done.**" (Acts 4:27-28) In fact, God orders the steps of all men and controls their very tongue. "The preparations of the heart in man, and the answer of the tongue are from the Lord." Prov. 16:1.

While God may do evil so that good may come of it, man my not do that same thing. Man cannot do evil (cause disease) in order that some good may come of it. That is the theory of vaccination. The ends cannot justify the means. We are forbidden to do evil in order to obtain some good end. Bad means corrupt the intended good. "And not rather, (as we be slanderously reported, and as some affirm that we say,) Let us do evil, that good may come? whose damnation is just." (Romans 3:8) Indeed, "whatsoever is not of faith is sin." (Romans 14:23)

A person is injected with a pathogen on the theory that the recipient's body will become immune to the disease. Even if that theory were correct, it would be a sin to inject a person with an antigen to cause an immune response. That is to "do evil that good may come." That is a sin. See Romans 14:23. But the good that is expected is a phantom; the medical theory of vaccination is fallacious. Job explains: "But ye are forgers of lies, ye are all physicians of no value." (Job 13:4)

      The gospel message is that those who have saving faith and are thus justified will live by that faith. Their faith is a living faith, not a dead faith. "For therein is the righteousness of God revealed from faith to faith: as it is written, The just shall live by faith." Romans 1:17. See also Galatians 3:11. Indeed, God has a warning for those who purport to believe but who do not live by faith. "Now the just shall live by faith: but if any man draw back, my soul shall have no pleasure in him." (Hebrews 10:38) "Not every one that saith unto me, Lord, Lord, shall enter into the kingdom of heaven; but he that doeth the will of my Father which is in heaven." (Matthew 7:21) Faith brings obedience. It is special obedience wrought by God through faith that God imparts in the believer. "But now is made manifest, and by the scriptures of the prophets, according to the commandment of the everlasting God, made known to all nations for the obedience of faith." (Romans 16:26) We are called on to have nothing to do with evil. We are to avoid even the appearance of evil. We are to "abstain from all appearance of evil." 1 Thessalonians 5:22. Indeed, we are to reprove evil. "And have no fellowship with the unfruitful works of darkness, but rather reprove them." (Ephesians 5:11) Vaccination is an unfruitful work of darkness forged by lies. Christians are duty-bound to reprove the evil practice.

4 The Sacrament of Vaccination

Doctors who have practiced for years and have seen the ineffectiveness of and damage done by vaccines are at a loss to explain the practice. They realize that it is not based on science. When considering why such a practice would continue in the face of such damning evidence against it, they come to the only logical conclusion left; vaccination is a superstitious religious practice.

Robert S. Mendelsohn, M.D., (1926-1988) was a practicing pediatrician for 30 years and a professor of pediatrics at the University of Illinois College of Medicine. He wrote a syndicated newspaper column and appeared on over 500 television and radio shows. In his book *Confessions of a Medical Heretic*, he characterized the medical profession as akin to a religious cult. Dr. Mendelsohn criticized the flu shot as a "farce." Dr. Mendelsohn called the alleged swine flu epidemic of 1976 a "fiasco." He portrayed doctors as powerful priests of a primitive and mysterious religion with arcane doctrines that the laity cannot understand. The central ethic of the religion is dishonesty. Dr. Mendelsohn states that "[t]he doctor is taught in his seminary, which he calls a medical school, to never tell the truth to patients."[86] Dr. Mendelsohn viewed vaccination as akin to religious superstition, where the cult member is left in a worse state after the "sacrament" is injected into the arm.

> If you follow the sounds of medical-governmental drum-beating in favor of a "preventive" procedure, you'll more often than not find yourself in the midst of one of the Church's least safe and effective sacraments. For instance, with some immunizations the danger in taking the shot may outweigh that of not taking it![87]

The only way to properly understand the dangers of vaccination is to realize that it is the product of a so-called science that runs on lies and disinformation. The practice of vaccination is the product of a medical practice based on superstition and greed. Dr. Mendelsohn stated:

> Once you understand Modern Medicine as a religion, you can fight it and defend yourself much more effectively than when you think you're fighting an art or a science.[88]

Dr. Richard Moskowitz, M. D. reflected on the ineffectiveness and dangers of vaccines and could not come up with a rational explanation for the practice. How can one justify vaccinating the population with a vaccine only to find that most of those vaccinated become ill with the disease for which they were vaccinated? Add to that the often debilitating side effects of the vaccines, and you are left with no scientific justification for the practice. Dr. Moskowitz concluded that vaccination could only be explained by a mindset in the medical community that has been taken over by religious superstition where each vaccination is a sacrament. Vaccines are administered without regard to the fact that they have been proven ineffective and unsafe because the reason for the administration is not medical science but rather religious dogma.

The fact is that we have been taught to accept vaccination as a kind of involuntary Communion, a sacrament of our participation in the unrestricted growth of scientific and industrial technology, utterly heedless of the long-term consequences to the health of our own species, let alone to the balance of Nature as a whole. For that reason alone, the other side of the case urgently needs to be heard.

***

[W]ith all due respect, I cannot have faith in the miracles or accept the sacraments of Merck, Sharp, and Dohme and the Centers for Disease Control. I prefer to stay with the miracle of life itself, which has given us illness and disease, to be sure, but also the arts of medicine and healing, through which we can acknowledge and experience our pain and vulnerability, and sometimes, with the grace of God and the help of our friends and neighbors, an awareness of health and well-being that knows no boundaries. That is my religion; and while I would willingly share it, I would not force it on anyone.[89]

Olivier Clerc states in his book, *The New World Religion: How Beliefs Secretly Influence Medical Dogmas and Practices*:

[P]hysicians have taken the place of priests; vaccination plays the same role as baptism; the search for health has replaced the quest for salvation; the fight against disease has replaced the fight against sin; eradication of viruses has taken the place of exorcising demons; the hope of physical immortality (cloning, genetic engineering) takes priority over eternal life.⁹⁰

Clerc observes the replacement of actual science with false science driven by the desire for riches. The Bible warns that the love of money is the root of all evil. 1 Timothy 6:10. Christians are called on to be wary of false religious doctrines like vaccination that are cloaked in so-called science. "[K]eep that which is committed to thy trust, avoiding profane and vain babblings, and oppositions of science falsely so called. Which some professing have erred concerning the faith." 1 Timothy 6:20-21. Christians are marching their children into the pediatrician's office to take part in a dangerous ritual of vaccination without realizing they are engaging in a heathen religious practice that is cloaked in the garb of medical science.

Clerc traces the substitution of Christian values with heathen superstition to the adoption of Louis Pasteur's mythological germ theory that has given rise to the dangerous practice of vaccination.

> We traditionally associate the birth of modern medicine with the publication of the work of French biologist Louis Pasteur (1822-1895), the father of vaccines. This choice fits perfectly with my thesis, as it was with Pasteur that the progressive and systematic transference of Christian symbolism to medicine began.⁹¹

Brett Wilcox, in his book, *Jabbed*,⁹² argues that vaccines are a ritual of religion and not a medical treatment based on science. It is easy to accept Wicox's premise once one understands the fraud, corruption, and superstition surrounding vaccination. The practice of injecting poisons into the body to prevent disease can only be understood as a superstitious religious practice because the science that supports it only appears to do so because the studies have been designed to conceal vaccine dangers. At the same time, the studies are conducted to falsely portray benefit where there is none. Wilcox explains:

> Vaccines, on the other hand, are infallible in the sect practiced by vaccine believers and sociopaths. Their infallibility is proclaimed in the primary vaccine creed: "Vaccines are safe and effective." Questioning the creed is verboten as is legal redress against vaccine manufacturers. The creed is an essential part of the vaccine paradigm because, unlike other pharmaceuticals, vaccines are administered to healthy individuals. Parents wouldn't let medical professionals jab their healthy kids if they didn't have faith in the creed. Vaccines—the sacred cow of public health—are a golden calf to the sociopaths who manufacture and manipulate the faith of the human herd. And with over 250 vaccines in development, that calf is growing ever more golden. By 2020, profits from the global vaccine market are expected to swell from nearly $24 billion to $61 billion. Referring to vaccines as a sacred cow and a golden calf is apropos from both religious and etymological perspectives. "Vacc" in the word "vaccine" is from the Latin word "cow." The original "vaccine" was a preparation of the cowpox virus taken from infected cows and inoculated in humans with the belief that it would provide immunity to smallpox.[93]

Those who question the legitimacy of vaccination are treated like religious heretics. They are vilified and shunned. Doctors are defrocked from the medical priesthood by the medical boards. The believers are indoctrinated to fear the invisible contagion such that anyone who does not receive the sacrament of vaccination is excommunicated as posing a threat to the entire community. Few ever stop to consider that if the vaccines were effective, those vaccinated should have nothing to fear. But the fact that the vaccinated believers still fear infection from the unvaccinated (i.e., the unclean; untouchables) is an implicit acknowledgment that they understand that the vaccines do not work. Wilcox explains:

> The Unholy Trinity—the pharmaceutical industry, the medical establishment and government—has successfully convinced the faithful that abstaining from vaccinations puts the entire flock at risk of damnation in the form of lethal disease outbreaks. Under the bonds of such indoctrination, people who otherwise respect legal and religious freedom heartily endorse the use of scorn, shame, hostility, name calling, discrimination, loss of the right of public education, loss of parental rights, fines, and even imprisonment for those who refuse to inject any and all vaccines the indoctrinated impose upon the rest of the flock. Former pharmaceutical representative Brandy Vaughan, now an industry whistleblower, relates the following: "I've being called a murderer, told that I should be in jail, burned at the stake, that my child will kill other children on the playground, that he should be taken away from me." Such accusations protect believers against the uncomfortable realization that the sanctuary in which they worship may not be what it claims to be, that the data supporting their beliefs is more smoke and mirrors than it is science. Leaving the Church is not for the faint of heart. Just as churches often hide, falsify, or erase faith-destroying information from their congregants, the sociopaths who run The Church of Vaccinology routinely hide, falsify or erase faith-destroying information from the public. Thus,

the spotlight of truth must not only shine on vaccines, it must also shine on the people who profit from the deliberate spread of vaccine-related propaganda and misinformation.[94]

Dr. Paul Offit is the co-inventor of the rotovirus vaccine. He is an expert in vaccines and immunology and the Chief of Infectious Diseases at Children's Hospital of Philadelphia. Offit is also the Maurice R. Hilleman Professor of Vaccinology at the Perelman School of Medicine at the University of Pennsylvania. Dr. Offit gives an example of the kind of nonsense being preached by the priesthood of vaccinologists. When trying to justify injecting vaccines containing heavy metals like mercury and aluminum and other dangerous adjuvants and excipients into tiny babies, Offit stated that it was not the ingredient that is dangerous but the dosing of that ingredient. Offit stated that "you can overdose on water. People who drink large quantities of water during a short period of time have occasionally suffered seizures as they've exceeded their bodies ability to hold onto sodium. As Paracelsus, a chemist, once said, 'The dose makes the poison.'"[95]

While it is technically accurate that one can drink too much water, it is a strange and deceptive argument to make when discussing vaccine toxicology. Marco Cáceres was beside himself to understand how Offit could use such reasoning to justify injecting vaccines containing known poisons into babies.

> You can overdose on drinking too much water? We are supposed to take this as a scientific comparison of the effect of highly toxic chemicals and metals being injected into fatty tissue, and ultimately the bloodstream and brain? Repeatedly injected, without much pause, over the course of our lifetime, from the time we are a fetus in our mother's womb, through our infancy, teenage and adult years, and finally until we are elderly and in

the twilight of our years?

The first inclination is to chuckle and say, "He's kidding, right?" But no, Dr. Offit doesn't give the impression he's joking around. The quote from Paracelsus is one of his favorites, which he often uses in interviews. The man really believes it's solely about the dose, and that whether it's mercury or water (... or applesauce, for that matter), it all comes down to how much you consume or inject.[96]

It gets worse. Offit is on record saying that a baby's immune system could handle as many as 100,000 vaccine shots.[97] This is the same man who said that dosing was everything and that one can overdose on too much water. Like all snake oil salesmen, he changes his tune depending on the audience. According to Offit, you should be more concerned with your child drinking too much water than allowing a doctor to inject 100,000 vaccines containing toxic chemicals into your child. But when you understand that Offit is the co-patent holder for a vaccine against rotavirus, it is clear that he is being paid handsomely to say such strange things.

This was not an off-the-cuff statement by Dr. Offit. He posted the statement in an official newsletter sent out from the Children's Hospital of Philadelphia (CHOP), where he is the director of the CHOP Vaccine Education Center. Under the heading: "Myth 1: Getting so many vaccines will overwhelm my child's immune system" is found the following statement:

> Compared to what they typically encounter and manage during the day, vaccines are literally a drop in the ocean." In fact, Dr. Offit's studies show that in theory, healthy infants could safely get up to 100,000 vaccines at once.[98]

When he was confronted with that statement, Dr. Offit reaffirmed that he genuinely believed it to be true that a child could safely get 100,000 vaccines injected into him at once. Dr. Offit said:

> "The 100,000 number makes me sound like a madman. Because that's the image: 100,000 shots sticking out of you. It's an awful image," Offit says. "Many people — including people who are on my side — have criticized me for that. But I was naive. In that article, I was being asked the question and **that is the answer to the question."**[99]

Offit reaffirmed, **"that is the answer to the question."** He said he understood that he sounded like a madman. But he did not say he was exaggerating or using hyperbole. Instead, he explained that was the answer to the question and truly believed what he said. He is correct that saying such a thing makes him sound like a madman; but believing it makes him a madman.

J.B. Handley, Co-Founder of Generation Rescue, comments:

> Not only is Offit's comment insane, it's also wildly dangerous and untrue. 100,000 vaccines given to a baby would cause immediate death, every single time. How profoundly disrespectful to the THOUSANDS of parents for whom ONE vaccine caused death for their child. ONE!!
>
> Let's look at the Vaccine Injury Compensation Program website for a moment, just to further highlight how crazy Offit's comments really are. What does it tells us? It shows 11,970 claims of injury and 1,006 claims of death, in every case from ONE vaccine. Offit is saying a baby can

handle 100,000 of something that has killed, at a bare minimum, more than 1,000 Americans.[100]

Assuming a vaccine dose range between 0.5 ml and 2.0 ml we find that at the lowest dosage volume, 100,000 vaccines will equal a total of 50 liters or 13.2 gallons of vaccine solution, and at the upper range, it would be 200 liters or 52.8 gallons injected into a child. Please be mindful that those gallons of vaccines would contain such excipient ingredients including, but not limited to, formaldehyde (a carcinogenic embalming fluid), ethylmercury (neurotoxin), aluminum (neurotoxin), 2-phenoxyethanol (insecticide), MRC-5 cells (aborted fetal tissue causing autoimmune disorders), polysorbate 80 (causing an immune response that can include anaphylaxis) and polyethylene glycol (PEG) (can cause hypersensitivity including anaphylaxis).

But according to the high priest of vaccinology, Paul Offit, there would be no problem injecting gallons of vaccines containing such chemicals into an infant. He wears the white clerical garment and is called a doctor. He is part of the medical priesthood whom you are expected to believe without question, regardless of how inane is his opinion. You must have faith; most of all, you must be obedient. The man is a religious zealot dressed up as a doctor, he is a quack, as are all priests in the cult of vaccinology. Brett Wilcox probably says it best:

> Prepare to enter the Inner Sanctum of The Church of Vaccinology. Prepare to drink from the Holy Grail. Prepare to kiss the hand of the Patron Saint of The Church, the Reverend Doctor Paul Offit. One proclamation echoes within the sacred chambers far more than any other. It embodies the religion's central tenet, the core doctrine, the cosmic creed:
>
> "Vaccines are safe and effective."

So it is, so it has ever been, and so it will ever be. Amen and amen.

The Unholy Trinity—pharma, the medical establishment, and government—has uttered, published, and broadcast this statement with such repetition that merely thinking or hearing it induces society into a hypnotic response, effectively shutting down critical thought processes while turning on faith-based magical thinking. "Vaccines are safe and effective." In a religious context, this proclamation is a creed. In organizational terms, it's policy. In marketing, it's the hook. In social psychology, it's propaganda. In literary parlance, it's myth. In legal vernacular, it's fraud. In the art of mind control, it's described as conversational hypnosis or "sleight of mouth." Under oath, it's perjury. In short, it's bunk.[101]

5 The Truth about the Polio Vaccine

The most often cited success story for vaccines is the alleged eradication of polio by the polio vaccines. Similar to the smallpox vaccine success myth, the polio vaccine success story is a medical tale more akin to a religious superstition than scientific fact.

Polio is short for Poliomyelitis. It is a combination of the Greek words for gray (polio) and marrow (mulos) and inflammation (itis). It denotes the inflammation of the gray matter of the spinal cord. The first great polio outbreak was the 1916 Northeastern United States polio outbreak. 25,000 people were stricken, and 5,000 died.

The 1916 polio outbreak began in Brooklyn, New York. Dan Olmstead reveals that a contagious virus did not cause the polio outbreak.[102] The first indication was that it was food-born. That is because it began with many who came down with polio after consuming ice cream at a particular ice cream shop in Brooklyn. But the illness struck adults as well. The ice cream shop owner was struck with the disease, but recovered. It turns out that the sugar that was used in making the ice cream was tainted with arsenic. How did that happen?

The tainted sugar was shipped to New York from Hawaii. There was a sugar plantation in Hawaii that was having a hard time financially and needed a solution to cutting labor costs. The problem was that weeds were choking out the sugar cane. In 1913 C.F. Eckart, head of the Hawaii Sugar Planters Association experiment station was hired by the plantation owners to solve the problem. Olmstead explains:

> The root of the problem at Olaa was the rainfall on the windward volcanic slope of the Big Island, which could reach 200 inches a year and allowed weeds to overtake the crop itself. The manpower required to keep ahead of them over the two-year growing season threatened whatever profit the plantation might eke out.[103]

Eckart's solution was to use arsenic to kill the weeds. The benefit of arsenic is that it killed the weeds but did not harm the sugar cane. But the problem was that the arsenic would absorb into the soil and then be taken up by the sugar cane. Thus, the arsenic ended up inside the sugar cane. The havested sugar cane was contaminated with the arsenic. After the sugar cane was refined and shipped to New York, it was introduced into ice cream and candy goods made by companies along the Northeastern United States. The people, primarily small children, who ate the sweets would then be stricken with polio caused by the ingestion of the arsenic.

The next great polio epidemic was after the widespread use of the pesticide DDT began in 1945. In the Mid-1950's Physician Morton S. Biskind testified before Congress that polio resulted from central nervous system poison (CNS) and not a virus.[104] The principal poison being spread among the populace of the day was dichlorodiphenyltrichloroethane, commonly known as DDT. DDT was used during World War 2 to control mosquitoes. By 1945, DDT was available for public sale in the United States and began to be widely used.[105] The government and industry promoted it for use as an agricultural and household pesticide.

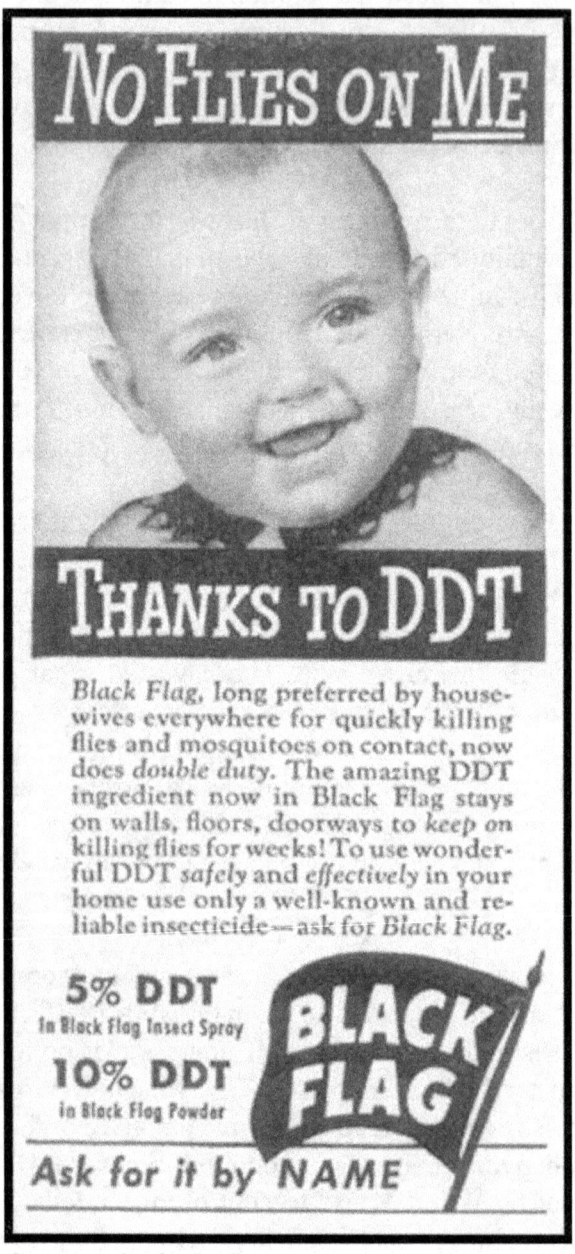

Source: Seth Anderson

Dr. Suzanne Humphries explains how in the 1940's and 50's DDT was thought to be safe:

> Insects were not just the bane of cattlemen and farmers throughout the world. Flies, in particular, were believed to spread polio outdoors and in the home. In response, fearful parents sprayed DDT on all their windowsills and sprinkled it on sandwiches in their children's lunch boxes. DDT in water was used to rinse clothes, bedding, and mattresses. It was thought to be a safe and effective insecticide—even safe enough to spray at public beaches and directly onto children in an effort to halt the spread of polio. [A DDT advertisement in the day said:] "Only a little fly you say? Yes...but what a dangerous monster! He can carry polio, and many other horrible disease germs, right into your home!"[106]

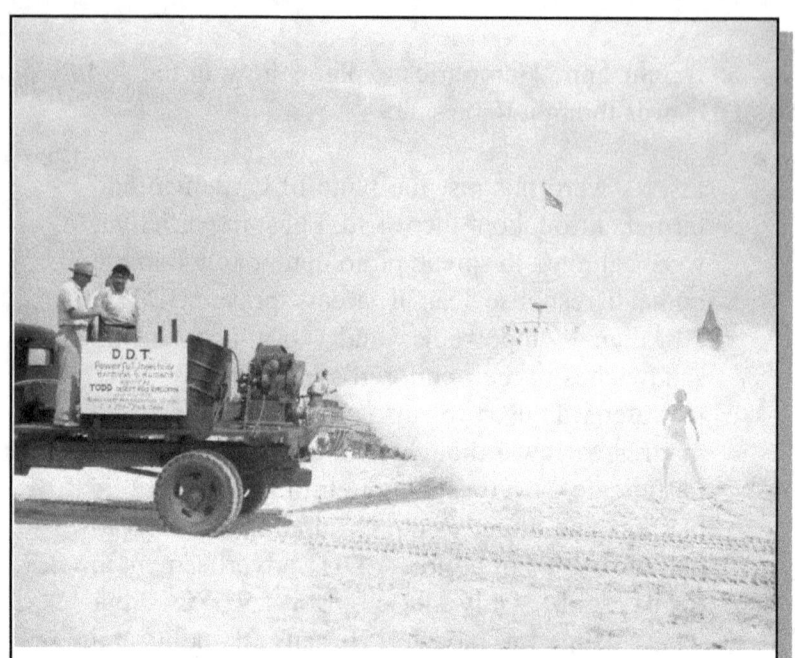

A beach on Long Island, New York is being sprayed with DDT on July 8, 1945. The new machine for spraying the insecticide is being tested for the first time. The beach goers have no fear of the DDT spray because they have been assured it is safe. The sign on the truck says: **"Powerful Insecticide Harmless to Humans."**

Dr. Humfrie's book, *Dissolving Illusions*, narrates the effects of DDT on a mosquito. The paralyzing effect on the mosquito is strikingly similar to that of a polio sufferer.

> [The]mosquito feels effects of DDT, gives frantic kick, leaps into air. As DDT enters nervous system and starts to paralyze muscles, mosquito seems to be trying to kick off paralyzing sensation. Paralysis of the nervous system affects the mosquito legs. The mosquito staggers, falls over, tries to push back onto its legs. It makes one last violent effort to rise but topples back onto its head. On its back

and almost completely paralyzed, the mosquito continues to battle against DDT but only succeeds in wiggling convulsively. It took DDT 45 minutes to knock the mosquito out completely.[107]

It is a myth that a virus causes polio. But that is the orthodox theory. Jim West explains that "[i]n developing countries, polio is blamed on poor sanitation. But in the United States, polio was blamed on lack of immunity due to good sanitation!"[108] Jim West found a direct correlation between the production of pesticides and the incidence of polio. West created the graph below that illustrates that "[v]irtually all peaks and valleys correlate with a direct one-to-one relationship with each pesticide as it enters and leaves the US market."[109] West further explains:

> Generally, pesticide production precedes polio incidence by 1 to 2 years. I assume that this variation is due to variations in reporting methods and the time it takes to move pesticides from factory to warehouse, through distribution channels, onto the food crops and to the dinner table.[110]

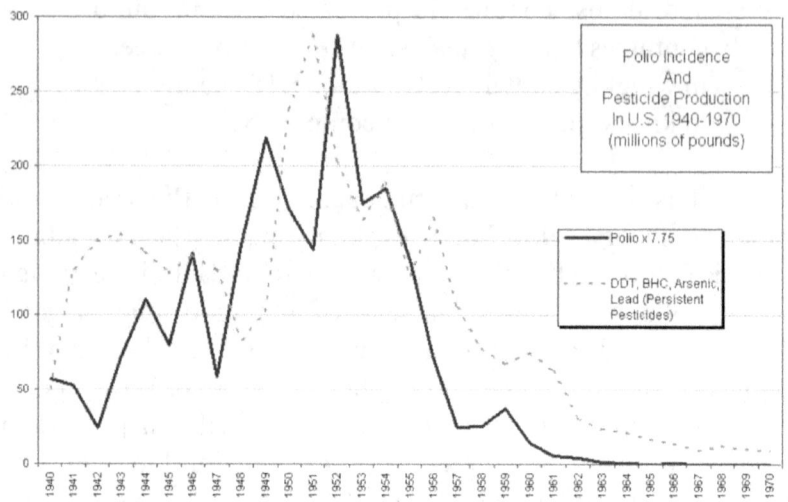

These pesticides represented in the graph are the major pesticides in use during the last major polio epidemic. West states:

> They persist in the environment as neurotoxins that cause polio-like symptoms, poliolike physiology, and were dumped onto and into human food at dosage levels far above that approved by the FDA. They directly correlate with the incidence of various neurological diseases called "polio" before 1965. They were utilized, according to Biskind, in the "most intensive campaign of mass poisoning in known human history."[111]

The graph shows that polio has no movement independent from pesticide movement. Yet, the virus theory for polio persists today. But one might argue that polio disappeared after the introduction of the polio vaccines. That is true, but the reduction in the incidence of polio after the introduction of the polio vaccines was not due to the effectiveness of the vaccines. Dr. Suzanne Humphries explains that there was a reduction in the use of dangerous pesticides like DDT at the time the polio vaccine was first introduced in 1955, and the criteria for reporting polio became more strict. [112]

The introduction of more strict criteria for reported polio upon the introduction of the polio vaccine had the effect of concealing vaccine-induced polio cases. After the polio vaccine was introduced, there were a significant number of vaccine-induced polio cases. But they were not reported as polio due to the strict requirements introduced for reporting a case of polio. Dr. Suzanne Humphries explains:

> In 1955, the year the Salk vaccine was released, the diagnostic criteria became much more stringent. If there was no residual paralysis 60 days after onset, the disease was not considered to be paralytic polio. This change made a huge difference in the documented prevalence of paralytic polio because most people who experience paralysis recover prior to 60 days.[113]

Recall the earlier outbreak of polio in 1916, which was caused by arsenic. Dr. Humprhies reveals that arsenic was a common ingredient in "therapeutic injections."

> After the removal of arsenic-containing pigments, arsenic poisoning resulted from medicines approved by the AMA in the form of supposedly therapeutic injections. Arsenic was used on fruits and vegetables in lead arsenate and calcium arsenate sprays, which resulted in human and animal ingestion. Washing or removing the outside contaminated layers of arsenic-treated produce was rarely recommended. Massive spray programs in the spring and at harvest are among the reasons why polio was once commonly referred to as summer diarrhea. Later, after cold storage for

produce was used to extend the shelf life, the programs extended into the winter.[114]

Polio vaccines are unsafe and ineffective. Research reveals that polio is not caused by a virus.[115] If a virus does not cause polio, how does the polio vaccine that allegedly has a live virus cause polio?[116] In 1957, Eleanor McBean explained:

> R. B. Pearson made an exhaustive study of the data and experiments that have been made with polio vaccines and summed up his finding as follows: "Hence, I believe **there was no virus in the vaccine used. It was just a solution of the toxins and acid end-products of the decomposed proteins used that caused all the paralysis.** The acids generated by cooked meat in Dr. Pottenger's cats (experiment that caused polio in the cats) affected the nerves first, and the acids formed in the decomposed proteins used in the vaccines affected the nerves first. It is the same thing and, no so-called 'virus' is connected with it." (From Infantile Paralysis, by Pearson.)[117]

In India, approximately 491,000 children were struck down with polio due to the polio vaccine.[118] To conceal the causal link between the polio vaccine and resulting polio, officials renamed polio non-polio acute flaccid paralysis (NPAFP). Every sentient being familiar with the facts knows the children are being paralyzed by polio and that the polio vaccine causes it. Still, medical and government officials have decided to play the game of relabelling the disease to protect pharmaceutical companies. The polio vaccines causing polio was known at least since 2017. Yet, with that knowledge, pharmacuetical companies persist in pushing their live polio oral vaccines in third world countries.

On September 24, 2019, the Children's Health Defense

Team reported that despite knowing that the oral live polio vaccines cause polio, "the Gates Foundation is 'pushing hard[119] to get the [new oral] vaccine into the field as soon as possible,' speculating that it will have a lower risk of transmitting vaccine virus—however, the Foundation cautiously notes that 'the only way to know for sure will be to use the vaccine.'"[120]

Stop and reflect on the recklessness of the Gates Foundation. They are pushing new oral polio vaccines into the field on nothing but speculation that the vaccines will work and knowing full well that the downside is the vaccines will cause polio. The Gates Foundation is perfectly comfortable experimenting with the children by using the vaccines to see if they will work. All the while, they know that many of the children will contract polio from their vaccine and be paralyzed for life. They are experimenting with children. That is an outrage!

Two months later, on November 25, 2019, the Associated Press reported: "Four African countries have reported new cases of polio linked to the oral vaccine, as global health numbers show there are now more children being paralyzed by viruses originating in vaccines than in the wild."[121]

Brian Shilhavy, the editor of Heath Impact News, wrote an article titled, *Big Pharma and Corporate Media Finally Admit the Oral Polio Vaccine is a Failure – Causes Polio Instead of Preventing.*[122] Shilhavy also included another article after his post from the Children's Health Defense Team explaining the causal link between polio vaccines and polio.[123]

The most notable aspect of Shilhavy's story is the evident coercion imposed on mothers forced to have their children vaccinated. Notice in the picture below that there are four heavily armed officers standing guard to ensure no resistance to the vaccine. Please make no mistake about it. This is a forced vaccination program that the Pakistani government is administering not to benefit children but rather the pharmaceutical companies. The government is the customer who buys the vaccines. The government then forces the vaccines on the populace. The deal with the government grants pharmaceutical companies immunity from any injuries caused by their unsafe and ineffective vaccines. If children develop polio from the vaccine, the pharmaceutical company's attitude is that it's too bad, so sad, for them. There is simply no compensation for the lifelong disability.

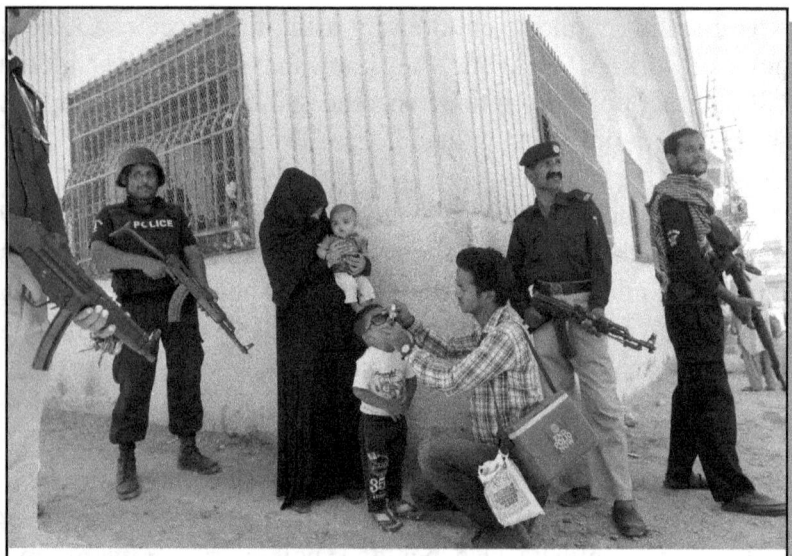

Photo by Asif Hassan/AFP taken during the 2016 Pakistan polio vaccine campaign. It shows the medical tyranny of forced vaccination under the protection of four heavily armed guards to ensure no resistance or interference.

6 Proof That the Measles Virus Does Not Exist

Children in the United States typically receive their mumps vaccination as part of the measles, mumps, and rubella (MMR) vaccine. The U.S. Centers for Disease Control and Prevention (CDC) advises children to receive their first dose between 12 and 15 months and their second between the ages of 4 and 6.[124] The CDC states that "[c]hildren can receive the second dose earlier as long as it is at least 28 days after the first dose."[125]

It has been proven in court that the alleged measles virus does not exist.[126] Dave Mihalovic, writing for Signs of the Times, reported:

> In a recent ruling, judges at the German Federal Supreme Court (BGH) confirmed that the measles virus does not exist. Furthermore, there is not a single scientific study in the world which could prove the existence of the virus in any scientific literature. This raises the question of what was actually injected into millions over the past few decades.

Not a single scientist, immunologist, infectious disease specialist or medical doctor has ever been able to establish a scientific foundation, not only for the vaccination of measles but any vaccination for infants, pregnant women, the elderly and even many adult subgroups.[127]

The case stems from a reward offered by German biologist Dr. Stefan Lanka. He offered 100,000 euros to anyone who could provide scientific evidence that the measles virus existed. Doctor David Bardens attempted to claim the prize after providing six studies published in a medical journal that allegedly proved the existence of a measles virus.[128] Stefan rejected his proof, and Barden sued. Barden initially won in the regional court in Ravensburg, South Germany. But that decision was overturned by the German Federal Supreme Court.

The BBC reported when Dr. Stefan lost in the first hearing.[129] But, strangely, it did not report on Dr. Stefan's victory on appeal to the German Federal Supreme Court. The Supreme Court decision is significant. Dave Mihalovic explained:

> Five experts have been involved in the case and presented the results of scientific studies. All five experts, including Prof. Dr. Dr. Andreas Podbielski who had been appointed by the OLG Stuttgart as the preceding court, have consistently found that **none of the six publications which have been introduced to the trial, contains scientific proof of the existence of the alleged measles virus.**
>
> In the trial, the results of research into so-called genetic fingerprints of alleged measles virus have been introduced. Two recognised laboratories, including the world's largest and leading genetic Institute, arrived at exactly the same results

independently. **The results prove that the authors of the six publications in the measles virus case were wrong, and as a direct result all measles virologists are still wrong today: They have misinterpreted ordinary constituents of cells as part of the suspected measles virus.**

Because of this error, during decades of consensus building process, normal cell constituents were mentally assembled into a model of a measles virus. To this day, an actual structure that corresponds to this model has been found neither in a human, nor in an animal. With the results of the genetic tests, all thesis of existence of measles virus has been scientifically disproved.

The authors of the six publications and all other persons involved, did not realise the error because they violated the fundamental scientific duty, which is the need to work "lege artis", i.e. in accordance with internationally defined rules and best practice of science. **They did not carry out any control experiments.** Control experiments would have protected authors and mankind from this momentous error. This error became the basis of belief in the existence of any disease-causing viruses. The expert appointed by the court, Prof. Dr. Dr. Podbielski, answering to the relevant question by the court, as per page 7 of the protocol explicitly confirmed that the authors did not conduct any control experiments.[130]

That court finding thoroughly impeaches the scientific claims that there is such a thing as a measles virus. The six publications are the foundational proof for the supposed existence of a measles virus relied on by doctors and scientist worldwide.

The refutation of those studies, in turn, refutes the alleged theory that a virus causes measles. Dave Mihalovic explains:

> The six publications submitted in the trial are the main relevant publications on the subject of "measles virus." Since further to these six publications there not any other publications which would attempt by scientific methods to prove the existence of the measles virus, the Supreme Court judgment in the measles virus trial and the results of the genetic tests have consequences: **Any national and international statements on the alleged measles virus, the infectivity of measles, and on the benefit and safety of vaccination against measles, are since then of no scientific character and have thus been deprived of their legal basis.**[131]

That means that the measles vaccine is a complete fraud. Another significant outcome was the acknowledgment that the measles vaccine causes many severe allergies and autoimmune reactions. Dave Mihalovic explains:

> Upon enquiries which had been triggered by the measles virus contest, the head of the National Reference Institute for Measles at the Robert Koch Institute (RKI), Prof. Dr. Annette Mankertz, admitted an important fact. This admission may explain the increased rate of vaccination-induced disabilities, namely of vaccination against measles, and why and how specifically this kind of vaccination seems to increasingly trigger autism.
>
> **Prof. Mankertz has admitted that the "measles virus" contains [a] typical cell's natural components (ribosomes, the protein factories of**

> the cell). **Since the vaccination against measles contains [the] "whole measles virus," this vaccine contains cell's own structures. This explains why vaccination against measles causes frequent and more severe allergies and autoimmune reactions than other types of vaccination.** The court expert Prof. Podbielski stated on several occasions that by the assertion of the RKI with regard to ribosomes in the measles virus, the thesis of existence of measles virus has been falsified.[132]

What the court decision reveals is that vaccines are based on fraud. The viruses the vaccines are supposed to fight do not exist. Indeed, the MMR vaccine, of which measles is a constituent element, is a dangerous scam. Mike Adams, writing for *Natural News*, reports that Merck fraudulently spiked blood samples to falsely show the efficacy of its measles, mumps, and rubella vaccine (MMR).

> According to two Merck scientists who filed a False Claims Act complaint in 2010 -- a complaint which was unsealed three years ago -- vaccine manufacturer Merck knowingly falsified its mumps vaccine test data, spiked blood samples with animal antibodies, sold a vaccine that actually promoted mumps and measles outbreaks, and ripped off governments and consumers who bought the vaccine thinking it was "95% effective."[133]

That lawsuit was followed by a 2012 antitrust class action lawsuit against Merck filed by Chatom Primary Care, based in Alabama.[134] The complaint alleges that Merck engaged in fraud by artificially inflating MMR vaccine efficacy test results, destroying evidence of falsified data, lying to the FDA, and threatening a virologist in Merck's vaccine division with jail if he reported the fraud to the FDA.[135]

It is not surprising that the MMR has been ineffective in the real world. Dr. Joseph Mercola reveals that "[i]n 2009, more than 1,000 people in New Jersey and New York came down with mumps. At the time, questions arose about the effectiveness of the vaccine as 77 percent of those sickened were vaccinated."[136]

7 The Emperor Has No Virus

The vaccine protocol is based on germ theory. Germ theory is the perfect scientific theory to control the masses. Many do not know that there is not a single study published in the history of medicine that has isolated a particle of virus that is capable of transmitting a disease from an ill person to a well person. The commonly accepted germ theory of illness spread by viruses is just a theory. It has never been proven. Indeed, there is significant evidence that it is wrong. The research paper written by Dr. Milton J. Rosenau, M.D., in 1919, stands as a refutation of the commonly accepted germ theory.[137]

Most people, and even most doctors, are ignorant of Dr. Resonau's experiments. Dr. Resenau conducted experiments during the height of the Spanish Flu epidemic. He wanted to establish the means by which influenza was spread. He took 100 healthy volunteers who agreed to be exposed to the Spanish Flu. They were exposed to influenza under controlled conditions but none of them contracted the flu.

Dr. Rosenau explained that his medical team "proceeded rather cautiously at first by administering a pure culture of bacillus of influenza, Pfeiffer's bacillus, in a rather moderate amount, into the nostrils of a few of these volunteers." None of the volunteers came down with the flu.

He next obtained the extractions from the lungs of recently deceased flu victims. He then lined up 19 volunteers and used an atomizer to spray the suspensions of the flu extractions into the noses and into the eyes, and back into the throats of 19 volunteers. None of the volunteers contracted the flu.

Dr. Rosenau then obtained material and mucous secretions from the mouth and nose and throat and bronchi of live persons who had the Spanish Flu and transferred that to 10 volunteers by spraying the infected phlegm directly "into each nostril and into the throat, while inspiring, and on the eye." None of the volunteers got sick.

Next, Dr. Resenau's team used cotton swabs to transfer infected "material directly from nose to nose and from throat to throat, using a West tube for the throat culture, so as to get the material not only from the tonsils, but also from the posterior nasopharynx." None of the 19 volunteers who received the infected swabs got sick.

Dr. Rosenau explains that "[o]ur next experiment consisted in injections of blood. We took five donors, five cases of influenza in the febrile stage, some of them again quite early in the disease. We drew 20 'c.c. from the arm vein of each, making a total of 100 c.c, which was mixed and treated with 1 per cent, of sodium citrate. Ten c.c. of the citrated whole blood were injected into each of the ten volunteers. None of them took sick in any way."

Dr. Rosenau was not done. "Then we collected a lot of mucous material from the upper respiratory tract, and filtered it through Mandler filters. While these filters will hold back the bacteria of ordinary size, they will allow 'ultramicroscopic' organisms to pass. This filtrate was injected into ten volunteers, each one receiving 3.5 c.c. subcutaneously, and none of these took sick in any way."

Dr. Rosenau thought perhaps that influenza was passed by direct human contact. So he had 10 volunteers engage in social contact with persons known to be infected with influenza.

> The volunteer was led up to the bedside of the patient; he was introduced. He sat down alongside the bed of the patient. They shook hands, and. by instructions, he got as close as he conveniently could, and they talked· for five minutes. At the end of the five minutes, the patient breathed out as hard as he could, while the volunteer, muzzle to muzzle (in accordance with his instructions, about 2 inches between the two), received this expired -breath, and at the same time was breathing in as the patient breathed out. This they repeated five times, and they did it fairly faithfully in almost all of the instances. After they had done this for five times, the patient coughed directly into the face of the volunteer, face to face, five different times. ... After our volunteer had had this sort of contact with the patient, talking and chatting and shaking hands with him for five minutes, and receiving his breath five times, and then his cough five times directly in his face, he moved to the next patient whom we had selected, and repeated this, and so on, until this volunteer had had that sort of contact with ten different cases of influenza, in different stages of the disease, mostly fresh cases, none of them more than three days old.
>
> We will remember that each one of the ten volunteers had that sort of intimate contact with each one of the ten different influenza patients. They were watched carefully for seven days—and

none of them took sick in any way.[138]

After failing to transmit influenza to any of the volunteers during his many experiments, Dr. Rosenau concluded that he did not know how influenza is contracted. "As a matter of fact, we entered the outbreak with a notion that we knew the cause of the disease, and were quite sure we knew how it was transmitted from person to person. Perhaps, if we have learned any thing, it is that we are not quite sure what we know about the disease."

Dr. Rosenau's experiments do not stand alone. Eleanor McBean reveals:

> Numerous experiments with germs conducted in the past have conclusively proven that bacteria does not and cannot produce disease in a healthy organism. Years ago, Dr. Pettenkofer, professor at the University of Vienna, came to the conclusion that germs alone do not produce pathology and for years defended his position from the lecture platform and in his writings. On more than one occasion he and his assistants swallowed the contents of glasses containing millions of living cholera germs. Dr. Thomas Powell of California, who is believed to have taken more germs than any other man, challenged his medical colleagues to produce a single disease by germ inoculation. He was inoculated with cholera germs, bubonic plague germs and bacteria of every description and which was fed to him in every kind of food, yet nothing happened. Read U.S. Government Bulletin "Hygienic Laboratory—Bulletin No. 123, Feb. 1921," for further proof on contagious diseases.[139]

8 The Spanish Flu of 1918

If the Spanish Flu was not a contagious virus, how did it spread to kill 20 million people? In preparation for WWI, a massive military vaccination experiment involving several prior developed vaccines, one being an anti-meningitis vaccine, took place in Fort Riley, Kansas.[140] It was no coincidence that the first "Spanish Flu" case was reported at Fort Riley, shortly after the first soldiers received their experimental vaccines. Dr. Sal Martingano, FICPA, explains:

> The fledgling pharmaceutical industry, sponsored by the 'Rockefeller Institute for Medical Research', had something they never had before – a large supply of human test subjects. Supplied by the U.S. military's first draft, the test pool of subjects ballooned to over 6 million men.
>
> Autopsies after the war proved that the 1918 flu was NOT a "FLU" at all. It was caused by random dosages of an experimental 'bacterial meningitis vaccine', which to this day, mimics flu-like symptoms. The massive, multiple assaults with additional vaccines on the unprepared immune systems of soldiers and civilians created a "killing

field". Those that were not vaccinated were not affected.

WWI U.S. soldiers were given 14 – 25 untested, experimental vaccines within days of each other, which triggered intensified cases of ALL the diseases at once. The doctors called it a new disease and proceeded to suppress the symptoms with additional drugs or vaccines.[141]

Dr. Martingano reveals that when WW1 ended sooner than expected, it left huge quantities of unused experimental vaccines. A government campaign generated fear among the people that the returning soldiers would spread diseases to their families. The campaign was effective because the soldiers who were pumped full of the experimental toxic vaccines came home as weak invalids. Their illnesses were, in reality, symptoms of being poisoned by the vaccines. But the government convinced the public that the soldiers had contracted diseases from Europe. And for that reason, citizens should be vaccinated for their own health and safety. The U.S. citizens lined up to be vaccinated with the same vaccines that made the soldiers ill. As a result, millions of civilians died in the same manner as the soldiers. That is what caused the great "Spanish Flu of 1918."

Eleanor McBean, in her 1977 book, *Swine Flu Exposed*,[142] gives her account of the "Spanish Flu."

> As has been stated before, all medical and non-medical authorities on vaccination agree that vaccines are designed to cause a mild case of the diseases they are supposed to prevent. But they also know and admit that there is no way whatsoever to predict whether the case will be mild or severe - even deadly. With this much uncertainty in dealing with the very lives of people,

it is very unscientific and extremely dangerous to use such a questionable procedure as vaccination.

Many vaccines also cause other diseases besides the one for which they are given. For instance, smallpox vaccine often causes syphilis, paralysis, leprosy, and cancer. (See the chapters on smallpox and plagues.) Polio shots, diphtheria toxin-antitoxin, typhoid vaccine, as well as measles, tetanus and all other shots often cause various other stages of disease such as post-vaccinal encephalitis (inflammation of the brain,) paralysis, spinal meningitis, blindness, cancer (sometimes within two years), tuberculosis, (two to twenty years after the shot,) arthritis, kidney disease, heart disease (heart failure sometimes within minutes after the shot and sometimes several hours later). Nerve damage and many other serious conditions also follow the injections.

When several shots are given (different vaccines) within a few days or a few weeks apart, they often trigger intensified cases of all the diseases at once, because the body cannot handle such a large amount of deadly poison being injected directly into the bloodstream. The doctors call it a new disease and proceed to suppress the symptoms.

When poison is taken by the mouth, the internal defense system has a chance to quickly eject some of it by vomiting, but when the poisons are shot directly into the body, bypassing all the natural safeguards, these dangerous poisons circulate immediately throughout the entire body in a matter of seconds and keep on circulating until all the cells are poisoned.

I heard that seven men dropped dead in a doctor's office after being vaccinated. This was in an army camp, so I wrote to the Government for verification. They sent me the report of U.S. Secretary of War, Henry L. Stimson. The report not only verified the report of the seven who dropped dead from the vaccines, but it stated that there had been 63 deaths and 28,585 cases of hepatitis as a direct result of the yellow fever vaccine during only 6 months of the war. That was only one of the 14 to 25 shots given the soldiers. We can imagine the damage that all these shots did to the men. (See the chapter on What Vaccinations Did to Our Soldiers.)

The first World War was of a short duration, so the vaccine makers were unable to use up all their vaccines. As they were (and still are) in business for profit, they decided to sell it to the rest of the population. So they drummed up the largest vaccination campaign in U.S. history. There were no epidemics to justify it so they used other tricks. Their propaganda claimed the soldiers were coming home from foreign countries with all kinds of diseases and that everyone must have all the shots on the market.

The people believed them because, first of all, they wanted to believe their doctors, and second, the returning soldiers certainly had been sick. They didn't know it was from doctor-made vaccine diseases, as the army doctors don't tell them things like that. Many of the returned soldiers were disabled for life by these drug-induced diseases.

Many were insane from postvaccinal encephalitis, but the doctors called it shell shock, even though many had never left American soil.

The conglomerate disease brought on by the many poison vaccines baffled the doctors, as they never had a vaccination spree before which used so many different vaccines. The new disease they had created had symptoms of all the diseases they had injected into the man. There was the high fever, extreme weakness, abdominal rash and intestinal disturbance characteristic of typhoid. The diphtheria vaccine caused lung congestion, chills and fever, swollen, sore throat clogged with the false membrane, and the choking suffocation because of difficulty in breathing followed by gasping and death, after which the body turned black from stagnant blood that had been deprived of oxygen in the suffocation stages. In early days they called it Black Death. The other vaccines cause their own reactions — paralysis, brain damage, lockjaw, etc.

When doctors had tried to suppress the symptoms of the typhoid with a stronger vaccine, it caused a worse form of typhoid which they named paratyphoid. But when they concocted a stronger and more dangerous vaccine to suppress that one, they created an even worse disease which they didn't have a name for. What should they call it? They didn't want to tell the people what it really was — their own Frankenstein monster which they had created with their vaccines and suppressive medicines. They wanted to direct the blame away from themselves, so they called it Spanish Influenza. It was certainly not of Spanish origin, and the Spanish people resented the implication that the world-wide scourge of that day should be blamed on them. But the name stuck and American medical doctors and vaccine makers were not suspected of the crime of this widespread devastation — the 1918 Flu Epidemic. It is only in recent years that researchers have been digging up the facts and laying the blame where it belongs.

Some of the soldiers may have been in Spain before coming home, but their diseases originated in their own home-based U.S. Army Camps. Our medical men still use that same dodge. When their own vaccines (required for travel) cause vaccine diseases abroad they use this as grounds for a scare campaign to stampede people into the vaccination centers. Do you remember the Hong Kong Flu and the Asian Flu and the London Flu scares? These were all medically-made epidemics mixed with the usual common colds which people have every year.

***

All the doctors and people who were living at the time of the 1918 Spanish Influenza epidemic say it was the most terrible disease the world has ever had. Strong men, hale and hearty, one day would be dead the next. The disease had the characteristics of the black death added to typhoid, diphtheria, pneumonia, smallpox, paralysis and all the diseases the people had been vaccinated with immediately following World War 1. Practically the entire population had been injected "seeded" with a dozen or more diseases — or toxic serums. When all those doctor-made diseases started breaking out all at once it was tragic.

That pandemic dragged on for two years, kept alive with the addition of more poison drugs administered by the doctors who tried to suppress the symptoms. As far as I could find out, the flu hit only the vaccinated. Those who had refused the shots escaped the flu. My family had refused all the vaccinations so we remained well all the time. We knew from the health teachings of Graham, Trail, Tilden and others, that people cannot contaminate the body with poisons without causing disease.

When the flu was at its peak, all the stores were closed as well as the schools, businesses — even the hospital, as the doctors and nurses had been vaccinated too and were down with the flu. No one was on the streets. It was like a ghost town. We [who didn't taken any vaccines] seemed to be the only family which didn't get the flu; so my parents went from house to house doing what they could to look after the sick, as it was impossible to get a doctor then. If it were possible for germs, bacteria, virus, or bacilli to cause disease, they had plenty of opportunity to attack my parents when they were spending many hours a day in the sick rooms. But they didn't get the flu and they didn't bring any germs home to attack us children and cause anything. None of our family had the flu — not even a sniffle— and it was in the winter with deep snow on the ground.

It has been said that the 1918 flu epidemic killed 20,000,000 people throughout the world. But, actually, the doctors killed them with their crude and deadly treatments and drugs. This is a harsh accusation but it is nevertheless true, judging by the success of the drugless doctors in comparison with that of the medical doctors.

While the medical men and medical hospitals were losing 33% of their flu cases, the non-medical hospitals such as BATTLE CREEK, KELLOGG and MACFADDEN'S HEALTH-RESTORIUM were getting almost 100% healings with their water cure, baths, enemas, etc., fasting and certain other simple healing methods, followed by carefully worked out diets of natural foods. One health doctor didn't lose a patient in eight years. The very successful health treatment of one of those drugless doctors who didn't lose any patients will be given in the other part of this book, titled VACCINATION CONDEMNED, to be published a little later.

If the medical doctors had been as advanced as the drugless doctors, there would not have been those 20 million deaths from the medical flu treatment.

There was seven times more disease among the vaccinated soldiers than among the unvaccinated civilians, and the diseases were those they had been vaccinated against. One soldier who had returned from overseas in 1912 told me that the army hospitals were filled with cases of infantile paralysis and he wondered why grown men should have an infant disease. Now, we know that paralysis is a common after-effect of vaccine poisoning. Those at home didn't get the paralysis until after the world-wide vaccination campaign in 1918.[143]

9 SARS-CoV-2 Virus Has Never Been Isolated

With all of the worldwide fervor over the COVID-19 pandemic, one might think that, certainly, the SARS-Cov-2 virus that causes COVID-19 has been isolated. That is not the case at all. A little known fact is that the alleged SARS-CoV-2 virus has never been isolated.

Incidentally, the CDC distinguishes between SARS-CoV-2 and COVID-19. The CDC states that SARS-CoV-2 is the virus that causes the disease COVID-19. COVID-19 means "coronavirus disease 2019" whereas SARS-CoV-2 means "severe acute respiratory syndrome coronavirus 2." But that distinction between the two acronyms is not commonly made by the public or the medical community.[144] Most equate SARS-CoV-2 and COVID-19 and use them interchangeably to describe the alleged infectious pathogen that is purported to be transmitted from one person to another.[145] Thus, this author will use those terms interchangeably to refer to the alleged pathogen.

The alleged SARS-CoV-2 virus has never been proven even to exist. Claims by governments and researchers to the contrary are simply false; they try to redefine what it means to isolate a virus and use obfuscatory language to conceal the deception. Please understand that the reported infections for SARS-CoV-2 among both unvaccinated and vaccinated persons are based on tests that are returning false-positive results.

Christine Massey is a biostatistician. On April 24, 2024, Christine Massey sent a Freedom of Information (FOIA) request to the CDC asking for any studies providing scientific evidence of the isolation of the alleged hantavirus proving that it causes illnesses it is purported to cause.[146] On May 10, 2024, Roger Andoh, acting as CDC/ATSDR FOIA Officer in the Office of the Chief Operating Officer, gave a sweeping response that the CDC has not conducted any controlled studies that purify and isolate the hantavirus or any other virus because the CDC does not perform such studies. Massey explains that "the 'experts' in the Division of High-Consequence Pathogens and Pathology have never obtained scientific evidence of purported 'viruses' existing in 'hosts' and causing the illness/symptoms that they are claimed to cause."[147] The CDC has confessed that it has never isolated, and thus has never scientifically proven, the existence of any virus.

Furthermore, there is not a single study of the alleged SARS-CoV2 virus being isolated or purified.[148] That can mean only one thing. Drs. Thomas Cowan and Andrew Kaufman succinctly concluded that "[t]he SARS-CoV2 virus does not exist."[149] On November 30, 2021, Christine Massey submitted an affidavit in a Canadian Federal Court averring that she has received responses to freedom of information (FOI) requests from Canadian and U.S. government agencies. She further stated that she had obtained records from FOI requests made by others to more than 138 institutions from 28 countries worldwide. Astoundingly, no institution was "able to cite even one record describing the isolation and purification of SARS-CoV-2 [the alleged virus purported to cause COVID-19]."[150] As of August 23, 2022, that number has expanded to 208 institutions in 35 countries. Yet still, none of the institutions "have provided or cited any record describing actual 'SARS-COV-2' isolation/purification."[151] The very existence of the SARS-Cov-2 virus seems to be a myth.

So, why, then are people testing positive for a non-existent SARS-CoV-2? A group of 22 highly respected scientists led by Pieter Borger, MSc, Ph.D., demanded a retraction of the report by Christian Drosten and Victor Corman that established the PCR test used worldwide for the SARS-CoV-2 virus. They cited "10 major scientific flaws at the molecular and methodological level" in the research that produced the SARS-CoV-2 PCR test. The scientists predicted that those flaws would result in false positive results. The most notable shortcoming of the research by Corman/Drosten was that the resulting SARS-COV-2 PCR test was arrived at without isolating the SARS-CoV-2 (COVID-19). How can one test for something that has not first been isolated? The scientists stated:

> The first and major issue [with the Corman/Drosten report] is that the novel Coronavirus SARS-CoV-2 (in the publication named 2019-nCoV and in February 2020 named SARS-CoV-2 by an international consortium of virus experts) is based on in silico (theoretical) sequences, supplied by a laboratory in China, because at the time neither control material of infectious ("live") or inactivated SARS-CoV-2 nor isolated genomic RNA of the virus was available to the authors. To date no validation has been performed by the authorship based on isolated SARS-CoV-2 viruses or full length RNA thereof. According to Corman et al.:

> "We aimed to develop and deploy robust diagnostic methodology for use in public health laboratory settings without having virus material available."[152] (endnotes deleted)

The alleged SARS-CoV-2 virus was identified in silico, meaning that it was created using a computer simulation. Essentially, the SARS-Cov-2 virus is a computer-generated theoretical virus that does not actually exist. The scientists concluded the obvious. A diagnostic test for SARS-CoV-2 is invalid if it is based on research without access to any actual virus material available on which to base the test.

Kary B Mullis invented the polymerase chain reaction (PCR) method, for which he won the 1993 Nobel Prize in Chemistry.[153] He died suddenly in August 2019, four months before the January 2020 publication of the Corman-Droster PCR test paper that formed the basis for the SARS-CoV-2 PCR test. Before his death, Mullis explained that with enough amplification the PCR test could be used to find almost anything. He said that "with PCR, if you do it well, you can find almost anything in anybody."[154] For that reason, Mullis cautioned that the PCR test should not be used to diagnose whether someone is ill. Mullis said that PCR is "a process that's used to make a whole lot of something out of something. That's what it is. It doesn't tell you that you're sick, and it doesn't tell you that the thing you ended up with really was going to hurt you or anything like that."[155] Thus, the inventor of the PCR test is on record stating that it is improper to use a PCR test to diagnose if someone is ill or infected with a virus.

The PCR COVID-19 test is done using reagents to extract a sample of RNA. An enzyme called reverse transcriptase converts the RNA to a complementary sequence of DNA. That DNA (called a primer) is replicated (amplified) many times over so the particular targeted DNA sequence in it can be detected. The more stages of replication the more likely the targeted sequence will be detected. Each time the DNA in the sample is amplified it doubles the number of molecules. The doubling is exponential after each cycle of amplification. But the number of cycles can vary from laboratory to laboratory. The probability of testing positive increases as a function of the number of cycles. The PCR cycles for a SARS-CoV-2 test from most laboratories are set at 40 cycles.[156]

Amandha Dawn Vollmer holds a Doctor of Naturopathic Medicine degree from the Canadian College of Naturopathic Medicine in Toronto and a Bachelor of Science in Agricultural Biotechnology. She has discovered that the test for SARS-CoV-2 is not actually testing for SARS-CoV-2. The polymerase chain reaction (PCR) test for SARS-CoV-2 is based on the research of German scientists Christian Drosten and Victor Corman who cobbled together the COVID-19 PCR test used worldwide to detect the SARS-CoV-2 virus. Amandha Vollmer discovered that the Corman/Drosten PCR test protocol adopted by the World Health Organization (WHO) to detect SARS-CoV-12 is actually testing for chromosome 8, which is present in everyone.[157] One of the primer sequences in the PCR test for SARS-CoV-2 that is promoted by the WHO is found in all human DNA. Essentially, we are the virus. That is why there is a 97% false positive rate on the COVID-19 PCR test. People are testing positive for SARS-CoV-2 because they're human.

ctccctttgttgtgttgt = The DNA sequence for the PCR test for SARS-CoV-2.[158]

ctccctttgttgtgttgt = Chromosome 8, which is present in all homo sapiens (humans).[159]

The false positive error is compounded because of the high PCR threshold cycle rates employed. Each amplification level exponentially increases the likelihood of detecting the presence of chromosome 8. The PCR test amplifies the test sample as an exponent of the number of cycles. Each cycle doubles the prior cycle. For example, if you start with a penny and each day you double the amount of money you had on the previous day, at the end of 28 days (cycles) you would have more than a million dollars. If you continued to double your money each day past the 28th day, you would have more than five billion dollars after 40 days (cycles). That is the kind of amplification that the PCR test performs. The CDC has recommended 40 cycles for the PCR test.[160] And most laboratories during the alleged pandemic were performing tests using that recommended 40-cycle standard. Anthony S. Fauci is the Director of the National Institute of Allergy and Infectious Diseases (NIAID). Dr. Fauci admitted that performing PCR tests to detect COVID-19 at 35 or more cycles will result in false-positives and the confidence in any such positive result for SARS-CoV-2 is "minuscule." Dr. Fauci stated:

> If you get a cycle threshold of 35 or more, the chances of it being replication-confident are minuscule...you almost never can culture virus from a 37 threshold cycle... someone does come in with 37, 38, even 36, you gotta say it's just dead nucleotides period.[161]

"Any test with a cycle threshold above 35 is too sensitive, agreed Juliet Morrison, a virologist at the University of California, Riverside. 'I'm shocked that people would think that 40 could represent a positive,' she said."[162]

Apoorva Mandavilli reported that experts with whom she conferred determined that "[i]n Massachusetts, from 85 to 90 percent of people who tested positive in July with a cycle threshold of 40 would have been deemed negative if the threshold were 30 cycles."[163] Dr. Michael Mina, an epidemiologist at the Harvard T.H. Chan School of Public Health, said about the Massachusetts findings that "I would say that none of those people should be contact-traced, not one,"*[164]*

The Portugal Court of Appeals in Lisbon agreed with the trial court, which granted a *writ of habeas corpus* on behalf of German tourists. The court of appeals ruled that German tourists were illegally detained by the Azores Regional Health Authority and ordered to be quarantined because the PCR test that was the basis of the detention is unreliable for detecting SARS-CoV-2. Peter Andrews reported that the Portuguese court cited a study conducted by "some of the leading European and world specialists," proving that the usual testing standard for a PCR test results in a SARS-CoV-2 false-positive result 97% of the time.[165]

The Portugal Court of Appeals in Lisbon, based upon a study by some of the leading European and world specialists, concluded that "[t]his means that if a person has a positive PCR test at a cycle threshold of 35 or higher (as in most laboratories in the USA and Europe), the chances of a person being infected are less than 3%. The probability of a person receiving a false positive is 97% or higher."*[166]*

The antigen tests are just as inaccurate and prone to false positives. Indeed, the FDA warned unequivocally that the antigen tests are inaccurate and give false positives. "The U.S. Food and Drug Administration (FDA) is alerting clinical laboratory staff and health care providers that false positive results can occur with antigen tests."[167]

Indeed, the FDA has now admitted that "all tests," for COVID-19, antigen and PCR, are inaccurate. The FDA states:

> The FDA reminds clinical laboratory staff and health care providers about the risk of false positive results with all laboratory tests. Laboratories should expect some false positive results to occur even when very accurate tests are used for screening large populations with a low prevalence of infection.[168]

Notice that the warning goes to "all laboratory tests," including both antigen and PCR tests. That astounding admission by the FDA has gone unreported by the major media outlets, even as many states, including Virginia, are issuing more draconian social distancing and masking orders based on those inaccurate false-positive COVID-19 test results.

The FDA explains the scope of the false positives using the antigen test. The following is guidance from the FDA:

> Remember that positive predictive value (PPV) varies with disease prevalence when interpreting results from diagnostic tests. PPV is the percent of positive test results that are true positives. **As disease prevalence decreases, the percent of test results that are false positives increase.**
>
> For example, a test with 98% specificity would have a PPV of just over 80% in a population with 10% prevalence, meaning 20 out of 100 positive results would be false positives.
>
> The same test would only have a PPV of approximately 30% in a population with 1% prevalence, meaning 70 out of 100 positive results would be false positives.
>
> This means that, in a population with 1% prevalence, only 30% of individuals with positive test results actually have the disease.[169]
>
> At 0.1% prevalence, the PPV would only be 4%, meaning that 96 out of 100 positive results would be false positives.

That is why there was a push for testing asymptomatic persons. The government knew that many would falsely test positive for COVID-19. The lockdowns, social distancing, and mask mandates are all based on the premise that those with no symptoms of COVID-19 can still spread the disease. But research has proven that there is no asymptomatic transfer of SARS-Cov-2, the alleged virus purported to cause COIVD-19.[170] The tyrannical overlords ignore such inconvenient studies. Once persons tested positive for COVID-19, they were tallied up as COVID-19 patients. Some who are ill with the flu may test positive for SARS-Cov-2.[171] That is why the flu disappeared during the 2020-2021 flu season.[172] All persons with the flu were counted not as flu cases but as COVID-19 cases.[173] They then used the COVID-19 scam to push the poisonous COVID-19 vaccines on the population and begin the actual killing. Their objective from the beginning was to force the toxic vaccines on the world population.[174]

10 The Lie of Asymptomatic Virus Spread

In the spring of 2020, a false premise was published far and wide that asymptomatic carriers of SARS-Cov-2, the alleged virus that purports to cause COVID-19, threatened to spread the alleged virus to others. Under that theory, someone who is not sick and feels no symptoms of illness could, nonetheless, spread the SARS-COV-2 virus to others. That was an unproven theory. But that theory was the basis upon which the world's governments shut down businesses and schools, mandated masks, required social distancing, and ultimately required mass COVID-19 vaccinations. The theory that a person could carry the SARS-CoV-2 virus without displaying symptoms and then spread it to others is now known to have been false.

The theory of the asymptomatic spread of SARS-CoV-2 was doubted by many. David Zweig explains that "[i]n June 2020, Dr. Maria Van Kerkhove, head of the World Health Organization's emerging diseases and zoonosis unit, said that transmission from asymptomatic people was 'very rare.'"[175] Allyson M Pollock, professor of public health at Newcastle University, posted an article in the British Medical Journal, likening the rarety of asymptomatic transfer of SARS-CoV-2 to finding a needle in a haystack. Dr. Pollock stated that "[s]earching for people who are asymptomatic yet infectious is like searching for needles that appear and reappear transiently in haystacks, particularly when rates are falling."[176] The governments of the world were well aware of the study conducted between May 14 and June 1, 2020, involving almost 10 million residents of Wuhan, China. That massive study found zero transmission of SARS-CoV-2 from asymptomatic carriers of the alleged virus.[177]

Unbeknownst to the general public is that from the outset the CDC and state governments had available a test that could have been used to determine if someone who tested positive for SARS-CoV-2 in a PCR test could spread the alleged virus to others. The world's governments kept that test secret because it undermined their asymptomatic premise for their oppressive measures. David Zweig explains:

> [A]s early as May and June of 2020, a test existed that, if it had been rolled out in medical centers and regular labs nationwide, could have enabled people to know for certain whether they were infectious or not. ... This raises serious questions for those in charge of the CDC, NIH, and NIAID for why resources were not allocated toward making this test broadly available.[178]

The federal and state governments knew about the test when they were locking down society. Indeed, in June 2021, the CDC published a study proving the efficacy of the new test for infectiousness.[179] But if you are a government locking people down, shutting down businesses, and masking people, on a false pretense, the last thing you want is to have your pretense be proven false. And that is just what the test would have done. David Zweig reveals how:

> And what they found does not match the narrative about a common threat of people walking around

without symptoms infecting others. For the majority of the pandemic only 4% of asymptomatic SARS-CoV-2 PCR-positive patients were shown to be infectious.[180]

Dr. Ralph Tayyar, an infectious diseases fellow at Stanford, explained:

"The probability of a kid in class who is not sick actually being infectious is very low," he said. Think about it this way: even if every single student in a school without symptoms was infected, 96 percent of them still weren't capable of transmitting to others. Yet, of course, most people without symptoms are not infected. Moreoer, just because 4 percent were technically capable of infecting others does not mean that in actuality they had sufficient amount of replicating virus to do so. We are talking about a subgroup of a subgroup of a subgroup.[181]

It gets worse, as the false positive COVID-19 PCR test rate from the beginning has been estimated to be as high as 97%. So we have a 97% population of false positive PCR results. That means that we have potentially 3% of the positive PCR positive test being infected with SARS-CoV-2, with only 4% of that 3% theoretically being able to pass on the alleged virus. That leaves us with an actual risk of spread among asymptomatic persons testing positive for SARS-CoV-2 at 0.12%. The risk goes down even further because that 0.12% only tells you that the person can potentially spread the alleged virus. A much smaller percentage of those have sufficient replication of the alleged virus in their system to spread the alleged it. Ultimately, the chance of an asymptomatic person spreading SARS-CoV-2 is minuscule. It is like finding a needle in a haystack.

The asymptomatic spread theory and the concealment of its falsity were done to ensure the success of the vaccination propaganda campaign. The goal from the beginning was a mass-vaccination program. The vaccines were the end goal. The vaccines are bioweapons to injure and kill people. That is not hyperbole. Dr. Michael Yeadon is the former Vice-President of Pfizer's allergy and respiratory research unit. He left Pfizer to found the biotechnology company, Ziarco, where he served as CEO. Ziarco was later sold to Novartis for $325 million. Dr. Yeadon has 32 years of experience designing drugs. He has maintained many close ties with insiders at Pfizer. In a May 8, 2023, interview with CHD, Dr. Yeadon had this to say about the COVID-19 vaccines:

> We are facing something much worse than an alleged virus. At the very least, these things that people that are being injected with, the injuries to people from these [inaudible] vaccines, I'm afraid, I wish I could tell you it was accidental. But it wasn't accidental. I spent 32 years in rational drug design. I know, and I knew, and wrote it before any of them had emergency use authorization, that they were dangerous. And I am afraid, and I am convinced and would say with my hand on the Bible, in front of a court, a judge, that these injections have been made to injure people, to maim and kill.[182]

Furthermore, Leading Reports reported on May 11, 2023, that Dr. Yeadon "claims that the COVID vaccines are bioweapons designed to kill billions of people as part of a depopulation agenda by the 'Deep State.'"[183]

11 Exosomes

An often identified culprit for disease is bacteria. But many will be surprised to learn that there has never been proven that any bacteria has ever caused a disease. Indeed, the entire germ theory is based on unproven assumptions. Dr. Thomas Cowan explains that bacteria are microbial patsies.

> [B]acteria are found at the site of disease for the same reason that firemen are found at the site of fires. Bacteria are the cleanup crew tasked with digesting and getting rid of dead and diseased tissues. Claiming that bacteria cause a certain disease is no more reasonable than claiming that firemen cause fires, especially as experimental evidence shows this to be false. Likewise, maggots on a dead dog are there to clean up dead tissue—no one would accuse the maggots of killing the dog. In fact, one therapy for necrotic tissue is maggot therapy (applying maggots to the wound). The maggots kill only the dead tissue; when there is only live tissue left to eat, they die off.[184]

The bacteria theory of disease had problems. Scientists

could not always find an offending bacterium for a disease. Louis Pasteur speculated that some pathogen was too small to be detected in a microscope. In the end, Pasteur admitted his germ theory of bacterial cause for disease was wrong. He acknowledged that his effort to prove his theory of bacterial contagion was a failure, He made a deathbed confession: "The germ is nothing; the terrain is everything." By terrain, he means the condition of a person who has been subjected to a stress or toxin in the environment causing the illness. A contemporary rival of Pasteur, Antoine Bechamp, advocated the terrain theory.

Dr. Cowen reveals that the eureka moment for scientists wedded to the germ theory came with the invention of the electron microscope;. The scientists could then see tiny "particles" at the disease site. They called these particles viruses, after the Latin word for toxin.

The concept of viruses causing diseases was just a hypothesis. You see, scientists only hypothesized that the "particles" they saw were disease causing viruses. The germ theory of diseases caused by viruses was based on that hypothesis. You might be surprised to learn that there has been no direct evidence of the existence of viruses. Derek M Yellon PhD, DSc, FRCP (Hon), FACC, FESC, FAHA, Professor of Molecular & Cellular Cardiology at University College London (UCL) explains:

> We already know that "viruses" began first as an idea in the early 1900's once it was discovered that bacteria were unable to be blamed for every disease and were also found regularly in healthy subjects. It was assumed that there must be something smaller than bacteria in the fluids causing disease. The concept of the "virus" came before there was ever any evidence submitted for the existence of this invisible entity. Over 100 years later, we still have no direct evidence as to the existence of

"viruses," only indirect evidence used to infer their existence.[185]

All studies, vaccines, and pharmaceuticals developed to fight viral infections are based on the assumption that viruses exist. Dr. Stefan Lanka explains that the theory that viruses cause disease has never been proven. Even more surprising is his revelation that there has never been the isolation of a virus in the history of medicine.

> The fact is and remains that a virus has never been isolated according to the meaning of the word isolation, and it has never been photographed and biochemically characterised as a whole unique structure. The electron micrographs of the alleged viruses, for example, really only show cellular particles from dying tissue and cells, and most photos show only a computer model (CGI – computer generated images). Because the involved parties BELIEVE that the dying tissue and cells transform themselves into viruses, their death is also regarded as propagation of the virus. The involved parties still believe this because the discoverer of this method was awarded the nobel Prize and his papers remain the reference papers on "viruses."[186]

If the so-called viruses seen in diseased cells are not viruses, what are they? Dr. Thomas Cowan reveals that they are exosomes. Exosomes, like bacteria, have been renamed "viruses" and made the patsies. Their function is to package up and expel toxins from the body. They are not viruses; they are not bad guys; they are good guys. They are the garbage collectors. But they find themselves falsely accused simply becaue they have been found at the scene of the disease. Dr. Cowan explains:

When a living organism is threatened in almost any way—through starvation, chemical poisoning, or electromagnetic effects—the cells and tissues have a mechanism for "packaging," "propagating" and releasing these poisons. Modern researchers have shown that exosomes have exactly the same attributes as "viruses." They are the same size, contain the same components, and act on the same receptors. HIV researcher James Hildreth, president and CEO of Meharry Medical College and former professor at Johns Hopkins, put it this way: "The virus is fully an exosome in every sense of the word." Exosomes are completely indistinguishable from what the virologists have been calling "viruses."[187]

Dr. Cowan explains that Exosomes do not attack cells, as is theorized with viruses under the germ theory. Instead, exosomes are created by your cells and expelled by your cells as those cells try to rid themselves of an environmental toxin. The exosomes are containers of toxins ejected from your cells.

Here's how exosomes work: let's say you have a poorly nourished organism, then you expose it to a common environmental toxin. The tissues and cells that are affected begin to produce, package, and secrete these poisons in the form of exosomes. This is a way of ridding the cells and tissues of substances that would do it great harm. The greater the exposure to toxic assaults, the more exosomes will be produced. Studies have shown that if one somehow stops the cells from producing and excreting these exosomes, then the cells and tissues, in fact the organism, will have a worse outcome. This research demonstrates that the production and excretion of exosomes is a crucial detoxification function of all cells and tissues.[188]

Exosomes also act as a warning system to the other cells. They send signals to the other cells that danger is afoot and they need to prepare for it. Exosomes are not a source of illness; they are a detoxification system. Dr. Cowan calls them "toxin gobbling messengers." Dr. Cowan likens them to "true firemen, obviously present in higher amounts in cases of disease, in which a higher burden of poisoning has occurred." But these beneficial exosomes have been made the bad guy, and called viruses because they contain toxins of which the body is trying to rid itself. Dr. Cowan concludes:

> The germ theory is wrong; the virus theory is wrong. Viruses are not here to kill us; in reality they are exosomes whose role is to provide the detoxification package and the communication system that allows us to live a full and healthy existence. A war on viruses is a war on life. It's clear that the misidentification of exosomes as viruses was a tragic mistake, one that it's about time we correct, once and for all.[189]

Although the germ theory was shown to be bankrupt and its primary champion eschewed it on his deathbed, it has been the religious dogma of modern medicine for two centuries. Why would that be? Because the governments of the world saw in that theory a way of controlling their population. As we have experienced during the COVID-19 scam-demic, the governments used the threat of the contagious disease to justify draconian lockdowns, social distancing, masking, tracking and tracing, relocation camps, and mandatory vaccinations. It was all based on the discredited germ theory.

12 Injecting Disease

Vaccines are "usually administered through needle injections."[190] Vaccine active ingredients are allegedly viruses or bacteria.[191] They are commonly called antigens. An antigen is defined as "a substance that enters the body and starts a process that can cause disease."[192] The injected antigen is usually attenuated or inactivated to reduce the risk of disease. The theory behind vaccines promoted to the public is to "stimulate a person's immune system to produce immunity to a specific disease, protecting the person from that disease."[193] In addition to the antigens, vaccines contain an adjuvant, which is intended to stimulate the immune response of the person. Adjuvants are typically heavy metals like mercury or aluminum, which are neurotoxic.[194] Many contaminants find their way into the vaccines from the manufacturing process, including, but not limited to, antibiotics, formaldehyde, and aborted fetal tissue.[195]

Vaccination is a strange medical practice where instead of the doctor trying to cure a person of a disease to make him well again, the doctor purposely infects a well person with a disease in the hope that his reaction to the infection will be less than it would otherwise be if he had contracted the disease through the environment. Vaccination is not without risk. There can be dire consequences to the practice. There are side effects to vaccination that the medical community calls adverse events that can range from soreness in the injection site to fever, paralysis, and even death. The expectation, which is often not realized, is that the vaccinated person will develop an immunity to the disease and be thus protected from future infection. Unlike natural immunity from a disease contracted from the environment, which is typically lifelong, the immunity from vaccination, if it is present at all, is fleeting, requiring booster shots.

Vaccines are not given as therapeutic medicine to treat a person who is ill with a disease. Vaccines are given to people who are well. To get vaccinated is to take on a spirit of fear and reliance on man rather than God.

> But when Jesus heard that, he said unto them, They that be whole need not a physician, but they that are sick." (Matthew 9:12)

> For God has not given us a spirit of fear, but of power and of love and of a sound mind" (2 Timothy 1:7).

Christians are religiously bound to care for their bodies as they are the temple of the Holy Spirit. It is a sin to defile our bodies by injecting them with the polluting poisons of vaccines. The consequent death and illness that flow from vaccination fulfill God's promise to destroy those who would defile their bodies through vaccination.

> Know ye not that ye are the temple of God, and that the Spirit of God dwelleth in you? If any man defile the temple of God, him shall God destroy; for the temple of God is holy, which temple ye are. (1 Corinthians 3:16-17)

> What? know ye not that your body is the temple of

the Holy Ghost which is in you, which ye have of God, and ye are not your own? For ye are bought with a price: therefore glorify God in your body, and in your spirit, which are God's. (1 Corinthians 6:19-20)

It is the wish of God that we prosper in our physical health. "Beloved, I wish above all things that thou mayest prosper and be in health, even as thy soul prospereth." 3 John 1:2. Vaccines are detrimental to health, and thus, it would violate God's command to be vaccinated. It is an established scientific fact that vaccines cause allergies and other ailments.

13   Poisonous Magic Potions

Merck is the largest vaccine manufacturer in the U.S. Merck claims to "make vaccines for 11 of the 17 diseases on the CDC's recommended immunization schedules."[196] Merck further claims it "distributed ~190M [vaccine] doses around the world in 2019."[197] Merck aspires "to be the premier research-intensive **biopharmaceutical** company."[198]

Another vaccine maker is Pfizer, which proclaims on its website that "[b]iotechnology is our foundation. Benefiting patients is our goal. Innovation, **pharmaceutical** development, and the most dedicated team of clinical researchers is how we do it."[199]

Jansen, a subdivision of Johnson & Johnson, is yet another U.S. pharmaceutical company that describes itself as making **pharmaceutical products**, including "vaccines to treat and cure infectious diseases."[200]

The most recent addition to the vaccine trade in the U.S. is Moderna, which considers itself a biotech company that it claims "has been named a top **biopharmaceutical** employer by Science for the past eight years."[201]

Notably, these companies all describe themselves as pharmaceutical companies. But when you read their websites, they claim to make medicines. Why do they not describe themselves as "medicine" companies? The reason is simple; they also make poisons, and poisons are not medicine.

Medicine means "Any substance, liquid or solid, that has the property of curing or mitigating disease."[202] It is derived from a Latin word "medicina, from medeor," meaning "to cure."[203]

Pharmaceutical, however, has a different, much more expansive definition. While pharmaceuticals can be medicines that cure, they can also be poisons that kill and injure.

Pharmaceutical is an adjective derived from the Greek word pharmacea, meaning "to practice witchcraft or use medicine; poison or medicine."[204] Indeed, the Greek word pharmakeia is translated in the English Bible as "witchcraft" and "sorcery." E.g., Galatians 5:20; Revelation 18:23. The Etymology Dictionary offers this: "from Late Latin pharmaceuticus 'of drugs,' from Greek pharmakeutikos, from pharmakeus 'preparer of drugs, poisoner.'"[205]

A supplier of a pharmaceutical is called a pharmacy. That noun is "directly from Medieval Latin pharmacia, from Greek pharmakeia 'a healing or harmful medicine, a healing or poisonous herb; a drug, poisonous potion; magic (potion), dye, raw material for physical or chemical processing.' This is from pharmakeus (fem. pharmakis) 'a preparer of drugs, a poisoner, a sorcerer' from pharmakon 'a drug, a poison, philter, charm, spell, enchantment.'"[206]

All of the pharmaceutical companies live up to their pharmaceutical billing by selling poisons that kill people. For example, Merck sold a product, Vioxx, to allegedly treat arthritis pain, knowing that it would kill many patients. Their studies showed that Vioxx caused patients to suffer heart attacks and die. Their studies showed that it increased heart attacks by 400% over the control group. Despite that danger, Merck pushed the poison for approval by the FDA. The New Atlantean reports Merck's efforts to get Vioxx approved by the FDA despite the studies showing that the drug killed people.

> Merck resorted to a public relations campaign that aggressively marketed the drug with the help of celebrity endorsements from the likes of Bruce Jenner before it was even approved, a standard of scientific review that revolved around obfuscating the intent of its studies, funding ghostwritten studies that painted the drug in a positive light, creating fake medical journals to laud the drug, and even working in tandem with the FDA to suppress scientific dissent by intimidating doctors who questioned the safety of the drug. Ultimately, the nefarious campaign behind getting Vioxx approved by the FDA would succeed.[207]

Merck falsely promoted Vioxx as safe and effective, knowing it would kill people. Predictably, Vioxx ended up causing 88,000 heart attacks and killing 38,000 people.[208] That is a death toll equivalent to fifteen (15) Pearl Harbors. The New England Journal of Medicine caught Merck altering its testing data by removing evidence in the data that Vioxx kills people.[209] As the body count mounted, the lawsuits followed, and Merck ended up paying $4.85 billion into a settlement fund, ending thousands of lawsuits.[210] Merck pled guilty to criminal charges for their "false statements about the drug's cardiovascular safety." Merck ended up paying $950 million to settle the criminal and civil charges brought against it by the U.S. Department of Justice.[211]

Pfizer acts more like a criminal enterprise. It has been described as "a rogue pharmaceutical corporation[] knowingly and deliberately put[ing] patients' lives at risk."[212] Pfizer's criminality in selling poisons to the public under the guise that they are safe medicines is breathtaking. For example, Pfizer peddled a dangerous antipsychotic drug, Geodon. Pfizer knew Geodon had a life-threatening side effect of altering the heart's rhythm, which posed the risk of sudden death.

Knowing this, Pfizer nonetheless mobilized an army of more than 250 psychiatrists nationwide to whom Pfizer paid handsome speaking fees to promote the deadly drug by convincing other doctors to employ Geodon for off-label use and switch their patients from other, safer drugs.[213] Geodon was just one of four poisonous drugs that in 2009 led to Pfizer paying the largest health care fraud fine in history, $2.3 billion.[214] That case uncovered evidence that Pfizer paid kickbacks to healthcare providers to induce them to prescribe their dangerous drugs. That is just the tip of the iceberg. Over the past 30 years, Pfizer has paid more than $4.7 billion to settle 34 civil and criminal settlements with the federal and state governments.[215]

Johnson & Johnson and its subsidiary Jansen have been sued repeatedly for injury and death caused by their pharmaceutical poisons. For example, it marketed off-label the antipsychotic drug Risperdal. The side effects of the drug included gynecomastia (abnormal breast tissue growth in males), type 2 diabetes, stroke, cardiac arrest, and death. The harm caused by that drug gave rise to 14,000 lawsuits against Johnson & Johnson and its subsidiary Jansen.[216] The U.S. Department of Justice prosecuted Johnson & Johnson and Jansen for their criminality in marketing Risperdal. Incidentally, Risperdal was only one of three drugs for which the DOJ was prosecuting Johnson & Johnson. The companies jointly pled guilty to criminal charges and paid $2.2 billion to settle the criminal and civil claims brought by the DOJ. The Justice Department stated that "the conduct at issue in this case jeopardized the health and safety of patients." The Justice Department stated the obvious in its press release about the criminal case settlement: the companies "put profit over patients' health."[217] That seems to be a pattern with all of the pharmaceutical companies.

On or about August 26, 2019, Johnson & Johnson was ordered to pay $572 million to the State of Oklahoma for fueling the opioid addiction crisis in that state.[218] The judge ruled that Johnson & Johnson engaged in deceptive marketing of its opioid drugs, Duragesic and Nucynta sold through its subsidiary Jansen Pharmaceuticals. Jack Fortier and Brian Mann reported for NPR that "Johnson & Johnson also profited by manufacturing raw ingredients for opioids and then selling them to other companies, including Purdue, which makes Oxycontin."[219] Purdue Pharmaceuticals was a co-defendant in the case. Purdue settled with the State of Oklahoma for $272 million.

Incidentally, Perdue Pharmaceuticals was shut down in 2020 and ordered to pay $8 billion in criminal penalties, forfeiture, and civil fines for fraud in its marketing of Oxycontin.[220] Purdue engaged in a scheme where it marketed its opioid products to more than 100 health care providers that Purdue knew were diverting opioids to addicts. Purdue used the traditional scheme of pharmaceutical companies to pay doctors through a doctor-speaker program to induce those doctors to write more prescriptions for Purdue's opioid products. The opioid crisis, fueled by the greed of pharmaceutical companies, reportedly killed 400,000 people from opioid overdoses.[221] According to the CDC, about half of those deaths were from Perdue Pharmacuetical's Oxycontin. Perdue is owned by the Billionaire Sackler family, who are supporters of Israel and large donors to Tel Aviv University. The Sackler School of Medicine in Tel Aviv is resisting a call to have the Sackler name removed from its school.[222]

Although it was clear early on that Oxycontin was addictive and dangerous, Purdue Pharmaceuticals continued to fraudulently market Oxycontin as a non-addictive pain killer knowing full well that the drug would kill people. "Purdue and three executives pleaded guilty in 2007 to federal charges of misbranding drugs and were ordered to pay $635 million."[223] As Purdue saw their profits drop in the U.S. as their criminal drug scheme was being exposed, they decided to move to Latin America, Asia, the Middle East, Africa and other regions. The Los Angeles Times reported in 2016:

> Prescriptions for OxyContin have fallen nearly 40% since 2010, meaning billions in lost revenue for its Connecticut manufacturer, Purdue Pharma. So the company's owners, the Sackler family, are pursuing a new strategy: Put the painkiller that set off the U.S. opioid crisis into medicine cabinets around the world. A network of international companies owned by the family is moving rapidly into Latin America, Asia, the Middle East, Africa and other regions, and pushing for broad use of painkillers in places ill-prepared to deal with the ravages of opioid abuse and addiction.[224]

Purdue Pharmaceuticals marketed its Oxycontin internationally through subsidiary companies and used the same deceptive marketing campaigns claiming it was safe and not habit-forming. The marketing was designed to overcome the deep-seated resistance of doctors who did not want to load up their patients on opioids because of the fear of addiction. The marketing campaign was designed to overcome the doctors' resistance it labeled "opiophobia." Purdue Pharmaceuticals was focused on making money no matter whom they destroyed. "The love of money is the root of all evil." 1 Timothy 6:10.

Moderna is the new pharmaceutical company on the block. The only product to make it to market in the history of that company as of 2023 has been its COVID-19 vaccine. That product has caused extensive death and injury. That is what pharmaceutical companies do best.

The pharmaceutical companies only care about making money; they do not care whom they injure and kill. Brett Wilcox reveals the sociopathic behavior of pharmaceutical companies. For example, in 1979, a series of sudden infant deaths could be attributed to DTP vaccines from Wyeth Pharmaceutical Company.[225] You would think the company would then recall the batch causing the deaths. But Wyeth did no such thing. Instead, Wyeth "senior management" instituted a policy memorialized in an August 27, 1979, memo that thereafter there would be a practice of "limiting distribution of a large number of vials from a single lot to a single state, county, or city health department."[226] Doing that ensured that the death from "hot lots" of DTP vaccines would be spread nationwide, the hope being that the deaths being less concentrated would thus be less noticeable. Wyeth understood that their DTP vaccines were killing children; their objective once the deadliness of their vaccine became known to the public was to ensure that the deaths were less noticeable so they would be less likely to be attributed to the DTP vaccine.

Brett Wilcox compares the behavior of Wyeth to drug dealers. "Drug dealers routinely kill for profit. Vaccine sociopaths have knowingly put at risk virtually every person on the planet to protect and increase their profits. Wyeth provided a disturbing example of sociopathy."[227]

Even scarier is that it is the policy of the U.S. Government to cooperate with the pharmaceutical companies in covering up any dangers posed by vaccines so that the population will not think that vaccines are unsafe or ineffective. This policy includes injecting dangerous vaccines into people's arms even though the pharmaceutical companies and the government know the vaccines will kill and injure the population. Below is a direct quote from the 1972 Executive Reorganization and Government Research of the Committee on Government Operations United States Senate:

> [E]ven when the contaminating virus was found to be oncogenic [cancer causing] in hamsters, the DBS [Division of Biologics Standards] and its expert advisory committee decided to leave existing stocks on the market rather than risk eroding public confidence by a recall. ... There has been a tendency on the part of certain higher government circles to play down any open discussion of problems associated with vaccines.[228]

Congress found that the pharmaceutical companies, with the cooperation of the Federal Government, intentionally allowed vaccines known to be contaminated with carcinogenic viruses to be left on the market and injected into people "rather than risk eroding public confidence by a recall" of the dangerous vaccines. That shocking finding was not isolated; it is part of a confidence game (a.k.a., a con game) designed to deceive the public into having confidence that vaccines are safe and effective when they are, in reality, dangerous and ineffectual. That is the behavior of sociopathic religious zealots. They will kill and harm people to keep the con game going and money rolling in.

For example, Congressman Percy Priest chaired a full investigation in 1956 of polio vaccine malfeasance by the pharmaceutical companies, including an instance where Cutter Pharmaceutical Company was making dangerous polio vaccines due to unsanitary and incompetent manufacturing practices that resulted in live polio viruses contaminating what was supposed to be an inactivated polio vaccine. Federal regulators knew the issue, but nothing was done to stop it. The Cutter vaccines caused children to be paralyzed with polio. Congressman Priest decided that the malfeasance should be covered up. The public should not be informed about the dangers of contaminated and dangerous polio vaccines that federal regulators allowed to be administered to children.

> [M]any responsible persons had felt that the public should be spared the ordeal of "knowledge about controversy." If word ever got out that the Public Health Service had actually done something damaging to the health of the American people, the consequences would be terrible. ... We felt that no lasting good could come to science or the public if the Public Health Services were discredited.[229]

The public is being conned into believing that vaccines are safe and effective when they are poisons that kill and injure. Brett Wilcox explains that the vaccine industry is nestled in a deceptive premise that vaccines are presumed safe and effective.

> How does the Unholy Trinity—the vaccine industry, medical establishment, and government—get away with calling vaccines "safe and effective" when the US Supreme Court has ruled that vaccines are "unavoidably unsafe?" The short answer is: it lies.[230]

So we see that these companies have chosen a word, pharmaceutical, to describe their businesses to include potions and poisons that are part of the curious dark arts of witchcraft. Indeed, vaccination is a practice embraced by those who worship Satan. For example, the Satanic Temple requires all attendees at their 2023 Satan Conference to be vaccinated and masked.[231] Satanists do not conform to the norms of society. But the vaccine requirement is not the Satanic Temple conforming to society; it is proof that society has conformed to the sorcery of Satanism by injecting poisons into their bodies. Those poisonous potions are made for them by pharmaceutical companies. And that is why pharmaceutical companies are not called medicine companies.

14 Unsafe and Ineffective Flu Vaccines

People are injected with more influenza vaccines than all other shots combined.[232] Lies drive the marketing to get the flu vaccine. The CDC falsely represents the number of people who die each year from the flu to scare the elderly into getting the flu shot. The CDC adds deaths from pneumonia to flu deaths to come up with a combined figure for flu and pneumonia deaths. For example, on April 6, 2023, the CDC reported on its "Influenza" page the mortality for 2021 as "Number of deaths: 41,917."[233] Even though it was on the "Influenza" page, the figure was reported under the heading "Influenza and pneumonia deaths." Interestingly, the CDC reveals that the total number of influenza-only deaths was reported to be 608. Thus, 99% of the deaths being reported as "influenza and pneumonia deaths" in 2021 were from pneumonia.

It is misleading to report the combined deaths from flu and pneumonia. That is because, as explained by Dr. David Rosenthal, director of Harvard University Health Service, the relationship between pneumonia and the flu is not unique.[234] Many other diseases can cause pneumonia.[235] People can die from pneumonia without ever having the flu. But because people typically do not die from influenza, the CDC has decided to hook the alleged flu deaths to pneumonia to scare the public into getting flu shots. Jon

Rappaport reported:

> In December of 2005, the British Medical Journal (online) published a shocking report by Peter Doshi, which spelled out the delusion and created tremors throughout the halls of the CDC. Here is a quote from Doshi's report:
>
> "[According to CDC statistics], 'influenza and pneumonia' took 62,034 lives in 2001—61,777 of which were attributable to pneumonia and 257 to flu, and in only 18 cases was the flu virus positively identified."[236]

The CDC used that sleight of hand until 2008, to announce that "every year ... about 36,000 people die from flu."[237] But that is twisting the truth because very few of those deaths are from the flu. The CDC had been doing that for years. On or about 2004, pediatrician Kenneth Stoller on behalf of the International Hyperbaric Medical Association, admonished the CDC about this deception and asked them to stop doing it.[238] On or before 2010, the CDC decided to change from saying that "every year ... about 36,000 people die from flu" to saying that "[e]ach year ... 36,000 people die from flu-related causes."[239] But, again, that is a lie. The 36,000 figure is coming from combining flu and pneumonia deaths. There is nothing unique about the relationship between the flu and pneumonia. It is misleading to call pneumonia a "flu-related cause" of death. People can die from pneumonia without ever having the flu. This is all done to fan the flames of fear to convince the uninformed masses to get a flu shot.

Glen Nowak, Ph.D., the Associate Director for Communications National Immunization Program in the CDC, gave a presentation in 2004 before the American Medical Association where he explained how the CDC uses the media to drum up demand for influenza vaccines.[240] His slide presentation is posted on the AMA website. In the presentation, he listed the media message that "Flu kills 36,000 per year" as the #2 predominant message pumped out from the CDC to the media during the week of September 21-28, 2003. That message, we now know, was a lie.

Dr. Novak's presentation states that his goal was "to broaden understanding and thinking about influenza vaccination communication– especially when it comes to greatly increasing coverage." He explained how the CDC will insert particular messages in the media to increase the uptake of the influenza vaccines for 2004-2005. One of his slides presents: "'Recipe' that Fosters Influenza Vaccine Interest and Demand." The recipe is a seven-step plan for "Generating Interest in, and Demand for, Flu (or any other) Vaccination." Dr. Novak's slide show was in 2004. The CDC has since evolved to now reporting the statistic for flu deaths under the heading: "influenza and pneumonia deaths." The CDC does not break out a separate report that only lists flu deaths because that puny number would not scare people into getting a flu vaccine.

Some of the pertinent slides that indicate the kind of messages that the CDC planned on feeding to the media are cut and pasted below:

> Medical experts and public health authorities publicly (e.g., via media) state concern and alarm (and predict dire outcomes)– and urge influenza vaccination.
>
> Framing of the flu season in terms that motivate behavior (e.g., as "very severe," "more severe than last or past years," "deadly")
>
> Continued reports (e.g., from health officials and media) that influenza is causing severe illness

and/or affecting lots of people– helping foster the perception that many people are susceptible to a bad case of influenza.

Visible/tangible examples of the seriousness of the illness (e.g., pictures of children, families of those affected coming forward) and people getting vaccinated (the first to motivate, the latter to reinforce)

References to, and discussions, of pandemic influenza–along with continued reference to the importance of vaccination.[241]

Below are the text in slides where Dr. Novak addresses some of the expected issues during the vaccine campaign.

Vaccination demand, particularly among people who don't routinely receive an annual influenza vaccination, is related to heightened concern, anxiety, and worry.

Effectively addressing parent concerns about a) the number and timing of vaccinations and b) thimerosal[242]

Some component of success (i.e., higher demand for influenza vaccine) stems from media stories and information that create motivating (i.e., high) levels of concern and anxiety about influenza.

The CDC is marketing to scare the public into getting an unsafe and ineffective flu shot. The CDC knows that the shot is almost worthless in protecting people from the flu. Yet, the CDC states:

Everyone 6 months and older in the United States should get an influenza (flu) vaccine every season with rare exception. CDC's Advisory Committee on Immunization Practices has made this "universal" recommendation since the 2010-2011 flu season.[243]

In his book, *Jabbed*, Brett Wilcox explains the worthlessness of the influenza vaccines.

> GSK tested Fluarix in 2 European countries during the 2006-2007 influenza season and found that 3.2 percent of the unvaxxed subjects came down with the flu or an "influenza-like illness" (ILI) while 1.2 percent of the subjects in the Fluarix group contracted the flu or an influenza-like illness. This equates to a 62.5% efficacy rate.

> The math used to obtain 62.5% is as follows: Divide 3.2 into 1.2 to get .375 or a 37.5% reduced incidence of flu in the treatment group. Subtract 37.5 from 100 to get an efficacy rate of 62.5%. This figure is not technically a lie, but it is absolutely deceptive. It gives the impression that Fluarix prevents the flu in 62.5% of people who get the jab. GSK knows full well that according to its own efficacy test that for every 100 people who are vaccinated with Fluarix, only 2 people derive any benefit (3.2 minus 1.2 equals 2). 2 out of 100 equals an absolute risk reduction or vaccine efficacy rate of 2% with a corresponding vaccine worthless rate of 98%.

> According to the 2015 meta-analysis conducted by the Cochrane Collaboration, the 98% worthless rate is fairly consistent among flu vaccine

recipients. The Collaboration reviewed 90 reports and found that on average flu jabs prevent 2.5% of people from coming down with an influenza-like illness and only 1.4% of people from contracting the flu. In other words, the flu jab is from 97.5% to 98.6% worthless.[244]

Wilcox points out that the above figures do not account for those who get sick because of the flu vaccine. The CDC adamantly states that "Flu vaccines CANNOT cause the flu"[245](emphasis in original). That is just another government lie. The inserts for Novartis' flu vaccine, FLUARIX, states that 16% of participants in its trial suffered flu-like symptoms within seven days of getting vaccinated.[246] So, how can the CDC and Novartis claim that the flu vaccine does not give one the flu? Simple, they do not count what happens within the first seven days of getting the shot. Novartis monitored the study subjects immediately after the vaccination. But they did not consider what happened in the first two weeks when calculating the efficacy of the vaccine. That two-week cut-out ensured that inconvenient evidence that showed that the vaccine was making people sick would not affect the efficacy statistics. The Novartis excluded the first two weeks of data after vaccination when calculating the vaccine efficacy because the first seven days showed a spike in flu-like symptoms among the test subjects. The study's raw data showed that for every two people helped by the vaccine, 16 were made sick from it. The vaccine is 8 times more likely to harm than help. Novartis did not count the 16% who came down with flu-like symptoms within the first week of the shot when reporting the vaccine's efficacy.

Adding insult to injury, almost half of the flu vaccines contain dangerous mercury. Congressman Bill Posey made the following statement on the floor of the House of Representatives in 2013.

Some believe that toxins like thimerosal, which is

50% ethylmercury, have played a role in the rise in autism and neurodevelopmental disabilities. In 2000 there was near universal agreement that mercury should be removed as a preservative for vaccines. Yet, today, nearly half of all annual flu vaccines, which are recommended for children and pregnant women, still contain mercury as a preservative—not simply trace amounts of mercury. It's 2013! Why are we still injecting ethylmercury into babies and pregnant women?[247]

Congressman Dan Burton submitted a report in the House of Representatives after a three-year investigation initiated by the Committee on Government Reform. Below is an excerpt from that report:

> The research is explicit that fetal brains are more sensitive than the adult brains to the adverse effects of methylmercury, which include:
>
> Severe brain damage
>
> Delayed achievement of developmental milestones
>
> Neurological abnormalities such as brisk tendon reflexes
>
> Widespread damage to all areas of the fetal brain, as opposed to focal lesions seen in adult tissue
>
> Microcephaly
>
> Purkinje [neuron] cells failed to migrate to the cerebellum
>
> Inhibition of both cell division and migration,

affecting the most basic process in brain development[248]

Knowing the dangers of mercury to an unborn child and that half of the flu vaccines contain mercury, the CDC still recommends that "[p]regnant women should receive a seasonal flu shot."[249] Russell Blaylock, M.D., a (retired) board-certified neurosurgeon, highly respected authority, and expert on brain damage caused by vaccines, stated: "I cannot think of anything more insane than vaccinating pregnant women."[250]

Lest you think that the mercury-free flu vaccine is safe, think again. The Medical Director and Chief Operating Officer of the Cleveland Clinic Wellness Institute, Daniel Neides, M.D., warns that the mercury-free flu vaccine is also dangerous. Dr. Neides posted the following article on January 6, 2017, on the Cleveland Clinic website.

> I am tired of all the nonsense we as American citizens are being fed while big business - and the government - continue to ignore the health and well-being of the fine people in this country. Why am I all fired up, you ask?
>
> I, like everyone else, took the advice of the Centers for Disease Control (CDC) - the government - and received a flu shot. I chose to receive the preservative free vaccine, thinking I did not want any thimerasol (i.e. mercury) that the "regular" flu vaccine contains.
>
> Makes sense, right? Why would any of us want to be injected with mercury if it can potentially cause harm? However, what I did not realize is that the preservative-free vaccine contains formaldehyde.

WHAT? How can you call it preservative-free, yet still put a preservative in it? And worse yet, formaldehyde is a known carcinogen. Yet, here we are, being lined up like cattle and injected with an unsafe product. Within 12 hours of receiving the vaccine, I was in bed feeling miserable and missed two days of work with a terrible cough and body aches.

My anger actually stems from a constant toxic burden that is contributing to the chronic disease epidemic. And yet the government continues to talk out of both sides of its mouth. We want our citizens to be healthy and take full advantage of the best healthcare system in the world (so we think), yet we don't treat our bodies with the love and attention they deserve.

***

Link to autism?

***

Slight detour. Why do I mention autism now twice in this article. Because we have to wake up out of our trance and stop following bad advice. Does the vaccine burden - as has been debated for years - cause autism? I don't know and will not debate that here. What I will stand up and scream is that newborns without intact immune systems and detoxification systems are being over-burdened with PRESERVATIVES AND ADJUVANTS IN THE VACCINES.

The adjuvants, like aluminum - used to stimulate

the immune system to create antibodies - can be incredibly harmful to the developing nervous system. Some of the vaccines have helped reduce the incidence of childhood communicable diseases, like meningitis and pneumonia. That is great news. But not at the expense of neurologic diseases like autism and ADHD increasing at alarming rates.

When I was in medical school in the late 1980s, the rate of autism was 1 in 1,000 children. For those born in the 1950's and 60's, do you recall a single student in your grade with an Individualized Education Program (IEP) for ADHD or someone with a diagnosis of autism? I do not.

As of 2010, the rate of autism in the U.S. escalated to 1 in 68 children. The deniers will simply state that we do a better job of diagnosing this "disorder". Really? Something (s) are over-burdening our ability to detoxify, and that is when the problems begin.

***

For those who want to dive in further, help me understand why we vaccinate newborns for hepatitis B - a sexually transmitted disease. Any exposure to this virus is unlikely to happen before our second decade of life, but we expose our precious newborns to toxic aluminum (an adjuvant in the vaccine) at one day of life.

And when they actually need the protection, many who have received this three-shot series in the first year of life will lack antibody protection--as immunity may not last.[251]

Two days after Dr. Neides posted that article, the Cleveland Clinic posted this response.

> Cleveland Clinic is fully committed to evidence-based medicine. Harmful myths and untruths about vaccinations have been scientifically debunked in rigorous ways. We completely support vaccinations to protect people, especially children who are particularly vulnerable. Our physician published his statement without authorization from Cleveland Clinic. His views do not reflect the position of Cleveland Clinic and appropriate disciplinary action will be taken.[252]

Did you notice the threat of disciplinary action? Well, the Cleveland Clinic acted and summarily fired Dr. Neides. There are many doctors who agree with Dr. Neides, but they keep their mouths shut because they know it will mean the end for their medical careers to criticize the safety or efficacy of vaccines.

In 2016, Dr. Nick Delgado made the astounding statement that he had spoken to some 500 doctors in the previous three years. He asked them privately if they would be willing to share their views on vaccinations. They told him, "No, I can't talk about it." Their response to his "Why not?" was "Because my license is at risk."[253]

Brett Wilcox recounts, "Andrew Wakefield, said that doctors tell him all the time that they'd like to speak up but are afraid of what it would do to their careers. Wakefield says he has little patience or tolerance for such people anymore. They took an oath to 'First Do No Harm,' and in remaining silent, they violate that oath and what it means to be a doctor."[254]

Del Bigtree, the producer of Vaxxed, described the situation of doctors being scared to speak out about the dangers of vaccines in an interview with ABC:

> The real sad thing is the [number] of doctors I've spoken to that say, "Del, I know that vaccines are causing autism, but I won't say it on camera because the pharmaceutical industry will destroy my career just like they did to Andy Wakefield." And that's where we find ourselves: being bullied by an industry that doesn't really care about our children.[255]

So, it is not just mercury that is dangerous to the mother and her unborn child. The other excipients in the flu vaccines cause severe adverse effects. Alexander Langmuir, former head of the CDC, was fired when he refused to say that people should get the flu vaccine. Langmuir said:

> I would not take the flu vaccine. My wife does not take the flu vaccine. No one should take the flu vaccine. And in fact when I was head of CDC, I wanted to make that as a public statement and I refused to say that you should take the flu vaccine. That's why I'm now professor at Harvard.[256]

FLUARIX is a flu vaccine that does NOT contain thimerosal.[257] Yet, the FLUARIX package insert lists the following adverse events experienced by people injected with the vaccine:

> Lymphadenopathy, tachycardia, vertigo, conjunctivitis, eye irritation, eye pain, eye redness, eye swelling, eyelid swelling, abdominal pain or discomfort, swelling of the mouth, throat, and/or tongue, asthenia, chest pain, feeling hot, injection site mass, injection site reaction, injection site warmth, body aches, anaphylactic reaction including shock, anaphylactoid reaction,

hypersensitivity, serum sickness, injection site abscess, injection site cellulitis, pharyngitis, rhinitis, tonsillitis, convulsion, encephalomyelitis, facial palsy, facial paresis, Guillain-Barré syndrome, hypoesthesia, myelitis, neuritis, neuropathy, paresthesia, syncope, asthma, bronchospasm, dyspnea, respiratory distress, stridor, angioedema, erythema, erythema multiforme, facial swelling, pruritus, Stevens-Johnson syndrome, sweating, urticarial, Henoch-Schönlein purpura, and vasculitis.[258]

15 COVID-19 Vaccine Scam

On or before August 23, 2021, the FDA announced that they do not know if the Pfizer-BioNTech or the Comirnaty COVID-19 vaccines worked to stop transmission. The FDA said it could only hope that the vaccines would do so.

> Most vaccines that protect from viral illnesses also reduce transmission of the virus that causes the disease by those who are vaccinated. While it is hoped this will be the case, **the scientific community does not yet know if the Pfizer-BioNTech COVID-19 Vaccine or Comirnaty will reduce such transmission.**[259]

The FDA lied. Before the FDA said, on or before August 23, 2021, they did not know if the Pfizer-BioNTech COVID-19 vaccines would reduce transmission, the CDC, on March 8, 2021, was already on record saying that fully vaccinated persons should be "mindful of the potential risk of transmitting the virus to others."[260] Indeed, the CDC was convinced that the COVID-19 vaccines did NOT work because it advised fully vaccinated residents of non-healthcare congregate settings to "quarantine for 14 days and be tested for SARS-CoV-2 following an exposure to someone with suspected or confirmed COVID-19."²⁶¹ The only reason to quarantine a fully vaccinated person exposed to COVID-19 would be if the vaccine does not prevent infection and does not prevent the transmission of COVID-19.

That means that while the FDA was claiming it was not sure if the Pfizer-BioNTech COVID-19 vaccine would reduce transmission, the CDC was already on record saying it was so sure it did not prevent transmission it was recommending quarantining for 14 days fully vaccinated persons who had been exposed to someone even suspected of having COVID-19. The left hand did not know what the right hand was doing. Which is worse, the deception by the FDA or the dystopian quarantining recommendation by the CDC?

The COVID-19 vaccine was supposed to prevent someone from getting COVID-19.²⁶² The whole purpose of the COVID-19 vaccine is to prevent COVID-19 infection. Indeed, that was the primary focus of the study that resulted in the Emergency Use Authorization (EUA) by the FDA for the Moderna and the Pfizer-BioNtech COVID-19 vaccines. But early in the COVID-19 vaccine program, on March 8, 2021, the CDC implicitly admitted that the COVID-19 vaccines are ineffective in preventing the infection and spread of COVID-19.²⁶³ On March 8, 2021, the CDC listed the following official recommendations for **fully vaccinated people**:

> For now, **fully vaccinated people** should continue to:
>
> ● Take precautions in public like **wearing a well-fitted mask and physical distancing**
> ● **Wear masks**, practice **physical distancing**, and adhere to other prevention measures when visiting with unvaccinated people who are at increased risk for severe COVID-19 disease or who have an

unvaccinated household member who is at increased risk for severe COVID-19 disease
- **Wear masks, maintain physical distance**, and practice other prevention measures when visiting with unvaccinated people from multiple households
- **Avoid medium- and large-sized in-person gatherings**
- **Get tested if experiencing COVID-19 symptoms**
- Follow guidance issued by individual employers
- Follow CDC and health department travel requirements and recommendations[264]

There is no way that if a person obtains immunity from COVID-19, as the vaccines were purported to do, the CDC would recommend that a person who is fully vaccinated continue to:

- **Wear a mask;**

- **Practice physical distancing;**

- **Avoid medium and large-sized in-person gatherings;**

- **Get tested if experiencing COVID-19 symptoms;**

- **Follow other prevention measures to stop the spread of COVID-19.**

The CDC claimed on March 8, 2021, that "a growing body of evidence suggests that fully vaccinated people are less likely to have asymptomatic infection and potentially less likely to transmit SARS-CoV-2 to others." Notice that the CDC used the terms "less likely" to be infected and "potentially less likely" to transmit

SARS-CoV-2. What do those unscientific weasel terms mean? The CDC was beginning a campaign of equivocation. The vaccines were proving ineffective. And the CDC was implicitly admitting it. The CDC said: "How long vaccine protection lasts and how much vaccines protect against emerging SARS-CoV-2 variants are still under investigation."

The CDC said they used the terms "less likely" to be infected and "potentially less likely" to transmit SARS-CoV-2 because they did not know at that time if the vaccines worked. But even that is a lie because they did know. The evidence was clear by that point that the vaccines offered no protection, and that is why the CDC continued to recommend that a vaccinated person still take precautions to prevent getting and spreading SARS-CoV-2. The CDC stated on March 8, 2021:

> Until more is known and vaccination coverage increases, some prevention measures will continue to be necessary for all people, regardless of vaccination status.[265]

That was a damning admission in light of the EUA authorization for the vaccines being based on the promise that the vaccines would **"prevent"** COVID-19. Indeed, on December 11, 2020, the FDA explicitly stated that it issued the EUA for the first COVID-19 vaccine from Pfizer-BioNTech "for the **prevention** of coronavirus disease 2019 (COVID-19) caused by severe acute respiratory syndrome coronavirus 2 (SARS-CoV-2)."[266]

The COVID-19 vaccines were promoted to the public as a preventive measure. But while the unofficial public pronouncements were that the COVID-19 vaccines were effective in preventing COVID-19, the CDC and FDA began the strange process of official equivocation about the effectiveness of the vaccines in preventing COVID-19. They very soon began to admit what they knew from the beginning. The vaccines were ineffective in preventing COVID-19.

The CDC described the "less likely" to be infected and "potentially less likely" to transmit SARS-CoV-2, "residual risk." Don't be fooled. Residual risk is a real risk. The CDC was admitting that the COVID-19 vaccines do not work. The CDC makes the astounding statement:

> The benefits of reducing social isolation and relaxing some measures such as quarantine requirements may outweigh **the residual risk of fully vaccinated people becoming ill with COVID-19 or transmitting SARS-CoV-2 to others.**[267]

That March 8, 2021, statement is proof that the CDC knew and admitted within the first three months of the COVID-19 vaccine programs that "fully vaccinated" people were at risk of "becoming ill with COVID-19 or transmitting SARS-CoV-2 to others." They knew that the vaccines did not work. Yet, the CDC kept up its vaccination campaign.

The CDC claimed that the residual risk is low for infection of a fully vaccinated person. But the claim that the residual risk is low makes no sense in light of the CDC's advice that a person should be monitored following any exposure to someone with "suspected or confirmed COVID-19."

> Fully vaccinated people who do not quarantine should still monitor for symptoms of COVID-19 for 14 days following an exposure. If they experience symptoms, they should isolate themselves from others, be clinically evaluated for COVID-19, including SARS-CoV-2 testing, if indicated, and inform their health care provider of their vaccination status at the time of presentation

to care.[268]

That advice would makes no sense unless the CDC had already established that vaccinated persons have, in-fact, been infected with SARS-CoV-2 after being vaccinated. Thus, to the satisfaction of the CDC, the vaccine had been proven to be ineffective in preventing COVID-19. Furthermore, the advice makes no sense unless the vaccine had been proven ineffective in preventing the spread of SARS-CoV-2. Indeed, the vaccine is so ineffective that the CDC recommended quarantining for 14 days a fully vaccinated person working in a jail or group home who had been exposed to someone suspected of having COVID-19.

> Fully vaccinated residents of non-healthcare congregate settings (e.g., correctional and detention facilities, group homes) should continue to quarantine for 14 days and be tested for SARS-CoV-2 following an exposure to someone with suspected or confirmed COVID-19. This is because residential congregate settings may face high turnover of residents, a higher risk of transmission, and challenges in maintaining recommended physical distancing.[269]

That advice to quarantine a fully vaccinated person who has been exposed to someone suspected of being infected with SARS-CoV-2 confirms that the CDC knew that the COVID-19 vaccines were ineffective against contracting and spreading SARS-CoV-2.

You only quarantine a person with a real risk of transmitting the disease. The fact that the CDC advised that a fully vaccinated person be quarantined upon being exposed to a person even suspected of having COVID-19 means that the CDC believed that a fully vaccinated person can be infected with SARS-CoV-2 and then spread that disease to others. That advice by the CDC testifies that the CDC believed at the early date of March 8, 2021, that the COVID-19 vaccines were ineffective in preventing the infection and spread of SARS-CoV-2.

The CDC knew that the COVID-19 vaccines had been proven to be ineffective. The CDC admitted that fact. The CDC explained that a "fully vaccinated" person can still become ill with COVID-19 and transmit SARS-CoV-2. The CDC stated that the only reason to relax some liberty restrictions for COVID-19 vaccine recipients is NOT that the vaccine is effective in preventing the infection and spread of SARS CoV-2 but to "improve COVID-19 vaccine acceptance and uptake" by the general public.

> Additionally, taking steps towards relaxing certain measures for vaccinated persons may help improve COVID-19 vaccine acceptance and uptake.[270]

The CDC admitted that the loosening of restrictions for fully vaccinated persons does not mean that those who have been vaccinated cannot still be infected with SARS-CoV-2 or spread the disease to someone else. The CDC only relaxed restrictions on vaccinated persons to encourage more people to get vaccinated. The CDC was clear that fully vaccinated persons can still get infected with SARS-CoV-2 and should remain on guard for the risk of transmitting the virus to others.

> Therefore, there are several activities that fully vaccinated people can resume now, at low risk to themselves, **while being mindful of the potential risk of transmitting the virus to others.**[271]

The CDC then completely lets the cat out of the bag with the following advice for fully vaccinated persons:

> Fully vaccinated people should not visit or attend

a gathering if they have tested positive for COVID-19 in the prior 10 days or are experiencing COVID-19 symptoms, regardless of vaccination status of the other people at the gathering.[272]

That advice from the CDC assumes two things.

1) Fully vaccinated persons can get infected with SARS-CoV-2.

2) Fully vaccinated persons can transmit SARS-CoV-2.

That CDC advice, given on March 8, 2021, proves that the CDC knew within three months of the vaccine program that the COVID-19 vaccines did not work.

After investigating a COVID-19 outbreak in Barnstable County, Massachusetts, where 74% of the 469 persons infected with COVID-19 were fully vaccinated, the CDC Director, Rochelle P. Walensky, MD, MPH, issued a statement on July 30, 2021.[273] In that news release Director Walensky admonished fully vaccinated persons to wear masks indoors because the COVID-19 vaccinations offer little or no protection against contracting COVID-19. A little-known fact is that those not listed among the fully vaccinated in the Barnstable outbreak may have been vaccinated, just not fully vaccinated. Many excluded from the fully vaccinated statistic were partially vaccinated, or their vaccination status was unknown.[274]

Furthermore, the CDC Director acknowledged in the July 30, 2021, Barnstable press release that "vaccinated people infected with Delta can transmit the virus."[275] Director Walensky revealed in the news release that the Barnstable outbreak was just one of many outbreaks the CDC was investigating nationwide. We have since learned that those other outbreaks nationwide were populated, for the most part, by those who had been fully vaccinated. Thus, the CDC and the medical establishment were fully aware by at least July 2021 that the COVID-19 vaccines do not prevent infection or spread. And, indeed, it was looking very much like the COVID-19 vaccines were causing illnesses. The alleged breakthrough cases were likely antibody-dependent enhancement caused by the vaccines.

Once the flames of COVID-19 fear were fanned, the population was primed to get their COVID-19 vaccines when they were rolled out on December 11, 2020. The ordinary people did not know the vaccines did not work and that they were dangerous. It is not that the government officials slowly learned after the vaccine rollout that the vaccines were ineffective and unsafe. They knew that from the beginning. They lied to the public. They are pretending that they only learned about the danger and ineffectiveness of the vaccines after their rollout. The purpose of the vaccines was to kill and injure. The officials behind the COVID-19 vaccine program are evil minions of the Devil who hate God. God reveals: "all they that hate me love death." Proverbs 8:36.

Dr. Deborah Birx was the U.S. Government Coronavirus Response Coordinator in the Trump Administration from February 27, 2020, until January 20, 2021. Dr. Birx was instrumental in pushing for COVID-19 vaccinations. On July 22, 2022, Neil Cavuto, a journalist for Fox News, "asked Dr. Birx why the unvaccinated should take the vaccine if it does not prevent COVID." Astonishingly, Dr. Birx started by recommending the COVID-19 vaccines but then admitted that she knew from the outset that the vaccines would not protect against infection. She said: "I knew these vaccines were not going to protect against infection, and I think we overplayed the vaccines. ... Let's be clear, 50% of the people that died from the Omicron surge were older vaccinated."[276]

While Dr. Birx knew the vaccines were ineffective in protecting against infection, she told the public a different story. She claimed that the COVID-19 vaccines were safe and effective while knowing they were not. On December 16, 2020, ABC News reported that Dr. Birx said:

> I understand how this vaccine was made. I understand the safety of the vaccine. And critically, I understand the depth of the efficacy of this vaccine. This is one of the most highly-effective vaccines we have in our infectious disease arsenal. And so that's why I'm very enthusiastic about the vaccine.[277]

She further stated on that day:

> I want to make it clear there's two very important sides to that equation. There is herd immunity, which would prevent community spread, and then there's absolute clarity on what people need, in an equity way, to prevent severe disease, hospitalizations and fatalities.[278]

One day earlier, on December 15, 2020, Laurence Smith of WDRB in Kentucky interviewed Dr. Birx. Her focus in the interview was on the steps needed to stop the spread of COVID-19. The key to stopping the spread of COVID-19, according to Dr. Birx, was to get as many people vaccinated as possible so that herd immunity could be achieved. She told Smith:

> While we have so much viral spread, it's really important to get control of this viral spread. ... And we can get to spring together by being vigilant now and being vaccinated when it's our turn. ... To truly achieve herd immunity, it's going to take through the summer and potentially even into the fall.

That's getting 70-80% of Americans immunized.[279]

She knew when she made those statements that the vaccines would not stop the spread of the alleged SARS-CoV-2 virus. Stopping the spread of a virus through herd immunity from a vaccine is premised on the theory that the vaccine will protect those in the herd against infection. Immunity is "[p]rotection against infectious disease."[280] By definition, immunity means a person can resist a particular infection.[281] If a person is immune from a disease, he is in a state where he "is not susceptible to [that] infection or disease."[282] If a person is immune to a disease, that disease does not affect that person; he will not become ill from that disease.[283]

But Dr. Birx's recent 2022 admission that she knew from the outset the vaccines would not protect against infection means that when she made the statements in 2020 about the COVID-19 vaccines providing immunity, she knew the vaccines would not protect against infection. She knew the vaccines were ineffective in stopping the spread of the alleged virus. That means that she intentionally lied on December 15th and 16th, 2020, when as Coronavirus Response Coordinator she claimed that the COVID-19 vaccines would give recipients immunity.

Why would Dr. Birx continue to recommend the COVID-19 vaccines during her July 22, 2022 interview when she knew from the beginning that "these vaccines were not going to protect against infection"? During her July 22, 2022 interview she justified the recommendation by changing the standard for the efficacy of the vaccines from preventing infection to reducing the severity of disease and hospitalizations. That is the pharmaceutical industry's tried and true bait-and-switch scheme. They sell to the public vaccines on the promise of preventing infection and the spread of disease. And when the vaccines are shown not to work, that evidence forces them to admit that the vaccines do not prevent disease. They then switch to a different efficacy standard of lowering the severity of the disease. That is the duplicitous game they are now playing with the COVID-19 vaccines.

Dr. Birx always knew that the COVID-19 vaccines would not work; they do not prevent infection, and she admitted they have been overplayed. Yet, knowing that, Dr. Birx still recommends today that people get vaccinated. "A double minded man is unstable in all his ways." James 1:8. As we have seen, the vaccines are not efficacious, even under the new phony efficacy standard. Indeed, the vaccines are driving the disease. People are getting very sick and suffering ADE from the vaccines.

President Joe Biden has repeatedly stated that the COVID-19 vaccines prevent the spread of SARS-CoV-2. Indeed, that was the alleged purpose of his unconstitutional executive orders requiring federal workers, federal contractors, and the private sector to receive the COVID-19 vaccine. In an October 7, 2021 speech Joe Biden stated:

> We still had more than a quarter of people in the United States who were eligible for vaccinations but didn't get the shot.
>
> And we know there is no other way to beat the pandemic than to get the vast majority of Americans vaccinated. It's as simple as that.
>
> And to — **to spread to our children, to spread throughout society and at our hospitals the risk of other variants** — it's all dangerous and obvious, but we're still not there.
>
> We have to beat this thing. So, while I didn't race to do it right away, that's why I've had to move toward requirements that everyone get vaccinated or I had the authority to do that. That wasn't my

first instinct.

My administration is now requiring federal workers to be vaccinated. We've also required federal contractors to be vaccinated. If you have a contract with the federal government, working for the federal government, you have to be vaccinated.

We're requiring active duty military to be vaccinated. We're making sure healthcare workers are vaccinated, because if you seek care at a healthcare facility, you should have the certainty that the pro- — **the people providing that care are protected from COVID and cannot spread it to you.**

The Labor Department is going to shortly issue an emergency rule — which I asked for several weeks ago, and they're going through the process — to require all employees [employers] with more than 100 people, whether they work for the federal government or not — this is within a — in the purview of the Labor Department — to ensure their workers are fully vaccinated or face testing at least once a week.

In total, this Labor Department vaccination requirement will cover 100 million Americans, about two thirds of all the people who work in America.

And here's the deal: These requirements are already proving that they work.

***

> But don't take it from me. Not from some, you know, liberal think tank this comes from. But here's what Wall Street is saying:
>
> Goldman Sachs, quote: "Vaccinations will have a positive impact on employment." **It means less spread of COVID-19, which will help people return to work.**[284]

On October 10, 2022, we found out that Pfizer never tested their vaccine for whether it would prevent transmission of the alleged SARS-CoV-2 virus. The CEO of Pfizer, Albert Bourla refused to testify before the European Parliament. Janine Small, President of International Markets at Pfizer testified in his stead. She testified before the European Parliament that Pfizer never tested their vaccine to determine if it would prevent the spread of the virus. At the hearing, Bob Roos, a Dutch European Parliament member, asked Small "was the Pfizer COVID vaccine tested on stopping the transmission of the virus before it entered the market?"[285] Small answered: "No. We had to really move at the speed of science to really understand what is taking place in the market."[286] That astounding admission hit the public like a bomb because it undermines the basis for vaccine mandates.

On May 16, 2021, Anthony Fauci appeared on CBS's "Face the Nation." The host, John Dickerson, interviewed him. During the interview, Dr. Fauci announced without equivocation that the COVID-19 vaccines are effective in stopping the spread of SARS-CoV-2. He stated that "even though there are breakthrough infections with vaccinated people ... [it is] not impossible but very, very low likelihood — that they're going to transmit it." He elaborated:

> When you get vaccinated, you not only protect your own health and that of the family but also you contribute to the community health by **preventing**

the spread of the virus throughout the community. ... In other words, **you become a dead end to the virus.** And when there are a lot of dead ends around, the virus is not going to go anywhere. And that's when you get a point that you have a markedly diminished rate of infection in the community.[287]

We now know Dr. Fauci's statements were not true because Pfizer never did any studies to determine the effectiveness of the vaccines in stopping the spread of SARS-CoV-2. There was simply no evidence from which Dr. Fauci could say otherwise. He was lying.

Indeed, we have proof that when he made those statements, he knew they were not true. We know that Fauci intentionally lied because four months earlier, on January 19, 2021, he said in an article that he knew the COVID-19 vaccines (and indeed all injectable vaccines) typically do not result in immunity that interrupts infection or transmission through mouth and nose. Mouth and nose (i.e., mucosal) transmission is the alleged means by which the COVID-19 virus is spread. Dr. Fauci was the co-author of the January 19, 2021 article in which he said:

> **Administration of parenterally administered vaccines alone typically does not result in potent mucosal immunity that might interrupt infection or transmission.** ... For these reasons, additional data regarding protection from infection should be generated as soon as possible.[288] (emphasis added)

His statement in the January 19, 2021 article was the opposite of his May 16, 2021 statement. There is no way to reconcile the two statements. Dr. Fauci lied to encourage people to get vaccinated, falsely telling them by doing so they would help others by stopping the spread of SARS-CoV-2. He knew what he was saying was a lie, and did not care who was injured by being injected with the ineffective and unsafe COVID-19 vaccines.

But that admission by Pfizer and Dr. Fauci's deception really miss the elephant in the room. That elephant in the room is the issue of whether the COVID-19 vaccines even prevents infection from the beginning. Pfizer did not test for whether the vaccine would prevent transmission because they knew to begin with that it would not stop infection. Pfizer knew that their COVID-19 vaccine was ineffective in doing what vaccines are supposed to do, provide immunity from infection. Pfizer's vaccine does not work and they know it.

Logically, if the vaccine cannot prevent transmission, that means it cannot prevent infection. In order for someone to spread the virus they must be infected from the begining. Thus, the key issue is stopping the infection. Of course, if the vaccine stops infection, it will necessarily stop the spread. Because if a person is not infected with a disease, he cannot transmit the disease; a person cannot spread something he does not have. All government officials knew from the beginning that the COVID-19 vaccines would not prevent infection and consequently would not prevent the spread of the virus.

Joseph Choi reported for The Hill the following December 3, 2020, statement from Pfizer CEO Albert Bourla:

> Pfizer chairman Albert Bourla told Dateline host Lester Holt that the pharmaceutical company was "not certain" if the vaccine prevented the coronavirus from being transmitted, saying, "This is something that needs to be examined."[289]

But just six weeks later, on January 13, 2020, the official Pfizer Twitter account strongly implied that, indeed, their vaccine does stop transmission of the SARS-Cov2 virus. "The ability to vaccinate at speed to gain herd immunity and stop transmission is our highest priority."[290]

To erase all doubt about Pfizer's public position, on June 8, 2021, Albert Bourla stated on Twitter: "Although data shows that severe #COVID19 is rare in children, widespread vaccination is a critical tool to help stop transmission."[291] Bourla later deleted that Tweet, but it was recovered using the Internet Archive Wayback Machine. Recall that Janine Small, President of International Markets at Pfizer, testified on October 10, 2022, before the European Parliament that Pfizer never tested their vaccine to determine if it would prevent the spread of the virus. Boural knew that and even said on December 3, 2020, that Pfizer was not sure if the vaccine prevented SARS-Cov2 from being transmitted, saying preventing transmission was something that needed to be examined. Yet, both Pfizer and its CEO, knowing that their vaccine was ineffective in preventing virus transmission, nonetheless had no qualms in lying to the public and misrepresenting it as effective. They are liars.

Senator Matthew Canavan, during an Australian Senate Education Employment and Legislation Committee hearing, asked the Australia Country Medical Director for Pfizer, Dr. Krishan Thiru, whether Pfizer tested its COVID-19 vaccine to determine if it could stop or reduce the transmission of the virus before its approval and rollout of the vaccine in 2020.[292] Dr. Thiru employed obfuscation in refusing to answer the question. Senator Canavan also asked Dr. Thiru on what evidence Pfizer Tweeted on January 13, 2020, that the Pfizer vaccine is intended to fulfill its high priority to gain herd immunity and stop transmission. Dr. Thiru again employed obfuscation in refusing to answer the question. Senator Canavan asked the Pfizer representative whether Pfizer CEO Albert Bourla's statement that widespread vaccination is a critical tool to help stop transmission was true. Dr. Thiru danced around the question but suggested in his answer that the Pfizer vaccine is NOT a critical tool to help stop the transmission of the SARS-CoV-2 virus.

Please understand that the SARS-CoV-2 virus does not actually exist. It has never been isolated.[293] Vaccinated people who are testing positive for SARS-CoV-2 do not actually have "breakthrough" COVID-19. They are testing positive for SARS-CoV-2 because the tests are rigged to provide false positive results.[294] The "breakthrough" patients actually are suffering from an autoimmune disease known as antibody-dependent enhancement (ADE) caused by the COVID-19 vaccines.[295] ADE is being falsely labeled as COVID-19, when in fact it is an autoimmune disease caused by the vaccine. Indeed, it seems that is the purpose of the vaccine; it is a kill shot.[296]

Please be mindful that the COVID-19 vaccines were authorized because they purportedly prevented infection and the spread of the disease. Dr. Hilary Marston of the National Institute of Allergy and Infectious Disease at the NIH, gave a presentation during an October 22, 2020 meeting of the Vaccines and Related Biological Products Advisory Committee.[297] That meeting was before the issuance of the EUAs for the COVID-19 vaccines. During her presentation, she explained that the primary endpoint for all COVID-19 vaccine studies was to prevent COVID-19. Below is one of her slides where it states: **"Primary Endpoint: Prevention of symptomatic COVID-19 disease (PCR confirmed)."**[298] The PCR tests for SARS-CoV-2, the alleged virus thought to cause COVID-19.

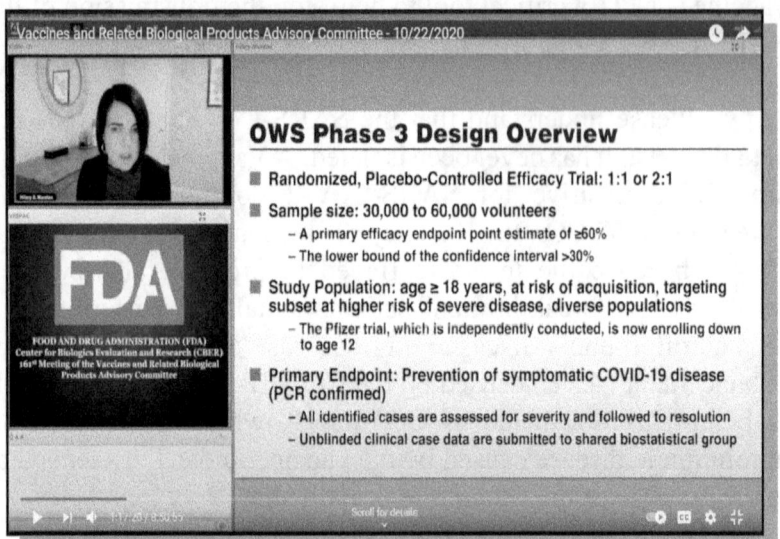

Indeed, the pertinent criteria announced by the FDA for the EUA granted to the Pfizer-BioNTech COVID-19 vaccine said nothing about lessening symptoms. The criteria for the EUA was simply that the vaccine may be effective in "preventing" COVID-19.

> Based on the totality of scientific evidence available to FDA, it is reasonable to believe that Pfizer-BioNTech COVID-19 Vaccine may be effective in **preventing COVID-19**, and that, when used under the conditions described in this authorization, the known and potential benefits of Pfizer-BioNTech COVID-19 Vaccine when used to **prevent COVID-19** outweigh its known and potential risks.[299]

And when on August 23, 2021, the FDA approved the substantially similar COMIRNATY (COVID-19 Vaccine, mRNA), it said nothing about lessening symptoms. The FDA only mentioned the alleged effectiveness of the approved vaccine to prevent COVID-19. The FDA stated that that "[t]he [approved] vaccine has been known as the Pfizer-BioNTech COVID-19 Vaccine, and will now be marketed as Comirnaty (koe-mir'-na-tee), for the **prevention of COVID-19** disease in individuals 16 years of age and older."[300]

When it became clear, though, that the vaccines were ineffective in preventing COVID-19, the standard for effectiveness had to be changed to something else. The standard for effectiveness is now no longer prevention of COVID-19 infection or preventing the spread of COVID-19. The standard has shifted to lessening the symptoms of COVID-19. It seems that the vaccine manufacturers and the CDC knew from the beginning that the COVID-19 vaccines would be ineffetive in preventing the spread of the disease. Indeed, as early as October 26, 2020, prior to the EUA issuance, Anthony Fauci, Director of the National Institute of Allergy and Infectious Diseases (NIAID), stated that preventing infection with COVID-19 was only a secondary endpoint. The primary purpose of the vaccine was not to prevent infection or spread but rather only to lessen symptoms.[301]

Dr. Fauci claimed at the time that preventing COVID-19 was only a secondary endpoint of the vaccines. He made that statement just four (4) days after his subordinate, Dr. Hilary Marston, gave a presentation during an October 22, 2020 meeting of the Vaccines and Related Biological Products Advisory Committee, where she explained that the **primary endpoint** of the COVID-19 vaccine trials was the **prevention** of COVID-19.[302] When people in government are conspiring to commit fraud, it is sometimes hard to keep everyone on the same sheet of music.

Before the FDA issuance of the EUA for the Moderna vaccine, Moderna Chief Medical Officer Tal Zaks stated on or before November 23, 2020: "our results show that this vaccine can prevent you from being sick, it can prevent you from being severely sick. **They do not show that it prevents you from**

potentially carrying this virus transiently and infecting others."[303] Yet, the basis on which the EUA was granted to Moderna was that it was allegedly effective in preventing infection. There was no basis for authorizing the EUA on the vaccine's ability to only lessen the symptoms of COVID-19, while not preventing infection. Moderna limited the measure of efficacy for their COVID-19 vaccine, in pertinent part, as follows: "**The primary efficacy endpoint was efficacy of the vaccine to prevent protocol-defined COVID-19 occurring** at least 14 days after the second dose in participants with negative SARS-CoV-2 status at baseline."[304] The EUA was based on the representation by Moderna that their study proved that the vaccine would prevent infection. But the Moderna's Chief Medical Officer Tal Zaks knew from the beginning that the vaccine was ineffective in preventing infection, and he said so.

The efficacy studies done for the EUA only measured the prevention of COVID-19. There was no publication of any studies that were the basis for EUA that measured lowering symptoms. For example, When you read page 35 of the Pfizer-BioNtech publication titled *Fact Sheet for Healthcare Providers Administering Vaccine*, it reveals that the only criterion reported for establishing the effectiveness of the COVID-19 vaccine is the subsequent infection rate in the study groups.[305] The study compared the COVID-19 infection rate among the vaccine group and the placebo group to come up with an effectiveness of 95% for the COVID-19 vaccine. The study announced that the "Vaccine Efficacy" was based upon a finding of the "First COVID-19 Occurrence From 7 Days After Dose 2."[306]

That fact sheet indicates that "FDA issued this EUA, based on Pfizer-BioNTech's request and submitted data. Although limited scientific information is available, based on the totality of the scientific evidence available to date, it is reasonable to believe that the Pfizer-BioNTech COVID-19 Vaccine **may be effective for the prevention of COVID-19** in individuals as specified in the

Full EUA Prescribing Information."[307]

On or about November 23, 2021, the FDA claimed that "[v]accinating children ages 5 years and older can help protect them from getting COVID-19, spreading the virus to others, and getting sick if they do get infected."[308] The FDA used the qualifying word "help," but the statement was intended to deceive people into believing that the vaccine would protect persons from being infected, getting sick, or spreading the alleged virus. It had become apparent by the time the FDA posted that statement that the vaccines did none of those things. On or about March 30, 2022, the CDC finally admitted in writing that the COVID-19 vaccines do not prevent infection. On its frequently asked questions page, the FDA posted the question: "Why should I get vaccinated if I might get COVID-19 anyway?" To which the FDA responded, in pertinent part: "Like all vaccines, COVID-19 vaccines are not 100% effective at preventing infection. Some people who are up to date with their COVID-19 vaccinations will get COVID-19 breakthrough infection."[309]

Since it has become clear that the COVID-19 vaccine does not prevent infection, the FDA has switched from saying that the COVID-19 vaccine will prevent infection to instead saying that "COVID-19 vaccination significantly lowers your risk of severe illness, hospitalization, and death if you get infected."[310] But people were prodded to get vaccinated to prevent infection. When that was seen not to be true, the FDA pivoted from preventing infection to claiming instead that "COVID 19-vaccines are effective at protecting people from getting seriously ill, being hospitalized, and dying."[311] But preventing serious illness, hospitalization, and death were not the efficacy criteria of the vaccine studies. The vaccine studies and approval under the EUA were based on the vaccine's purported ability to prevent COVID-19.

Ponder the sheer nonsense of measuring any medication's

efficacy by whether it lowers the risk of hospitalization or death. Even Kool-Aid could be touted by that low bar as a wonder drug. Indeed, the CDC has created a measure of efficacy that is almost impossible to verify. If one receives a COVID-19 vaccine and then gets sick from COVID-19 and survives, the doctor will claim that the person survived the bout from COVID-19 because of the vaccine. But that can never be known, and the doctor knows it. Indeed, suffering during any illness is subjective. After the person survives the alleged COVID-19 bout, he will be told by his doctor that it was a good thing he was vaccinated; otherwise, it could have been much worse. The doctor will convince the patient that the vaccine lowered the severity of the symptoms. But the doctor is just making it up. If the person is not hospitalized, the doctor will say the vaccine kept his patient out of the hospital. If the person is hospitalized, the doctor will lower the bar further and say the vaccine saved his life. It is a subjective game that the COVID-19 vaccine always wins. It is a medical scam.

This bait and switch strategy was brought to light publically when on January 30, 2021, Andrew Court reported for The Daily Mail that "Democrat Rep. Stephen Lynch has tested positive to COVID-19 after receiving both shots of the Pfizer vaccine."[312] In a that news article it was explained that the reason that Rep. Lynch was infected with COVID-19 after being vaccinated is that "Pfizer's vaccine does not necessarily prevent COVID-19 infection, but is said to be 95 percent effective in stopping the serious symptoms that are caused by the coronavirus."[313]

Pfizer-BioNtech announced that their COVID-19 vaccine was 95% effective in "preventing" COVID-19. They did NOT announce that it was 95% effective in reducing symptoms of COVID-19. The FDA allowed the EUA of the Pfizer COVID-19 vaccine because the COVID-19 vaccine study claimed a 95% effectiveness in "preventing" the recipients from getting COVID-19 after they had been vaccinated.[314] Indeed, the FDA states the reason for the EUA of the Pfizer-BioNtech COVID-19 vaccine was that it is theorized to be effective in "preventing" the SARS-CoV-2 infection. The FDA explicitly states:

> Pfizer-BioNTech COVID-19 Vaccine is authorized to **prevent** coronavirus disease 2019 (COVID-19) caused by severe acute respiratory syndrome coronavirus 2 (SARS-CoV-2) in individuals 16 years of age and older.[315]

The argument that the COVID-19 vaccines lessen symptoms is a smokescreen. The report from Britain's Chief Scientific Adviser, Patrick Vallance, proves it. In July 2021, he stated that 40% of all COVID-19 patients being admitted to hospitals with COVID-19 are fully vaccinated.[316] That fact alone proves that the COVID-19 vaccines do not lessen symptoms. Persons are admitted to the hospital when they have severe symptoms. The fact 40% of those being hospitalized for COVID-19 are fully vaccinated indicates that the patients are suffering severe symptoms and thus the vaccines do not lessen the symptoms. You cannot have droves of vaccinated people jamming into hospitals after coming down with COVID-19 and maintain that the vaccines lessen symptoms.

Indeed, the FDA explicitly stated on or before August 20, 2021, that it did not know if the Pfizer-BioNTech COVID-19 vaccine reduces symptoms. The FDA has stated that the Pfizer-BioNtech COVID-19 vaccine has been authorized under the EUA hoping that it will **"prevent"** COVID-19 and NOT in the hope it will reduce the severity of COVID-19.

> To date, only a small number of severe cases have occurred during the study, which makes it **difficult to evaluate whether the vaccine reduces the severity of COVID-19.** Pfizer-BioNTech COVID-19 vaccine is **authorized to prevent**

coronavirus disease 2019 (COVID-19) caused by severe acute respiratory syndrome coronavirus 2 (SARS-CoV-2) in individuals 16 years of age and older.[317]

The CDC has expressed hope that the COVID-19 vaccines will prevent infection, but the evidence is that the vaccines do no such thing. The CDC claims that a person who is vaccinated is unlikely to be infected with COVID-19, but then they give the following guidance, which suggests that they know that the likelihood of a vaccinated person getting COVID-19 is significant:

> Fully vaccinated people who have come into close contact with someone with COVID-19 should be tested 3-5 days following the date of their exposure and wear a mask in public indoor settings for 14 days or until they receive a negative test result. They should isolate if they test positive.[318]

That advice indicates that the CDC has no confidence in the efficacy of the COVID-19 vaccines in preventing the disease.

CDC Director, Dr. Rachelle Walensky has even less faith in the COVID-19 vaccines. She revealed that not only do the vaccines not lessen the symptoms, but NPR reports that "Walensky noted that data from Israel suggests 'increased risk of severe disease amongst those vaccinated early.'"[319]

Writing for Roll Call, Emily Kopp reported on July 30, 2021, that data presented at a confidential congressional briefing showed that "[u]p to 15 percent of deaths in May were among vaccinated people."[320]

A government report from Public Health England reveals that persons who have been vaccinated are six (6) times more likely to die from the delta variant of the SARS-COV-2 than those who are unvaccinated.[321] The report shows that 26 out of 4,087 fully vaccinated persons died from the variant. Whereas 34 out of 35,521 unvaccinated persons died from the variant.[322] That is a 665% greater death rate among the vaccinated group. So much for lessening symptoms.

If it has now been shown that the vaccine is truly ineffective in "preventing" a vaccine recipient from getting COVID-19, it should be announced as ineffective. The vaccine should be taken off the market. Apparently, that will not happen. Instead, there is now being announced a new criterion for effectiveness that was never studied. And that new criteria is lessening of symptoms. But that is also a deception because the data proves the vaccines don't do that either. This bait and switch strategy for vaccines has been around since the 1800's. Dr. Suzanne Humphries reveals that "[w]hen it was clear that the smallpox vaccine was not able to prevent disease, the medical profession tried to justify vaccination by changing the goal posts from lifelong 'perfect' immunity to "milder disease.'"[323] Dr. Humphries revealed that bait and switch from immunity to milder symptoms was used to justify getting ineffective pertussis and influenza vaccines in 2013.

The CDC seems incapable of telling the truth. After it went through all the machinations to change the criteria from preventing infection and spread to lessening symptoms, it is now faced with vaccines that nobody wants. Why would anyone get vaccinated against COVID-19 if the vaccine does not prevent the infection or spread of the illness? Faced with that reality, what did the CDC decide to do? It seems the CDC is hoping that most will forget that the COVID-19 vaccines do not prevent infection or spread because the CDC is now going back to claiming that is what the COVID-19 vaccines will do.

The agency is like a snake oil salesman hawking his wares without much thought to the reality of what it says. As we have seen above, the CDC knows the COVID-19 vaccines do not prevent COVID-19. Yet, on or before March 17, 2023, the CDC posted on its website that "COVID-19 vaccination is recommended for everyone ages 6 months and older in the United States for the **prevention** of COVID-19."[324] You read that correctly. The CDC is now touting the COVID-19 vaccines as preventatives against COVID-19, while knowing they do no such thing. Below is a cropped screenshot from the CDC website.

> Recommendations for COVID-19 vaccine use
>
> Groups recommended for vaccination
> COVID-19 vaccination is recommended for everyone ages 6 months and older in the United States for the prevention of COVID-19. There is currently no FDA-approved or FDA-authorized COVID-19 vaccine for children younger than age 6 months.

The CDC is suddenly changing its tune and is now saying that the COVID-19 vaccines prevent COVID-19. But the medical community and the general public understand that the COVID-19 vaccines do NOT prevent a person from getting COVID-19. For example, in an October 27, 2022, article in Medical News Today, which incidentally was medically reviewed for accuracy by Meredith Goodwin, M.D., FAAFP, Helen Miller explains what everyone now knows:

> The COVID-19 vaccine does not prevent COVID-19. A person who is fully vaccinated can still contract the SARS-CoV-2 virus, which causes COVID-19, and may go on to develop the disease.[325]

What is the point of getting a vaccine that does not prevent the disease? Miller explains that the purpose of the vaccine is not to prevent COVID-19 but rather to "strengthen immunity against the virus and help prevent serious illness, hospitalization, and death."[326] That is what the CDC had previously said. But the CDC is now stating that the COVID-19 vaccines do not just prevent serious illness from COVID-19, but any degree of the disease; the CDC claims now that the COVID-19 vaccines prevent COVID-19, which is false.

It gets worse. On or before December 22, 2022, the CDC posted a statement that "COVID 19-vaccines are effective at preventing severe illness from COVID-19 and **limiting the spread of the virus** that causes it."[327] One of the vaccines that the CDC recommends is the Pfizer-BioNTech COVID-19 vaccine. Pfizer-BioNTech is on record in testimony before the EU Parliament that it never tested its vaccine for whether it would prevent the spread of the virus. Indeed, it has been proven that none of the COVID-19 vaccines prevent the spread of SARS-CoV-2. But the pathological liars at the CDC say that the ineffective COVID-19 vaccines prevent the spread of SARS-CoV-2. Below is a cropped screenshot from the CDC website.

> **Ensuring COVID-19 Vaccine Safety in the US**
>
> Updated Dec. 22, 2022   Español | Other Languages   Print
>
> **Vaccine Safety and Monitoring**
>
> - COVID-19 vaccines were developed using science that has been around for decades.
> - COVID-19 vaccines are **safe**, and meet the Food and Drug Administration's (FDA's) rigorous scientific standards for safety, effectiveness, and manufacturing quality.
> - **COVID 19-vaccines are effective** at preventing severe illness from COVID-19 and limiting the spread of the virus that causes it. ←
> - Millions of people in the United States have received COVID-19 vaccines.
> - COVID-19 vaccines are **monitored** by the most intense safety monitoring efforts in U.S. history.
>
> CDC recommends COVID-19 vaccines for everyone ages 6 months and older, and boosters for everyone 5 years and older, if eligible.
>
> - Children and teens ages 6 months–17 years
> - Adults ages 18 years and older

Dr. John Campbell, Ph.D., was incredulous at what the CDC said on its website. He could not believe that the CDC said that the COVID-19 vaccines prevent the spread of the SARS-CoV-2 virus that causes COVID-19 because the evidence clearly establishes that the vaccines do no such thing. Dr. Campbell sated:

> [COVID-19] vaccines are safe, according to the Centers for Disease Control. [That statement] was taken from their website not an hour ago. ... "COVID 19 vaccines are effective at preventing some severe illness from COVID-19 and limiting the spread of the virus that causes it."[328]

Dr. Campbell then sardonically states:

> Now, you might have thought that COVID vaccination has minimal if any effect for any period of time at preventing the spread of COVID-19. You might have thought that; I might have thought that, but, hey, we're both wrong because the CDC states here in black and white, taken from their website not an hour ago that, and I've made a note. Note: "and limiting the spread of the virus that causes it."[329]

Dr. Campbell then exhales as he tries to stop laughing before he continues to speak in exasperated disbelief.

> This is the CDC. This is the CDC on Tuesday, the 28th of March 2023, saying the COVID vaccine prevents the spread of COVID-19.[330]

Dr. Campbell then drops his head in his hands in shock and disbelief at what he has just read on the CDC website. He continues then to sarcastically explain the incredible statements by the CDC:

> That's what it says. It prevents the spread of COVID-19! That's what they say on their website, today! And we can't argue with it, it must be right because it's on the CDC website. So, there we go, make a note of that. The vaccine prevents the spread.[331]

Dr. Campbell then shakes his head as he says in an exasperated, cynical, mocking tone: "Unbelievable! Because I thought it didn't really prevent the spread but there you go. [You] can't be right all the time. So that's what they're saying."[332]

On or before March 2021, Johns Hopkins said that an effective vaccine "will protect someone who receives it by lowering the chance of getting COVID-19." But that the "more important" benefit of the COVID-19 vaccines was that they are "highly efficacious at preventing serious illness, hospitalization and death."[333] On July 28, 2022, the Johns Hopkins article was updated to include the following statement: "Johns Hopkins Medicine views the FDA-approved mRNA vaccines from Pfizer and Moderna as highly effective at preventing serious disease, hospitalization, and death from COVID-19."[334]

The authors of that Johns Hopkins article knew with certainty when they wrote that statement it is not true that the COVID-19 vaccines were "highly effective at preventing serious disease, hospitalization, and death from COVID-19" because it had become quite evident by the time that they wrote that that the vast majority of the people dying from COVID-19 were vaccinated.

Johns Hopkins is an elite medical center at the forefront of the medical establishment and has medical data from governments worldwide at its fingertips. The UK has monthly mortality data regarding deaths from COVID-19 that are regularly published and made available online. That data revealed a steady rate of COVID-19 deaths among the vaccinated population each month. It is more accurate to describe those people as persons who tested positive for SARS-CoV-2 before dying because SARS-CoV-2 does not exist. The UK data shows that during the 21 months between April 1, 2021, and December 31, 2022, 86% of the COVID-19 deaths in the UK were among those vaccinated against COVID-19.[335] Clearly, it is not true that the COVID-19 vaccines are "highly effective at preventing serious disease, hospitalization, and death from COVID-19." when 86% of those who are dying with COVID-19 have gotten the COVID-19 vaccine.

Johns Hopkins has followed the CDC lead and has now changed its tune regarding the efficacy of the COVID-19 vaccines in preventing COVID-19 and the spread of the virus that causes it. The change is subtle but real. On or before November 1, 2022, the same article cited above was again updated to place highlights around a statement that "evidence continues to indicate that getting a COVID-19 vaccine is the best protection against getting COVID-19, whether you have already had COVID-19 or not."[336] Johns Hopkins further now states that "[g]etting vaccinated provides greater protection to others since the vaccine helps reduce the spread of COVID-19." But we know that both statements are not true.

Johns Hopkins has gone from saying that the COVID-19 vaccines merely "lower the chance of getting COVID-19" to saying with certainty that "getting a COVID-19 vaccine is the best protection against getting COVID-19." That flies in the face of the evidence that has now become so apparent. Adding insult to injury, Johns Hopkins now says that the vaccine "helps reduce the spread of COVID-19." The evidence is now in. It is clear that the vaccines do no such thing. Indeed, Pfizer-BioNTech is on record admitting they never even tested their COVID-19 vaccine to determine whether it would reduce the spread of COVID-19.

In the same article in which Johns Hopkins states that the COVID-19 vaccines help reduce the spread of COVID-19, Johns Hopkins implicitly acknowledges that the vaccines do no such thing. In the article, Johns Hopkins explains that it follows the CDC's recommendation for those vaccinated to wear masks and remain physically distant from others in all of their facilities. If the vaccines effectively prevented the spread of SARS-CoV-2, no such steps would be necessary to prevent the transmission of the alleged virus.

16   COVID-19 Vaccines are Ineffective

On August 26, 2022, the CDC claimed that "[h]ospitalization rates among unvaccinated adults were 3.4 times as high as those among vaccinated adults."[337] But the report's published statistics reveal that 44.1% of persons hospitalized during the period spanning June 20, 2021–May 31, 2022 were fully vaccinated:

> Among hospitalized nonpregnant patients in this same period, 39.1% had received a primary vaccination series and 1 booster or additional dose; 5.0% had received a primary series and ≥2 boosters or additional doses.[338]

According to the CDC published statistics, 44.1% (39.1% + 5.0%) of those hospitalized between June 20, 2021 and May 31, 2022, for COVID-19 had been fully vaccinated and received at least one COVID-19 booster shot. Please understand that those statistics are manipulated to inflate the numbers for COVID-19 unvaccinated patients while deflating the numbers for COVID-19 vaccinated patients.[339]

In a report of Los Angeles County, California, COVID-19 deaths and hospitalizations, it was revealed that the CDC classified

COVID-19 hospitalizations and deaths of fully vaccinated persons only if those persons are hospitalized or die 14 days or more after the final dose of a COVID-19 vaccine.[340]

The CDC also decided that someone who dies or is hospitalized after receiving a COVID-19 vaccine will nonetheless be listed as an unvaccinated death or hospitalization if that person died less than 14 days after receiving the first dose of a two-dose series (Moderna and Pfizer) or the first dose of a one dose administration (Johnson & Johnson) or if they cannot determine when the person was vaccinated when referencing the California Immunization Registry.

All other cases falling outside those parameters will be considered partially vaccinated. Partially vaccinated persons would be those who died or were hospitalized ≥14 days after receiving the first dose and <14 days after the second dose in a 2-dose series.

How are partially vaccinated persons treated statistically by the CDC? The CDC states:

> For the purpose of this surveillance, a vaccine breakthrough infection is defined as the detection of SARS-CoV-2 RNA or antigen in a respiratory specimen collected from a person ≥14 days after they have completed all recommended doses of a U.S. Food and Drug Administration (FDA)-authorized COVID-19 vaccine.[341]

Dr. Joseph Mercola explains:

> The CDC is also playing with statistics in other ways to create the false and inaccurate impression that unvaccinated people make up the bulk of infections, hospitalizations and deaths. For example, we now find out the agency is counting

anyone who died within the first 14 days post-injection as unvaccinated.

Not only does this inaccurately inflate the unvaccinated death toll, but it also hides the real dangers of the COVID shots, as the vast majority of deaths from these shots occur within the first two weeks. Now their deaths are counted as unvaccinated deaths rather than being counted as deaths due to vaccine injury or COVID-19 breakthrough infections![342]

***

In other words, if you've received one dose of Pfizer or Moderna and develop symptomatic COVID-19, get admitted to the hospital and/or die from COVID, you're counted as an unvaccinated case. If you've received two doses and get ill within 14 days, you're still counted as an unvaccinated case.

The problem with this is that over 80% of hospitalizations and deaths appear to be occurring among those who have received the jabs, but this reality is hidden by the way cases are defined and counted. A really clever and common strategy of the CDC during the pandemic has been to change the definitions and goalposts so it supports their nefarious narrative.[343]

A breakthrough case is a person who is deemed to be infected with COVID-19 only after being fully vaccinated 14 days or more after receiving all recommended COVID-19 vaccine doses. That means that a partially vaccinated person is NOT listed among the breakthrough cases. That, in turn, means that a partially vaccinated person diagnosed with COVID-19 is NOT listed among the breakthrough COVID-19 cases. Thus, the CDC treats partially vaccinated persons as being unvaccinated COVID-19 cases statistically.

Another confounding factor explained by Dr. Mercola is that to "count as a confirmed vaccinated individual, you must send your vaccination card to your primary care physician's office and have them add it to your electronic medical record. If you got the shot at a pharmacy, you'll need to verify that they forwarded your proof of vaccination to your doctor. Primary care offices are then responsible for sharing their patients' immunization data with the state's immunization information system. Patient-recorded proof of vaccination is only accepted for influenza and pneumococcal vaccines, not COVID-19 injections. What this all means is that, say you got the shot several weeks ago at a drive-through vaccination clinic and get admitted to the hospital with COVID symptoms. Unless your COVID shot status has actually been added into the medical system, you will not be counted as 'vaccinated.'"[344] This all has the effect of artificially inflating the unvaccinated COVID-19 infection tally while showing a misleadingly reduced breakthrough infection rate for those vaccinated.

Likely, the deaths and hospitalizations suffered by those vaccinated for COVID-19 are not because the vaccines have failed to protect those who were vaccinated but rather because the vaccines are causing the deaths and hospitalizations through what is called antibody-dependent enhancement (ADE).[345] Indeed, that is the conclusion of renowned virologist and Nobel Prize Laureate Prof. Luc Montagnier.[346]

The CDC is trying to keep a lid on antibody-dependent enhancement (ADE). ADE can happen many months after vaccination, but ADE can sometimes manifest early. For example, 35 nuns received COVID-19 vaccines, and within two days, 28 nuns fell ill and tested positive for COVID-19, with two nuns dying during those two days.[347] A third nun also died days later. That is clear evidence of ADE within days of being vaccinated. Such evidence of early-onset ADE is information the CDC does not want to be known. And so, from now on, those cases will be listed as unvaccinated COVID-19 cases.

The CDC is trying to bury their statistical sleight of hand down a memory hole. The above language from the CDC that a COVID-19 breakthrough infection is limited to a COVID-19 diagnosis from a person ≥ 14 days after they have completed all recommended COVID-19 vaccines that had been posted on the CDC website on or before September 3, 2021, at the URL cited in the endnote has been deleted from the CDC website. But Washoe County (Nevada) Health District quotes that deleted CDC language on its COVID-19 Facts page.[348]

The CDC is playing a game of trying to obfuscate the ADE cases (which the CDC calls breakthrough COVID-19 cases) suffered by vaccinated persons while continuing to inflate the alleged COVID-19 cases suffered by the unvaccinated population. The false narrative of a killer SARS-CoV-2 virus causing COVID-19 disease has been generated by two principle methods. 1) false-positive PCR tests which can be manipulated into reporting an artificially high number of false-positives by altering the cycle threshold (CT value), and 2) inflating the case count by a broad definition of what is a COVID-19 case, such as listing a positive PCR test as a COVID-19 case, even if the person never experienced any symptoms. But it seems that inflation strategy began to backfire.

It was becoming an embarrassment to the FDA, CDC, and the vaccine makers because their COVID-19 inflation efforts began to present a very high number of breakthrough infections (which are really ADE cases) for vaccinated persons. To address this, the CDC announced new rules for reporting breakthrough cases of vaccinated persons that they do not apply to unvaccinated persons. First, the CDC instructed local health officials, when reporting breakthrough COVID-19 infections for vaccinated persons, to "submit only specimens with Ct value ≤28 to CDC for sequencing."[349] But the CDC left standing its recommended cycle threshold of 40 cycles for testing unvaccinated patients.[350] Even Anthony Fauci admitted that a cycle threshold more than 35 in a PCR test would return a meaningless false postive test result.[351]

To further lower the reported numbers of breathrough cases, the CDC announced that "[a]s of May 1, 2021, CDC transitioned from monitoring all reported vaccine breakthrough cases to focus on identifying and investigating only hospitalized or fatal cases due to any cause."[352] Neither of these two new strategies were applied to the unvaccinated reporting. There are now different rules for reporting vaccinated COVID-19 cases and unvaccinated COVID-19 cases. The effect is to lower the reported number of vaccinated COVID-19 breakthrough cases while continuing the stratagem of inflating the reported unvaccinated COVID-19 cases. Dr. Joseph Mercola summarizes the consequences of the CDC's data manipulation.

> It's not just the CDC's definition of a breakthrough case that skews the data. Even more egregious and illogical is the fact that the CDC even has two different sets of testing guidelines — one for vaccinated patients and another for the unvaccinated.
>
> Since the beginning of the pandemic, the CDC has recommended a PCR test cycle threshold (CT) of 40. This flies in the face of scientific consensus, which has long been that a CT over 35 will produce 97% false positives, essentially rendering the test useless.

In mid-May 2021, the CDC finally lowered its recommended CT count, but only for patients who have received one or more COVID shots. So, if you have received a COVID injection, the CDC's guidelines call for your PCR test to be run at a CT of 28 or less. If you are unvaccinated, your PCR test is to be run at a CT of 40, which grossly overestimates the true prevalence of infection.

The end result is that unvaccinated individuals who get tested are FAR more prone to get false positives, while those who have received the jab are more likely to get an accurate diagnosis of infection.[353]

Reporting for *Off Guardian*, Kit Knightly explains how the CDC manipulates data to prop up vaccine efficacy while keeping the COVID-19 scare going. In a series of examples, she describes how under similar circumstances one could be reported as a COVID-19 case when unvaccinated but not reported as a COVID-19 case when vaccinated under the CDC reporting standards.

> Person A has **not been vaccinated**. They test positive for COVID using a PCR test at 40 cycles and, despite having no symptoms, they are officially a "COVID case". [But the person would NOT be a COVID case if he were **vaccinated**.]

> Person B has been **vaccinated**. They test positive at 28 cycles, and spend six weeks bedridden with a high fever. Because they never went into a hospital and didn't die they are NOT a COVID case. [But the person would be reported as a COVID case if he were **not vaccinated**.]

Person C, who was also **vaccinated**, did die. After weeks in hospital with a high fever and respiratory problems. Only their positive PCR test was 29 cycles, so they're not officially a COVID case either. [But the person would be reported as a COVID case if he were **not vaccinated**.][354]

Even those efforts by the CDC to manipulate the data cannot mask the ineffectiveness of the COVID-19 vaccines. With those numbers, how can anyone say that the COVID-19 vaccines effectively stop COVID-19 infection? The major takeaway from these statistics is that massive numbers of vaccinated people are being hospitalized for illnesses attributed to COVID-19. In reality, they are suffering diseases stemming from antibody-dependent enhancement (ADE) caused by the COVID-19 vaccines.

One might argue that the reason that so many vaccinated people are being hospitalized for COVID-19 compared to the unvaccinated is that the population of vaccinated people is greater. But when we look at death rates from COVID-19 and adjust for population, we find that, in fact, those who are vaccinated are dying at a greater rate from COVID-19 than those who are unvaccinated. A former reporter for the New York Times, Alex Berenson, analyzed the official data from the UK government comparing the death rate of those who had been vaccinated with a COVID-19 vaccine with those who remained unvaccinated.[355] He made a startling discovery. Those who had been vaccinated are dying at more than twice the rate of those who remained unvaccinated.[356]

Below is a chart that illustrates the difference in the death rates. The chart reflects a comparison of deaths per 100,000 vaccinated persons against the deaths per 100,000 of unvaccinated persons. The graph shows that vaccinated persons are dying at more than twice the rate of unvaccinated persons. Berenson observed that "overall deaths in Britain are running well above normal."[357] That means that the higher number of deaths among vaccinated persons are an aberration that can only be explained by the variable: vaccination. That, in turn, means that there must be a causal link between vaccination and a higher death rate. Berenson drew the only logical conclusion from that data: **"I don't know how to explain this other than vaccine-caused mortality."**[358]

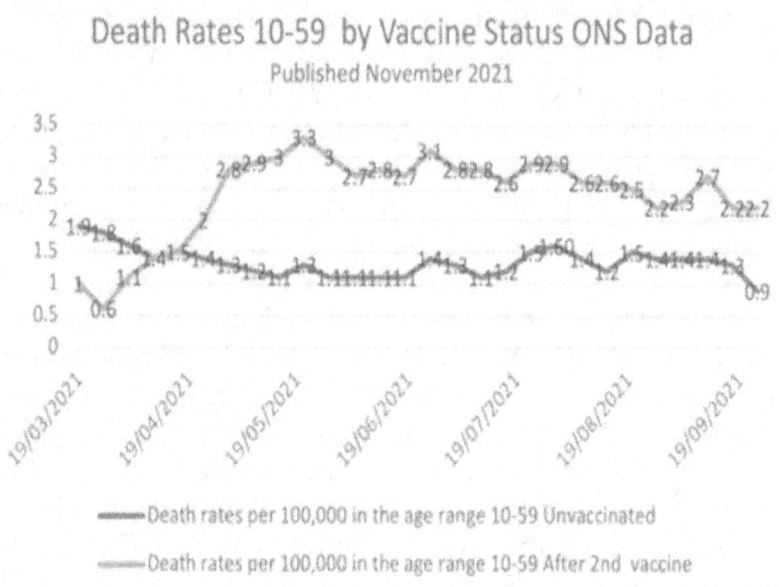

This author looked at the data in the Excel spreadsheet[359] prepared by the UK Government and did a little calculating of my own. My calculations confirm the findings of Alex Benson. Interestingly, the data further shows that across the board the unvaccinated die at a lower rate than the population as a whole. It seems that the unvaccinated are healthier than the general population.

This author found the exact opposite when I looked at the death rate of the vaccinated population. Those who are vaccinated with the COVID-19 vaccine die at a greater rate than the population as a whole. This suggests that the vaccinated population is less healthy than the general population. This data confirms the research done regarding childhood vaccination. Children who receive childhood vaccinations are significantly less healthy than their unvaccinated counterparts.[360]

I took the averages of the deaths per week during the reporting period from January 8, 2021, to September 24, 2021 reported by the UK Government. I found that the average per week mortality rate was 14.6 per 100,000 persons for unvaccinated persons. Multiplying that figure by 52 weeks we arrive at a yearly mortality rate of **0.76%**. That is lower than the average mortality rate of 0.94% for England as a whole.

But when this author looked at the average per week mortality rate for those who received two COVID 19 vaccination shots I found that 26.58 persons out of 100,000 persons who received two doses died per week on average. That is an average yearly mortality rate of **1.4%**. That mortality rate far exceeds the average mortality rate for England of 0.94%.

This author found that on average per week 18.09 persons per 100,00 persons who received one dose of the vaccine died within 21 days of the first dose of the COVID vaccine. That matches the average yearly mortality rate of 0.94% for England.

But what was most remarkable was the mortality rate measured for those who died 21 or more days after the first dose of the COVID-19 vaccine. This author found that on average 30.04 per 100,000 persons died per week who received one dose of the COVID-19 vaccine when their deaths happened 21 days or more after the first dose of the COVID-19 vaccine. That translates to an average yearly mortality rate of **1.6%** for those who make it 21 days or more after the first shot of the COVID-19 vaccine. That is far above the average mortality rate in England of 0.94%.

In conclusion, the official data from the UK Government shows that those vaccinated with two doses of the COVID-19 vaccine have a mortality rate of **1.4%**, which is almost twice the mortality rate (**0.76%**) of those who are unvaccinated. The average death rate for the entire English population, which includes vaccinated and unvaccinated, is 0.94%. Thus, the unvaccinated die at a lower rate than the general population. In contrast, the vaccinated persons die at a greater rate than the general population.

When one realizes that the persons who die after the first shot are not around to get a second shot, one can reasonably conclude that the data for the post-second shot mortality rate understates the deadliness of the COVID-19 vaccines. That is a problem because the standard for reporting vaccine deaths is to report only those deaths 14 days or more after receiving the second shot as deaths of vaccinated persons. A person who only receives one COVID-19 shot or who dies within 14 days of the second shot is considered to be unvaccinated. Those persons fall in the unvaccinated column even though the persons received one or even two vaccination shots. The UK data in this report is unusual in that it separately reports those who died after the first shot.

Dr. Günter Kampf, a Professor at the University Medicine Greifswald, Institute for Hygiene and Environmental Medicine, wrote an article published in *The Lancet* explaining that official government data shows that COVID-19 is being spread mainly through those who have received a COVID-19 vaccination. Dr. Kampf explains:

> In Germany, the rate of symptomatic COVID-19 cases among the fully vaccinated ("breakthrough infections") is reported weekly since July 2021 and was 16.9% at that time among patients of 60 years and older. This proportion is increasing week by week and was 58.9% on 27. October 2021 [...] providing clear evidence of the increasing

relevance of the fully vaccinated as a possible source of transmission.[361]

Below is a chart showing the "[v]accination rates and proportions of fully vaccinated people among symptomatic COVID-19 cases (≥60 years) in Germany between 21 July and 27 October 2021 based on the weekly reports from the Robert Koch-Institute."[362]

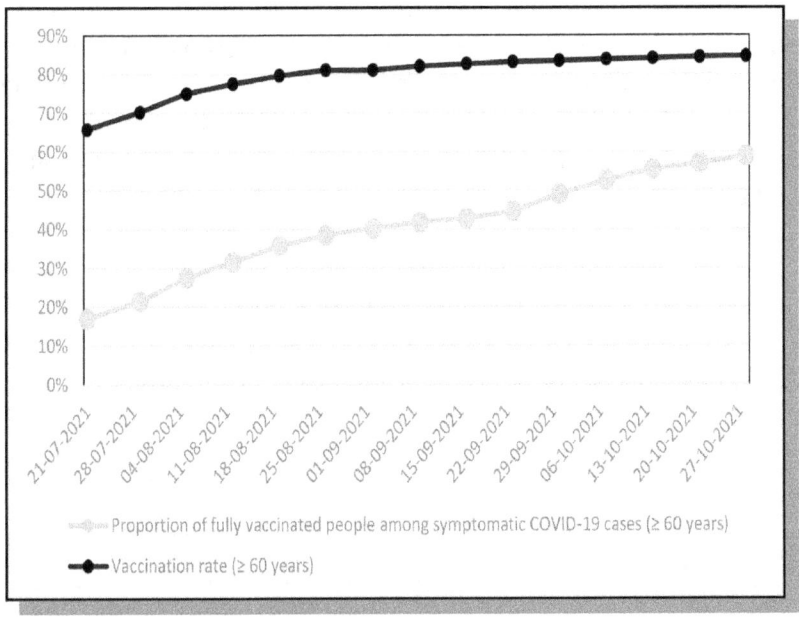

The report upon which the above statistics are based is from the Robert Koch Institute.[363] "The Robert Koch Institute (RKI) is the [German] government's central scientific institution in the field of biomedicine."[364] RKI is tasked with the identification, surveillance, and prevention of diseases to provide the German government with a scientific basis for health-related political decision-making.

Dr. Kampf explains that the RKI study reveals that in Germany, as of October 2021, 58.9% of the symptomatic COVID-19 cases among those ≥ 60 years old are from vaccinated persons. That suggests that the vaccines are driving the infection.

The chart below illustrates that the German data set from the Koch Institute revealed that there were 4,206 cases of the Omicron variant of COVID-19 in Germany between 21 July and 27 October 2021. Of those 4,206 reported cases, 4,020 infected people were fully vaccinated (2,883) or both fully vaccinated and boosted (1,137) (2,883 + 1,137 = 4,020). Only 186 of the reported Omicron COVID-19 cases were unvaccinated. Thus, more than 95% of Germany's reported Omicron COVID-19 variant infections were people who were fully vaccinated or both fully vaccinated and boosted.

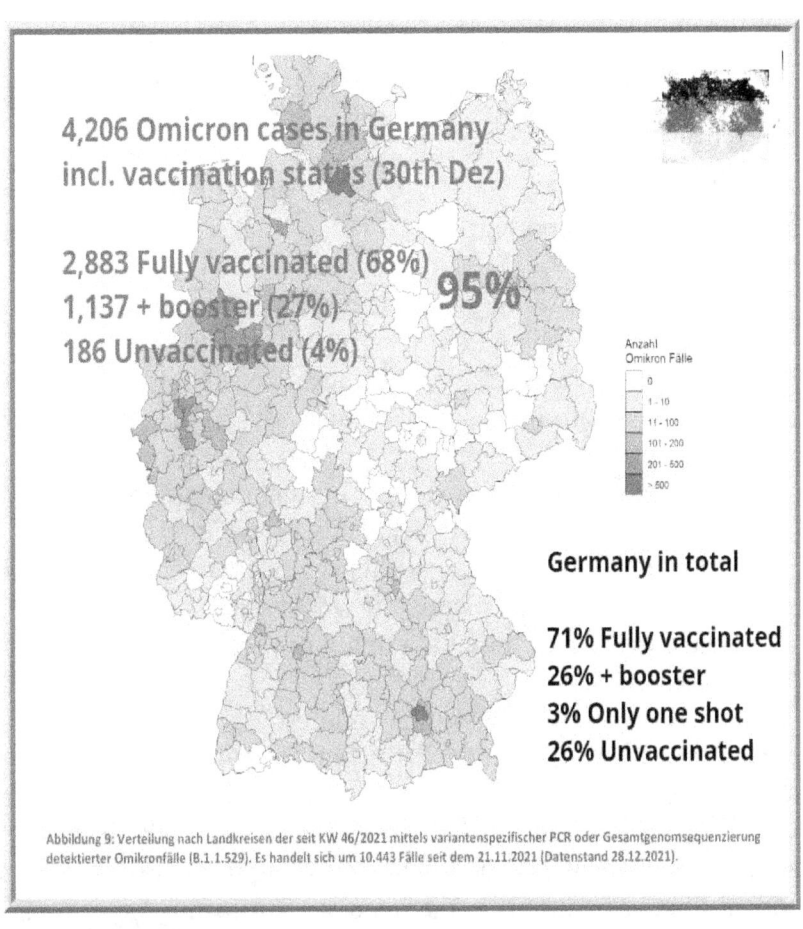

Abbildung 9: Verteilung nach Landkreisen der seit KW 46/2021 mittels variantenspezifischer PCR oder Gesamtgenomsequenzierung detektierter Omikronfälle (B.1.1.529). Es handelt sich um 10.443 Fälle seit dem 21.11.2021 (Datenstand 28.12.2021).

The Delta and Omicron variants of COVID-19 seem to be cover stories to explain away ADE being suffered by COVID-19 vaccine recipients. There is no other reasonable explanation for the fact that RKI has reported that more than 95% of all the Omicron variant cases in Germany are from those who have received two or more doses of the COVID-19 vaccine.[365] Notably, there is no reporting category for those who received only one (1) dose of the COVID-19 vaccine.[366] It is, therefore, likely that single-dose recipients have been included in the "unvaccinated" group. Thus it appears that the vaccines are driving the Omicron variant of COVID-19. Omicron bears all of the hallmarks of ADE, but there is a complete media blackout of ADE. And so, the vaccinated persons diagnosed with COVID-19 are not being described as ADE cases but instead are being mischaracterized as breakthrough Omicron variant cases.

On December 21, 2021, Ethan Huff, writing for NEWSTARGET reported:

> "It appears to be grossly negligent to ignore the vaccinated population as a possible and relevant source of transmission when deciding about public health control measures," Kampf says.
>
> To continue calling the current situation a "pandemic of the unvaccinated" is simply false, Kampf warns. In reality, this is a pandemic of the vaccinated, as the plandemic would already be over had everyone chosen to remain unvaccinated.[367]

Dr. Kampf does not address antibody-dependent enhancement (ADE), which is the actual cause of the illnesses among those vaccinated. What is truly happening is that the vaccinated are suffering the symptoms of antibody-dependent enhancement (ADE). The patients reporting to the hospital with severe illnesses caused by the vaccines are testing positive for COVID-19, thus being labeled as COVID-19 breakthrough cases. In reality, they are suffering from the ADE side effects of the vaccine itself.

The vaccine makers are scamming the public when they claim their vaccines work. Moderna, for example, reported to the FDA that their studies showed a 94.1% efficacy for their Moderna COVID-19 mRNA vaccine. But that figure is the relative risk reduction and not the total (absolute) risk reduction. The total risk reduction for the Moderna vaccine is only 1.25%. That means that one can expect that there will be a reduction of 1.25% in COVID-19 infections in the population after being vaccinated.

Thus you would have to vaccinate 10,000 persons to protect the 125 people at risk from COVID-19. That means that the federal government is needlessly paying to vaccinate 9,875 out of every 10,000 persons. Such a massive vaccine program to protect so few people only benefits the vaccine makers. And when one realizes that the vaccine is driving ADE, which the medical community is reporting as COVID-19, it explains perfectly why the data shows that more vaccinated persons are being infected and hospitalized with COVID-19 than unvaccinated persons.

When a vaccinated person is diagnosed with COVID-19 it is called a breakthrough case. Even with the efforts of the CDC to under-report COVID-19 breakthrough cases involving vaccinated persons, while at the same time inflating the unvaccinated COVID-19 infection numbers, the data shows a growing trend of vaccinated persons being infected, hospitalized, and dying from COVID-19. While the data shows that the vaccines are ineffective, the federal and state governments are still pushing COVID-19 vaccines as safe and effective. For example, the State of Maryland Department of Health vaccine information website states:

> Vaccines are an effective and critical tool to bring the pandemic under control by helping to prevent infection, serious illness, hospitalization and death due to COVID-19. **Although there are cases of people who become sick after they are fully vaccinated, cases where fully vaccinated people are hospitalized or die from COVID-19 are rare and vaccines remain the best way to prevent COVID-19 and its complications.**[368]

The problem with that statement is that it is not true. Writing for the Gateway Pundit, Joe Hoft revealed that the state government statistics from the Maryland Department of Health (MDH) contradict the above statement.[369] The MDH data showed that "[b]etween Sept 22, 2021, and Oct 10, 2021, Maryland had an additional 21,864 Covid-19 cases [of] which 7,233 or 33.1% of the cases were classified as breakthrough cases. ... During this same period, Maryland lost 259 citizens to Covid-19. Of those 259 souls, 77 or 29.7% were fully vaccinated."[370] The MDH has the temerity to claim that it is rare for fully vaccinated people to be hospitalized or die from COVID-19, when its own statistics show that a significant plurality of the population dying from COVID-19 are those who have been vaccinated.

None other than the former CDC Director, Robert Redfield, refuted the false claim made by the State of Maryland Department of Health that it is rare for a fully vaccinated person to die from COVID-19. On or about October 25, 2021, Redfield responded to a question from Martha MacCallum on FOX News about Colin Powell's recent death that his family states was caused by the COVID-19 vaccine:

> I hear a lot of times people feel it's a rare event that fully vaccinated people may die. I happen to be the senior advisor to Governor Hogan in the state of Maryland. In the last 6-8 weeks, more than 40 percent of people who died in Maryland were fully vaccinated."[371]

Jim Hoft explained that "Andy Owen, a spokesperson for the Maryland Department of Health had a different claim that from Sept. 1 to Oct. 15, only about 30% of Marylanders who died of confirmed COVID-19 were fully vaccinated."[372]

Whether it is 30% or 40%, is really of no import. The fact that any vaccinated persons, let alone such a significant plurality of vaccinated people, are being diagnosed as having COVID-19 and dying from it is stark proof that the COVID-19 vaccines are ineffective. Assuming those deaths are actually from ADE caused by the COVID-19 vaccines proves that the vaccines are also unsafe. But what is really disturbing is that in the face of such evidence that a significant number of persons vaccinated with COVID-19 vaccines are dying, state health authorities claim that "cases where fully vaccinated people are hospitalized or die from COVID-19 are rare and vaccines remain the best way to prevent COVID-19 and its complications."[373] That is an unconscionable lie.

That kind of deception by state health officials is being played out all over the country. Hoft explains:

> In Pennsylvania, the acting Sec. of Health Alison Beam stated at a news conference at Lancaster General Hospital, "With nearly seven million Pennsylvanians fully vaccinated, the data makes it clear: the vaccines are safe and effective at preventing severe illness from Covid-19."
>
> However, recent analysis of cases and deaths between September 15 and Oct 4 show that in 132k cases, 26.1% of them were classified as breakthrough and 305 (26.5%) deaths out of a total of 1,153 were in fully vaccinated people. But Sec. of Health Alison Beam makes no mention of that.[374]

Hoft cites a UK Government Health report showing "that between week 37 and week 40 of 2021, there was a total of 2,805 COVID-19 deaths and 2,136 or 76.1% were fully vaccinated. These deaths happened within 28 days of a positive Covid-19 test."[375] Yet, in the face of that data, the British Government health officials still promote the COVID-19 vaccines as effective in preventing COVID-19, and they claim that the COVID-19 vaccines provide a high level of protection against death from COVID-19.[376] The UK Government dares to recommend the COVID-19 vaccines despite official UK Government statistics that reveal that those who had been vaccinated are dying at more than twice the rate of those who remained unvaccinated.³⁷⁷

On or about July 27, 2021, Dr. Anthony Fauci, Director of the National Institute of Allergy and Infectious Diseases (NIAID), and member of the White House coronavirus task force, said

> When you look at the virus in the nasal pharynx of a vaccinated person who gets a breakthrough infection with [the] delta [variant of COVID-19], it is exactly the same as the level of virus in a unvaccinated person who is infected. That's the problem.³⁷⁸

On or about August 7, 2021, CDC Director Rochelle Walensky stated the following during a CNN interview:

> Our vaccines are working exceptionally well. They continue to work well for Delta with regard to severe illness and death, they prevent it. **But what they can't do anymore is prevent transmission.**³⁷⁹ (emphasis added)

That was a retraction of Walensky's earlier mistaken claim in March 2021 that vaccinated people almost never carry COVID-19.

The Washington Post reported on an internal document from the CDC:

> It cites a combination of recently obtained, still-unpublished data from outbreak investigations and outside studies showing that vaccinated individuals infected with delta may be able to transmit the virus as easily as those who are unvaccinated.³⁸⁰

On or about April 9, 2021, the Prime Minister of England, Boris Johnson, advised persons that they may not meet indoors with vaccinated persons. He admitted that the vaccines do not prevent transmission of COVID-19. He responded to a question that he read out loud during a briefing:

> "Can I now meet my friends and family members indoors if they are vaccinated?" There I am afraid the answer is no, because we're not yet at that stage, we're still very much in the world where you can meet friends and family outdoors, under the rule of six, or two households. And even if your friends and family members may be vaccinated, the vaccines are not giving 100% protection and that's why we need to be cautious. We don't think that they [COVID-19 vaccines] entirely reduce or remove the risk of transmission.[381]

That was not a slip of the tongue or a mistake. Johnson's opinion was based on the data coming from the British health authorities. On or about October 23, 2021, The Prime Minister emphatically repeated that the COVID-19 vaccine "doesn't protect you against catching the disease, and it doesn't protect you from passing it on."[382] Johnson, curiously, went on to promote the COVID-19 vaccine booster, even though the first course of the vaccine has been proven ineffective in preventing infection and the spread of the disease. He trumpeted the new mantra justifying the vaccine booster; it is supposed to lessen the symptoms of COVID-19.

The VAERS system contains hard data on the harm being caused by the COVID-19 vaccines. It is run by the CDC, which is part of the executive branch of government. President Biden is the chief of the executive branch. VAERS is his system. When he issued his order, he and his federal health officials knew that the COVID-19 vaccines were injuring and killing people. A rational

President would have put a halt to the death and injury. But instead, President Biden accelerated the injections by mandating them for executive branch workers.

President Biden's claim that "[t]he vaccines are safe, highly effective,"[383] is provably false. The CDC and the vaccine manufacturers are on record admitting that the COVID-19 vaccines do not prevent the spread of COVID-19. Indeed, before the EUA authorization by the FDA of the Pfizer-BioNtech vaccine, the Daily Mail reported that on or before December 4, 2020, "Pfizer CEO [Albert Bourla] admits he is 'not certain' their COVID-19 shot will prevent vaccinated people from spreading the virus."[384]

As cited above, Moderna Chief Medical Officer Tal Zaks is on record saying that the Moderna vaccine can prevent someone from getting sick from COVID-19 but that there is no evidence that it can prevent someone receiving the vaccine from carrying the virus and infecting others.[385]

The predictions of Moderna and Pfizer have proven correct. A very high percentage of new COVID-19 cases are from vaccinated persons. Britain's Chief Scientific Adviser Patrick Vallance claimed in July 2021 that he mistakenly said that 60% of people being admitted to hospital with COVID-19 are fully vaccinated. He later clarified that he meant to say that 60% of those admitted for COVID-19 to the hospital are unvaccinated.[386] Please don't miss the significance of that admission. It means that the England health authorities recognize that 40% of COVID-19 hospitalizations are from fully vaccinated persons.

There are many anecdotal examples of fully vaccinated persons being subsequently infected with COVID-19. For example, it was reported by COVID Legal USA on March 12, 2021, that there was a COVID-19 infection outbreak at the Cottonwoods Care Centre retirement facility in Kelowna, British

Columbia, even though 82% of the residents were fully vaccinated. Eight out of the twelve COVID-19 confirmed cases were fully vaccinated persons.[387] That means that 66% of confirmed COVID-19 cases were from those who were fully vaccinated.

In a complaint filed in a federal lawsuit, the plaintiffs made the following common-sense observation:

> [T]he logic for the COVD-19 vaccines breaks down when one considers the Defendants' theory of asymptomatic spread. For over a year now, these Defendants and state-level public health authorities have told the American public that SARS-CoV-2 can be spread by people who have none of the symptoms of COVID-19. If that is the case, then a vaccine that merely reduces symptoms yields no benefits - the virus spreads anyway. If that is not the case, and asymptomatic spread is not real, then asymptomatic individuals do not need to be vaccinated with a vaccine that neither prevents infection with SARS-CoV-2 nor prevents its transmission.

What is the point of any employer vaccine mandate when the COVID-19 vaccines have now been proven to be ineffective? There is no reason to get the vaccine if prevention of infections and spread is the objective. Furthermore, there is no justification to require those who are not vaccinated to wear masks, get tested, social distance, and not travel since they are no more likely to spread the alleged SARS-CoV-2 virus than those who are fully vaccinated.

Because it became clear early on that the COVID-19 vaccines did not prevent the spread of SARS-CoV-2, the CDC found it necessary to issue a press release on March 8, 2021, saying that fully vaccinated Americans must "continue to take these COVID-19 precautions when in public."³⁸⁸ That included wearing masks, staying six feet apart from other people, and avoiding large crowds.

Indeed, the COVID-19 infection rate for vaccinated persons has gotten so out of hand that on July 27, 2021, the CDC had to change its guidance because of the alleged spreading of COVID-19 by vaccinated persons. NBC News reported:

> The Centers for Disease Control and Prevention issued new guidance on Tuesday recommending indoor mask use in areas with high transmission rates after new data suggested fully **vaccinated individuals are not just contracting Covid-19 but could potentially infect others.**
>
> CDC Director Rochelle Walensky said recent studies had shown that those **vaccinated individuals who do become infected with Covid have just as much viral load as the unvaccinated, making it possible for them to spread the virus to others.** Based on that finding, Walensky said the CDC is also recommending that all school children wear masks in the fall.³⁸⁹ (emphasis added)

Emily Kopp, writing for Roll Call, reported that a confidential congressional briefing revealed that "[t]here are 35,000 symptomatic breakthrough cases each week." Kopp concluded that vaccinated persons can be "superspreaders" of SARS-CoV-2.

> The newly released report showing that vaccinated people can still be superspreaders drove the recent decision by the CDC to once again recommend masks for vaccinated people indoors where case

counts are high or substantial.[390]

On August 6, 2021, the CDC published a report that 346 out of out of 469 COVID-19 cases (74%) in a breakout in Barnsdale County, Massachusetts, were of people who were fully vaccinated.[391] The COVID-19 vaccines are proving to be ineffective in preventing infection.

Dr. Nina Pierpont (MD, Ph.D.), has a BA in biology from Yale University, MA and Ph.D. in population biology/evolutionary biology/ecology from Princeton University, and MD from Johns Hopkins University School of Medicine. Dr. Pierpont has been a Clinical Assistant Professor of Pediatrics at Columbia University's College of Physicians & Surgeons. She is currently in private practice in upstate New York, specializing in behavioral medicine. Dr. Pierpont reviewed the available data, principally from three scientific studies, and concluded that COVID-19 vaccine mandates have no justification because "current vaccines do not prevent transmission of SARS-CoV-2."[392]

Pfizer CEO Albert Bourla, in his attempt to sell the public on their COVID-19 vaccine booster during a news interview, let the cat out of the bag by stating: "We know that two doses of the vaccine offers very limited protection if any."[393] When Pfizer realized the implications of that admission, it immediately filed a copyright claim on that interview and took steps to purge it from the internet. I was able to track down the video of the interview at the Instagram link found in the endnote.[394]

99% of the University of California football team and staff were fully vaccinated.[395] There are approximately 143 players and staff on that team.[396] But on November 13, 2021, it was announced that the team had to cancel its upcoming football game with USC because 47 players and staff members on the University of California football team had tested positive for COVID-19. Many of them were symptomatic for COVID-19, which is why the entire team was tested. That is a 33% COVID-19 infection rate for a single group of fully vaccinated persons. The COVID-19 vaccines are not just ineffective; it seems that the vaccines are driving the infection. It is more likely that the players and coaches are suffering from antibody-dependent enhancement caused by the vaccine.

Indeed, COVID-19 vaccinations are detrimental to the USA's counter-drug mission. For example, on December 25, 2021, Carol Rosenberg and Aishvarya Kavi reported for *The New York Times* that the USS Milwaukee was supposed to deploy to intercept drug traffickers in the Caribbean, but the ship could not do so because of a Covid-19 outbreak onboard the ship.[397] The 105-man crew of the vessel was 100% vaccinated against COVID-19. That is a clear example that the COVID-19 vaccines are ineffective in preventing COVID-19. What was really going on aboard the ship likely was that the sailors were suffering from antibody-dependent enhancement (ADE) caused by the vaccines themselves. The vaccines were making the sailors sick. Oddly, the USS Milwaukee incident comes on the heels of active-duty troops in the Army and Navy being fired because they refused to get vaccinated under President Biden's vaccination mandate for the armed services. Perfectly healthy soldiers and sailors were relieved of duty for exercising their rights to refuse to take experimental vaccines that have now been demonstrated to be both unsafe and ineffective. All the while, the readiness of the armed services is being detrimentally impacted by the growing occurrence of ADE among the soldiers and sailors caused by the mandated vaccines.

On November 10, 2021, U.S. District Court Judge T. Kent Wetherell, II, issued an opinion wherein he denied a request from a plaintiff for a preliminary injunction. He ruled against the doctor requesting a religious exemption. Nonetheless, in the course of rendering his opinion, the judge ruled:

[T]the evidence I have shows the vaccine is

"leaky" and "nonsterilizing" in that **it does not prevent transmission of the virus, nor does it protect vaccinated persons from contracting the virus**. ... [T]he evidence before the court from plaintiff's medical experts suggest **that vaccinated persons actually transmit the virus at a higher rate than unvaccinated**. ... [T]he vaccines are unnecessary for persons who have previously had COVID because **natural immunity provides equivalent or greater protection against severe infection than the vaccines**. ... [T]he irrefutable evidence in this case shows that vaccines simply do not accomplish the purpose of the policy that it's aimed at achieving; that is, "keeping everyone safer," because, again, **they do not protect people from contracting the virus**, nor do they prevent people from getting the virus.[398] (emphasis added)

So prevalent were the breakthrough cases of COVID-19 that the CDC announced that beginning on May 1, 2021, it would no longer monitor or report any breakthrough cases that did not result in hospitialization or death.[399] The CDC and its pharmaceutical overlords could not allow people to use official government statistics to prove that the COVID-19 vaccines are ineffective.

U.S. Senator for Massachusetts, Edward Markey, saw through the CDC's subterfuge. In an official letter of inquiry he demanded to know why the CDC would no longer continue to monitor the breakthrough cases.[400] Senator Markey noted the obvious fact that breakthrough cases are a good measure of COVID-19 vaccine effectiveness. He said that 43.4% of the new COVID-19 infections in Massachusetts were among those who were vaccinated. Notably, Senator Markey asked the CDC: "Is the effectiveness of COVID-19 vaccines decreasing in light of these breakthrough cases?" The answer is clear. Indeed, the evident affirmative answer to that question is why the CDC decided to stop reporting breakthrough COVID-19 cases. The CDC's decision not to report COVID-19 breakthrough cases among the vaccinated population was indicative of a conspiracy between it and the pharmaceutical companies to cover up of the ineffectiveness of the COVID-19 vaccines.

The Expose investigative news service explained that in March 2022, the UK Health Security Agency (UKHSA) announced that starting on April 1st 2022, they would no longer publish the vaccination status of Covid-19 cases, hospitalizations and deaths in England.[401] The UKHSA did that because the reported data showed that the unvaccinated population was suffering fewer hospitalizations and deaths from COVID-19 than those who had recieved the COVID-19 vaccine. Of course, that was not the reason given by the UKHSA. Instead, the UKHSA claimed this was because the UK Government had ended free universal Covid-19 testing, which affected their "ability to robustly monitor Covid-19 cases by vaccination status."[402] But that was a lie.

The Expose revealed the lie of the UKHSA by looking at the statistics from another UK Government agency. The Office for National Statistics (ONS), had published data on deaths by vaccination status.[403] That was the very data that the UKHSA said would no longer be available. *The Expose* reporters examined the ONS data starting from the beginning of April 2022 through the end of May 2022. *The Expose* found the shocking truth that between April 1, 2022, and May 31, 2022, 4,647 of the 4,935 total deaths from COVID-19 during that period were among the vaccinated population. That means that 94% of the COVID-19 deaths in the UK during April and May 2022 were among those vaccinated against COVID-19.

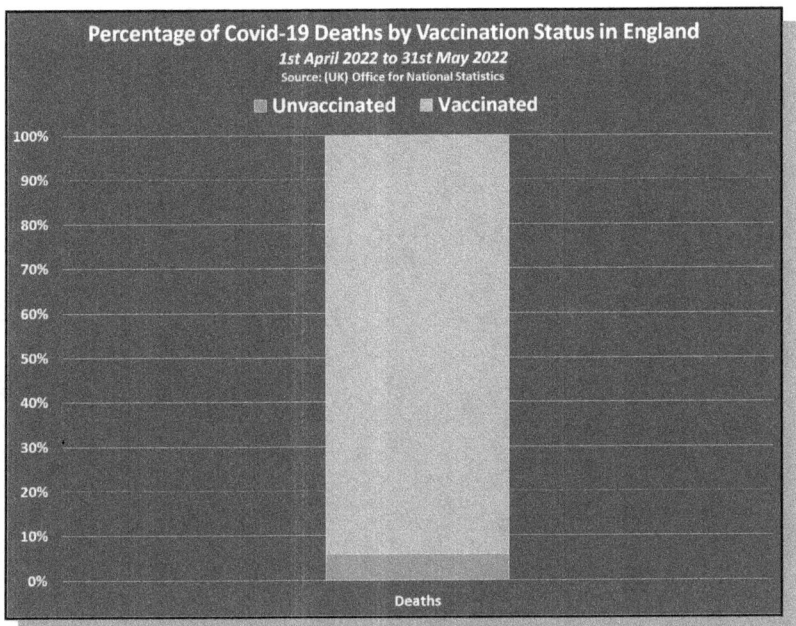

The statistics revealed another shocking detail. It seems that the more shots, the more deadly the vaccines are. Those who received three COVID-19 shots accounted for 4,215 of the 4,647 total deaths among the vaccinated population. That means that those that received three COVID-19 shots accounted for 90% of the vaccinated COVID-19 deaths during April and May 2022. See the graphic below from *The Expose*.

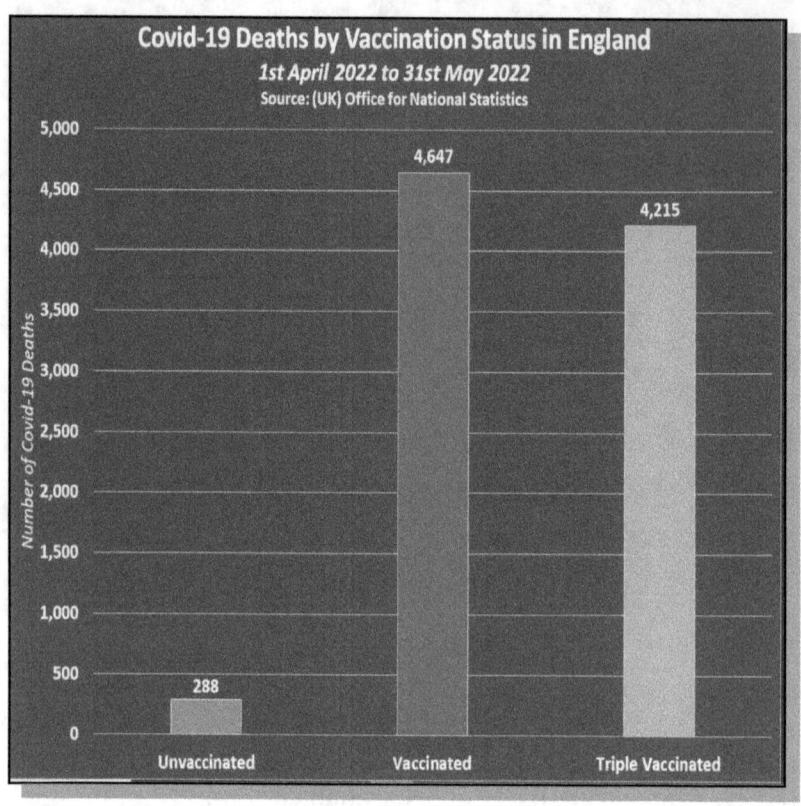

As stated by *The Expose* investigators, "[t]hese aren't the kind of figures you would expect to see if the Covid-19 injections really are up to 95% effective at preventing death, are they?" Indeed, that is likely why the UKHSA decided to stop giving separate statistics revealing the deaths and hospitalizations of vaccinated and unvaccinated persons in the UK.

On March 26, 2023, *The Expose* issued an updated report showing that in the 21 months between April 1, 2021, and December 31, 2022, 86% of the COVID-19 deaths in the UK were among those vaccinated against COVID-19.[404] Those statistics go beyond simply proving that the COVID-19 vaccines are ineffective. Those statistics suggest causation; they suggest antibody-dependent enhancement; the vaccines are dangerous.

The State of Vermont has had a very similar experience to that of England. The Vermont Daily Chronicle reported that 76% of COVID-19 deaths in the State of Vermont during September 2021 were of persons who had received COVID-19 vaccinations.[405] Yet, the State of Vermont Department of Public Health claims that "[v]accines are the best tool we have to protect ourselves against COVID-19, especially from severe illness, hospitalization and death."[406]

In Antwerp, Belgium, 100% of the hospitalized "COVID cases" are fully vaccinated persons. The Hall Turner Radio Show reported that "CEOs and medical directors of Antwerp hospitals met this week and the mood was worrying. They're having another COVID outbreak, but this time, ALL the patients . . . are fully vaccinated."[407] Kristiaan Deckers, Medical Director of the Antwerp GZA, remarked that "the question is whether the vaccines will still work."[408] It was further reported:

> Other officials, who asked to not be named for fear of retribution were far more candid. Said one CEO "Either the vaccines just don't work or, worse, it is the vaccines themselves causing COVID in these people. But if we are publicly quoted as stating the obvious, we will be driven out of our jobs and out of our profession. There is an almost cult-like zeitgeist that no one is allowed to say anything against the vaccines, even if they don't work or are hurting people.[409]

Data from the government health authorities in Scotland showed that the fully COVID-19 vaccinated accounted for 89% of COVID-19 deaths, whilst also accounting for 77% of COVID-19 hospitalizations, and 65% of alleged COVID-19 cases from October 9 through November 5, 2021.[410] According to the data from Public Health Scotland, for December 18, 2021, to January 14, 2022, the COVID-19 case rate was 2.5 times greater for those who received two COVID-19 vaccinations than those who were unvaccinated.[411] Over that same period, there was a 5% greater hospitalization rate for those who had received two COVID-19 vaccines than those who were unvaccinated.[412] From December 11, 2021, to January 7, 2022, there was a 55% greater mortality rate from COVID-19 for those who received two doses of the COVID-19 vaccine compared to those who were unvaccinated.[413]

That was hard data from the health authorities in Scotland. Apparently, someone was not pleased with those revelations. And so, Public Health Scotland deleted the report from the internet. The report from Public Health Scotland, from December 18, 2021, to January 14, 2022, was formerly found at the link in the endnote at the end of this sentence.[414] The report is now gone. But this author found the report using the internet archive Wayback machine. The archive link for the report is at the end of this sentence.[415]

Public Health Scotland has taken further action to conceal the death and destruction caused by the COVID-19 vaccines. On February 16, 2022, Public Health Scotland announced that "[f]rom 16 February 2022, Public Health Scotland (PHS) will no longer report COVID-19 cases, hospitalisations, and deaths by vaccination status on a weekly basis. PHS will continue to provide updates from the latest scientific analyses and reports on the effectiveness of COVID-19 vaccines. ... While PHS has stated that the data in the report should not be used as a measure of vaccine effectiveness, PHS is aware of inappropriate use and misinterpretation of the data when taken in isolation without fully understanding the limitations described below."[416]

The Scottish health authorities are taking their toys and going home. They don't think that the public is playing nice with their raw data comparing deaths and hospitalizations of the unvaccinated with the vaccinated population. And so, rather than continue to provide it, they are simply shutting down the flow of information revealing the death and destruction caused by the COVID-19 vaccines.

The government health authorities claim that the data is being inappropriately misinterpreted.[417] I don't think it is inappropriately misinterpreting the data when one concludes that the COVID-19 vaccines are ineffective and dangerous after reading that there is a 55% greater mortality rate from COVID-19 for those who received two doses of the COVID-19 vaccine compared to those who were unvaccinated.

That disturbing statistic may be something that the government of Scotland does not want known, but it is not an inappropriate interpretation to say that it reveals that the COVID-19 vaccines are unsafe and ineffectual.

Below is a graph prepared by Steve Kirsch[418] from the actual Scotland Pubic Health authorities data.[419] This is the information that Public Health Scotland is trying to conceal from the public. Please understand that this data represents COVID-19 per 100,000. The data clearly shows that the vaccinated population did much worse.

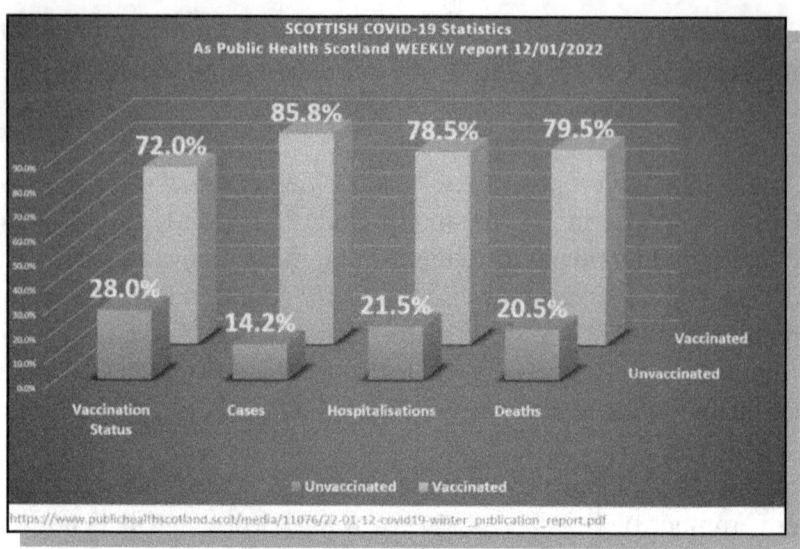

The Public Health Scotland (PHS) COVID-19 Winter Statistical Report dated 12 January 2022 reveals that those who received 2 COVID-19 shots died at a 59% greater rate than those who were unvaccinated. More striking is what a chart in the report reveals when COVID-19 deaths of all persons who received 1, 2, and 3 doses of the COVID-19 vaccine are compared to the unvaccinated persons.[420] When the vaccinated population of those who received 1, 2, and 3 shots is added together, we find that their death rate from COVID-19 was 3.56 times that of the unvaccinated population. Public Health Scotland will no longer provide this information because it reveals that the vaccines are unsafe and ineffective.

We are seeing antibody dependent enhancement (ADE) caused by the vaccine being reported throughout the world, not as

ADE, but rather as COVID-19. ADE being reported as COVID-19 was not unexpected. As noted above, Pfizer explained that ADE will usually be presented as having "severe or unusual manifestations of COVID-19."[421] Thus, what is being announced as "breakthrough" cases of COVID-19 are actually cases of ADE caused by the COVID-19 vaccines. For example, *The Expose* news site reported on the government statistics from Canada[422] showing that the vaccinated population of Canada account for 89% of all COVID-19 cases, 86% of all COVID-19 hospitalizations, and 90% of all COVID-19 deaths.

COVID-19 *Cases* in Canada: Between June 6, 2022 and July 3, 2022 in Canada, "the unvaccinated population accounted for just 11% of Covid-19 cases ... whilst **the vaccinated population accounted for 89%**, 74% of which were among the triple and quadruple jabbed."[423]

COVID-19 *Hospitalizations* in Canada: Between June 6, 2022 and July 3, 2022 in Canada, "the unvaccinated population accounted for just 14% of Covid-19 hospitalisations ... whilst **the vaccinated population accounted for 86%**, 75% of which were among the triple and quadruple jabbed."[424]

COVID-19 *Deaths* in Canada: Between June 6, 2022 and July 3, 2022 in Canada, "the unvaccinated population accounted for just 10% of Covid-19 deaths ... whilst **the vaccinated population accounted for 90%**, 87% of which were among the triple and quadruple jabbed."[425] See the graphic below from *The Expose*.

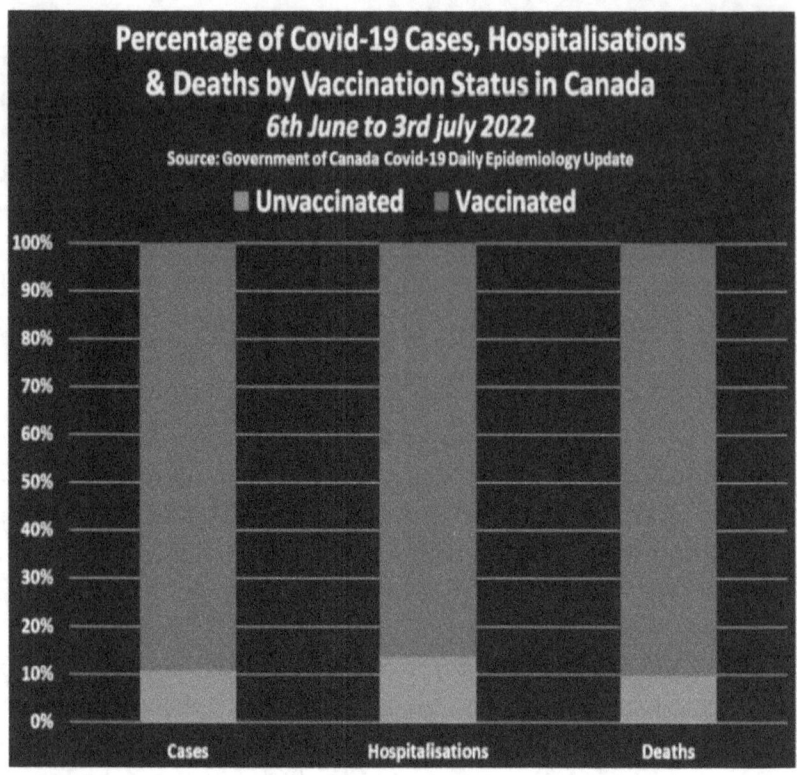

That manifest danger from the COVID-19 vaccines is in the face of evidence that the COVID-19 vaccines are ineffective. There is study,[426] after study,[427] after study,[428] after study[429] proving that vaccinated individuals can still test positive for COVID-19 and manifest illnesses associated with COVID-19. The United Kingdom Health Security Agency COVID-19 Vaccine Surveillance Report published on October 21, 2021, reveals that "[i]n individuals aged greater than 30, the rate of a positive COVID-19 test is higher in vaccinated individuals compared to unvaccinated."[430] But that statement from the British Government understates the ineffectiveness of the COVID-19 vaccinations. Indeed, when looking at the population from 18 years old and up, we find that the infection rate among the vaccinated population is significantly higher than the infection rate for the unvaccinated population. The British Government report reveals that over a monitoring period spanning week 38 to week 41 of 2021, the COVID-19 case rate for the vaccinated group over 18 years old was significantly more than the case rate for the unvaccinated group. There were 5,871 cases of COVID-19 for every 100,000 vaccinated persons more than 18 years old. In contrast, there were only 3,584 COVID-19 for every 100,000 unvaccinated persons more than 18 years old.[431] The workforce would fall largely in the over 18-year-old age bracket. Those statistics mean that a vaccinated person in the workforce is more likely to be infected with COVID-19 than an unvaccinated person.

The method used by the vaccine makers for reporting the efficacy of the COVID-19 vaccines (relative risk reduction) is to subtract the percentage of infected vaccinated persons from the percentage of infected unvaccinated persons and divide that number by the percentage of infected unvaccinated persons (U-V/U). Using that formula, and applying it to the UK government data, this author calculated that the actual effectiveness of the COVID-19 vaccines in the real world is minus-64%.[432] That means that a vaccinated person is 64% more likely to catch COVID-19 than an unvaccinated person.[433]

That calculation of minus-64% COVID-19 vaccine efficacy was from the official reported data of the UK Health Security Agency.[434] That minus-64% means that the immune system of the person who is vaccinated is so debilitated by the vaccine that, on a percentage basis, he is 64% more likely to be infected with COVID-19 than an unvaccinated person. That is data from week 42 of 2021. The UK Health Security Agency data shows that when comparing the number of persons with COVID-19 per 100,000 vaccinated persons to the number of persons with COVID-19 per 100,000 unvaccinated persons, the vaccinated group has significantly higher rate of COVID-19 cases than the unvaccinated group. That indicates that over time the vaccines have a negative efficacy. The COVID-19 vaccines make a person more susceptible to COVID-19. Recall that the efficacy of the COVID-19 vaccines have been calculated to drop at an average rate of 5% per week.[435] As time passes, the likelihood of COVID-19 infection (or more likely, antibody-dependent enhancement (ADE)) increases for the vaccinated persons.

The null hypothesis in a recent study was that areas with low vaccination rates drive the ongoing surge of new COVID-19. The study disproved that null hypothesis. That study by S. V. Subramanian from the Harvard Center for Population and Development Studies published on the NIH website concluded that "increases in COVID-19 are unrelated to levels of vaccination across 68 countries and 2,947 counties in the United States."[436] The study determined that the COVID-19 vaccines are not effective. While the study disproved the null hypothesis, one finds that the data goes beyond showing ineffectiveness of the COVID-19 vaccines. The data showed a positive correlation between vaccine rate and infection rate. The data indicate that COVID-19 vaccines are driving the infection. For example, the study presented data showing that U.S. counties with higher COVID-19 vaccine rates had higher rates of COVID-19 cases. The study states:

> Of the top 5 counties that have the highest percentage of population fully vaccinated (99.9–84.3%), the US Centers for Disease Control and Prevention (CDC) identifies 4 of them as "High" Transmission counties. Chattahoochee (Georgia), McKinley (New Mexico), and Arecibo (Puerto Rico) counties have above 90% of their population fully vaccinated with all three being classified as "High" transmission. Conversely, of the 57 counties that have been classified as "low" transmission counties by the CDC, 26.3% (15) have percentage of population fully vaccinated below 20%.[437]

206

When looking at the country-level data, the reader finds the same correlation. In disproving the null hypothesis, the study determined there was no relationship between the percentage of the population fully vaccinated and new COVID-19 cases. The study concluded that the COVID-19 vaccines are ineffective. But the data goes beyond showing the vaccines are ineffective. The study shows that vaccines cause a higher rate of COIVD-19 infection. The study showed that the higher the COVID-19 vaccine rate in a country, the higher is its COVID-19 infection rate. The study reveals that "[i]n fact, the trend line suggests a marginally positive association such that countries with higher percentage of population fully vaccinated have higher COVID-19 cases per 1 million people." Thus, the vaccines seem to drive the COVID-19 infection. The study states:

> At the country-level, there appears to be no discernable relationship between percentage of population fully vaccinated and new COVID-19 cases in the last 7 days. In fact, the trend line suggests a marginally positive association such that countries with higher percentage of population fully vaccinated have higher COVID-19 cases per 1 million people. Notably, Israel with over 60% of their population fully vaccinated had the highest COVID-19 cases per 1 million people in the last 7 days. The lack of a meaningful association between percentage population fully vaccinated and new COVID-19 cases is further exemplified, for instance, by comparison of Iceland and Portugal. Both countries have over 75% of their population fully vaccinated and have more COVID-19 cases per 1 million people than countries such as Vietnam and South Africa that have around 10% of their population fully vaccinated.[438]

What accounts for the phenomenon of vaccines that offer

no protection? Some think that the answer has been found in a massive study involving approximately 620,000 U.S. Veterans who received COVID-19 vaccines. The researchers determined that "[t]he proportionate reduction in infection associated with vaccination declined for all vaccine types, with the largest declines for Janssen followed by Pfizer-BioNTech and Moderna."[439]

The decline in protection for the Johnson & Johnson (Janssen) COVID-19 vaccine was significant. The protection from COVID-19 dropped from 88% protection against COVID-19 in March 2021 down to 3% protection, just five months later in August 2021. The protection from infection for Pfizer-BioNTech dropped from 91% in March to 50% in August. The Moderna vaccine protection dropped from 92% in March to 64% in August. The vaccines' problem is that they only provide a few months of protection before that protection drops precipitously. What is the point of getting a vaccination that offers only a few short months of protection?

But the waning vaccine efficacy is not why the risk of COVID-19 infection is the same for the vaccinated as it is for unvaccinated. The data indicates that the risk of COVID-19 is actually worse for the vaccinated who are more than 30 years old. It is not that the vaccines are ineffective that is the reason for the COVID-19 infections among the vaccinated; the vaccines drive an illness called antibody dependent enhancement (ADE). ADE is being reported as COVID-19 because the patients are testing positive for COIVD-19.

In October 2021, the U.S. FDA issued an EUA for a COVID-19 vaccine for children five years and older, and the U.S. CDC recommended that EUA COVID-19 vaccine for those children. On March 8, 2022, Florida State Surgeon General Joseph Ladpapo, M.D., Ph.D., contradicted the U.S. CDC and officially recommended against giving the COVID-19 vaccine to healthy children 5 to 17 years old.[440] He made that recommendation based on the limited risk that COVID-19 posed to the young compared to the "higher than anticipated severe adverse events occurred among those receiving the COVID-19 vaccine" in clinical trials.[441] He revealed the troubling fact that the COVID-19 vaccines have no long-term immunity benefit. They don't work as advertised. Dr. Ladpapo explained that a "study conducted out of New York determined that COVID-19 vaccine efficacy declined 84%, from 68% to 12%, over a span of two months for children aged 5 to 11."[442] He further stated that the "same study determined that COVID-19 vaccine efficacy declined 40%, from 85% to 51%, over a span of two months for adolescents ages 12 to 17."[443] Despite that evidence, in June 2022, the FDA authorized a COVID-19 vaccine for children older than six months, and the U.S. CDC recommended that vaccine for those children.[444]

After pushing millions to get vaccinated, the CDC has now implicitly acknowledged that vaccines do not have any beneficial effect on preventing the infection or spread of COVID-19. On September 23, 2022, the CDC guidance was updated to note that **"vaccination status is no longer used to inform source control, screening testing, or post-exposure recommendations."**[445]

The "breakthrough infections" from the alleged COVID-19 virus did not surprise government officials or pharmaceutical companies. It is well known within the field of immunology that no vaccines provide lasting immunity. Thus, the hope of attaining herd immunity through vaccination is propaganda based on mythology.

We now have confirmation that the propaganda coming out of the CDC and FDA claiming that the COVID-19 vaccines were safe and effective was a lie. The Depatment of Health and Human Services (HHS) Secretary Robert F. Kennedy Jr., who oversees both the CDC and the FDA, made statements on August 5, 2025, that, in effect, revealed that previously published FDA and CDC claims that the COVID-19 vaccines are safe and effective were misleading.

On August 5, 2025, the Department of Health and Human Services (HHS) announced that it was cancelling 22 mRNA projects worth $500 million.[446] Incidentally, the CDC and FDA are component agencies within HHS. The reason for the project cancellations was that an extensive review of the data showed that the mRNA vaccines were ineffective against COVID-19. "The data show these vaccines fail to protect effectively against upper respiratory infections like COVID and flu."[447]

Furthermore, HHS Secretary Robert F. Kennedy Jr. said that the mRNA vaccines cause undue risk to the health of the patients. "After reviewing the science and consulting top experts at NIH [the National Institutes of Health] and FDA [Food and Drug Administration], HHS has determined that mRNA technology poses more risk than benefits for these respiratory viruses."[448] Notably, Secretary Kennedy stated that the mRNA vaccines have the effect of prolonging a pandemic through antigenic shift that drives mutations of the alleged virus with those mutations escaping the vaccine's alleged protection. Thus, the mRNA COVID-19 vaccines made the pandemic worse.

The HHS press release was backed by research. The press release cited 656 peer-reviewed scientific papers establishing that the mRNA vaccines are dangerous to the health of the recipients.[449] There were an additional 70 peer-reviewed papers cited by HHS that established not only that the mRNA vaccines were ineffective but that they drove vaccine-resistant variants, exacerbating the COVID-19 epidemic. The vaccines were not just ineffective; they made the pandemic worse.

Catherine J Frompovich interviewed Stanford Research Immunologist Dr. Tetyana Obukhanych, Ph.D. Frompovich asked Dr. Obukhanych the following: "Vaccinated children are coming down with the same infectious diseases for which they have been fully vaccinated. Why do you think vaccine 'immunity'— if we can call it that—is so short lived and not adequate?" Dr. Obukhanych gave the following revealing answer:

> We would expect that vaccinated individuals would not be involved (or very minimally involved) in any outbreak of an infectious disease for which they have been vaccinated. Yet, when outbreaks are analyzed, it becomes apparent that most often this is not the case. Vaccinated individuals are indeed very frequently involved and constitute a high proportion of disease cases.
>
> I think this is happening because vaccination does not engage the genuine mechanism of immunity. Vaccination typically engages the immune response—that is, everything that immunologists would theoretically "want" to see being engaged in the immune system. But apparently this is not enough to confer robust protection that matches natural immunity. Our knowledge of the immune system is far from being complete.[450]

Marcella Piper-Terry is a vaccine researcher, the mother of a daughter recovering from autism, and the founder of VaxTruth.org, who came to the same conclusion arrived at by Dr. Obukhanych.

> There is no such thing as vaccine-induced herd immunity. It doesn't exist. It never has. The vast majority of adults have ZERO immunity from vaccines and we have not been having huge outbreaks of disease. Let's please just stop talking about how we're going to lose herd immunity if we stop vaccinating. We can't lose what we've never

had.[451]

Vaccine-induced herd immunity is the mythology behind vaccine mandates. The tyranny of mandates is based on something that is not real. Brett Wilcox explains that vaccine-induced herd immunity is like a superstitious religious belief.

> Whereas the vaccines-are-safe-and-effective dogma assures parents and patients that vaccines safely prevent disease, the doctrine of herd immunity persuades parents and patients that they have a social obligation to vaccinate, that those who fail to vaccinate are "free loaders"—people who freely reap the benefits of vaccines while failing to assume their share of vaccine risks. The two doctrines have now combined in an irrational yet powerful third doctrine: vaccines protect vaccine recipients but only if everyone else vaccinates. Thus, the unvaccinated have morphed from free loaders into diseased and filthy child abusers, child killers, and murderers. It is this third doctrine that vaccine believers and sociopaths wield to justify discrimination, mandatory vaccination, and just plain nasty behavior.
>
> By comparison, ancient believers once threatened to kill non-believers to help them see the value of converting to the religion of their more righteous oppressors. Modern vaccine believers believe their salvation lies in the conversion and baptism by vaccination of all of humanity. Thus, believers view the unvaccinated not only as vectors of disease but also as the indispensible key to their own salvation from the ever-threatening hell of infectious disease.[452]

17 COVID-19 Vaccines Are Dangerous

Vaccines are largely ineffective and unsafe. Indeed, it is an established medical fact that the COVID-19 vaccines not only do not prevent illness, they cause illness. Please be mindful that the COVID-19 vaccines were authorized because they purportedly prevented infection and the spread of the disease.

Dr. Peter McCullough, M.D., is an American cardiologist. He is one of the most highly respected and published cardiologists in the U.S. Dr. McCullough, M.D., was vice chief of internal medicine at Baylor University Medical Center and a professor at Texas A&M University. He is editor-in-chief of the journal Reviews in Cardiovascular Medicine and Cardiorenal Medicine. Dr McCullough is an internationally recognized kidney and cardiovascular authority. He has more than 1000 publications. In fact, Dr. McCullough is reputed to be the most cited medical doctor on COVID-19 treatments at the National Library of Medicine, with more than 600 citations. Dr. McCullough has testified before Congress. Dr. McCullough is a medical expert on vaccines. Indeed, he has chaired more than two dozen vaccine safety monitoring boards for the FDA, and National Institute for Health.[453] Dr. McCullough's expert medical opinion is that the COVID-19 vaccines are unsafe and ineffective.[454]

Dr. McCullough was once one of the most published and cited authors in the medical community. Since he has come out explaining the dangers of the COVID-19 vaccines, Baylor and Texas A&M have cut ties with him. He has had his research revealing the dangers of the COVID-19 vaccines suddenly unpublished and deleted.[455]

Dr. Peter McCullough, M.D., gave an informative presentation at the 2022 United Healthcare Summit.[456] During his presentation, Dr. Mcullough cited the sweeping research by the World Council For Health (WCH) that revealed the dangers of the COVID-19 vaccines. This author decided to check his claims about the WCH research findings. I discovered that he was correct. My research took me beyond the WCH findings. It includes some surprising facts and evidence, which will be shocking to some, about the COVID-19 vaccines.

The World Council For Health (WCH) extensively studied the world databases on the COVID-19 vaccine injuries. The WCH studied the WHO VigiAccess, CDC VAERS, EudraVigilance, and UK Yellow Card Scheme to determine whether the COVID-19 vaccines are safe.[457] On June 11, 2022, the WCH announced its results. The WCH found that the databases revealed more than 40,000 deaths linked to the COVID-19 vaccines and called for an immediate recall of those vaccines.[458]

Those reported deaths are just the tip of the proverbial iceberg. Dr. Katrina Lindley explains the deficiency in the reports:

> [S]uch systems of passive surveillance result in significantly fewer ADR [adverse drug reaction] reports than active surveillance reporting. As a result, the actual number of adverse events that occurred in temporal relation to Covid-19 injections is likely to be much higher than revealed by the available official data.[459]

The under-reporting in the databases is quite significant. Indeed, it is exponential. For example, because the VAERS database relies on passive reporting, it suffers from a systemic flaw known to HHS. That flaw is that the VAERS database under-reports the vaccine adverse events by a factor of 100. A Harvard study of the VAERS database that HHS commissioned revealed that "fewer than 1% of vaccine adverse events are reported."[460] That statistical finding in the Harvard study has been confirmed to be accurate in a subsequent scientific study.[461]

The underreporting in VAERS has been verified in other studies. The Journal of the American Medical Association (JAMA) reported that the Vaccine Adverse Events Reporting System (VAERS) reports that occurrence of anaphylaxis from the COVID-19 Vaccines is "4.7 cases/million Pfizer-BioNTech vaccine doses administered and 2.5 cases/million Moderna vaccine doses administered, based on information through January 18, 2021."[462] In a March 30, 2021 posting, the CDC reported similar statistics alleging that "[a]naphylaxis after COVID-19 vaccination is **rare** and occurred in approximately 2 to 5 people per million vaccinated in the United States based on events reported to VAERS."[463] (bold emphasis in original)

The problem with the reports from JAMA and the CDC is that they are contradicted by another, more recent, March 8, 2021 report from JAMA. That study of Mass General Brigham (MGB) employees receiving COVID-19 vaccines, was published by the JAMA reveals that "severe reactions consistent with anaphylaxis occurred at a rate of 2.47 per 10,000 vaccinations."[464]

Elizabeth A. Brehm, wrote a letter on behalf of the Informed Consent Action Network (ICAN) to Dr. Rochelle P. Walensky, the Director of the Centers for Disease Control and Prevention.[465] Brehm pointed out that the MGB study reveals that the VAERS is under-reporting the accounts of anaphylaxis from the COVID-19 vaccines by a factor of between 50 and 120 times.

215

ICAN complained that "[t]he underreporting of anaphylaxis by the CDC and VAERS is particularly troubling because it is mandatory for medical providers to report anaphylaxis after any COVID-19 vaccine to VAERS."[466] The most salient point in the letter from ICAN is the revelation from the MGB study that "the rate of reporting [of COVID-19 vaccine anaphylaxis adverse reactions] still appears to be only around 0.8 to 2 percent of all cases of anaphylaxis." The ICAN letter goes on to point out the obvious:

> This raises serious concerns regarding (1) under-reporting of other serious adverse events following COVID-19 vaccination, and (2) adverse events following other vaccines for which there has not been the same push to report adverse events. The anaphylaxis study highlights the urgency of the ongoing, well-known problem with adverse event reporting post-vaccination.[467]

The MGB and WCH studies confirm the previous study done by Harvard that indicated that "fewer than 1% of vaccine adverse events" are reported in the VAERS system. Thus, you can multiply any statistic from the VAERS system by 100, and you will have a better idea of the actual number for that category of adverse events. Thus, deaths reported under VAERS would likely be subject to the same under-reporting as would anaphylaxis. As with anaphylaxis, we can expect that only 1% of all deaths from COVID-19 vaccines are being reported in the VAERS system.

The CDC-run Vaccine Adverse Events Reporting Service (VAERS) is a passive reporting system. It relies, for the most part, on reporting of practitioners of adverse events from vaccines. Keep in mind that the VAERS data discloses correlation and it does not prove causation. But that does not mean that the COVID-19 vaccine did not cause the adverse event; it simply means that the causation has not yet been proven with scientific certainty. But the VAERS data establishes probable cause to believe that the

COVID-19 vaccines are responsible for a significant plurality of the reported adverse events.

The adverse events listed in VAERS have not been clinically proven to have been caused by the listed vaccine. But we can reasonably infer that those who died within 48 hours of the onset of illness after the vaccination died from the vaccine. Megan Redshaw determined that of those VAERS reported as having died after receiving the COVID-19 vaccine, 19% died within 24 hours of vaccination, 27% died within 48 hours of vaccination, and 41% died after becoming ill within 48 hours of vaccination.[468] We will consider that 41% figure of temporal proximity as establishing a reasonable belief that the COVID-19 vaccines were the cause of those deaths.

It is fair to infer that a very high percentage of those who showed symptoms within 48 hours of receiving the vaccine and later died did so from the vaccine. VAERS reported that of July 15, 2022, there were 29,635 deaths attributed to COVID-19 vaccines. 41% of 29,635 is 12,150. Thus, one can reasonably conclude there is probable cause to believe that 12,150 persons died from the COVID-19 vaccine. Understanding that the VAERS system only reports 1% of the actual deaths, we find that the deaths from the COVID-19 vaccines are 1,215,000 people as of July 15, 2022.

The World Council For Health (WCH) noted that the Polio Vaccine was recalled in less than one year after ten reported deaths, yet the Covid-19 vaccine, with 29,635 associated deaths, has not been recalled after two years.[469] The WCH concluded that "[t]here is sufficient evidence of adverse events relating to Covid-19 vaccines to indicate that a product recall is immediately necessary."[470] The WCH came to that conclusion based on the associated deaths reported as of July 15, 2022, in VAERS being approximately 29,635. But the argument for an immediate recall becomes more compelling when one considers that there is probable cause to believe that the number of deaths caused by the COVID-19 vaccines is actually closer to 1.2 million (12,635 x .41 = 12,150) x 100 = 1,215,000.[471]

Similar numbers were arrived at by other researchers. VAERS is a database that reports adverse events associated with vaccines. The appearance of an adverse event in the database does not prove that the vaccine caused the adverse event. Because the VAERS database reports correlation and does not prove causation, we are left to extrapolate causation from the numbers reported in the VAERS database. Researchers led by Dr. Scott McLachlan, Ph.D., determined that the vaccine caused 86% of deaths reported in VAERS.[472] Dr. Jessica Rose, Ph.D., and her team of researchers studied the U.S. VAERS database and determined that VAERS underreported adverse events, including deaths, from the COVID-19 vaccines by a factor of 41. That means the actual adverse events, including deaths, associated with the COVID-19 vaccines are 41 times greater than reported in the VAERS system.[473]

Dr. Rose is a Canadian researcher with a Bachelor Degree in Applied Mathematics and a Master's degree in Immunology from Memorial University of Newfoundland. She also holds a Ph.D. in Computational Biology from Bar Ilan University and two Post Doctoral degrees: one in Molecular Biology from the Hebrew University of Jerusalem and one in Biochemistry from the Technion Institute of Technology.

Assuming the VAERS system underreports adverse events by 41-fold, and the COVID-19 vaccine caused 86% of the deaths reported in VAERS, we can determine the actual number of deaths caused by the COVID-19 vaccines.[474] As of September 23, 2022, the VAERS database reported that 31,214 persons died after being vaccinated with a COVID-19 vaccine. Although the U.S. Government keeps the VAERS database, it also includes deaths from COVID-19 vaccinations in other countries. Approximately 50% of the deaths reported in VAERS are from other countries.

That means approximately 15,000 persons died in the U.S. alone from COVID-19 vaccines.

We will start with the 15,000 U.S. figure. Multiplying that figure by 41 we arrive at 615,000. But only 86% of that number can be said to have died from the vaccine. Multiplying 615,000 by .86, we arrive at a final figure of 528,900 as the number of persons who died from the COVID-19 vaccines in the U.S. as of September 23, 2022. If we apply that formula to the total of U.S. and overseas reported deaths in VAERS, we arrive at a figure of 1.1 million deaths caused by the COVID-19 vaccines as of September 23, 2022. That is very close to the estimated 1.2 million deaths caused by the COVID-19 vaccines as of July 15, 2022, which was arrived at above using a different calculation method and assumptions.

As of July 28, 2022, there have been more adverse event reports in VAERS for the COVID-19 vaccines than all other 70+ vaccines combined during the entire 32 year history of the VAERS database. Of the total 2.2 million adverse event reports in VAERS over the last 32 years, 1.3 million of those reports were for adverse events from the COVID-19 vaccines in the past 19 months.[475]

Megan Redshaw also revealed that the VAERS data shows "[t]here were 77 reports of Guillain-Barré Syndrome with 55% of cases attributed to Pfizer, 40% to Moderna and 10% to J&J."[476] Recall that the VAERS database only reflects 1% of actual injuries. Thus, as of April 8, 2021, we can reasonably infer that there have been 7,700 cases of Guillain-Barré Syndrome correlated to COVID-19 vaccines. Guillain-Barré is an autoimmune disorder that causes a person's immune system to damage the body's nerves. This autoimmune response causes severe muscle weakness and sometimes paralysis. The paralysis can be transitory, but it can also be permanent.

Only Janssen (J&J) mentions Guillain-Barré Syndrome in

its fact sheet as a risk from its COVID-19 vaccine.[477] Guillain-Barré Syndrome is not mentioned as an adverse event outcome in either of the COIVD-19 vaccine fact sheets provided to recipients and caregivers from Moderna or Pfizer-BioNTech.[478] But Guillain-Barré Syndrome was listed by the FDA among the possible "adverse event outcomes" being monitored during the COIVD-19 vaccine trials. A slide from a presentation by Steve Anderson, Director of Biostatistics and Epidemiology for the FDA, at the October 22, 2020 Vaccines and Related Biological Products Advisory Committee meeting lists Guillain-Barré Syndrome as one of the possible adverse event outcomes being monitored by the FDA during the COVID-19 vaccine trials.[479] The slide can be seen in the chapter in this book on antibody-dependent enhancement. They knew what to look for because they knew what they were seeing. The slide was shown for only a split second before it disappeared from view, and Dr. Anderson made no mention of it. No doubt they discovered Guillain-Barré Syndrome in all the vaccines, but only Janssen would admit to it.

Why focus only on VAERS data of deaths and Guillain-Barré Syndrome? That is because death and Guillain-Barré Syndrome were the two events that caused the swine flu vaccine to be abruptly pulled from the market. Recall that the swine flu vaccine was administered to 40 million people over a 10 week period in 1976. That vaccine program was stopped within 10 weeks because 25 people died and 500 people developed Guillain-Barré Syndrome.[480]

Guess what else Dr. Anderson listed on his slide among the possible adverse event outcomes from the COVID-19 vaccine trials? — "Deaths."[481] As I said earlier, they knew what to look for because they knew what they were seeing. They were not going to waste their time looking for things that they did not expect to find. And they could not avoid seeing people drop dead. The FDA and the vaccine makers knew that the COVID-19 vaccines would kill people. That revelation in the flashed slide seemed to be inadvertent because the slide with that information disappeared within a split second with no comment on it from Dr. Anderson. Almost certainly, the adverse event outcome of 'deaths" were found during the COVID-19 vaccine studies because we see COVID-19 vaccine deaths happening throughout the country. But death is not listed as an adverse event in the COVID-19 vaccine fact sheets provided to the recipients and caregivers from the vaccine makers.

The swine flu vaccine program is generally recognized as a "debacle" of epic proportions because of the debilitating injuries and deaths caused by it. But we have the same thing happening with the COVID-19 vaccines but on an exponentially greater level, and yet the COVID-19 vaccines are still being promoted as safe.

The deaths from the COVID-19 vaccines in the U.S. are exponentially greater than the deaths from the swine flu vaccine (25). The same goes for the cases of Guillain-Barré Syndrome from the COIVD-19 vaccine (7,700) versus the swine flu vaccine (500). Those figures are from the early date of April 8, 2021, which was only four months into the COVID-19 vaccine program. No doubt, the cases have continued to mount. Comparing the death rate for the COVID-19 vaccine to the swine flu vaccine, we find that the COVID-19 vaccine is 1,000 times more deadly than the disastrous swine flu vaccine.

So, why was the swine flu vaccine withdrawn from the market, and the exponentially more dangerous COVID-19 vaccine is being promoted as safe and effective? The difference is that the swine flu vaccine was introduced in 1976. That was before Congress passed the National Vaccine Injury Act (NVIA) of 1986. That law granted pharmaceutical companies immunity for injuries caused by their vaccines. The Public Readiness and Emergency Preparedness Act (PREP Act), which authorizes the Countermeasures Injury Compensation Program (CICP) to provide benefits to injured parties, gives pharmaceutical companies even more liability protection than the NVIA. The COVID-19 vaccines presently fall under the PREP Act (CICP).

There is simply no incentive for pharmaceutical companies or government regulators to ensure that vaccines are safe so long as they fall under the protection of the CICP or NVIA. The claims that vaccines are safe and effective are part of a deceptive theater; those behind the curtain know the truth, while the mesmerizing magic show beguiles the audience.

The CDC and the mainstream media persistently promote the COVID-19 vaccines like circus barkers drawing in the suckers to their destruction. President Biden characterizes the COVID-19 vaccines as "safe, free, and effective vaccines."[482] When, on September 9, 2021, President Biden announced his vaccine requirement for federal workers he said: "The vaccines are safe, highly effective."[483]

The President's Executive Order 14043 of September 9, 2021, mandating COVID-19 vaccinations for federal workers, must be considered in light of the carnage that was already known to have been caused by the COVID-19 vaccines by the time he issued the order. As of August 13, 2021, there were reported in the HHS Vaccine Adverse Event Reporting System (VAERS) 13,068 deaths correlated to the COVID-19 vaccines.[484] The Pfizer-BioNTech COVID-19 vaccine accounted for 9,024 of those deaths.[485] A research team from the American Frontline Doctors (AFLD) found that the VAERS database indicates that the total reported vaccine deaths in the first quarter of 2021 represents a 12,000% to 25,000% increase in vaccine deaths, year-on-year.[486] The AFLD determined that there were more deaths (approx. 4,000) from the COVID-19 vaccines reported in VAERS in the first four months of 2021 than deaths reported in VAERS for all other vaccines combined (1,529) over the ten year period from 2009 to 2019.[487] The AFLD research team determined that COVID-19 Vaccines have caused 99% of all reported vaccine deaths in

2021.[488] All other vaccines combined account for the remaining 1% of vaccine deaths. The carnage caused by the COVID-19 vaccines was known when President Biden issued his vaccine mandate for federal workers.

Dr. McCullough explains that the COVID-19 experimental vaccine is "the largest application of a biological product with the greatest amount of morbidity and mortality in the history of our country."[489]

Dr. McCullough details the malfeasance of the government regulatory agencies. "With this program, there is no critical event committee, there is no data-safety monitoring board, and there's no human ethics committee. Those structures are mandatory for all large clinical investigations, and so the word that's really used for what's going on is malfeasance, that's wrongdoing of people in authority."[490]

In an interview, Dr. McCullough gave listeners some perspective on just how dangerous the COVID-19 vaccines are. He explains that "[a] typical new drug at about five deaths, unexplained deaths, we get a black-box warning, your listeners would see it on TV, saying it may cause death," McCullough said. "And then at about 50 deaths it's pulled off the market."[491]

Dr. McCullough juxtaposes that with what he has been able to gather from confidential sources that "[w]e think we have 50,000 dead Americans. Fifty thousand deaths. So we actually have more deaths due to the vaccine per day than certainly the viral illness by far. It's basically propagandized bioterrorism by injection."[492] That statement regarding 50,000 deaths was made on June 11, 2021, which was less than six months after the COVID-19 vaccine rollout.

There is a government database that, unlike VAERS, is not public. That database is found in the Centers for Medicare and

Medicaid Services (CMS). A whistleblower, who is a computer programmer with subject matter expertise in the healthcare data analytics field, has filed a sworn affidavit in a lawsuit that the CMS data collated with VAERS data shows 45,000 deaths from COVID-19 vaccines.[493] The affiant stated under oath on July 13, 2021, the following:

> It is my professional estimate that VAERS (the Vaccine Adverse Event Reporting System) database, while extremely useful, is under-reported by a conservative factor of at least 5. On July 9, 2021, there were 9,048 deaths reported in VAERS. I verified these numbers by collating all of the data from VAERS myself, not relying on a third party to report them. In tandem, I queried data from CMS medical claims with regard to vaccines and patient deaths, and have assessed that the deaths occurring within 3 days of vaccination are higher than those reported in VAERS by a factor of at least 5. This would indicate the true number of vaccine-related deaths was at least 45,000. Put in perspective, the swine flu vaccine was taken off the market which only resulted in 53 deaths.[494]

Dr. McCullough's estimate of 50,000 deaths and the CMS expert's estimates of 45,000 deaths from the COVID-19 vaccines may yet still be exponentially under reporting because the sources are relying on government data. Such data suffers from under reporting. The VAERS data study commissioned by HHS concluded that the under reporting in VAERS was by a factor of 100. The VAERS system was only capturing 1% of the adverse events.

The HHS-funded Harvard study revealed that the VAERS data represents only 1% of the total adverse events.[495] As of July 28, 2022, there have been more adverse event reports in VAERS for the COVID-19 vaccines than all other 70+ other vaccines combined during the entire 32 year history of the VAERS database. Of the total 2.2 million adverse event reports in VAERS over the last 32 years, 1.3 million of those reports were for adverse events from the COVID-19 vaccines in the past 19 months.[496]

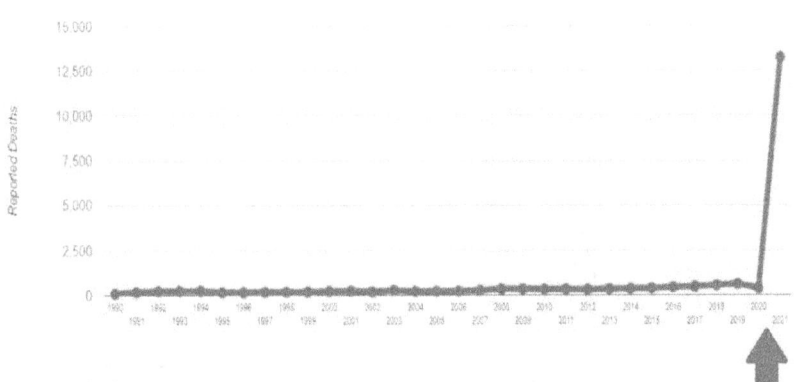

FDA authorizes emergency use COVID-19 Vaccines

The Expose reported that "[t]he UK Medicine Regulator has confirmed that over a period of nineteen months the Covid-19 Vaccines have caused at least 5.5x as many deaths as all other available vaccines combined in the past 21 years."[497] But when measuring the lethality of the COVID-19 vaccines side-by-side against all other vaccines over the same 19-month period, it was found that the COVID-19 vaccine caused 7,402% (74x) more deaths than all other vaccines combined during that 19-month period.[498] As we saw with the German government statistics, the deaths from vaccines is vastly under-reported. But such under-reporting should be across the board for all vaccines. And so, the statistics about the relative number of deaths should be somewhat accurate. Based on those relative statistics, the COVID-19 vaccines are 74 times more deadly than all other vaccines combined. The below graphic is from *The Expose*.

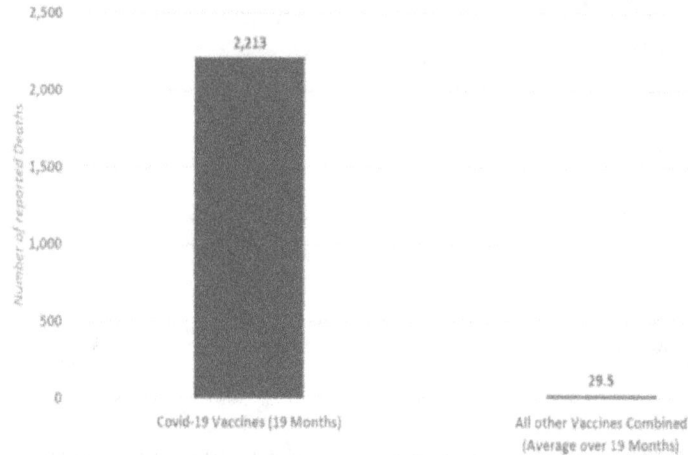

Reported Deaths due to Covid-19 Vaccination from Jan 21 to July 22 (19 Months) vs Average Number of Deaths due to all other Vaccines Combined over a 19 Month Period
Source: UK Medicine and Health Care product Regulatory Agency (MHRA) Yellow Card Report

On July 19, 2021, America's Frontline Doctors (AFLDS) filed a motion seeking immediate injunctive relief in the Alabama Federal District Court to stop the Emergency Use Authorization (EUA) of the experimental COVID-19 injections. The plaintiffs averred the following facts in their certified complaint about the relative dangers of the COVID-19 vaccines:

> According to data extracted from the Defendants' Vaccine Adverse Events Reporting System ("VAERS"), 99% of all deaths attributed to vaccines in the first quarter of 2021 are attributed to the COVID-19 Vaccines, and only 1% are attributed to all other vaccines. The number of vaccine deaths reported in the same period constitutes a 12,000% to 25,000% increase in

vaccine deaths, year-on-year.⁴⁹⁹

Why are the COVID-19 vaccines so harmful? Dr. Robert Malone has the answer. Dr. Malone is a medical doctor and a world-famous infectious disease expert. Dr. Malone has close to 100 peer-reviewed publications and published abstracts and has over 11,477 citations of his peer reviewed publications. **Most notably, Dr. Malone is the inventor of the mRNA technology used by Pfizer-BioNTech and Moderna in their COVID-19 vaccines.**⁵⁰⁰ Vaccines using mRNA technology are not like conventional vaccines, which use weakened forms of the virus. An mRNA vaccine uses only part of the virus's genetic code. An mRNA vaccine carries code into the body, where it enters cells. The mRNA instructs those cells to create spike proteins that are associated with SARS-CoV-2 (the alleged virus that causes COVID-19). These spike proteins are recognized by the immune system, which then attacks them. **Dr. Malone has stated that the spike proteins generated by the cells through the mRNA code are cytotoxic.**⁵⁰¹ That means that the spike proteins are toxic to living cells. Thus, the COVID-19 mRNA vaccines made by Pfizer-BioNTech and Moderna allowed under the EUA cause the body to create spike proteins that kill the cells in the body. That cytotoxicity is the cause of the many adverse events being reported in VAERS. Malone explained that he is a regulatory professional and has connections with persons in senior positions in the FDA. On or about June 13, 2021, Malone stated that he alerted those senior officials in the FDA to the cytotoxicity of the spike protein being generated by the mRNA vaccines "months-and-months ago."⁵⁰²

With damning data establishing within the first month that the COVID-19 vaccines are unsafe, the mainstream media quickly sprung into action to do the bidding of the CDC and report that "initial safety data shows everything is going well."⁵⁰³ For example, Karen Weintraub reported on January 28, 2021, for *USA Today* the following false information:

Everyone who experienced an allergic response has been treated successfully, and no other serious problems have turned up among the first 22 million people vaccinated, according to the Centers for Disease Control and Prevention.[504]

I don't know about you, but I would say that 104 permanent disabilities, 273 life-threatening events, 11 birth defects, 722 hospitalizations, 2,056 visits to the emergency room, and 329 deaths within the first month of the COVID-19 rollout would fall into the category of "serious problems." Indeed, the deaths associated with the COVID-19 vaccines, as reported in VAERS, had exploded to 33,011, and hospitalizations had soared to 186,726 by December 16, 2022.[505] To put those figures into perspective, a typical new drug receives a black box warning after five unexplained deaths. If the deaths raise to 50 the drug is pulled off the market. Yet within one month there were 329 deaths attributed to the COVID-19 vaccines, yet *USA Today* runs a story claiming that the COVID-19 vaccines are "not causing large numbers of unusual or dangerous results."[506] So, how does *USA Today* address those deaths? They dismiss them as not being caused by the vaccine. Weintraub writes:

> Vaccinated people have suffered major health crises and even death within a few days of receiving a shot, but the rate of those events is no higher than would be expected in the general population and cannot be connected to the vaccine, the review found.[507]

That is a complete lie. There is simply no way to reconcile that statement with the fact that there have been more adverse event reports in VAERS for the COVID-19 vaccines than all other 70+ other vaccines combined during the entire 32 year history of the VAERS database.

Interestingly, the CDC and *USA Today* credit the reports of minor responses and allergic reactions as being caused by the vaccines when the person is treated and recovers. But when the person dies or is seriously injured "it cannot be connected to the vaccine." *USA Today* puts the VAERS data in its report; it is there for all to see. But *USA Today* spins the data to the CDC's and mainstream media's preconceived conclusion that the COVID-19 vaccine is safe and effective. Keep in mind this article (more like cheerleading) was early on and floated to minimize the early data of injuries and death and encourage people to be vaccinated.

The same VAERS reporting system that faithfully reports minor injuries is suddenly deemed by *USA Today* not sufficient to conclude that serious injury or death is caused by the vaccine. What a scam. It's a game of heads I win, tails you lose. With that kind of approach, it is easy for *USA Today* to misrepresent that "[a]lthough it's never possible to prove something is completely safe, data from these tracking systems suggests the vaccines are not causing large numbers of unusual or dangerous results."[508]

Keep in mind that conclusion is in the face of an acknowldegment in the *USA Today* report that "[t]he problems in slightly more than 1,000 of those [9,000 VAERSS] reports were considered serious."[509] *USA Today*'s claim that the COVID-19 vaccines are "not causing large numbers of unusual or dangerous results" was refuted, even at that early stage, by the VAERS data. But *USA Today* tried to put a favorable spin on the incriminating data.

Dr. Denis Rancourt, Ph.D., is a former tenured full professor of physics at the University of Ottawa, who has published more than one hundred articles in leading science journals. Dr. Rancourt took the all-cause mortality increases by country and correlated them to the vaccine rollouts in each country. He was able to extrapolate a death rate for the COVID-19 vaccines. In his February 9, 2023 report he concluded that approximately 13 million people have died worldwide from the COVID-19 vaccines.[510] That figure includes 330,000 deaths in the United States alone. He used robust criteria to establish causation based on the Loannidis criteria of experiment, temporality, and consistency.

While the CDC plays down the hazards of the COVID-19 vaccines, others have taken notice of the VAERS raw data that proves the vaccines are dangerous. For example, on February 15, 2023, the Florida Department of Health issued a health alert to doctors and the public regarding the dangers of the COVID-19 vaccines. Florida health officials are concerned about the significant increase in adverse events reported in VAERS during the COVID-19 vaccine campaign. Some may try to argue that the increase in adverse events was because there was a 400% increase in vaccinations due to the COVID-19 vaccination campaign. The problem is that the Florida Department of Health recorded a troubling 1,700% spike in vaccine adverse events during the 2021 COVID-19 vaccine campaign. In addition, the life-threatening adverse events exploded to an increase of 4,400% during the COVID-19 vaccine program. That means the COVID-19 vaccines are four (4) times more harmful and eleven (11) times more life-threatening than any other vaccine. Below is a chart posted by the Florida Department of Health showing the disturbing spike in reported adverse events.[511]

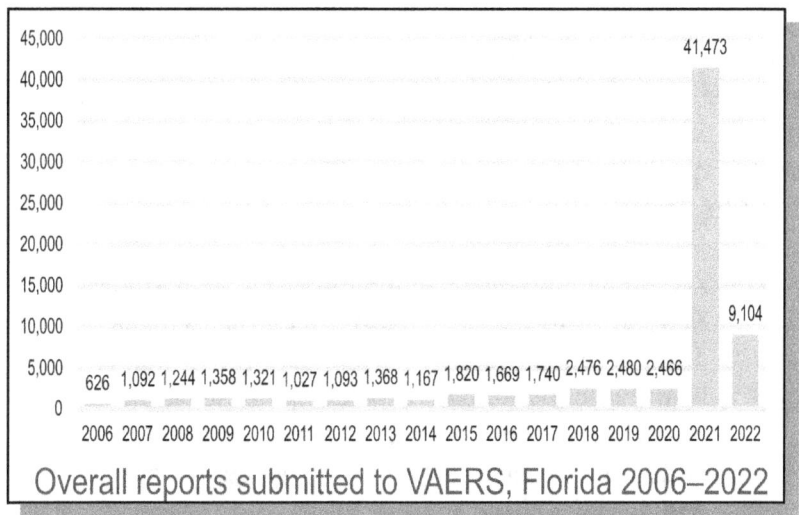

Overall reports submitted to VAERS, Florida 2006–2022

This spike in adverse events prompted Florida Surgeon General, Joseph Ladapo, M.D., to write a letter to Robert M. Calif, MD, Commissioner, U.S. Food and Drug Administration (FDA), and Rochelle P. Walensky, Director, Centers for Disease Control and Prevention (CDC). General Ladapo stated:

> [A]academic researchers throughout our country and around the globe have seen troubling safety signals of adverse events surrounding this vaccine. Their concerns are corroborated by the substantial increase in VAERS reports from Florida, including life-threatening conditions. We have never seen this type of response following previous mass vaccination efforts pushed by the federal government. Even the HINI vaccine did not trigger this sort of response. In Florida alone, we saw a 1,700% increase in reports after the release of the COVID-I9 vaccine, compared to an increase of 400% in vaccine administration for the same period. The reporting of life threatening conditions increased 4,400%.[512]

What was unusual (and refreshing) was that General Ladapo implied that the CDC and the FDA were restricting and diminishing the rights and liberties of U.S. citizens by restricting transparency in the medical community and failing to communicate the risks of the COVID-19 vaccines. He called on them to stop it.

> As a father, physician, and Surgeon General for the State of Florida, I request that your agencies promote transparency in health care professionals to accurately communicate the risks these vaccines pose. I request that you work to protect the rights and liberties that we are endowed with, not restrict, and diminish them.[513]

The Florida Department of Health's health alert did not simply note the correlation between the increase in adverse events and the rollout of the COVID-19 vaccines. The Florida health officials were positing that the COVID-19 vaccines are unsafe. In support of that position, they cited specific research studies that have found that the COVID-19 vaccines cause serious health problems.

> According to a study,[514] mRNA COVID-19 vaccines were associated with an excess risk of serious adverse events, including coagulation disorders, acute cardiac injuries, Bell's palsy, and encephalitis. This risk was 1 in 550 individuals, which is much higher than other vaccines.

> A second study,[515] found increased acute cardiac arrests and other acute cardiac events following mRNA COVID-19 vaccination.

> Additionally,[researchers in an article in The Journal of the American Medical Association[516]]

assessed the risk of thromboembolic and thrombocytopenic events related to COVID-19 vaccines and found preliminary evidence of increased risk of both coronary disease and cardiovascular disease.

CDC spokesman Nick Spinelli tried to do damage control and responded to General Ladapo's letter that the Florida Department of Public Health's conclusions were misleading because the data was missing context.[517] He then threw up the smokescreen argument that the VAERS system shows correlation and not necessarily causation. While that statement is true, he is hiding the ball. He conceals that correlation often gives reasonable belief for causation, particularly when there is a temporal relationship between the vaccine and the injury. To say that it cannot be proven that someone dies from a vaccination when they have a heart attack after getting a vaccine is, on its face, accurate. But when there is a pattern of such deaths, and there is no other reasonable cause, it is fair to say that one should be careful about deciding to receive the vaccine. VAERS is not irrelevant, but the CDC argues that VAERS data is only coincidental because there is no sure proof of causation.

The CDC is playing a misleading game. Most of the VAERS reports are submitted by medical professionals who have looked at the circumstantial evidence and determined that there is probable cause (i.e., reason to believe) that the vaccine in question caused the sickness or death they are reporting. It is like a witness who tells police that he heard a gunshot and saw John Doe running from a room carrying a smoking gun. The witness enters the room to see Tom Thumb dead on the floor with a bullet hole in his head. The police would clearly have probable cause to arrest John Doe for the murder of Tom Thumb. But would those facts be enough to prove John Doe's guilt beyond a reasonable doubt? What if John Doe's defense is that Tom Thumb put the gun to his head to commit suicide, and he tried to grab the gun to prevent the suicide, and Tom Thumb suddenly pulled the trigger? John Doe claims he ran from the scene with the gun to report the suicide to the police. If that is true, then John Doe is not guilty of murder. Of course, there is the matter of what other evidence there is in the case and whether the jury believes John Doe's defense.

There is a difference between probable cause to arrest and proof of guilt at trial beyond a reasonable doubt. And that is what the CDC is obfuscating. The CDC is conflating what is necessary to stop the vaccine program, which is equivalent to what is needed to arrest John Doe, with what is required to prove the vaccines cause death and injury, which is equivalent to what is necessary to prove John Doe murdered Tom Thumb.

Just as there is probable cause to arrest John Doe for the murder of Tom Thumb, so also there is probable cause to stop the COVID-19 vaccinations because there is probable cause from the VAERS data showing that the vaccines are unsafe. Just as further investigation will be necessary to prove that John Doe is guilty of murder, so also, further investigation will be necessary to establish with scientific certainty that the vaccines are causing the death and destruction as reported in the VAERS system.

Another important point the CDC is not revealing is that the reported deaths and injuries are just the tip of the proverbial iceberg. Dr. Katrina Lindley explains that the VAERS data under-reports fatalities and injuries because VAERS is a passive reporting system. The reality is that "systems of passive surveillance result in significantly fewer ADR [adverse drug reaction] reports than active surveillance reporting."[518] Consequently, "the actual number of adverse events that occurred in temporal relation to Covid-19 injections is likely to be much higher than revealed by the available official data."[519] But the CDC will not mention that truth.

The CDC is just plain lying about the dangers of the

COVID-19 vaccines. Another CDC spokesman said in an email sent to the media, "COVID-19 vaccines have undergone—and continue to undergo—the most intense vaccine safety monitoring in U.S. history."[520] That is a lie. But the CDC spokesman goes further. He states that "[c]linical research has demonstrated the safety and effectiveness of the recommended COVID-19 primary series vaccines, as well as the recommended updated vaccines."[521] That is another lie. It seems that the CDC is staffed with pathological liars.

Indeed, the deception about the COVID-19 vaccines is so clear and egregious that on December 12, 2022, the Governor of Florida called for a grand jury investigation to bring criminal charges against the officials and companies involved in the death and destruction caused by the vaccines. Arek Sarkissian, reporting for Politico, revealed:

> [Florida] Gov. Ron DeSantis on Tuesday asked the Florida Supreme Court to empanel a grand jury to investigate "wrongdoing" linked to the Covid-19 vaccines, including spreading false and misleading claims about the efficacy of the doses.
>
> Most of the medical community, including the Centers for Disease Control and Prevention, the FDA and Johns Hopkins, have emphasized that the Covid vaccine is safe and effective in preventing the virus and protecting against serious symptoms.
>
> But DeSantis said during a live-streamed round table discussion with Florida Surgeon General Joseph Ladapo that it's against Florida law to mislead the public, especially when it comes to drug safety. He sought to undermine the efficacy of the Covid vaccine and claimed that vaccine manufacturers such as Moderna have made a

fortune on Covid-19 mandates.

"I think people want the truth that I think people want accountability," DeSantis said. "You need to have a thorough investigation into what's happened with the shots."

In a petition to the state Supreme Court asking for the grand jury, the DeSantis administration said that the "pharmaceutical industry has a notorious history of misleading the public for financial gain" and the grand jury will probe "the development, promotion, and distribution of vaccines purported to prevent COVID-19 infection, symptoms, and transmission."[522]

The Florida Governor stated in his petition that government officials and pharmaceutical companies misled the public about the safety and efficacy of the COVID-19 vaccines. The deception caused people to decide to get the vaccines which caused them injuries. The injuries were foreseeable because government officials and manufacturers knew that the vaccines were dangerous. For example, while the pharmaceutical companies claimed there was no causal link between their vaccines and myocarditis, they knew at the time from their studies and other published studies that, in fact, their vaccines caused myocarditis. The gravamen of the charges in the *Petition For Order To Empanel a Statewide Grand Jury* are as follows:

> Florida law prohibits fraudulent practices, including the dissemination of false or misleading advertisements of a drug and the use of any representation or suggestion in any advertisement relating to a drug that an application of a drug is effective when it is not. § 499.0051(11), Fla. Stat. The pharmaceutical industry has a notorious

history of misleading the public for financial gain. 42 Questions have been raised regarding the veracity of the representations made by the pharmaceutical manufacturers of COVID-19 vaccines, particularly with respect to transmission, prevention, efficacy, and safety. An investigation is warranted to determine whether the pharmaceutical industry has engaged 1n fraudulent practices. The people of Florida deserve to know the truth.[523]

Sucharit Bhakdi, M.D., is a retired doctor. He is a microbiologist and an expert in immunology. He was a post-doctoral researcher at the Max Planck Institute of Immunobiology and Epigenetics and at The Protein Laboratory in Copenhagen. He was appointed associate professor at the Institute of Medical Microbiology at Giessen University. He was named chair of Medical Microbiology at the University of Mainz. Dr. Bhakdi has published over three hundred articles on immunology, bacteriology, virology, and parasitology, for which he has received numerous awards and the Order of Merit of Rhineland-Palatinate.[524]

Alex Newman, the Senior Editor of The New American magazine, interviewed Dr. Bhakdi.[525] During the interview, the world-renowned microbiologist warned that the COVID-19 virus hysteria is based on lies. The COVID "vaccines" are set to cause a global catastrophe and decimation of the human population. He explains that the PCR test has been abused to artificially inflate the danger of COVID-19 and produce fear in an unscientific way.

Dr. Bhakdi expects massive, deadly clotting and immune system responses that will destroy the human body. During a previous Fox News interview, Dr. Bhakdi warned of impending doom from the vaccines. He calls for criminal prosecutions of the people responsible for the vaccine injuries and death and an immediate halt to the global vaccine experiment.

18   CDC Changes the Definition of Vaccine

The CDC and the vaccine makers understood from the beginning that the COVID-19 mRNA vaccines were ineffective in protecting persons from COVID-19. As the ineffectiveness of the COVID-19 injections in providing immunity was becoming increasingly clear, the CDC realized that the injections did not meet the definition of a vaccine. Indeed, in a Motion for a Preliminary Injunction against HHS filed on July 19, 2021, the plaintiffs alleged:

> [T]he "Pfizer-BioNTech COVID-19 Vaccine" and the "Moderna COVID-19 Vaccine" do not meet the CDC's own definitions. They do not stimulate the body to produce immunity from a disease. They are a synthetic fragment of nucleic acid embedded in a fat carrier that is introduced into human cells, not for the purpose of inducing immunity from infection with the SARS-CoV-2 virus, and not to block further transmission of the virus, but in order to lessen the symptoms of COVID-19. No published, peer-reviewed studies prove that the "Pfizer-BioNTech COVID-19 Vaccine" and the "Moderna COVID-19 Vaccine" confer immunity

or stop transmission.[526]

The lawyers for HHS realized that the plaintiffs were correct. They advised their clients at the HHS component agency, the CDC, that they needed to fix that problem. So many of the laws protecting pharmaceutical companies from liability required that their injections be vaccines. They needed to change the very definition of a vaccine to include an injection that is ineffective in producing immunity to the disease.

The CDC defines immunity as "[p]rotection from an infectious disease. If you are immune to a disease, you can be exposed to it without becoming infected."[527] So far, so good. Up until September 2021, the CDC's definition of "vaccine" was "[a] product that stimulates a person's immune system to produce immunity to a specific disease, protecting the person from that disease."[528] So it was understood by all before September 2021 that a vaccine "stimulates a person's immune system to produce immunity." And immunity means "[p]rotection from an infectious disease. If you are immune to a disease, you can be exposed to it without becoming infected."

> ## CDC Definitions Prior to September 2021
>
> ### Definition of Terms
>
> Related Information and Materials
>
> Let's start by defining several basic terms:
>
> **Immunity:** Protection from an infectious disease. If you are immune to a disease, you can be exposed to it without becoming infected.
>
> **Vaccine:** A product that stimulates a person's immune system to produce immunity to a specific disease, protecting the person from that disease. Vaccines are usually administered through needle injections, but can also be administered by mouth or sprayed into the nose.
>
> **Vaccination:** The act of introducing a vaccine into the body to produce immunity to a specific disease.
>
> **Immunization:** A process by which a person becomes protected against a disease through vaccination. This term is often used interchangeably with vaccination or inoculation.

Notice that the CDC defines immunization as only obtained "through vaccination." That implies no natural immune protection from a disease once a person recovers. The CDC implicitly pushes the fallacy that the only efficacious immunization is through vaccination. The CDC misleadingly portrays vaccination, inoculation, and immunization as synonyms.

But in September 2021, the CDC made a notable change. The CDC changed the definition of vaccine to mean instead "[a] preparation that is used to stimulate the body's immune response against diseases."[529] Now, the definition of a vaccine includes a vaccine that merely "stimulates the body's immune response" without actually producing any protection from disease. Now, a vaccine can be ineffective in providing any protection in preventing infection; it only needs to stimulate the body's immune response regardless of whether that stimulation is effective in protecting against disease.

> **CDC Definitions After September 2021**
>
> **Definition of Terms**
>
> **Immunity:** Protection from an infectious disease. If you are immune to a disease, you can be exposed to it without becoming infected.
>
> **Vaccine:** A preparation that is used to stimulate the body's immune response against diseases. Vaccines are usually administered through needle injections, but some can be administered by mouth or sprayed into the nose.
>
> **Vaccination:** The act of introducing a vaccine into the body to produce protection from a specific disease.
>
> ➡ **Immunization:** A process by which a person becomes protected against a disease through vaccination. This term is often used interchangeably with vaccination or inoculation.
>
> **Related Pages**
> See the Vaccine and Immunization Glossary of Terms

Notice that the CDC maintains that immunization is only through vaccination. The CDC even recommends that those who have recovered from COVID-19 still receive a COVID-19 vaccine. "Getting a COVID-19 vaccine after having COVID-19 provides added protection against the virus that causes COVID-19."[530] Such advice impeaches the germ theory upon which vaccines are based. The whole purpose of a vaccine is to replicate natural immunity by injecting an antigen to stimulate the immune system to protect against future infection. Why get a vaccine when a person has already recovered from the illness and fulfilled the immunity requirement? Vaccinating a person who has recovered from the illness that is the target of the vaccine makes no scientific sense. But it does make perfect Machiavellian genocidal sense.

The Cleveland Clinic did a study that concluded that "[i]ndividuals who have had SARS-CoV-2 infection are unlikely to benefit from COVID-19 vaccination."[531] That study does not stand alone. Other studies confirm the results. The CDC recommendation for someone who has recovered from COVID-19 to be vaccinated against COVID-19 is dangerous quackery. Studies have shown that children with natural immunity from COVID-19 and then received a COVID-19 vaccine had their immunity from COVID-19 go negative after five months.[532] That means the children who already had natural immunity were more susceptible to the COVID-19 infection after getting the vaccine. Thus, the vaccine harms the patient who already has natural immunity. That harm is caused by vaccine-induced antibody-dependent enhancement.[533]

In an email response to a news inquiry, a spokesman for the CDC stated: "while there have been slight changes in wording over time to the definition of 'vaccine' on the CDC's website, those haven't impacted the overall definition. ... The previous definition…could be interpreted to mean that vaccines were 100% effective, which has never been the case for any vaccine, so the current definition is more transparent."[534]

The real reason for the changed definition is that since the mRNA vaccines have been such a spectacular failure, a change in the definition was necessary to account for that failure. For the CDC to claim that changing the meaning of vaccine from "stimulates a person's immune system to produce immunity" to "stimulate the body's immune response against diseases" is only a slight change that does not impact the definition is dissimulation of the first order.

If the new definition was not a change, then why do it? There is a world of difference between producing immunity and simply responding to a disease. Under the new definition, the body's response could be, and as we have seen with the mRNA vaccines, has been, ineffective in fighting off the disease. Before the definition change, a vaccine was required to offer immunity from the disease; now, all that is needed is for the vaccine to prompt the body's immune system to respond to the disease. Indeed, the body could respond to the disease with a cytokine storm (a.k.a., antibody-dependent enhancement), which may kill the patient, as we have seen with mRNA COVID-19 vaccines. Now, the ineffectiveness of vaccines is built into the definition.

The CDC's redefinition of vaccine is part of the Orwellian newspeak, where our language is being altered to meet the ideological needs of the Zionist ruling class. The power of the these international communists is pervasive. For example, within a little more than a month of introducing the mRNA COVID-19 vaccines, Merriam-Webster Dictionary changed the definition of vaccine to accommodate the ineffective and dangerous new vaccines. That was approximately eight months before the CDC vaccine definition changed.

Before January 18, 2021, the Merriam-Webster Dictionary definition of vaccine was given as:

> [A] preparation of killed microorganisms, living attenuated organisms, or living fully virulent organisms that is administered to **produce or artificially increase immunity to a particular disease.**[535]

But sometime between January 18, 2021, and January 26, 2021, Merriam-Webster changed the definition to remove the requirement that a vaccine must **"produce or artificially increase immunity to a particular disease."** The new definition only requires the vaccine to **"stimulate the body's immune response against a specific infectious agent or disease."** Thus an injection can be ineffective in producing immunity as long as it stimulates the body's immune response. That stimulation of the body's immune response could be quite detrimental, as when the stimulation causes illness due to antibody-dependent enhancement. The new vaccine definition, in pertinent part, states:

> [A] preparation that is administered (as by injection) to **stimulate the body's immune**

response against a specific infectious agent or disease: such as ... an antigenic preparation of a typically inactivated or attenuated (see ATTENUATED sense 2) pathogenic agent (such as a bacterium or virus) or one of its components or products (such as a protein or toxin) ... a preparation of genetic material (such as a strand of **synthesized messenger RNA**) that is used by the cells of the body to produce an antigenic substance (such as a fragment of virus spike protein).[536]

Now, an injection can be a vaccine if it merely stimulates the body's immune response and does not "produce or artificially increase immunity to a particular disease." The Merriam-Webster change was an acknowledgment that the COVID-19 mRNA vaccines are ineffective in producing or increasing immunity to COVID-19. This definition change is evidence that they knew from the beginning that the mRNA COVID-19 vaccines would not stop infection or spread of COVID-19; it would only "stimulate the body's immune response."

Indeed, the Merriam-Webster Dictionary even adds the new mRNA technology to its definition. Merriam-Webster defines a biological weapon (i.e., bioweapon) as "a harmful biological agent (as a pathogenic microorganism or a neurotoxin) used as a weapon to cause death or disease usually on a large scale."[537] An injection that stimulates the body's immune system to attack itself is a bioweapon. That is what the COVID-19 vaccine does. The new definition of vaccine means that if an injection causes harm by stimulating the body's immune system to attack itself through antibody-dependent enhancement, it is still a vaccine. Thus, any bioweapon (e,g,, COVID-19 injection) can masquerade as a vaccine. Since the new definition of a vaccine includes within it the characteristics of a bioweapon, the manufacturers and all who administer the bioweapon are protected from liability by the Public Readiness and Emergency Preparedness Act (PREP Act), which authorizes the Countermeasures Injury Compensation Program (CICP) that grants pharmaceutical companies and medical professionals liability protection for vaccines made and administered under an emergency use authorization(EUA).

19 Increased All-Cause Mortality

Vaccine manufacturers often try to obscure their vaccines' dangerousness by arguing that correlation does not necessarily mean causation. That bare statement is true. The correlation is not causation argument offers some logical cover when there is an allegation that a vaccine caused an adverse event or a death. The correlation is not necessarily causation argument can be made in any individual case of death without scientific confirmation that the vaccine caused the death. The vaccine makers often argue a myriad of co-factors for the deaths.

But we must key in on the word "necessarily." While correlation does not "necessarily" prove causation, correlation can nonetheless be convincing evidence of causation where no other variables can explain the adverse event or death. There is a statistic that saps the persuasiveness of the correlation is not necessarily causation argument. The all-cause mortality statistic for an entire population makes it difficult to conceal the deaths caused by a population-wide vaccine program. The occurrence of events (deaths) spread over a large population after the occurrence of an independent variable (vaccination) administered to that same population raises a stronger inference of causation than a single occurrence of an event (death) after a single prior independent variable (vaccination).

The Bradford-Hill criteria are used to determine if there is a causal relationship between a presumed cause and an observed effect. Five Bradford-Hill criteria pertinent to showing if vaccines cause adverse events indicate a causal relationship between COVID-19 vaccinations and excess deaths.[538] 1) Consistency in the reported association between vaccinations and deaths by different authorities at different locations. 2) The association between vaccinations and deaths is strong, involving large populations. 3) There is a specific association between vaccinations and deaths rather than some other factor. 4) There is a temporal relationship between vaccinations and deaths, such that the deaths follow after the vaccinations. 5) It is biologically plausible that vaccinations are causing the deaths.[539]

All-cause mortality covers the gambit of people who die from all causes. A significant increase in all-cause mortality indicates that something acted on the population to bring about that increase. Thus, if a vaccine is dangerous and causes widespread death, the increased deaths will appear in the all-cause mortality rate. Suppose the only change in population behavior is vaccination. In that case, a subsequent increase in deaths would be convincing evidence that the vaccine caused those deaths. The correlation between the population-wide vaccine program and the increased deaths from all causes is compelling evidence that the vaccine is the independent variable causing the deaths since there is no other variable that would explain the excess deaths.

A February 2023 study that compared the average monthly all-cause mortality rate for the years 2016-2019 to the monthly all-cause mortality for the first nine months of 2022 found that the countries that vaccinated their population for COVID-19 during 2021 saw a 0.105% increase in the monthly all-cause mortality rate for every one percent increase in people being vaccinated in that country.[540] That is a direct correlation between COVID-19 vaccines and increased deaths across many countries. More COVID-19 vaccines result in more deaths.

The study looked at the all-cause mortality for the first nine months of 2022 and compared it to the vaccination uptake in 31 European countries by the end of 2021. The 31 countries studied were the EU member states, plus Norway, Iceland, Liechtenstein, and Switzerland. The researchers determined the correlation between vaccination uptake and the mortality rate was significant. It "implies that the mortality increases the higher the vaccination uptake. Specifically, it shows that a one percentage point increase in 2021 vaccination uptake is associated with an increase in 2022 monthly mortality by 0.105 percent."[541]

The vaccine uptake for the COVID-19 vaccines for the countries ranged from Bulgaria, with 27.7% of the country vaccinated, to Portugal, with 83.1% of the population vaccinated. All countries, except Bulgaria, vaccinated more than 50% of their people.

The 0.105% increase in mortality for every one percent increase in vaccinations represents a 10.5% increase in all-cause mortality among the vaccinated population. To understand the significance of the 10.5% increase in all-cause mortality in Western Europe's vaccinated population, we must consider that the background mortality rate from all causes in most Western countries is approximately 1% per year.[542] Eurostat reported that "the number of deaths per 1,000 persons was estimated at 10.4 in the EU in 2019."

For simplicity's sake, we will use 1% as the base mortality rate for Western Europe. That means that year in and year out, approximately 1% of the population in Western Europe die each year. Thus, the statistics from the February 2023 study showing an increase in the all-cause mortality rate of 0.105% for every percentage increase in vaccine uptake indicates that the COVID-19 vaccines are correlated with a rise of 10.5% in all-cause mortality in Western Europe. Assuming a base rate of about 1%, that means there is a death rate of 1.105% for the vaccinated population.

Looking at the U.S, we find the same increase in the mortality rate correlated to the rollout of the COVID-19 vaccines. But U.S. death statistics for 2020, in particular, must be looked at with suspicion. That is because the CDC has been caught fudging the mortality data. For example, The Guardian reported that the CDC was caught over-counting COVID-19 deaths.[543] Once the CDC was confronted with the over-count, it claimed to have corrected it and attributed it to a "coding logic error." Oddly, no "coding logic error" had ever happened before the COVID-19 "pandemic." Usually, a coding error would result in the missed recording of statistics. It is rather suspicious that the "coding logic error" resulted in an artificial increase in COVID-19 deaths.

Also, the CDC has massaged the COVID-19 death data to under-report the vaccinated deaths from COVID-19 by listing vaccinated deaths as unvaccinated deaths. Add to that the efforts made by the CDC to prevent effective treatments like hyrdroxychloroquine and ivermectin for flu-like illnesses while locking down and masking people and administering dangerous and ineffective treatments such as remdesivir, midazolam, and ventilation. It is no wonder that the death rate increased in 2020. With those cautions in mind we will look at what seems to be an increase in mortality in the U.S. after the introduction of the COVID-19 vaccines.

Because of the anomalous government actions during the 2020 "pandemic" and the untrustworthiness of the mortality rates reported by the CDC that year, we will use the average mortality rates in the U.S. from 2015 to 2019. We will compare the average mortality rate from 2015-2019 to the death rates after the introduction of the COVID-19 vaccines to obtain the delta. The average annual mortality rate for 2015-2019 was 0.86%.[544] That means an average of 0.86% of the U.S. population died annually between 2015 and 2019.

The Organisation for Economic Co-operation and Development (OECD) is an intergovernmental organization with 38 member countries. It keeps data on mortality for those countries, which includes the U.S. The data shows a significant increase in all-cause mortality in the U.S. after the rollout of the COVID1-19 vaccines.[545]

That website only provides U.S. all-cause death numbers for 2020, 2021, and 2022. To give the raw death numbers meaning, we must be able to compare them to the deaths for prior years. As noted earlier, the average death rate reported by the CDC for the years 2015 to 2019 was 0.86%.[546] But that number is unhelpful in comparing it to the raw death numbers reported by the OECD. In order to compare the average mortality rate for 2015-2019 to the mortality rate for 2020, 2021, and 2022, we must convert the raw numbers provided by the OECD to a percentage.

The OECD website lists the all-cause deaths and reveals that the 2020 all-cause mortality rate in the U.S. was 1.04%. That figure was arrived at by dividing the all-cause deaths reported by the OECD (3,441,118)[547] by the mid-year U.S. population reported by the U.S. Census Bureau on June 30, 2020 (331,509,617).[548] The OECD website lists the all-cause deaths reveals that the 2021 all-cause mortality rate in the U.S. was 1.04%. That figure was arrived at by dividing the all-cause deaths reported by the OECD (3,457,525)[549] by the mid-year U.S. population reported by the U.S. Census Bureau on June 30, 2021 (332,028,282).[550] The OECD website lists the all cause deaths and reveals that the 2022 all-cause mortality rate in the U.S. was 0.981%. That figure was arrived at by dividing the all-cause deaths reported by the OECD (3,270,300)[551] by the mid-year U.S. population reported by the U.S. Census Bureau on June 30, 2022 (333,282,419).[552]

Thus we find an increase in the mortality rate in the U.S. in 2020 of 0.18% (1.04%−0.86% = 0.18%). Recall that 2020 saw some strange and anomalous actions and reporting of deaths by the CDC, so the numbers cannot be relied upon. What is really interesting is that after the rollout of the COVID-19 vaccines in 2021, we see the same increase in mortality of 0.18% (1.04%−0.86% = 0.18%). You would expect the mortality rate to decrease if you assume the vaccines are effective due to the massive vaccine program. Instead, we find continued carnage at the same rate as 2020. Then, in 2022, we find that there was a continuation of the excess deaths but at a slightly slower clip of 0.12% (0.98%−0.86% = 0.12%).

The 2021 0.18% increase over the 0.86% death rate represents an astounding 20% increase in the mortality rate in the U.S. during 2021. The 2022 0.12% increase over the 0.86% death rate represents a 14% increase in the mortality rate in the U.S during 2022. **What that means in real numbers is that there have been approximately 997,589 excess U.S. deaths correlated to the rollout of the COVID-19 vaccines during 2021 and 2022.**[553] Again, correlation does not necessarily mean causation. But the statistics from the UK where the vaccinated death rate can be compared to the unvaccinated death rate, strengthens the causation argument.

When we focus on the statistics from the UK, the inference of causation becomes clearer. That is because the UK Office for National Statistics (ONS) breaks down its death statistics by vaccination status. Thus, we can compare the all-cause death rate of the vaccinated population against the all-cause death rate for the unvaccinated population and find out from where the excess deaths are coming.

The investigative journalists at *The Expose* examined the official death data from the UK Office for National Statistics (ONS). On March 21, 2023, *The Expose* reported that between

January 1, 2021, and May 31, 2022, the all-cause mortality rate among those who had received a COVID-19 vaccine was 1.36%. But the all-cause mortality rate for those who had not received any COVID-19 vaccine was 0.58%. The mortality rate among the COVID-19 vaccinated population is more than double that of the unvaccinated population. *The Expose* reported:

> 44.48 million people had received at least one dose of a Covid-19 vaccine in England, and 606,537 of those people had sadly died. This, therefore, equates to 1 in every 73 [which is a 1.36% mortality rate for] Covid-19 vaccinated people having sadly died by the 1st of June 2022.
>
> 18.9 million people had not received a single dose of a Covid-19 vaccine in England, and 109,891 of those people had sadly died. This, therefore, equates to 1 in every 172 [which is a 0.58% mortality rate for] unvaccinated people having sadly died by the 1st of June 2022.[554]

The above data presents total all-cause mortality of 1.130% for both vaccinated and unvaccinated combined between January 1, 2021, and May 31, 2022. There were 716,428 total deaths (606,537 vaccinated + 109,891 unvaccinated = 716,428 total deaths). The total vaccinated and unvaccinated population was 63.38 million (44.8 million vaccinated + 18.9 million unvaccinated = 63..38 million total population). That results in a total mortality rate of 1.130% (716,428 ÷ 63.38 million = 1.130%).

The UK's base mortality rate for 2019 and prior was less than 1%. But for simplicity's sake, we will use 1% for the base mortality rate for the UK. Assuming a base mortality rate of 1%, that means there has been about a 13% increase in total mortality in the UK between January 1, 2021, and May 31, 2022, after the rollout of the COVID-19 vaccines. That increased mortality is attributable entirely to the vaccinated population because the unvaccinated population had a mortality rate of approximately 0.58%, which is far below the approximate 1% total expected mortality rate for Wester European countries. *The Expose* explains:

> The official figures unfortunately confirm that mortality rates per 100,000 are the lowest among the unvaccinated population in every single age group in England. And the data reveals the gap between the unvaccinated and vaccinated populations in terms of mortality rates is widening by the month.[555]

When you break out just the vaccinated group, we find a mortality rate of 1.36%. Comparing that to the expected base mortality rate of approximately 1%, we see a whopping 36% increase in mortality among the vaccinated population. *The Expose* comes to the ineluctable conclusion:

> There is no other conclusion that can be found for the fact mortality rates per 100,000 are the lowest among the unvaccinated other than that the Covid-19 injections are killing people.[556]

To put that in perspective, a study of 1,118 unique armed conflicts spanning 193 countries between 1990 and 2017 found that the increase in civilian mortality during a war is 81.5 per 100,000 population.[557] That is an increased mortality rate of 0.0815% during a war. That increased war mortality is due to a break-down in infrastructure that increases communicable and non-communicable diseases, respiratory infections, maternal, neonatal, and nutritional diseases, respiratory infections and tuberculosis, enteric infections, and maternal and neonatal disorders, increased cardiovascular diseases, diabetes and kidney diseases, neoplasms, and digestive diseases, etc.

During a war, the civilian mortality rate increases by 0.0815%. Assuming the background mortality rate in the European Union of approximately 1%, we arrive at a total civilian mortality rate during a war in Europe of approximately 1.0815%. The COVID-19 vaccines are inferred to cause a greater mortality increase of 10.5% among the vaccinated population of Western Europe. That suggests that the COVID-19 vaccines had a devastating effect on the population of Europe. The inference from the all-cause mortality statistics is that the COVID-19 vaccines caused the mortality rate to increase in the vaccinated population to 1.105% which is more than what would be expected in the civilian population during a war.

According to the European Centre for Disease Prevention and Control, as of March 2023, approximately 330 million persons in the EU have received at least two doses of a COVID-19 vaccine.[558] Ordinarily, about 3.3 million of those people would die from all different causes each year. But extrapolating a death rate of 0.105% increase in the monthly all-cause mortality rate for every one percent of the persons vaccinated, we can expect that an additional 10.5%, or 346,500 persons will have died from the COVID-19 vaccine in 2022.

While correlation does not "necessarily" mean causation when the correlation across so many different countries only shows a rise in mortality, the inference of causation is robust. It certainly raises to the level of at least probable cause. Dr. John Campbell, Ph.D., opined that the correlation from the February 2023 study was so strong that he declared it a "slam dunk."[559]

Mathematician Igor Chudov conducted a separate study and analyzed the correlation between COVID-19 booster shots and the rise in all-cause mortality across approximately 29 countries (including the USA). He used the average weekly mortality rates of 2017-2019 to establish the baseline and compared it to the weekly mortality increase during weeks 10 to 35 in 2022. On

August 30, 2022, Chudov announced his findings.[560] He was shocked by what he found. He discovered an almost linear correlation between the rate of COVID-19 booster shots and a rise in national mortality rates. The P value for the correlation was 0.0002. A P value that is below 0.05 is considered statistically significant. A P value that is 0.0002 is considered to be an ironclad correlation that could not be by random coincidence.

Chudov was careful to say that he was merely reporting the correlation. Chudov stated that the proper interpretation "is that there is an EXTREMELY PROMINENT RELATIONSHIP between boosters and deaths in 2022." (emphasis in original). The correlation showed: "More boosters – more deaths!" Chudov concluded:

> Despite my stating clearly that I uncovered a *correlation*, not a *causation*, I personally believe that boosters ARE a cause of increased mortality. There are many reasons to believe this to be highly likely.[561] (italics and emphasis in original)

Igor Chudov conducted another analysis of UK data. This time it was limited to UK mortality data. He analyzed the unique data from the UK, which tracked the COVID-19 vaccinated population. The UK Government has data where it collects and reports weekly excess mortality by vaccination status.[562] To arrive at the excess mortality, the UK government used the average mortality rate between 2015 to 2019 as their base mortality rate.

The UK Government tracks the vaccination rates among quintiles that rank a population according to economic disparities. Igor Chudov downloaded and analyzed the May to September 2022 UK Government data. He found a direct correlation between an increase in the vaccination rate and an increase in the excess death rate.

The lowest rank of the five quintiles was the most economically deprived and was found to have the lowest vaccine rate of 79.40%. That lowest quintile was shown to have an excess death rate of 7.85%. There was a steady increase in the death rate as the vaccination rate increased with the economic status of the quintile. The highest excess death rate of 12.55% was found at the highest quintile, with a COVID-19 vaccine rate of 93%. When you look at the chart below, you can see a steady increase in the death rate as there is an increase in the vaccination rate.

Deprivation Level	Vaccination Rate %	Excess Mortality %
Most Deprived	79.4%	7.85%
More Deprived	84.5%	9.22%
Median	88.7%	11.36%
More Wealthy	91.1%	12.37%
Most Wealthy	93.0%	12.55%

As you can see from the above chart, there is a direct correlation between the COVID-19 vaccination rate and the mortality rate. More COVID-19 vaccines mean more deaths. Chudov analyzed those statistics and found that the R^2 was 0.9471. That means that the increase in the COVID-19 vaccination rate explains 95% of the increase in the death rate across the quintiles.

Chudov further calculated the P value for the statistics to be 0.0052. That means there is only a 0.5% chance that the increase in the death rate correlated to the increase in the vaccine rate was due to chance. Chudov plotted the data on a chart, illustrating the obvious correlation between increased COVID-19 vaccination and deaths. Chudov concluded that "this makes a very strong case that excess mortality in the UK in May-Sep 2022 is caused by Covid vaccines."[563]

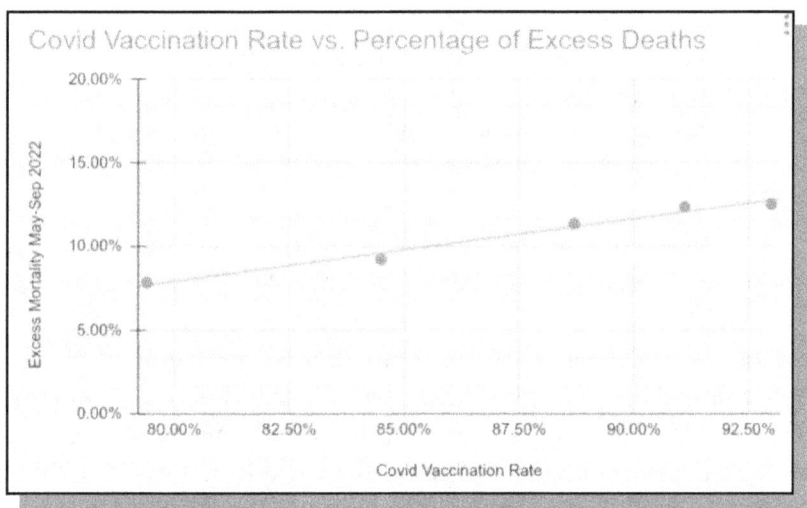

Chudov also uncovered evidence from another statistician showing a significant drop in the UK birthrate in 2022 compared to 2021. The statistician did some digging and found a correlation between the increase in the COVID-19 vaccination rate and a decline in the birth rate.[564] That correlation was based on the UK deprivation statistics. The study showed that the proportion of women giving birth in the two wealthier quintiles of the UK population, which had the higher COVID-19 vaccination rate, dropped in 2022. But the proportion of women giving birth in the two more deprived quintiles of the population, which had a lower vaccination rate, increased in 2022. That was notable because it is the reverse of the historical precedent between 2017 and 2020, where the two higher quintiles had a steadily growing proportion of mothers giving birth, and the two most deprived quintiles had a steadily reduced proportion of mothers giving. That suddenly flipped in 2022, directly correlating to the COVID-19 vaccination program and a reduced overall birth rate. Chudov suggested that the COVID-19 vaccines are acting as a depopulation scheme. Chudov commented:

> We have an interesting situation: Covid vaccines appear to cause a decline in birth rate, and at the same time, an increase in the death rate. A decline in births and a simultaneous increase in deaths is called depopulation. So, is Covid vaccine a depopulation vaccine?[565]

Up to this point, we have been comparing total all-cause mortality differences. But the devastating effect of the vaccines can be seen more clearly when looking at just the sliver of increase in excess deaths from all causes. For example, according to official government data from the Australian Organisation for Economic Co-Operation and Development (OECD), the increase in excess deaths became exponential upon the rollout of the COVID-19 vaccines in 2021. *The Expose* reports that "the Australian Government confirms the first 38 weeks of 2021 saw a shocking 1,452% increase in excess deaths following the rollout of the COVID-19 injections compared to the same period in 2020."[566] *The Expose* limited its analysis to the first 38 weeks of 2020, 2021, and 2022 because it only had official government statistics for excess death data available for the first 38 weeks of 2022.

When comparing the excess deaths during the first 38 weeks of 2022, when the vaccine rollout was in full swing, compared to the first 38 weeks of 2020, during the height of the alleged COVID-19 pandemic, *The Expose* discovered a whopping 5,162% increase in excess deaths in 2022 compared with 2020.

By 2022, the nation was hit by a devastating blow,

with a shocking 5,162% increase in excess deaths in the first 38 weeks of the year following the repeat rollout of the COVID-19 injections compared to the first 38 weeks of 2020, at the alleged height of the pandemic.[567]

If the vaccines were effective, you would expect just the opposite. You would expect that there would be more excess deaths during the height of the COVID-19 pandemic, with the number dropping into negative territory after the protective effect of the vaccines saving lives during 2021 and 2022. But in (the first 38 weeks of) 2021, after the COVID-19 vaccine rollout, there was a whopping 1,452% increase in excess deaths over (the first 38 weeks of) 2020 pandemic levels. And there was an explosion of 5,162% increased excess deaths in (the first 38 weeks of) 2022 over the excess death rate during (the first 38 weeks of) 2020, which was the height of the alleged COVID-19 pandemic. That can mean only one thing. The COVID-19 vaccines are killing people.

Denis Rancourt, Ph.D., is an accomplished interdisciplinary scientist and physicist and a former tenured Full Professor of Physics and lead scientist, originally at the University of Ottawa. Dr. Rancourt studied all-cause mortality for the years beginning in 2020. He concluded, "[t]here was no pandemic causing excess mortality."[568] He explained that the 2020 excess mortality was the result of a "multi-pronged state and iatrogenic attack against populations, and against societal support structures, which caused all the excess mortality, in every jurisdiction."[569] He attributed the rise in all-cause mortality starting in 2021 to the COVID-19 vaccines. He stated, "we quantified many instances in which a rapid rollout of a dose in the imposed vaccine schedule was synchronous with an otherwise unexpected peak in all-cause mortality." Dr. Rancourt determined that the vaccines killed 3.7 million people in India alone. He further determined:

In Western countries, we quantified the average all-ages rate of death to be 1 death for every 2000 injections, to increase exponentially with age (doubling every additional 5 years of age), and to be as large as 1 death for every 100 injections for those 80 years and older. We estimated that the vaccines had killed 13 million worldwide.[570]

Dr. Rancourt conducted a later study that was published on September 17, 2023.[571] The Data from that extensive research study involved 17 countries, which comprised 9.10% of the worldwide population and 10.3% of the worldwide COVID-19 injections. The study showed a significant rise in all-cause mortality that synchronized with the rollout of the COVID-19 vaccines. The researchers concluded that "[i]t is unlikely that the rise in all-cause mortality (ACM) coinciding with the rollout and sustained administration of COVID-19 vaccines in all 17 countries could be due to any cause other than the vaccines."[572] The study deduced that the 13.25 billion COVID-19 vaccine injections worldwide caused a statistically inferred increase of 17 million worldwide deaths from all causes as of September 2, 2023. The researchers stated: "This would correspond to a mass iatrogenic [caused by medical treatment] event that killed (0.213 ± 0.006) % of the world population (1 death per 470 living persons, in less than 3 years)."[573]

We have more than statistical inference of causation. There is medical proof that the COVID-19 vaccines are killing people. Renowned cardiologist Dr. Peter McCullough, Yale epidemiologist Dr. Harvey Risch, and former Senior Pandemic Advisor to the Secretary of Health and Human Services, Paul E. Alexander, Ph.D. along with other doctors and researchers, conducted a study to determine the causal link between the reported COIVID-19 vaccine deaths in VAERS and the COVID-19 vaccine. They reviewed 325 autopsy cases and one necropsy case of persons who died after receiving a COVID-19 vaccine. The doctors determined that "[a] total of 240 deaths (73.9%) were independently adjudicated as directly due to or significantly contributed to by COVID-19 vaccination."[574] The average time in which the persons died after vaccination was 14.3 days. The study proves causation; it attests that COVID-19 vaccines are killing people. A pre-print of the study was posted on The Lancet website on July 5, 2023, pending peer review.[575] But after a high volume of downloads, after only 24 hours, The Lancet removed the pre-print from its website. The coverup continues.

20 Prion Disease

Dr. Peter McCullough called the COVID-19 vaccines bioterrorism.[576] That was not hyperbole. Other highly respected doctors share that opinion. Dr. Barthelow Classen likens the COVID-19 vaccines to bioweapons. Dr. Barthelow Classen, M.D., has published a report revealing that the Pfizer-BioNTech COVID-19 vaccine uses an RNA sequence known to cause prion diseases such as Alzheimer's and amyotrophic lateral sclerosis (ALS).[577] Dr. Classen states that "[t]he current analysis indicates Pfizer's RNA based COVID-19 vaccine contains many of these RNA sequences that have been shown to have high affinity for TDP-43 or FUS and have the potential to induce chronic degenerative neurological diseases."[578] Dr. Classen reveals that the manifestation of the disease may take many years after the vaccination to develop in the vaccine recipient.

Other researchers have confirmed the findings of Dr. Classen. Jeff Childers reports a study revealing that COVID-19 vaccines have been shown to cause mad-cow disease.[579] That study "cited three previous studies from 2020 and 2021 finding a link between the mRNA jabs and prion diseases like Mad Cow."[580] The researchers identify the prion disease as a virulent kind of mad-cow disease, which Childers calls "Turbo Mad Cow."

Dr. Classen opines that the mRNA COVID-19 vaccines have the earmarks of bioweapons that are purposely designed to harm.

> Many have raised the warning that the current epidemic of COVID-19 is actually the result of a bioweapons attack released in part by individuals in the United States government. Such a theory is not far fetched given that the 2001 anthrax attack in the US originated at Fort Detrick, a US army bioweapon facility. Because the FBI's anthrax investigation was closed against the advice of the lead FBI agent in the case, there are likely conspirators still working in the US government. In such a scenario the primary focus of stopping a bioweapons attack must be to apprehend the conspirators or the attacks will never cease. Approving a vaccine, utilizing novel RNA technology without extensive testing is extremely dangerous. The vaccine could be a bioweapon and even more dangerous than the original infection.[581]

Dr. Stephanie Seneff, Ph.D., who is a senior research scientist at MIT Computer Science and Artificial Intelligence Laboratory, opines that "[g]iving young people COVID vaccines will likely cause an 'alarming increase in several major neurodegenerative diseases.'"[582] Dr. Seneff elaborated:

> [B]oth the mRNA vaccines and the DNA vector vaccines may be a pathway to crippling disease sometime in the future. Through the prion-like action of the spike protein, we will likely see an alarming increase in several major neurodegenerative diseases, including Parkinson's

disease, CKD, ALS and Alzheimer's, and these diseases will show up with increasing prevalence among younger and younger populations, in years to come.[583]

Dr. Seneff affirms the opinion of Dr. Classen that it takes years before the prion disease causes degeneration of the brain sufficient for a diagnosis of permanent brain damage.

Unfortunately, we won't know whether the vaccines caused this increase because there will usually be a long time separation between the vaccination event and the disease diagnosis.[584]

Dr. Seneff explains how the delay in the manifestation of brain damage works to the advantage of pharmaceutical companies. She said it is "very convenient for the vaccine manufacturers, who stand to make huge profits off of our misfortunes — both from the sale of the vaccines themselves and from the large medical cost of treating all these debilitating diseases."[585]

21 Myocarditis

Peter McCullough, M.D., and Dr. Jessica Rose, Ph.D., researched the sudden appearance of myocarditis in young people. Dr. McCullough is a highly-published world-renowned cardiologist, and Dr. Rose is a Canadian researcher with a Bachelor's Degree in Applied Mathematics and a Master's degree in Immunology from Memorial University of Newfoundland. She also holds a Ph.D. in Computational Biology from Bar Ilan University and two Post Doctoral degrees: one in Molecular Biology from the Hebrew University of Jerusalem and one in Biochemistry from the Technion Institute of Technology. Drs. McCullough and Rose determined that the COVID-19 vaccines caused myocarditis. While their study focused on young people, their conclusions also apply to the population as a whole. The October 1, 2021, McCullough & Rose report revealed the following startling facts.

> Within 8 weeks of the public offering of COVID-19 products to the 12-15-year-old age group, **we found 19 times the expected number of myocarditis cases in the vaccination volunteers over background myocarditis rates for this age group.**[586]

The VAERS system only reports about 1% of the actual adverse events.[587] VAERS is a reporting system that shows correlation. Further analysis is required to prove causation. Drs. McCullough and Rose did that further analysis and opined that the VAERS data indicates a cause and effect between the vaccinations and teenage myocarditis. Their report indicates: "It is noteworthy that 'Vaccine-induced myocarditis' was in fact used as the descriptor by medical professionals as the reason for the myocarditis in the VAERS database."[588] Their report labeled the myocarditis caused by the vaccines "COVID-19-Injection-Related Myocarditis (CIRM);" the report concluded:

> Thus, due to both the problems of under-reporting and the known lag in report processing, this analysis reveals a strong signal from the VAERS data that the risk of suffering CIRM [COVID-19-Injection-Related Myocarditis] – especially males is unacceptably high. Again, children are not a high-risk group for COVID-19 respiratory illness, and yet they are the high-risk group for CIRM.[589]

The McCullough & Rose report caused quite a stir in the medical community. After the preliminary draft of their report was peer-reviewed and approved for publication, it was posted by the publisher on its NIH website. Shortly thereafter, the publisher, Elsevier, without giving a reason, suddenly withdrew the publication. Dr. McCullough is reportedly pursuing legal action against Elsevier for its unlawful actions.

In its guidance dated October 4, 2022, the U.S. CDC recommended COVID-19 vaccines for all persons over six months old.[590] That is a bizarre recommendation when viewed in light of a January 25, 2022, study published in the Journal of the American Medical Association (JAMA).[591] That study was conducted by the FDA and CDC using the VAERS data. The study confirmed the findings of Drs. Rose and McCullough. The joint CDC/FDA study showed that the incidence of autoimmune heart disease (myocarditis) among those vaccinated against COVID-19 was 13,200% higher than among the unvaccinated.[592]

On October 7, 2022, Dr. Ladpapo, M.D., Ph.D., in his capacity as Florida Surgeon General, contradicted the U.S. CDC and announced that the risks of COVID-19 vaccines outweigh the benefits for 18 to 39-year-old males. He came to that conclusion based on a scientific study of the mortality risk of the COVID-19 vaccines. That study "found there is an 84% increase in the relative incidence of cardiac-related death among males 18-39 years old within 28 days following mRNA vaccination."[593]

Dr. Toby Rogers points out that "Pfizer's clinical trial in kids was intentionally undersized to hide harms. This is a well-known trick of the pharmaceutical industry. The FDA even called them out on it earlier this summer and asked Pfizer to expand the trial, and Pfizer just ignored them because they can."[594] Dr. Rogers explains the trick: "To put it simply, if the rate of particular adverse outcome in kids as a result of this shot is 1 in 5,000 and the trial only enrolls 1,518 in the treatment group then one is unlikely to spot this particular harm in the clinical trial. Voilà "Safe & Effective (TM)".[595]

Another trick vaccine makers use is to have a brief period to monitor test participants for adverse events. Pfizer only followed cohort 1 for two months and cohort 2 for 17 days for adverse events. But many adverse events take much longer to show up. Dr. Rogers observed: "As the old saying goes, 'you can have it quick or you can have it done right, but you cannot have both.' Pfizer chose quick."[596]

Such short observation periods acts to conceal the harm done to the heart. Dr. Rogers explains that "the harms of myocarditis from these shots will likely unfold over the course of years." The Pfizer study seemed designed to conceal the danger of myocarditis. For example, "they estimate 'excess' (read: caused by the shot) myocarditis using data from the private 'Optum health claim database' instead of the public VAERS system."[597] That is odd indeed. Why use a private database and eschew using the government-administered VAERS database? There was something in the VAERS system that Pfizer and the FDA did not want known.

Drs. Peter McCullough and Jessical Rose found out why the FDA and Pfizer steered clear of the VAERS database. Drs. McCullough and Rose revealed how the VAERS database showed a substantial cause and effect relationship between the COVID-19 vaccines and myocarditis.[598]

That information reported by McCullough and Rose was in the VAERS database and was known to the FDA when it authorized the use of the unsafe and ineffective COVID-19 vaccines for children 5 through 11 years of age. That seems to be why the FDA and Pfizer steered clear of the VAERS data and instead used the private data from Optum Health.

Another fact that the McCullough & Rose report revealed was that the incidence of myocarditis among teenagers is much worse than even the raw statistics obtained from the Vaccine Adverse Events Reporting Service (VAERS) indicate. The report states:

> Because of the spontaneous reporting of events to VAERS, we can assume that the cases reported thus far are not rare, but rather, just the tip of the iceberg. Again, under-reporting is a known and serious disadvantage of the VAERS system.[599]

Myocarditis can cause irreversible heart damage. Once the heart muscle is damaged, it cannot be repaired by the body. It is a devastating condition. Dr. Rogers explains that "over the course of several years many of those children will die. Dr. Anthony Hinton ('Consultant Surgeon with 30 years experience in the NHS') points out that myocarditis has a 20% fatality rate after 2 years and a 50% fatality rate after 5 years."[600] One person observed: "You can't have 'mild myocarditis' — in the same way you can't be 'a little bit pregnant.'"[601] Dr. Aaron Kheriaty, M.D., stated that "there is no such thing as "mild" myocarditis. Inflammation of the heart is always medically serious. Anyone attempting to minimize it is not giving medical information but selling something."[602] The Associated Press (AP) tried to debunk the seriousness of vaccine induced myocaditis and contacted Dr. Kheriaty. He told the AP that "'mild myocarditis' is like saying 'mild heart attack [myocardits is] always medically serious, even on the mild end of the spectrum."[603]

On November 16, 2021, this author received the fact check inquiry from the Associated Press (AP). I wrote an article about vaccine-induced myocarditis. The article was titled: *The FDA and Pfizer Concealed Evidence That COVID-19 Vaccines Will Cause Myocarditis in Children.*[604] In that article, I explained how severe myocarditis could be. The AP claimed that my contention that myocarditis is a dangerous heart condition was "not correct." The AP claimed that it had "gotten confirmation from Dr. Eric Adler and Dr. Leslie Cooper, professors of medicine and practicing cardiologists, that most myocarditis cases are indeed mild or asymptomatic."

The AP experts' opinion raises an issue. How can a doctor know to look for myocarditis if it is asymptomatic? It would seem that the only time that asymptomatic myocarditis would be detected is after the person suddenly and unexpectedly dies or is hospitalized. Otherwise, if the patient is asymptomatic, there is no complaint for the doctor to examine the patient for myocarditis. It seems that asymptomatic myocarditis is a very serious and perilous condition indeed. That is why we have an epidemic of young people with asymptomatic myocarditis who are dying suddenly.

I replied in an email to the inquiry by asking: "Have you spoken with Dr. Anthony Hinton? He is a surgeon with 30 years' of experience. He opines that "myocarditis has a 20% fatality rate after 2 years and a 50% fatality rate after 5 years?" I also emailed the AP the following additional information.

> Myocarditis is caused by vaccine induced blood clotting. The mechanism for the COVID-19 vaccine causing myocarditis and other organ damage is blood clotting caused by the spike protein generated by the cells coded with the mRNA from the COVID-19 vaccine. Dr. Charles Hoffe, M.D., explains in straightforward terms how the mRNA COVID vaccines cause the body to create the spike proteins that in turn cause widespread microscopic blood clotting.
>
> Dr. Hoffe reveals that when someone is given an mRNA vaccine, "it is literally collected by your lymphatic system and fed into your circulation. So these little packages of messenger RNA — and by the way, in a single dose of a Moderna vaccine, there are 40 trillion mRNA molecules that are injected into your arm ... they go into your blood stream in these little packages that are designed to be absorbed into your cells."[605]
>
> Dr. Hoffe reveals that the absorption of the mRNA is most notable in the capillary networks, which are the tiniest blood vessels in the body. Because they are so small, the blood slows down while flowing through the capillaries. The little packages of mRNA from the vaccine are absorbed into the cells around the blood vessels (the vascular

endothelium). There, the mRNA packages are absorbed, and the body goes to work reading the mRNA code. The blood vessel cells (the endothelium) begin manufacturing trillions and trillions of COVID spike proteins. There are 40 trillion mRNA packets per vaccine dose; each of those gene packets can produce many, many spike proteins.

The theory behind the mRNA COVID-19 vaccines is that your body will recognize the spike protein created by your cells as a foreign protein and make antibodies against it. Theoretically, you are then protected against COVID-19. But Dr. Hoffe explains the problem with how the mRNA acts in the body. The spike proteins are jutting from the cell walls in the very tiny capillaries in the body and block the blood flow.

> In a virus — in a coronavirus — that spike protein becomes part of the viral capsule — like the cell wall around the virus called the viral capsule. But it's not in a virus — it's in your cells. So therefore it becomes part of the cell wall of your vascular endothelium — which means that these cells that line your blood vessels, which are supposed to be smooth so that your blood flows smoothly, now have these little spiky bits sticking out. So it is absolutely inevitable that blood clots will form — because your blood platelets circulate around in your blood vessels — and

> the purpose of blood platelets is to detect a damaged vessel and block that vessel to stop bleeding. So when the platelet comes through the capillary, it suddenly hits all these COVID spikes that are jutting into the inside of the vessel — it is absolutely inevitable that a blood clot will form to block that vessel. That's how platelets work.

Dr. Hoffe is presently treating patients suffering from COVID-19 vaccine injuries. He reveals the health dangers of mRNA vaccines.

> So the most alarming thing about this is that there are some parts of your body — like your heart and your brain, and your spinal cord and your lungs, which cannot regenerate — when those tissues are damaged by blocked vessels, they are permanently damaged. So I now have 6 people in my medical practice who have reduced effect tolerance, which means they get out of breath much more easily than they used to....literally what's happened to them is they have plugged up thousands of tiny capillaries in their lungs — and the terrifying thing about this is....that once you block off a significant number of blood vessels in your lungs, your heart is now pumping against a much greater resistance to

trying and get the blood through your lungs — a condition called pulmonary artery hypertension. A condition of high blood pressure in your lungs because the blood can't get through because so many of the vessels are blocked. People with pulmonary artery hypertension usually die of right sided heart failure within three years.

So the huge concern about this mechanism of injury is that these shots are causing permanent damage — and the worst is yet to come. Some tissues in your body like intestine and liver and kidneys that can regenerate to quite a good degree — but brain and spinal cord and heart muscle and lungs do not. When they are damaged, it's permanent — like all these young people who are now getting myocarditis from these shots — they have permanently damaged hearts — it doesn't matter how mild it is, they will not be able to do what they used to be able to do....but with each successive shot, the damage will add and add and add. It's going to be cumulative because you are getting progressively more damaged capillaries.

I also pointed the AP to the following information from the

Myocarditis Foundation:

> A rare form of heart disease, myocarditis develops when the heart muscle becomes inflamed and enlarged, thus weakening the heart. Naturally, the risk of sudden death for people with myocarditis is a reason for concern.[606]

I further supplied the AP with a link to a published article and emiled the AP the following quote from the article:

> Immediate complications of myocarditis include ventricular dysrhythmias, left ventricular aneurysm, CHF, and dilated cardiomyopathy. The mortality rate is up to 20% at 1 year and 50% at 5 years. Despite optimal medical management, overall mortality has not changed in the last 30 years.[607]

The AP contacted Michael Kang, the author of the article I had sent them; and Kang claimed that I had misrepresented the figures in the article. I did not misrepresent anything. I simply quoted the passage from Michael Kang's article. The AP had orignally emailed this author and asked me for further evidence supporting my article about myocarditis; and I gave it to them. Quoting Kang's own words does not constitute misrepresentation. Kang stated that his article was written "as a general review of viral myocarditis and does not pertain to vaccine induced myocarditis."[608] The AP reported:

> With regards to the myocarditis death rate, Kang said his article was referencing the most severe forms of myocarditis. Those numbers pertain to smaller, older studies, in which patients had extreme forms of the disease, "not what we are seeing with the covid19 vaccine," Kang said in an email.[609]

How can Kang say that somehow the conclusion in his article, which is based on "overall mortality" statistics that he said in the article have "not changed in the last 30 years" do not apply to myocarditis induced by the COVID-19 vaccines? What study has he done to distinguish virus-induced myocarditis (the subject of his article) from COVID-19 vaccine-induced myocarditis? And when you read his article in context, his statistics were clearly about the "overall mortality" for myocarditis and not the most severe forms of myocarditis, as Kang now claims. Indeed, he describes his statistics as "overall mortality" rates for myocarditis.

In the context of the quote about mortality, Kang begins discussing acute myocarditis, which he describes as the "first two weeks," which he distinguishes from chronic myocarditis, which he describes as "lasting more than 2 weeks." Acute in the context of the article means "immediate," it does not mean severe. His article addresses three phases of myocarditis "acute, subacute, or chronic." Subacute is between acute and chronic, and is a temporal measure.

Interestingly, Kang's article undermines one of the premises of the AP fact-check, that myocarditis does not result in permanent heart damage. Kang states in his article:

> Myocarditis begins with the direct invasion of an infectious agent and its subsequent replication within or around the myocardium causing myonecrosis. **This leads to the destruction of the cardiac tissue** from the infiltration and replication of the infectious agent.[610] (endnotes omitted)

Once heart tissue is destroyed, it cannot regenerate. The AP fact check conflated the issue by framing it as whether someone can recover from myocarditis. Certainly someone can recover from myocarditis. Myocarditis is inflammation of the heart. That inflammation often causes damage to the heart tissue. The issue is

275

not whether one can recover from myocarditis but whether when the heart is damaged by myocarditis, can the body repair that damage. The answer to that question is no. Other organs in the body can repair themselves; the heart and brain cannot repair themselves. Once the heart tissue is damaged, that damage is permanent.

The AP fact check cites Dr. Eric Adler, who states, "[t]hough dead heart tissue is indeed felt to be non-recoverable there are lots of examples of damaged hearts that recover to normal function over time or with medical therapy."[611] A heart that is damaged is quite simply not the same as it was before the damage. Just because some people can make it by and exist with a damaged heart does not mean it is a minor life inconvenience. Especially when those who do not recover sometimes die. And indeed, many do not get treatment because the onset of the damage kills them before they can receive medical care; they just die suddenly. The AP article downplays the dangers of myocarditis, seemingly to offset the concern of getting myocarditis from the COVID-19 vaccine. The argument of the AP seems to be that myocarditis is not all that bad, so don't worry if the COVID-19 vaccine causes it. That approach is reckless.

When Kang discussed severe forms of myocarditis, he said that "[p]atients with severe disease have a poor prognosis without a transplant."[612] That is dire indeed! Contrast that with what Kang said about mild myocarditis: "Patients with mild myocarditis usually have a good outcome."[613] And what does he think is a good outcome? He states, "[t]he long-term prognosis was usually good, with a 3 to 5-year survival ranging from 56 to 83%, respectively." He meant that the survival rate was 83% after 3 years dropping to 56% after 5 years.

Thus, according to Kang, mild myocarditis outcome is "usually good" because 83% survive for 3 years and 56% survive after 5 years. That is only just a little bit better than the "overall mortality" of "50% at 5 years."

It seems that Kang's fancy dancing cannot get him out from underneath the statistics for "overall mortality" for myocarditis that is "20% at 1 year and 50% at 5 years." He pointed out that "[d]espite optimal medical management, overall mortality has not changed in the last 30 years." But suddenly, when he is called on the carpet, Kang maintains that those rock-solid numbers with a 30-year pedigree have no applicability to COVID-19 vaccine-induced myocarditis.

This dangerous effect of the COVID-19 vaccines is well known to the vaccine makers and the FDA. The AP fact-check article did not mention the information I provided from Dr. Hoffe, Dr. Hinton, or the Myocarditis Foundation. Instead, the AP focused on Michael Kang. It was as though once the AP found someone who would cave in and agree with their premise, no further fact-checking was necessary. The AP gave the impression that my article was based solely on the statistics in Kang's article. But that is not the case and is not what I said. I cited Kang, along with Dr. Hoffe and Dr. Hinton. But the AP steered clear of those other doctors.

In a December 6, 2021 interview with Bret Weinstein, world-renowned cardiologist Dr. Peter Mcullough revealed that the usual rate of myocarditis in a given year in the United States is 640 cases. In 2021, VAERS reported 11,000 cases of myocarditis associated with the COVID-19 vaccines. That represents a 17-fold increase in myocarditis due to the COVID-19 vaccines. He further revealed that approximately 13% of myocarditis cases involve permanent damage to the heart. He also stated that the CDC and FDA were reprehensibly reckless when they falsely claimed that myocarditis caused by the COVID-19 vaccine was rare and mild.

> I was on national TV in June when the FDA and CDC reviewed myocarditis. And they said two

things that I think were completely incorrect from a public health perspective. I'm trained in public health. At this point time my career I have over 650 publications in the National Library of Medicine and Pubmed. I'm an editor of a major cardiology journal, former editor of another journal, I'm the principal editor of my own textbook. I am in academic medicine right now and anybody you're talking to on COVID-19, I imagine I'm probably at the top of the academic pile, right now, of scholarship.

I can tell you those two statements by our public health officials who are junior to me in their scholarship and accomplishments, both of those statements I think are reprehensible and reckless. They said that myocarditis is mild. And they said it was rare. Well it wasn't mild then because 90% of the kids are in the hospital. By regulatory standards, anything that causes hospitalization, as you know, is a serious adverse event. It's never classified as mild, never!

And then they said it was rare because they took 200 cases and they divided by the universe and people who got the vaccine. Well, we can't do that in safety because we didn't assess everybody from myocarditis, so we don't know if it's rare. And when we see a signal like this in safety pharmacovigilance we use the term, tip of the iceberg. So I was on national TV saying, listen it's not mild because the kids are being hospitalized, and two, it's not rare, it's the tip of the iceberg. And boy was I right. Being at now 11,000 cases in VAERS. And you're right, it's underreported.

And interestingly, it's who reports it. There's a paper that's published in the American College of Pediatrics that asked the question in 2016 who reports to VAERS. And you know who reports to VAERS? The answer was about about 14% of the time it's actually the patient or the patient's family that reports to VAERS. 86% of the time it's another entity that actually really was concerned that the product, in this case, the vaccine, caused the problems. That means doctors, nurses, people [who] administered the vaccine, and pharmaceutical companies who receive this and they're concerned about their products. So I have to tell you this VAERS data is real. And I've heard people say that "oh anybody can report things to VAERS." I filled out the various sheets, But I'll tell you every single page says "warning," This falsification is punishable by imprisonment or federal fines. I tell you right now the VAERS system 11,000 cases. That's serious, and the number almost certainly is going to be much larger.[614]

Vaccine-induced myocarditis is widespread, affecting athletes' ability to continue competing in their sport. For example, Free West Media reported on April 2, 2022, that 15 tennis players dropped out of the Miami Open due to unexplained illnesses.[615] Fans and the news media were baffled and unable to explain the weird turn of events. Two favorites to win the tournament, Paula Badosa and Jannik Sinner, dropped out after becoming "unwell." Badosa was soon to be ranked third in the world.

Jannik Sinner could only compete for 22 minutes before he bent over on the court and could not continue. His opponent, Francisco Cerundolo described it as very strange. Free West Media offered no analysis about what caused the sudden wave of resignations from the tournament from physical infirmities.

None of the withdrawals or retirements have been attributed by the media to vaccine injury. Indeed the mainstream media is not discussing the reasons for the withdrawals and retirements from the tournament.[616] Some of the stated injuries suggest that some of the withdrawals and retirements were not from the vaccine. Some of the reasons given were "foot injury," "thigh injury," and "low back injury." Oddly there were three withdrawals or retirements for "abdominal injuries," which could mean anything from a muscle pull to intestinal discomfort. But some reasons for the withdrawals and retirements from the tournament raise suspicion that they were caused by vaccine injury. For example, M. Vondrousova withdrew due to a "viral illness," C. Tauson retired due to "heat illness," V. Azarenka retired due to "personal reasons."

One of the common side effects of the COVID-19 mRNA vaccines is blood clotting, which often causes muscle and joint pain, which could be masked by being reported as an "injury" to a muscle or joint.

J.D. Rucker, writing for The Liberty Daily, was not so reticent to comment on the cause of the Miami Open carnage. J.D. Rucker opined:

> Nobody is pointing to the obvious. All of the players must be "fully vaccinated" [against COVID-19] in order to compete. Just as we've noted for several months, most major sports have been hit with "inexplicable" medical conditions popping up in young and otherwise healthy athletes, including our report that three cyclists fell in March alone.[617]
>
> Folks, this is the [COVID-19] jab. There is no

other viable possibility, especially when we consider how even the CDC and other agencies have acknowledge the Covid "vaccines" cause increases in heart problems for young people, including myocarditis, pericarditis, and heart attacks.

There has never been as much gaslighting and propaganda geared towards covering up the truth than with these [COVID-19] injections. Leaders across the country and around the world have so much wrapped into the vaccines, one has to wonder who's pulling the strings. Some of it is personal; any politician who comes out with the truth about the jabs will be pushed out of office faster than Will Smith's exit from Hollywood's elite club. The same is true for journalists. Corporate media is just as invested and possibly even more complicit in spreading the lies.

But it may be worse than that. Like so many things we've witnessed over the last three years, there appears to be a coordinated effort to suppress the truth. Pandemic Panic Theater is still in action despite the odd February push by Democrats to lift most face mask and vaccine mandates. There are already talks of 5th and 6th jabs even as the 4th jab gets rolled out in the United States.

Is this all part of The Great Reset agenda? Is it all about control? Depopulation? The answer to all three questions is very likely, "Yes."

These [COVID-19] injections are dangerous. Athletes across the globe are falling. Average people are experiencing horrible adverse reactions.

Tens, perhaps hundreds of thousands of people are dying from them. It could even be millions; the data is so obscured. All the while, politicians and corporate media are pretending it all away is if there's nothing to see here.[618]

Retsef Levi, Ph.D., is the J. Spencer Standish (1945) Professor at the MIT Sloan School of Management. He is a specialist in operations research, which concerns safety and quality in the manufacture of biological drugs and health policy. After analyzing the death and destruction caused by the COVID-19 vaccines, most notably the significant spike in myocarditis among the young, Dr. Levi issued a formal statement calling for the cessation of all such vaccines:

> I'm filming this video to share my strong conviction that at this point in time all covid mRNA vaccination programs should stop immediately. They should stop because they completely failed to fulfill any of their advertised promise regarding efficacy. And more importantly, they should stop because of the mounting and undisputable evidence that they caused unprecedented level of harm, including the death of young people and children.[619]

22 Killing Children to Save Them

The FDA's 242-page manual titled *Communicating Risks and Benefits: An Evidence-Based User's Guide* explains that the "number needed to treat" (NNT) is one of the three most important statistics for describing the risk and benefits of any drug or vaccine.[620] Toby Rogers, Ph.D., explains that the CDC and the FDA violated their own standards and the fundamental norms of science by not revealing the NNT when reviewing the Emergency Use Authorizations (EUA) and Biologics License Application from Pfizer-BioNTech when reviewing its COVID-19 vaccine for use in children ages 5 to 11.

Dr. Rogers explains that the pharmaceutical industry hates talking about NNT. They hate talking about NNT even more when it comes to COVID-19 vaccines because the NNT is so high that the COVID-19 vaccines could not pass any honest risk-benefit analysis.[621]

The NNT can be reported for any number of variables, such as deaths, ICU admissions, hospitalizations, etc. Taking death as an example, the death NNT for 5 to 11 year-olds from COVID-19 would tell the researchers and the public how many children need to be vaccinated to prevent a single death from COVID-19.

The lower the risk from the disease, the higher the NNT. Children ages 5 to 11 are at extremely low risk of hospitalization, ICU admission, or death from COVID-19. Indeed, there were no hospitalizations, ICU admissions, or deaths in either the vaccine group or the control group in the Pfizer-BioNTech trials involving 5 to 11 year-olds. Dr. Rogers explains:

> [The NNT] is calculated by dividing 1 by the Absolute Risk Reduction. But there was no risk reduction in hospitalizations, ICU admissions, nor death for 5 to 11 year olds. So if one remembers grade school math, 1/0 is "undefined" since one cannot divide by zero.
>
> This means one could vaccinate every child age 5 to 11 in the U.S. and not prevent a single hospitalization, ICU admission, or death from coronavirus — according to Pfizer's own clinical trial data as submitted to the FDA.
>
> It appears Pfizer was not even trying to conduct a responsible clinical trial of its mRNA shot in kids ages 5 to 11. Pfizer submitted an EUA application to the FDA showing no health benefit in children ages 5 to 11 and the FDA's Vaccines and Related Biologics Products Advisory Committee approved it anyway, 17 – 0 with 1 abstention.[622]

Dr. Rogers assumed a very generous 80% efficacy in preventing hospitalizations and deaths of 5 to 11-year-olds. He extrapolated that efficacy rate from the FDA claim that Pfizer-BioNTech has an 80% efficacy rate for COVID-associated hospitalizations for ages 20+ years old. The FDA used that 80% figure to estimate the efficacy rate for the Pfizer-BioNTech COVID-19 vaccine for 5 to 11-year-olds. Using the FDA's very optimistic benefit of the Pfizer-BioNTech COVID-19 vaccine, Dr.

Rogers calculated the death NNT for children 5 to 11 years old.

Dr. Rogers used the optimistically reported efficacy of 80% from the FDA and applied that figure to the reported fatalities for COVID-19 for 5 to 11-year-olds and calculated the death NNT for the Pfizer-BioNTech COVID-19 vaccine was 630,775. That means that the vaccine must be given to 630,775 children to save one child.

But that astronomical death NNT does not tell the whole story. We must compare that death NNT to the death risk from the vaccine. Dr. Rogers used the nearest age group vaccine risk data (12 to 15-year-olds) available and applied that data to the 5 to 11-year-olds. This is known as immuno-bridging of data. The VAERS data under-reports adverse events by a factor of 100. But Dr. Rogers multiplied the reported death numbers by a more conservative 41 times. By doing that, he determined that there were 5,248 deaths in the 12-15-year-old age group from the COVID-19 vaccines. Dr. Rogers compared the death rate to the death NNT and concluded:

> Simply put, the Biden administration plan would kill 5,248 children via Pfizer mRNA shots in order to save 45 children from dying of coronavirus.
>
> **For every one child saved by the shot, another 117 would be killed by the shot.**
>
> The Pfizer mRNA shot fails any honest risk-benefit analysis in children ages 5 to 11.

***

The Biden Administration, the FDA, and the CDC claim they "follow the science" and yet they violate their own standards and scientific norms in order to exaggerate the benefits and hide the harms from vaccines.

The FDA refused to calculate an [NNT], not because it forgot, but because agency officials knew the number and corresponding side effects are so high it would destroy the case for mRNA vaccines in children this age.[623] (emphasis added)

23 Sudden Adult Death Syndrome

The ADE and myocarditis suffered by vaccine recipients is causing them to unexpctedly die in large numbers. The sudden deaths of young people in the prime of health cannot be ignored. Edward Dowd, in his book, "Cause Unknown," *The Epidemic of Sudden Deaths in 2021 and 2022*, reveals that in 2006, a systematic review was done of sudden cardiac death by young athletes over a period of 38 years.[624] Experts at the Division of Pediatric Cardiology at the University Hospital of Lausanne, Switzerland, looked at the data on deaths between 1966 and 2004. They found that there were 1,101 total cases of sudden cardiac deaths over that period. That amounts to an average rate of 29 sudden cardiac deaths per year.

Fast forward to 2021 and 2022, and we find that the rate of cardiac deaths among young athletes exceeds 29 deaths per "month." Indeed, Dowd reveals that not a single month during 2021 and 2022 had fewer than 29 cardiac deaths among young athletes. For example, in December 2021, there were 90 deaths, and about the same number the next month.[625]

The prevalence of those deaths is forcing the hand of the media to report on them. But the mass media is trying to conceal the cause of the sudden deaths of thousands of young people by labeling the deaths sudden adult death syndrome (SADS). It is sometimes also called sudden arrhythmic death syndrome (SADS). The medical establishment and the media engage in all sorts of conjecture, including blaming the sudden premature deaths on a genetic condition.[626] But they do not ever mention the elephant in the room, the COVID-19 vaccines, as a suspected cause for the deaths. Ethan Huff, writing for Natural News, explains:

> In an attempt to explain away the rash of deaths occurring in otherwise healthy-seeming adults who got "vaccinated" for the Wuhan coronavirus (COVID-19), the medical establishment has coined a new term called "Sudden Adult Death Syndrome," or SADS, that it is pretending appeared out of nowhere with no explanation.[627]
>
> Much like Sudden Infant Death Syndrome (SIDS), which was also made up out of thin air to explain away infant deaths caused by vaccines, SADS is being called a "mystery" condition that could strike anyone at any time for no apparent reason.[628]

It is quite strange that the apparent culprits, the COVID-19 vaccines, are not even mentioned in the major media. They report the sudden premature deaths and essentially leave the readers to guess why young people are keeling over dead in the prime of their lives. Ethan Huff explains the obvious:

> They will never admit to it, but the sudden rise in SADS directly coincides with the unleashing of Operation Warp Speed, which has turned hundreds of millions of Americans into deadly spike protein factories. These spike proteins are ripping apart their cardiovascular systems and leaving them prone to early death.[629]

24 How the Vaccine Makers Scammed the Public

The 94.1% efficacy result for the Moderna COVID-19 mRNA vaccine reported by the FDA is misleading because they are not telling you that it is a relative risk reduction and not an absolute (total) risk reduction.[630] The vaccine manufacturers used misleading statistics to report the effectiveness of their vaccines. The vaccine manufacturers and often persons running studies, including the study of 620,000 veterans discussed earlier in this book, are reporting the relative efficacy of the COVID-19 vaccines.

In the Moderna study, the subsequent COVID-19 infection rate for the vaccinated group was 0.079%. The COVID-19 infection rate for the placebo group was 1.33%. That means that the rate of those who were infected by COVID-19 after receiving the vaccine was reduced by 1.25% as compared to those who were infected by COVID-19 after receiving a placebo (1.33% − 0.079% = 1.25%). Thus, the vaccine has an absolute efficacy of 1.25%. One can expect that there will be a reduction of 1.25% in COVID-19 infections in the population after being vaccinated. Out of a group of 10,000 people who are vaccinated with the Moderna mRNA COVID-19 vaccine, there will be approximately 125 fewer illnesses from COVID-19.

But that is not how Moderna reported the results. Instead of a 1.25% efficacy rate, which is the absolute (total) efficacy rate, the FDA review indicates that Moderna reported a 94.1% efficacy rate, which is a relative efficacy rate.[631] The relative efficacy rate is misleading because it gives the false impression that out of 10,000 people, 9,410 people would be protected from getting COVID-19. How did Moderna come up with the 94.1% figure? They divided the rate of subsequent COVID-19 infection in the vaccinated group (0.079%) by the rate of subsequent COVID-19 infection in the placebo group (1.33%) and then subtracted that difference (0.059) from one (1) to arrive at (0.941) to arrive at 94.1%. After rounding, the FDA reported the interim effectiveness for the Moderna mRNA COVID-19 vaccine of 94.1%. But that is not the absolute (total) efficacy, which is what people want to know. That 94.1% figure is a relative risk reduction, which is different from a absolute (total) risk reduction.

The false impression given by that figure is that the vaccine will effectively protect 9,410 out of 10,000 people from COVID-19. In reality, 9,867 are at no risk of getting COVID-19 (10,000 − 133 = 9,867). That means that out of every 10,000 people vaccinated with the COVID-19 vaccine, it will only prevent 125 people from becoming ill from COVID-19 (133 - 8 = 125). According to the study, a total of only 133 people out of every 10,000 are at risk to get COVID-19, and the vaccine will protect 125 of those 133 people. When the relative efficacy rate of 94.1% is reported, most people do not understand that it ignores the 9,867 people out of 10,000 who are at no risk of getting COVID-19 and do not need to be vaccinated. Thus, the true efficacy rate is the absolute efficacy rate. The absolute efficacy rate takes into account the entire population of people. The absolute (total) efficacy rate for the vaccine is only 1.25 % (125 people out of 10,000). That is the efficacy rate the public should have been informed about, and not 94.1 %, which gives the false impression that the vaccine will protect 9,410 people out of 10,000.

Dr. Ron Brown of the University of Waterloo explains that Moderna's and Pfizer-BioNTech's reporting of their vaccine's relative efficacy rate (a.k.a. risk reduction) is misleading to the public.[632] Researchers often use relative risk reduction, but it should not be announced to the public as the vaccine's efficacy because it always gives an elevated sense of the vaccine's efficacy.[633] The public was thus given an artificially inflated impression of effectiveness of the COVID-19 vaccinesis.[634] Dr. Brown stated that absolute risk reduction should be given to clinicians and the public. Indeed, in a draft advisory, the FDA stated that relative risk reduction should never be given to the public without also mentioning the absolute risk reduction.[635] The FDA explained, "that research suggests that consumers do not understand relative frequencies." The FDA explained that "[c]onsumers may also find the efficacy or risk probability described as a relative frequency harder to comprehend and more favorable as compared to the absolute frequency."[636] The concern of the FDA is that the consumer will view the benefit from a vaccine much greater than it is in reality if they are only informed of the relative efficacy rates. The FDA recommended that the public always be given the absolute efficacy rate.

Dr. Brown states that "selective reporting of vaccine efficacy measures can cause a type of outcome reporting bias that misrepresents health information disseminated to the public."[637] Dr. Brown presents an example in an article he prepared to show how misleading relative risk reduction can be. Dr. Brown explains how a risk reduction of only 1% can be sold to the public as a risk reduction of 50%:

> [The figure below] shows an example of a vaccine clinical trial for an infectious disease. The vaccine and placebo groups in Figure 1 each have 100 randomly assigned individuals with no history of infection, and an event is defined as the incidence of infection among all individuals during the

course of the trial. The percentage of events in the vaccine group is the experimental event rate (EER) or the risk of infection in the vaccine group (1/100 = 1%), and the percentage of events in the placebo group is the control event rate (CER) or the risk of infection in the placebo group (2/100 = 2%). Absolute risk reduction (ARR) is the disease risk difference between the placebo and vaccine groups, i.e., the CER minus the EER (2% - 1% = 1%). The ARR is also known as the vaccine disease preventable incidence (VDPI). Relative risk reduction (RRR) or vaccine efficacy (VE) is the reduced risk from vaccination, the ARR or VDPI, relative to or divided by the risk in unvaccinated individuals, the CER (1%/2% = 50%)

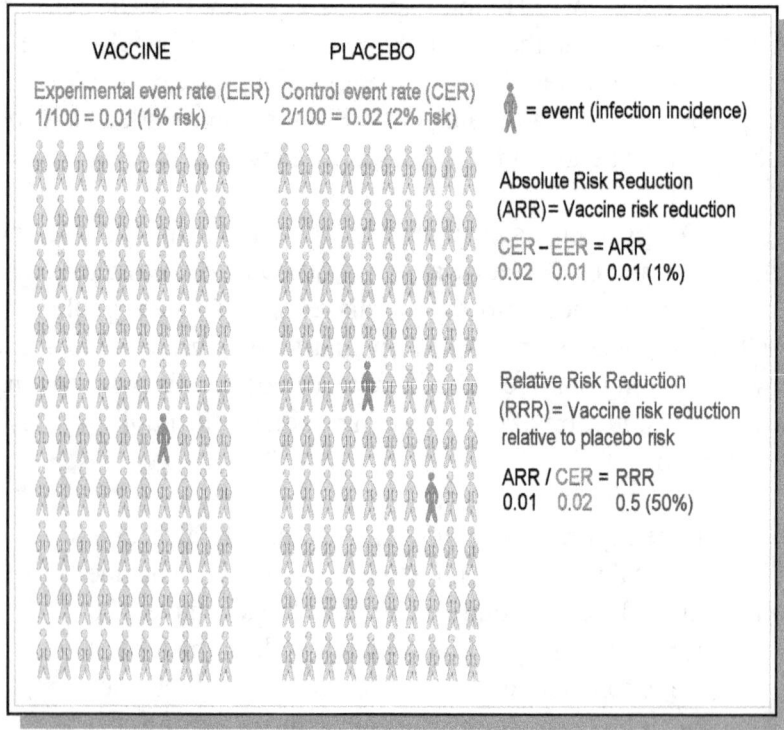

The same issue explained above with the Moderna report, Dr. Brown found in the Pfizer-BioNTech study. He explains how the absolute risk reduction of the Pfizer-BioNTech COVID-19 vaccine of 0.7% tells a very different story from the much-publicized relative risk reductions of 95.1% for that vaccine. While the relative efficacy rate was widely publicized, the absolute efficacy rate was not shared with the public.

The COVID-19 vaccines are unsafe and ineffective. As we have seen, the manufacturers and some insiders in the federal regulatory agencies knew before the EUA was issued that the vaccines would not prevent COVID-19 infections. If that is the case, why did the FDA give them EUA status? The vaccines were given EUA status based on the clinical studies performed by the vaccine manufacturers. An objective review of the data in the studies and the protocols reveals that they were rigged to falsely show that the vaccines were effective.

Dr. David Martin reveals that Moderna concealed the evidence that their vaccine was ineffective by waiting 14 days to perform a confirmatory RT-PCR test on the test subjects.[638] They reported that the Moderna study shows that within 7 days of both the first and the second vaccinations, the group receiving the Moderna COVID-19 vaccines displayed greater systemic symptoms of COVID-19 than the control group.[639] But Moderna ignored those systemic COVID-19 symptoms by reporting them not as symptoms of COVID-19 caused by the vaccine but systemic adverse reactions to the vaccine.

Moderna avoided reporting the COVID-19 systemic symptoms caused to the vaccine recipients within 7 days of receiving the first and the second vaccinations as being "confirmed COVID-19 cases" by not testing the vaccine recipients with the RT-PCR test during that time. By not performing the RT-PCR test, Moderna was able to report the COVID-19 symptoms during that 7 day period under a category of "systemic adverse reactions" to the vaccine instead of "systemic symptoms" of COVID-19 caused by the vaccine that were confirmed COVID-19 cases. Moderna did not do any confirmatory RT-PCR tests on the test subjects until 14 days following the second vaccination. Thus, by waiting until 14 days after the second vaccination to conduct the confirmatory RT-PCR tests, Moderna was able to report that their vaccine was 94.1% (interim results were 94.5%) effective in preventing COVID-19.

The FDA reported that Moderna limited the measure of efficacy for their COVID-19 vaccine as follows: "The primary efficacy endpoint was efficacy of the vaccine to prevent protocol-defined COVID-19 occurring at least 14 days after the second dose in participants with negative SARS-CoV-2 status at baseline."[640]

What is a confirmed COVID-19 case? Moderna defined it thusly in its study submitted to the FDA:

> For the primary efficacy endpoint, the case definition for a confirmed COVID-19 case was defined as:
> • At least TWO of the following systemic symptoms: Fever (=38°C), chills, myalgia, headache, sore throat, new olfactory and taste disorder(s), or
> • At least ONE of the following respiratory signs/symptoms: cough, shortness of breath or difficulty breathing, OR clinical or radiographical evidence of pneumonia; and
> • NP swab, nasal swab, or saliva sample (or respiratory sample, if hospitalized) positive for SARS-CoV-2 by RT-PCR.[641]

Notice in the chart below the systemic symptoms for

COVID-19 (**fever, chills, myalgia, and headache**) were significantly greater within 7 days of the second vaccination. But Moderna did not perform any confirmatory RT-PCR test during that period. Consequently, those systemic symptoms of COVID-19 were reported not as systemic symptoms of COVID-19 caused by the vaccine that were confirmed COVID-19 cases but as "systemic adverse reactions" to the vaccine.

Moderna reported that an astounding **81.9%** of the vaccinated group aged 18-64 years old suffered systemic adverse events after the second vaccination. That is more than double the systemic adverse events occurring in the placebo group. Even more telling is that **17.4%** of the vaccinated group aged 18-64 years old suffered grade 3 systemic adverse events after the second vaccination. A grade 3 adverse event is defined as a severe adverse event. That is more than eight (8) times the grade 3 severe systemic adverse events in the placebo group. Furthermore, 10 people in the vaccine group suffered a grade 4 systemic adverse event. A grade 4 adverse event is a life-threatening adverse event. That is more than five (5) times the rate of the placebo group's grade 4 systemic adverse events.

Table 23. Frequency of Solicited Systemic Adverse Reactions Within 7 Days Following Either the First or Second Dose of Vaccine, Participants Age 18-64 years, Solicited Safety Set[a]				
Adverse Reaction	Vaccine Group Dose 1 n/N (%)	Placebo Group Dose 1 n/N (%)	Vaccine Group Dose 2 n/N (%)	Placebo Group Dose 2 n/N (%)
Any Systemic	6503/11405 (57.0)	5063/11406 (44.4)	8484/10358 (81.9)	3967/10320 (38.4)
Grade 3	363/11405 (3.2)	248/11406 (2.2)	1801/10358 (17.4)	215/10320 (2.1)
Grade 4	5/11405 (<0.1)	4/11406 (<0.1)	10/10358 (<0.1)	2/10320 (<0.1)

The chart below is from the Moderna COVE Study Group and published in the New England Journal of Medicine.[642] I annotated it to indicate certain percentages and circle the "systemic symptoms" of COVID-19 as defined by Moderna but reported by Moderna as "systemic adverse events."

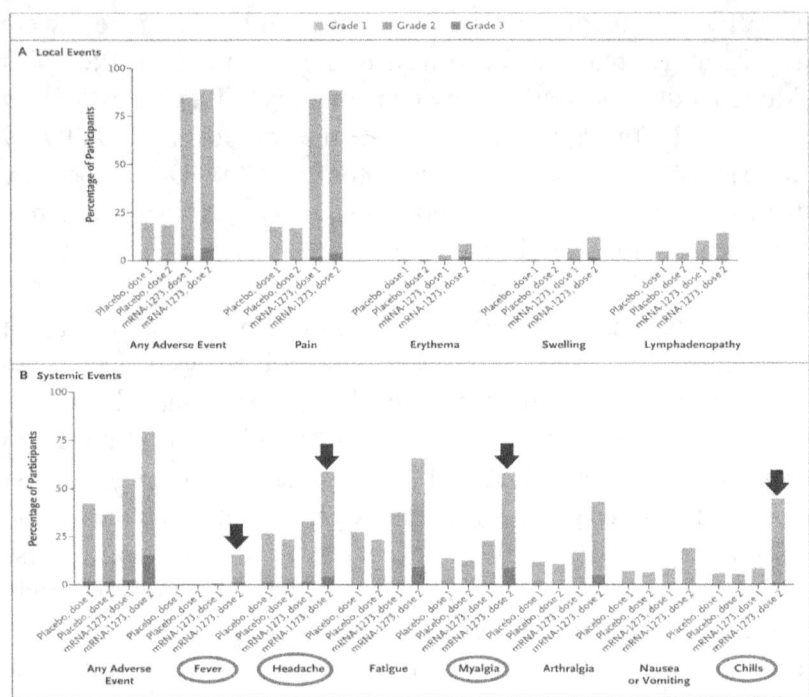

Shown is the percentage of participants who had a solicited local or systemic adverse event **within 7 days** after injection 1 or injection 2 of either the placebo or the mRNA-1273 vaccine. The above chart was provided by the Moderna COVE Study Group and published in the New England Journal of Medicine. It was annotated by Edward Hendrie with arrows to indicate the percentages for participants suffering adverse events from the second COVID-19 vaccine dose for systemic symptoms and red circles indicating the systemic symptoms of COVID-19 as defined by Moderna.

For the primary efficacy endpoint of preventing COVID-19, Moderna defined, in pertinent part, the case definition for a **confirmed COVID-19 case** in their report presented to the FDA to obtain Emergency Use Authorization (EUA) as:
• At least TWO of the following systemic symptoms: Fever (=38°C), chills, myalgia, headache, sore throat, new olfactory and taste disorder(s), and
• Positive test for SARS-CoV-2 by RT-PCR.

Notice that within **7 days** a significantly greater percentage of the COVID-19 vaccine recipients displayed COVID-19 **"systemic symptoms"** (circled in red) than the placebo group. But they were not reported as COVID-19 infections because no RT-PCR test was done to confirm them as COVID-19 cases. By not performing the RT-PCR test the symptoms could be reported under a category of **"systemic adverse reactions"** to the vaccine instead of **"systemic symptoms"** of COVID-19 caused by the vaccine that were confirmed COVID-19 cases. Moderna did not do any RT-PCR tests until **14 days** following the second vaccination. Thus, by waiting until **14 days** after the second vaccination to conduct the RT-PCR tests, Moderna was able to report that their vaccine was 94.1% effective in preventing COVID-19.

Peter Doshi, Ph.D., is Associate Professor of Pharmaceutical Health Services Research at the University of Maryland School of Pharmacy. He is also a senior editor at the British Medical Journal (aka, BMJ).

Dr. Doshi wrote an opinion in the BMJ wherein he criticized the Pfizer COVID-19 safety and efficacy trials. He noted several irregularities in the study. Dr. Doshi explains:

> All attention has focused on the dramatic efficacy results: Pfizer reported 170 PCR confirmed covid-19 cases, split 8 to 162 between vaccine and placebo groups. But these numbers were dwarfed by a category of disease called "suspected covid-19"—those with symptomatic covid-19 that were not PCR confirmed. According to FDA's report on Pfizer's vaccine, there were **"3410 total cases of suspected, but unconfirmed covid-19 in the overall study population, 1594 occurred in the vaccine group vs. 1816 in the placebo group."**
>
> With 20 times more suspected than confirmed cases, this category of disease cannot be ignored simply because there was no positive PCR test result. Indeed this makes it all the more urgent to understand. A rough estimate of vaccine efficacy against developing covid-19 symptoms, with or without a positive PCR test result, would be a **relative risk reduction of 19%** (see footnote)—far below the 50% effectiveness threshold for authorization set by regulators.[643]

You read that correctly; there were 3,410 cases of suspected COVID-19 with no indication in the report whether or not they were tested. The report only indicated that the participants were not confirmed to be COVID-19 via a PCR test. It gets worse. That information was not revealed in the 92-page report filed by Pfizer-BioNTech. Dr. Doshi reveals:

> There is a clear need for data to answer these questions, but Pfizer's 92-page report didn't mention the 3410 "suspected covid-19" cases. Nor did its publication in the New England Journal of Medicine. Nor did any of the reports on Moderna's vaccine. The only source that appears to have reported it is FDA's review of Pfizer's vaccine.[644]

One can reasonably infer that the reason Pfizer did not reveal the 3,410 cases of suspected COVID-19 is that the revelation of that data would undermine the safety and efficacy of the COVID-19 vaccine under study.

Dr. Doshi was also troubled by the unusually unbalanced and unexplained numbers of people excluded from the efficacy analysis. There were five (5) times more people lost in the vaccine group due to protocol deviations than the control group. 311 were excluded from the vaccine group vs. 60 on placebo. Dr. Doshi was perplexed:

> What were these protocol deviations in Pfizer's study, and why were there five times more participants excluded in the vaccine group? The FDA report doesn't say, and these exclusions are difficult to even spot in Pfizer's report and journal publication.[645]

Not mentioned by Dr. Doshi was that in the Pfizer trial, as in the Moderna trial, those that had suspected COVID-19 within seven (7) days of vaccination were not publically reported by Pfizer. The FDA auditors found that data. The FDA explained that "[s]uspected COVID-19 cases that occurred within seven (7) days after any vaccination were 409 in the vaccine group vs. 287 in the placebo group."[646] You read that correctly; there were more suspected COVID-19 cases within seven (7) days in the vaccinated group than in the placebo group. They manifested clinical symptoms of COVID-19. They got ill from the vaccine. Those persons were likely not given confirmatory COVID-19 PCR tests and thus were left in the suspected category, just as was done in the Moderna trial. That way, Pfizer could be sure not to contradict their desired outcome of preventing COVID-19. But the suspected COVID-19 cases within seven (7) days were not reported by Pfizer in their published reports. The government auditors were left to guess that "[i]t is possible that the imbalance in suspected COVID-19 cases occurring in the seven (7) days postvaccination represents vaccine reactogenicity with symptoms that overlap with those of COVID-19."[647] But that is just a guess by the auditors, as Pfizer, apparently, provided no explanation.

There is a reason that Moderna and Pfizer did not PCR test those who showed symptoms of COVID-19 within seven (7) days of vaccination. They knew the results would likely be positive. Indeed, that is what we see in the real world. For example, 35 nuns received the COVID-19 vaccine, and within two days, 28 nuns fell ill and tested positive for COVID-19, with two of the nuns dying during those two days.[648] A third nun also died days later. That is clear evidence of ADE within days of being vaccinated. It is the very evidence that both Moderna and Pfizer sought to conceal in their studies.

The Canadian Covid Care Alliance (CCCA) scrutinized the Pfizer data and confirmed Dr. Doshi's findings. The CCCA found that the relative risk reduction reported by Pfizer was inaccurate. The CCCA discovered:

> The Pfizer trials DID NOT test all participants for COVID-19. Instead, they instructed their investigators to test only those with a COVID-19

symptom and left it up to their discretion to decide what those were.[649]

That means that asymptomatic infection would have been missed entirely. A high level of subjectivity was introduced to the study. An investigator had the ability to sway the results. The lack of objective, systematic testing made the results unreliable.[650]

"The basis for the Emergency Use Authorization was the Confirmed COVID cases of 8 vs 162, which meant a Relative Risk Reduction of 95%. But **when dealing with such a small number of cases, any change can impact the results significantly.**" The inoculated group lost **80** persons to follow up. The placebo group lost **86** persons to follow up. There were **1,594** persons in the inoculated group that were suspected of having COVID-19 but were not tested. There were **1,816** persons in the placebo group that were suspected of having COVID-19 but were not tested. Those numbers render the reported 95% efficacy meaningless. The CCCA explains:

> **Lost to follow up** means **they lost touch with those subjects** and can't confirm whether they got sick or not. They don't know.
>
> **Suspected, but unconfirmed** means these people were **symptomatic for COVID-19**, but were never tested. (Discretion for testing was left up to the investigator.)
>
> The fact that the Lost to Follow Up and Suspected but Unconfirmed numbers are higher - and here they are even significantly higher - than the End Point numbers means that **this data is unreliable. The study should not have been accepted in this state.** In normal scientific practice they should have returned to investigate further.[651]

The improprieties in the study inflated the RRR. When the excluded numbers are factored back into the equation, the true RRR was actually 19% and not the reported 95%. Thus the study actually proved that the vaccines were ineffective. And that is just what we see in the real-world results after the EUA was granted. Below is a chart from the CCCA illustrating how the failure to test the suspected cases of COVID-19 affected the results.

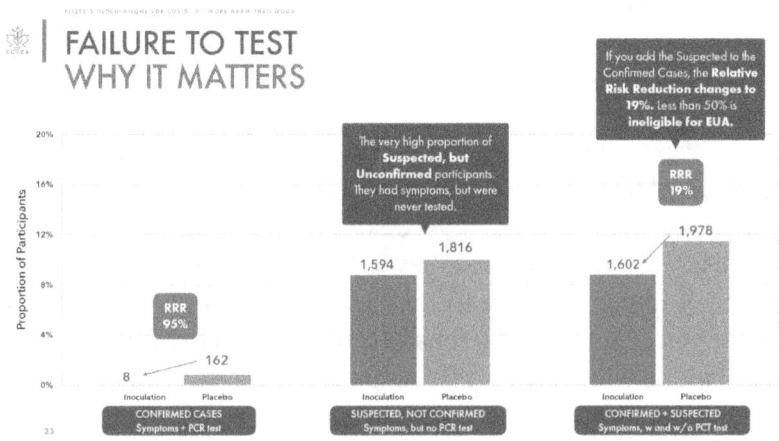

Dr. Doshi was further troubled by the fact that the adjudication committee for the Pfizer adjudication committee consisted of three Pfizer employees. The study could hardly be unbiased when it is being run by Pfizer employees being paid by the company that is banking on a favorable outcome.

Brook Jackson, a whistleblower who helped run one of Pfizer's clinical trials, revealed that the Pfizer trials were rigged. Vaccinated individuals who had COVID-19 were not being tested for COVID-19 to conceal the vaccine's ineffectiveness.[652] Both Moderna and Pfizer concealed data showing injuries caused by their vaccines. For example, injuries caused by the vaccines were concealed and not reported by the scheme of removing those in the trials who were vaccine injured. For example, 302 vaccinated subjects were dismissed from one of the Pfizer study groups. Another stratagem is for the principal medical investigator (PI) to aggressively reclassify each serious complication as unrelated to the vaccines.[653] For example, in one Pfizer study group, 21 vaccinated study participants died, but their deaths were reported as being "unrelated to the vaccines."[654] The pharmaceutical companies set parameters for the trials that avoided long-term follow-up on study participants. Thus, preventing the reporting of incriminating safety data. Adding insult to injury, the pharmaceutical companies refused to pay for medical treatment for the injured trial participants, as they had initially contracted to do.

Pfizer has been caught lying about the severity of the injuries suffered by trial participants during its COVID-19 vaccine trials. And medical doctors are so afraid of attributing vaccine injuries to the vaccines that they will resort to saying the patients are crazy rather than get to the cause of the injury. Maddie de Garay is an example. U.S. Senator Ron Johnson tweeted the plight of Maddi de Garay. "After being part of a Covid vaccine trial for 12-15 year-olds, Maddie has been to the ER 9 times and hospitalized 3 times for a total of 2 months. Doctors even wanted to put her in a mental hospital saying her symptoms were caused by anxiety."[655] Pfizer is doing all it can to cover up Maddie's injuries and others like her. Young Maddie has lost bowel and bladder control and lost the ability to walk and is now bound to a wheelchair, yet Pfizer listed her adverse reaction to their vaccine as "functional abdominal pain."[656]

Twelve-year-old Maddie de Garay volunteered for the Pfizer vaccine trial. Her mother, Stephanie de Garay, explained that Maddie volunteered for the Pfizer vaccine trial "to help everyone else, and they're not helping here. Before Maddie got her final dose of the vaccine, she was healthy, got straight As, had lots of friends, and had a life." Megan Redshaw reported on Maddie for The Defender:

Upon receiving the second shot, Maddie immediately felt pain at the injection site and over the next 24-hours developed severe abdominal and chest pain, de Garay said at the press event. Maddie told her mother it felt like her heart was being ripped out through her neck, and she had painful electrical shocks down her neck and spine that forced her to walk hunched over.

Maddie's parents took her to the emergency room as instructed by the vaccine trial nurse administrator. Her labs were taken, she was checked for appendicitis, given an IV with medicine and sent home. The diagnosis in the discharge summary read "adverse effect of vaccine initial encounter." Maddie's condition continued to worsen. Over the next two and a half months her abdominal, muscle and nerve pain became unbearable, her mother said.

She developed gastroparesis, nausea and vomiting, erratic blood pressure, memory loss, brain fog, headaches, dizziness, fainting, seizures, verbal and motor tics, menstrual cycle issues, lost feeling from the waist down, lost bowel and bladder control and had an nasogastric tube placed because she lost her ability to eat.[657]

Below is Maddie de Garay's vaccine card introduced as an exhibit as part of her Mother's, Stephanie de Garay's, public comment to the FDA as a supporting document to prove that Maddie was in the trial and got the actual vaccine. It is posted on the FDA website.[658]

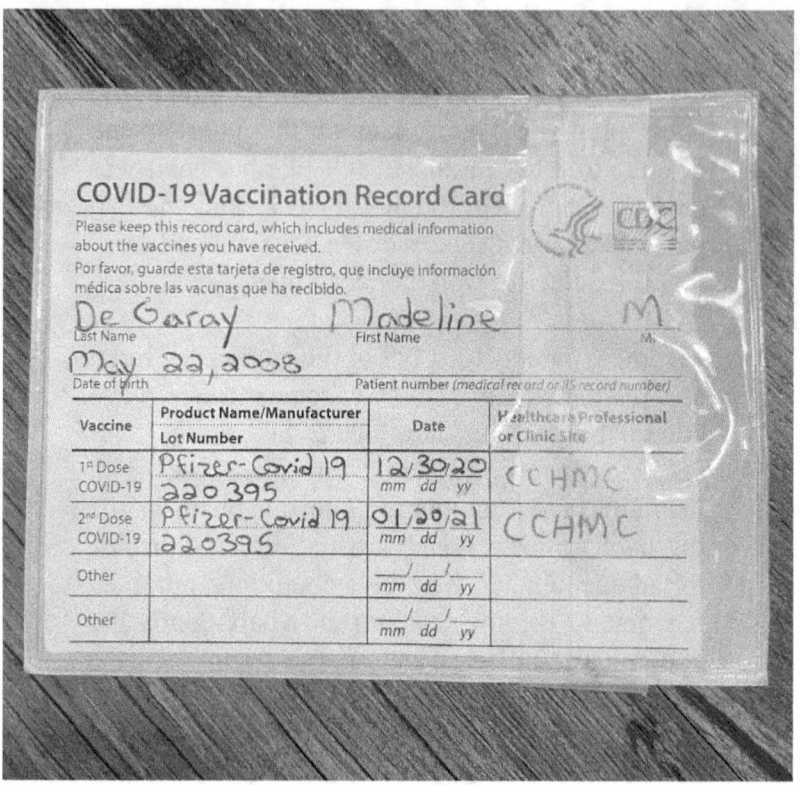

The Canadian Covid Care Alliance studied the raw data from the Pfizer COVID-19 trials. The researchers found that data hidden in the report proves that vaccinated persons are more likely to suffer physical harm and death from the vaccine compared to unvaccinated persons.[659]

PFIZER TRIALS DID NOT PROVE SAFETY THEY PROVED HARM

	ILLNESS			DEATHS	
	BNT162b2	Placebo	Risk Change	BNT162b2	Placebo
Efficacy	77	850	-91%	20	14
Related Adverse Event	5,241	1,311	+300%		
Any Severe Adverse Event	262	150	+75%		
Any Serious Adverse Event	127	116	+10%		

These are the results of Pfizer's own randomized control trial.
LEVEL 1 EVIDENCE OF HARM.

Pfizer published its study results on November 30, 2020, but four months earlier, on or before July 22, 2020, the U.S. government had already placed a $1.95 billion order for the Pfizer COVID-19 vaccine.[660] At that time Pfizer had just begun to enter its late-stage, 30,000-person study. The study had not begun and no data had even been generated. But recall, Pfizer ran the study and was able to rig it to say what they wanted it to say. The skids were greased. There were 1.95 billion reasons for making sure the Pfizer COVID-19 vaccine study showed safety and efficacy. "The love of money is the root of all evil." 1 Timothy 6:10.

Amazingly, the financial deals were being struck when the U.S. government did not know what it was buying. Indeed, the dose level has not even been determined because the late-stage trials have not been conducted. On July 22, 2020, Jared S. Hopkins and Chris Wack, writing for the Wall Street Journal, reported, "Pfizer and BioNTech said they expect to seek emergency use authorization or some form of regulatory approval as early as October."[661] To do that meant that the favorable results from the testing must have been baked into the study. Hopkins and Wack noted that "[v]accines typically take years to develop and prove they work safely, and many fail during the process."[662] But in July of 2020, Pfizer confidently expected "approval as early as October." So was the FDA, as the Federal Government had already agreed to pay billions of dollars to buy the untested vaccine. Hopkins and Wack explain that "[t]he U.S. Food and Drug Administration has the authority to quickly authorize drugs and vaccines on an emergency basis."[663] The deal with Pfizer is not the only drug vaccine deal signed. Hopkins and Wack explain:

> As part of its Operation Warp Speed program, the U.S. has already struck agreements with other vaccine developers to secure doses, including a $1.2 billion deal with AstraZeneca PLC for at least 300 million doses of a vaccine developed by University of Oxford researchers. A $1.6 billion agreement with Novavax Inc. will fund clinical studies of its experimental vaccine and establish large-scale manufacturing of doses."[664]

How were the vaccine manufacturers cutting the time for development so drastically? Simple, they were ramping up the manufacturing of their vaccines as they were testing them. I kid you not. Hopkins and Wack revealed that in July 2020, "Covid-19 vaccine developers are also combining phases of studies and studying their vaccines at the same time they are ramping up manufacturing capabilities, industry and health officials say."[665] That means that the pharmaceutical companies already manufactured the same vaccine that they had not yet finished testing for safety and efficacy. Pfizer Chief Business Officer John Young admitted this. Young stated: "This is unprecedented, and that is the only way you can really move at this kind of speed—is to do so many stages over your development and manufacturing process in parallel, rather than doing them sequentially."[666] Pfizer is not financially stupid. This was not a gamble; this was a sure thing. The fix was in, and Pfizer knew it. With the COVID-19 vaccines, the drug companies were expecting favorable results from their trials. And, as we now know, they got them. Of course, they did. They preordained the favorable results. The pharmaceutical companies are experts in those kinds of shenanigans. And they expected a big pay-off. They were not disappointed. In 2021 alone, Pfizer hauled in $36.8 billion in sales for its COVID-19 vaccine. That made the Pfizer COVID-19 vaccine the most profitable pharmaceutical product over a one year period in the history of pharmaceuticals.[667]

Johnson & Johnson began planning to manufacture their COVID-19 vaccine within the first few months of the alleged COVID-19 pandemic. Matt Grossman reported on March 30, 2020, for The Wall Street Journal that "Johnson & Johnson said it would try to scale its global manufacturing capabilities to make more than 1 billion doses of a Covid-19 vaccine by the end of next year."[668] That was well before they even began human testing their vaccine.

In a July 16, 2020, Wall Street Journal article, it was revealed that J&J had invested in "manufacturing sites" and "filling sites" and everything necessary to deliver one billion vaccines. That was after their initial March 2020 plans and still before their vaccine had even undergone human testing. J&J did not even know if their vaccine would cure or harm the patient. Why would J&J spend millions of dollars building manufacturing facilities for an untested vaccine? Because they knew that the vaccine would be approved. The skids were greased, and it didn't care if the vaccine was safe or effective; it knew that the vaccine would be allowed under an EUA, which protected J&J from civil liability for injuries caused by the vaccine. The July 16, 2020, Wall Street Journal article reveals:

> Johnson & Johnson ... said Thursday it plans to begin the first human studies of its experimental coronavirus vaccine next week, as it races to make the shot available starting early next year.

The New Brunswick, N.J., company's initial study will aim to enroll more than 1,000 healthy adults, starting first in Belgium on July 22 and then the following week in the U.S. Researchers will assess the vaccine's safety and ability to induce an immune response, J&J Chief Scientific Officer Paul Stoffels said Thursday on a conference call with analysts. The company also plans studies in additional countries.

The more definitive testing will take place as soon as September. J&J said it is still having discussions with the U.S. National Institutes of Health for a large phase 3 clinical trial that could begin in late September, which would test whether the vaccine protects people from Covid-19, the disease caused by the new coronavirus.

J&J could get an answer about whether the vaccine safely prevents Covid-19 by the end of the year, Dr. Stoffels said. If successful, the company expects the shot to become available in early 2021, and J&J plans to manufacture up to one billion doses by the end of next year.

"We have the manufacturing sites, we have the filling sites, we have everything that's needed to deliver that one billion vaccines" next year, Dr. Stoffels said.[669]

It has been now confirmed that the COVID-19 vaccines from Moderna, Pfizer-BioNtech, and Johnson & Johnson (Janssen) do not prevent COVID-19. The vaccines were authorized to be used on an emergency basis to prevent COVID-19, but they have been shown not to do that. So, the pharmaceutical companies just changed the rules for what it means to be effective. Now the standard is no longer whether the vaccine prevents COVID-19 but, instead, whether it lessens the symptoms of COVID-19. When Democrat Rep. Stephen Lynch tested positive to COVID-19 after receiving both shots of the Pfizer vaccine, the Daily Mail explained that "Pfizer's vaccine does not necessarily prevent COVID-19 infection, but is said to be 95 percent effective in stopping the serious symptoms that are caused by the coronavirus."[670]

Moderna knew from the outset that their vaccine would not prevent COVID-19. A careful reading of Moderna's study indicates that its vaccine likely causes COVID-19. Indeed, there have been many reported cases since the use of both the Moderna and Pfizer-BioNtech vaccines were authorized under the FDA's EUA where the recipient of a COVID-19 vaccination became subsequently ill from COVID-19 and the COVID-19 illness was determined to have been caused by the COVID-19 vaccination.

The insiders seemed to have known from the beginning that the COVID-19 vaccines would not prevent COVID-19 and very likely cause COVID-19. Before either vaccine was authorized, Anthony Fauci explained that reducing symptoms of COVID-19 was the "primary endpoint" of the vaccines. Fauci said that getting rid of the virus through immunity was only a "secondary endpoint." On October 28, 2020, Carol Crist, writing for WebMD, summarized Dr. Fauci's argument as meaning that "with reduced severe symptoms, the coronavirus would pose a lower threat as a pandemic. Then scientists could focus on developing a solution that would reach the full goal of preventing initial infection."[671]

On October 29, 2020, Dr. Fauci explained: "If the vaccine also allows you to prevent initial infection that would be great," Fauci said. "But what I would settle for, and all my colleagues would settle for, is the primary endpoint, which is to prevent clinically recognizable disease. That's what we hope happens."[672]

Dr. Fauci said that reducing symptoms of COVID-19 was the "primary endpoint" of the COVID-19 vaccines and not the prevention of COVID-19. But Fauci's statement is contradicted by the FDA. The FDA reported that the primary efficacy endpoint when reviewing the data in deciding whether to grant Moderna's petition to obtain an Emergency Use Authorization (EUA) for their COVID-19 vaccine was its ability to prevent COVID-19. The FDA review states that **"[t]he primary efficacy endpoint was efficacy of the vaccine to prevent protocol-defined COVID-19."**[673] The protocol-defined COVID-19 included a positive PCR test for SARS-CoV-2, the alleged virus purported to cause COVID-19.

Moderna, J&J, and Pfizer-BioNtech got their COVID-19 vaccines authorized by the FDA under EUAs based on their alleged effectiveness in preventing COVID-19. They then promoted the vaccines to the public on that basis. When the vaccines are increasingly proving ineffective in preventing COVID-19, they just change the standard for success to lessening symptoms. They knew full well that the FDA could not approve an EUA for lessening symptoms and nobody would take a vaccine that would not prevent the targeted disease. So they used the classic bait and switch strategy with a willing accomplice in the FDA.

25 Food Allergies

Vinu Arumugham, in an article written for the Journal of Developing Drugs, reveals that "Nobel Laureate Charles Richet demonstrated over a hundred years ago that injecting a protein into animals or humans causes immune system sensitization to that protein."[674] What does that mean for the person receiving the vaccine? Arumugham explains that "[s]ubsequent exposure to the protein can result in allergic reactions or anaphylaxis."[675] Thus, food proteins injected into a person through a vaccine can have the effect of causing a subsequent allergic reaction by that person who subsequently eats food that contains the food proteins in the vaccine.

Vaccines are the source of the explosion in food allergies in the United States. Indeed, there are more than 15 million Americans who suffer from life-threatening food allergies. Arumugham reveals how this happens.

> Vaccines contain adjuvants such as pertussis toxins and aluminum compounds that also bias towards allergy. Adjuvants also increase the immunogenicity of injected food proteins. This combination of atopic children and food protein injection along with adjuvants contributes to

millions developing life-threatening food allergies.

That means that vaccines can cause food allergies. Arumugham reveals that this scientific fact of vaccine-induced allergies "has since been demonstrated over and over again in humans and animal models."[676] Vaccines contain food proteins derived from chicken eggs, casein, gelatin, soy, agar, peanut oil, etc. Those ingredients sound innocent enough. And if they were eaten they would not be harmful and, indeed, would be nutritious. But when those same ingredients are injected into a human body, in a significant number of cases, a person develops an allergic reaction or even anaphylaxis to that food protein.

The allergic reaction is caused because accompanying the food protein is an adjuvant whose purpose is to stimulate the body's immune response to the antigen. The problem is that the stimulated immune response is not limited to the antigen. The body also develops an immune response to the food proteins in the vaccine. The stimulated immune response to the food protein causes an allergic reaction to the food when consumed.

For example, casein is a phosphoprotein derived from milk. Trace amounts of casein are often found in vaccines. Indeed, the DTaP children's vaccine is cultured using bovine casein as a medium. There has been an explosion of people who have developed allergies to milk. According to the American College of Allergy, Asthma, and Immunology, "cow's milk is the most common food allergy in children under the age of 5."[677] It is probable that milk allergies in young children are a direct result of the stimulated immune response to the bovine casein in the DTaP vaccine.

Anaphylaxis caused by peanuts is the leading cause of death among food allergies. Brett Wilcox, in his book, *Jabbed*, reveals that "[a]ccording to Heather Fraser, author of *The Peanut Allergy Epidemic*, the explosion of peanut and many other allergies in recent years is linked to the use of peanut oil in vaccines."[678]

Robyn Charron scrutinized the evidence gathered in Heather Fraser's book, *The Peanut Allergy Epidemic*. She concluded that Fraser was correct. The explosion in peanut allergies directly results from vaccinations. Charon states:

> A lot of people might be surprised to know that there are food oils in injectable vaccines. In the 1930s there was cottonseed oil in vaccines, followed by a short-lived spate of cottonseed oil allergies of about a decade that quietly went away with a change in formula. In the 1960s and 1970s a flu vaccine used peanut oil as an adjuvant to make a smaller amount of influenza antigen elicit a bigger antibody response from the immune system. From 1950-1980 an injectable penicillin was suspended in peanut oil to allow for a slow release of penicillin while the body metabolized the oil. The occasional anaphylactic death from subsequently eating peanuts made headlines.[679]

Charron explains how the oil used in a vaccine doesn't need to be peanut oil to cause a peanut allergy. Oils in vaccines that are closely related to peanut oil cause peanut allergies. Charron identifies the use of castor oil in the original formula of the Vitamin K shot given to newborns as causing peanut allergies because castor oil is known to cross-sensitize immune systems to peanut oil. When the Vitamin K injection was reformulated in 2006 to replace castor oil with lecithin derived from soybean and egg that only exacerbated the resulting food allergies because soybean and peanuts have molecular weights that cause cross-reactivity. The soybean oil in the vaccine is sensitizing some babies to peanuts. Charron further explains how the bacterial Hib vaccine causes peanut allergies:

It is now known that the structure and weight of the Hib bacteria proteins are very similar to the structure and weight of the peanut protein, which leads to cross reactivity to peanuts and tree nuts. We are, essentially, creating anaphylactic babies in the same manner researchers create anaphylactic mice: administering a peanut-like protein fused to adjuvant bacterial toxin.[680]

Shockingly, that fact regarding vaccine-induced allergies has been known by the scientific community for more than one hundred years, but the pharmaceutical companies, which largely fund the medical schools, keep physicians, most notably pediatricians, in the dark about it. Indeed, medical doctors are only given a few hours of instruction on vaccines during medical school. Physicians are ill-equipped by their medical training to assess the safety of vaccines. That ignorance is by design.

26   Toxic Excipients

Vaccines contain excipients that are added to the antigen. According to the CDC, only the antigen is considered the "active ingredient."[681] But that does not mean that the excipients do not serve an active function. And it does not mean that the exipients do not actively affect the injected patient. Excipients are often toxic and cause long-term adverse health effects, including severe immunological and brain disorders. The excipients fall into three basic categories: 1) adjuvants, 2) preservatives, and 3) stabilizers.[682] Adjuvants are designed to stimulate the immune response to the antigen in the vaccine. Preservatives prevent degradation and contamination. Stabilizers help keep the vaccines potent during storage.

There are also trace chemicals and materials found in the vaccines. For example, vaccines often contain antibiotics that are used to prevent contamination of bacteria during manufacturing. Vaccines contain cell culture materials used to grow the antigen, such as egg protein and aborted fetal tissue. The trace chemicals are often dangerous, although they may be listed as "inactive ingredients." For instance, the CDC describes toxins found in vaccines, such as formaldehyde, which is used to inactivate viruses, "inactive ingredients."[683] Formaldehyde is a dangerous toxic chemical that disrupts cellular functions and is cytotoxic (causes cell death).[684] Please understand that the CDC does not test the vaccines to determine what ingredients are in them. The CDC simply takes the vaccine manufacturers at their word and republishes the ingredients found in the vaccine package insert.

Vinu Arumugham discovered that "there are no specifications limiting allergen content in vaccines approved for use in the United States." What does that mean for vaccine patients? It means that no safe level has been established for any allergens contained in vaccines. Those who make vaccine excipients such as sorbitol and Polysorbate 80 are not limited in any way by government regulations as to the residual allergens contained in their injectable grade products. Arumugham made the disturbing discovery that "[s]ince there are no limits, suppliers do not test for allergens in production. Further, residual allergens that may be present in the excipients are not even listed in the vaccine package inserts." Thus, there is no way for a doctor to know all of the excipient ingredients in the vaccine being injected into his patient. The doctor (and the patient) are literally flying blind. Each new vaccine injection poses a risk of the patient developing food or other allergies.

Aluminum

A common adjuvant is aluminum.[685] Indeed, the CDC lists aluminum, aluminum hydroxide, aluminum phosphate, aluminum sulfate, or aluminum hydroxyphosphate sulfate as ingredients in 27 vaccines.[686] Aluminum is a dangerous neurotoxin and carcinogen. Research has established that "[t]he adverse neurologic, hematopoietic, skeletal, respiratory, immunologic, and other effects associated with excessive aluminum (Al) exposures are well known."[687]

Research has proven that the neurological effects of aluminum include "impairment on neurobehavioral tests for psychomotor and cognitive performance and an increased incidence of subjective neurological symptoms."[688] Indeed, "studies clearly identify the nervous system as the most sensitive target of aluminum toxicity."[689] In studies involving "intramuscular administration of aluminum hydroxide or aluminum phosphate vaccine adjuvants in rabbits, increased levels of aluminum were found in the kidney, spleen, liver, heart, lymph nodes, and brain (in decreasing order of aluminum concentration)."[690]

Pediatrician Dr. Paul Thomas explains:

Aluminum, the adjuvant in most vaccines, is the largest and most powerful trigger of autoimmunity. There's an entire book about it called, *Vaccines and Autoimmunity*, edited by Schoenfeld. There are hundreds of articles pointing to this issue. That's just a small piece. ... [Y]our baby's born, and the first thing they do is give your baby a hepatitis B vaccine with a huge dose, 250 mcg. of aluminum, TEN TIMES THE MAXIMUM TOXIC DOSE, according to the FDA. [The FDA] has had an active policy up since 2000 stating not to exceed 5 micrograms/Kg/day of parenteral aluminum. ... And this is also where mandatory vaccine laws are just harmful.[691] (emphasis in original)

Mercury

In 1999, the U.S. Food and Drug Administration (FDA) determined that mercury in childhood vaccines, in the form of thimerosal, exceeded FDA guidelines for mercury exposure. But it was not taken out of childhood vaccines in the U.S. until 2001.[692] Mercury is a known neurotoxin. The mercury safety standards were determined by measuring methylmercury. But the mercury in thimerosal metabolizes in the body as ethylmercury. The FDA had no safety guidelines for ethylmercury. The FDA did not know what to do, so they correctly required vaccine companies to reduce or eliminate the use of thimerosal in vaccines. The CDC identifies thimerosal as a preservative. Mercury is an effective preservative because it kills bacteria; indeed, it is a heavy metal poison that kills all cells on contact, including the brain cells of infants, as it courses through their fragile bodies. It is still being used in vaccines. While thimerosal has been removed from childhood vaccines, according to the CDC, it remains an ingredient in influenza, tetanus, and Diptheria vaccines.[693]

Eli Lilly, the thimerosal patent holder, contracted for a safety study on thimerosal. The study was determined later to be fraudulent. Researchers H.M. Powell and W.A. Jamieson, both Lilly employees, published the fraudulent study, which the FDA still cites on its website today as proof that thimerosal is safe. The FDA speaks with a forked tongue. It removed thimerosal from childhood vaccines because of mercury toxicity, but it still claims it is safe. That is because thimerosal remains in other vaccines, some of which have since ended up on the childhood vaccine schedule (e.g., the influenza vaccine). The FDA presently states:

> Prior to introduction of thimerosal in the 1930's, data were available in several animal species and humans providing evidence for its safety and effectiveness as a preservative (Powell and Jamieson 1931). Since then, thimerosal has been the subject of numerous studies ... and has a long record of safe and effective use preventing bacterial and fungal contamination of vaccines, with no ill effects established other than minor local reactions at the site of injection.[694]

That is a lie. Thimerosal has devastated children's lives, causing lifelong autism and digestive disorders. But the FDA does not stop there. As of 2016, the FDA had posted on its website the following details about the Powell and Jamieson study:

> The earliest published report of thimerosal use in humans was published in 1931 (Powell and Jamieson 1931). In this report, 22 individuals received 1% solution of thimerosal intravenously for unspecified therapeutic reasons. Subjects received up to 26 milligrams thimerosal/kg (1 milligrams equals 1,000 micrograms) with no reported toxic effects, although 2 subjects demonstrated phlebitis or sloughing of skin after local infiltration. Of note, this study was not specifically designed to examine toxicity; 7 of 22 subjects were observed for only one day, the specific clinical assessments were not described, and no laboratory studies were reported.[695]

That statement was removed from the FDA website some time after 2016. Technically what the FDA says about the Powell and Jamieson study is true. But what is not explained is why "7 of 22 subjects were observed for only one day." 7 of the 22 subjects were observed for only one day because they died that day![696] You read that correctly. 7 out of the 22 subjects died the day they were injected with thimerosal. But the table for the study did not reflect that the study subjects had died. Most of the remaining study patients died by the end of the second day.[697] Those facts were not revealed until 2002. Powell and Jamieson knew before the human studies that thimerosal was toxic because they had done animal studies. A significant number of the animals died from mercury poisoning.[698]

What is reprehensible is that the FDA has known since at least 2002 that the Powell and Jamieson 1931 study was fraudulent. In 2002 an Eli Lilly whistleblower revealed the fraud.[699] But the FDA still cites that scam study as proof that injecting toxic mercury into people is safe.

The FDA knows that the mercury in thimerosal causes

autism because in 1999 Thomas M. Verstraeten, M.D., from the CDC, NIP, Division of Epidemiology and Surveillance Vaccine Safety and Development Branch, did a retrospective study involving 400,000 children and determined that those who received vaccines containing thimerosal were 7.6 times more likely to suffer from autism.[700] More than 165 studies have focused on thimerosal, which found it to be harmful. Dr. Brian Hooker, M.D., reports:

> 16 [of those 165 studies] were conducted to specifically examine the effects of Thimerosal on human infants or children with reported outcomes of death; acrodynia; poisoning; allergic reaction; malformations; auto-immune reaction; Well's syndrome; developmental delay; and neurodevelopmental disorders, including tics, speech delay, language delay, attention deficit disorder, and autism.[701]

Polyethylene Glycol

Both the Moderna and the Pfizer/BionTech COVID-19 mRNA vaccines contain lipids, which have polyethylene glycol (PEG) as part of the lipid ingredients.[702] While PEG is not strictly an adjuvant, it allegedly enhances the effect of mRNA vaccines by helping the mRNA access cells. PEG has been proven to cause hypersensitivity reactions.[703] A hypersensitivity reaction is an exaggerated or inappropriate immune response that can include anaphylaxis.[704] "The Anaphylaxis is a medical emergency because it can lead to an acute, life-threatening respiratory failure."[705] Indeed, as of March 5, 2021, "at least 1,689 recipients of the Pfizer and Moderna injections have reported anaphylactic or serious allergic reactions."[706] The anaphylaxis was predictable. Prior research documented the detrimental effects of PEG on drug delivery. On September 25, 2020, Robert Kennedy, Jr., warned the FDA and NIH about the dangers of PEG in the (at that time) proposed mRNA vaccines.[707] No action was taken by the FDA, NIH, Moderna, or Pfizer to mitigate the risk inherent in the mRNA vaccine PEG excipients.

Polysorbate 80

Polysorbate 80 is an excipient contained in the Johnson & Johnson (aka Janssen) COVID-19 vaccine.[708] It is also an ingredient in the following vaccines: DtaP-IPV, Hep B influenza Meningaogoccal, Pneumococcal, Rotavirus, Tdap, Shingles.[709] Polysorbate 80 is used in vaccines as a surfactant that allows the antigen to evenly dissolve in the excipient vaccine ingredients. Polysorbate 80 is manufactured from food sources such as coconut, palm, sunflower, tapioca, wheat, corn, etc. That sounds safe enough, but Vinue Arumugham explains that it is impossible to guarantee that these products from which the polysorbate 80 is derived do not contain residual allergen proteins. Polysorbate 80 has been proven to cause hypersensitivity reactions.[710] A hypersensitivity reaction is a type of exaggerated or inappropriate immune response that can include anaphylaxis.[711] "The Anaphylaxis is a medical emergency because it can lead to an acute, life-threatening respiratory failure."[712] Indeed, CNBC reported that "[t]wo trial participants suffered severe allergic reactions shortly after getting Johnson & Johnson's Covid-19 vaccine."[713]

Brett Wilcox, in his book, *Jabbed*, deconstructs the FDA's argument that the ingredients in vaccines are safe.

> "Vaccine Ingredients," [is] a subject of utmost importance, because vaccines are chemical concoctions produced by pharmaceutical companies and the simple truth is that nature did not arrange for the ingredients in vaccines to be injected into the blood streams of humans or any other creature. So what exactly does the FDA have

to say about vaccine ingredients?

"A vaccine is made-up of various ingredients and each ingredient present in a vaccine is there for a specific reason. Different ingredients have different roles in a vaccine, and vaccines licensed for use in the United States are demonstrated to be safe and effective before they are used by the public."

But enough said. The FDA has decreed that vaccines include "various ingredients" and each ingredient is there "for a specific reason" accomplishing "different roles." And, since the FDA pronounces vaccines "to be safe and effective," any sane parent or patient would be a fool not to conclude that all of those unnamed ingredients are also "safe and effective."

Let's test that theory using FDA's logic. Formaldehyde, ethylmercury, aluminum, 2-phenoxyethanol, MRC-5 cells, peanut oil, polysorbate 80, and potassium chloride, are a few of the dozens of ingredients found in vaccines. Formaldehyde—embalming fluid—is defined as a carcinogen, but when placed in vaccines, it miraculously becomes safe and effective. Ethylmercury and aluminum are neurotoxins and are synergistically neurotoxic when ingested, but when injected they change into something that's "safe and effective." 2-phenoxyethanol is an insecticide. Humans are not insects, but somehow injecting humans with this insecticide is "safe and effective." Potassium chloride is used in lethal injections to shut down the heart and stop breathing, but when injected into babies it's "safe and effective." Of course, the dosage in vaccines is a small fraction of a lethal dosage, but less of a poison does not equal safe, it equals less toxic. MRC-5 cells are cells from aborted human fetuses. Foreign proteins—human or otherwise—can result in a host of medical problems including autoimmune disorders when ingested, but when injected, they're "safe and effective."[714]

Foreign Proteins

Anaphylaxis has been a known side effect of vaccines since 1913. Indeed, the less severe anaphylaxis, an allergic reaction, is so predictable and prevalent that it should be considered a design feature of vaccines. Eleanor McBean explains the debilitating effects of injecting foreign proteins into the bloodstream through vaccination.

> All vaccines and serums are foreign proteins and therefore a virulent poison. If any protein enters the body illegitimately, through any channel other than the digestive tract, it becomes a strong poison. Proteins in themselves cannot be used by the body—they first require to be broken up by the various processes of digestion into Amino Acids before they become useful as a nutrient to the organism and can be taken into the blood stream to be used as building materials. Injections of therapeutic serums in human beings and animals result in impairment and great injury to some of the most vital organs—heart, lungs, liver, kidneys, nerves etc.[715]

> ANAPHYLAXIS or SERUM POISONING or DISEASE, sometimes called SERUM SHOCK, are the terms being used to indicate the harmful after-effects of vaccination. We cannot tell in

advance of the inoculation the amount of damage which will be done in any particular individual, whether he will die of anaphylaxis, be severely damaged for life or throw it off with a minimum amount of harm to himself. The degree of injury done to the organism may have no immediate noticeable effect but will find expression eventually, especially if the harmful practice is continued. It may result in constitutional debility, degeneration, chronic disease, and death. Some of the symptoms following vaccination and resulting in Serum Sickness are: Fever, Glandular Enlargement, Urticaria, Leucopenia, Leukotaxis, Sciatica, Phlebitis, Pain and Tenderness of the Joints, Paralysis, Heart Failure, Collapse and Death.[716]

Eleanor McBean wrote that in 1957. She was revealing what scientists, government agencies, and pharmaceutical companies have known with certainty since 1913; injecting protein into the bloodstream acts as a poison that causes anaphylaxis (i.e., serum poisoning). A less severe anaphylaxis is typically called an allergic reaction.

Sasha Latypova is a former pharmaceutical executive with 25 years of experience in clinical trials, clinical technologies, and regulatory approvals. She owned and managed several contract research organizations doing work for more than 60 pharmaceutical companies worldwide, including, but not limited to, Pfizer, Johnson and Johnson, Novartis, AstraZeneca, and GSK. Latypova reveals that vaccines work in the exact opposite way as we're told they do. She states that it's impossible to make a vaccine that does anything but poison somebody.[717] She states that "vaccines prime our bodies to react badly to anything that's injected into us, including benign substances like milk or egg proteins. Hence the proliferation of allergies, such as allergies to milk, eggs, wheat, peanuts, etc."[718]

Latypova explains that "this has been known since 1913, when Charles Richet—a French physiologist and self-proclaimed eugenicist—won a Nobel Prize for figuring out that injecting animals with toxins primes them for harmful or deadly reactions if they encounter the same toxins in the environment, even in small amounts. He called these reactions 'anaphylactic' reactions, but said that these reactions also included allergies."[719] Latypova explains that, "[i]t's impossible to vaccinate for anything. And Richet has demonstrated it conclusively and was given Nobel Prize for it ... because he figured out how to poison everyone by sensitizing them to the most commonly occurring things in their environment."[720] Vinu Arumugham confirms Latypova's findings; he explains in a research paper:

> Nobel Laureate Charles Richet demonstrated over a hundred years ago that injecting a protein into animals or humans causes immune system sensitization to that protein. Subsequent exposure to the protein can result in allergic reactions or anaphylaxis. This fact has since been demonstrated over and over again in humans and animal models. The Institute of Medicine (IOM) confirmed that food proteins in vaccines cause food allergy, in its 2011 report on vaccine adverse events. The IOM's confirmation is the latest and most authoritative since Dr. Richet's discovery. Many vaccines and injections contain food proteins. Many studies since 1940 have demonstrated that food proteins in vaccines cause sensitization in humans. ... Vaccines contain adjuvants such as pertussis toxins and aluminum compounds that also bias towards allergy. Adjuvants also increase the immunogenicity of injected food proteins. This combination of atopic children and food protein

> injection along with adjuvants, contributes to millions developing lifethreatening food allergies.[721]

The Nobel Prize Foundation describes the standard view of the theory behind vaccination.

> Our immune system protects us from attacks by microorganisms and poisonous substances. After experiencing an attack, the immune system learns to defend itself against new attacks—we become immune. One of the ways this is used is with vaccinations, when a low dosage of an infectious substance provides immunity.[722]

That is the standard theory of vaccination. But the Nobel Prize Foundation explains that Charles Richet discovered that vaccines have the opposite effect. Vaccination actually makes one sicker.

> Through studies involving dogs, Charles Richet demonstrated an opposite effect in 1902. After an initial low dose of a substance, a new dose some weeks later could produce a severe reaction. He called the phenomenon anaphylaxis. The result had important implications for our understanding of allergies.[723]

Charles Richet was a eugenicist. He was part of the same eugenics philosophy shared by Bill Gates. Eugenicists think that the earth is overpopulated, and thus it is proper to poison people through vaccination to keep the population in check. Vaccination is the most ingenious way of poisoning because it is slow-acting and brings on death over a long time through a series of disabling diseases that are difficult to trace to their source–vaccines. The government agencies propped up seemingly to protect the public in actuality act as gatekeepers for the pharmaceutical companies to conceal the dangerousness of vaccines and their causal link to life-shortening diseases.

The medical profession and governments know that vaccines contain harmful poisons. Their protestations to the contrary are simply lies. Indeed, adverse reactions to vaccines are listed in the ICD-CM as "poisoning." **Poison is "a substance that through its chemical action usually kills, injures, or impairs an organism."**[724] As we have seen, the vaccine ingredients contain excipients like aluminum, formaldehyde, antibiotics, Polyethylene Glycol, and polysorbate 80 that are neurotoxic and carcinogenic. The adverse events from vaccines sometimes result in death. Most survive the vaccinations only to have a lifetime of health issues. But the poisons in the vaccines are so slow-acting that most do not realize that their allergies, heart conditions, autism, infertility, cancer, and neuromuscular diseases are caused by vaccines. The medical establishment knows the vaccine ingredients are poisonous, and they say so in their billing codes, known as the International Classification of Diseases Clinical Modification (ICD-CM).

The CDC explains:

> [ICD-9-CM and] ICD-10-CM—the International Classification of Diseases, [Ninth and] Tenth Revision[s], Clinical Modification—[...are] based to code and classify medical diagnoses. [ICD-9-CM and] ICD-10-CM [...are] based on [ICD-9 and] ICD-10, the system[s] used to code and classify mortality data from death certificates.[725]

The modern trend in the ICD-CM is away from specifying the specific vaccine that caused the poisoning instead to identifying the vaccine under a generic category of vaccines. For example, "poisoning by tetanus vaccine" under the ICD-9-CM has been swept into the generic category of "Poisoning by other bacterial vaccines" under the ICD-10-CM. "Poisoning by measles vaccine" under the ICD-9-CM has been swept into the generic category of "Poisoning by other viral vaccines" under the ICD-10-CM. The ICDM-9-CM has specific code listings for poisoning by tetanus, diphtheria, measles, poliomyelitis, tuberculosis, typhoid, paratyphoid, cholera, pertussis, smallpox, typhus, yellow fever, and rabies vaccines. Many of those specific ICD-9-CM listings have been recategorized into general categories under the ICD-10-CM. Below are a few examples:

ICD-9-CM Diagnosis Code 978.4: **Poisoning by tetanus vaccine.**[726]
ICD-9-CM Diagnosis Code 978.4 converts approximately to 2025 ICD-10-CM T50.A92A **Poisoning by other bacterial vaccines**, intentional self-harm, initial encounter.[727]

ICD-9-CM Diagnosis Code 978.5: **Poisoning by diphtheria vaccine.**[728]
ICD-9-CM Diagnosis Code 978.5 converts approximately to 2025 ICD-10-CM T50.A92A **Poisoning by other bacterial vaccines**, intentional self-harm, initial encounter.[729]

ICD-9-CM Diagnosis Code 979.4: **Poisoning by measles vaccine.**[730]
ICD-9-CM 979.4 converts approximately to: 2025 ICD-10-CM Diagnosis Code T50.B91A (effective October 1, 2024): **Poisoning by other viral vaccines**, accidental (unintentional), initial encounter.[731]

ICD-9-CM Diagnosis Code 979.5: **Poisoning by poliomyelitis vaccine**.
ICD-9-CM Diagnosis Code 979.5 converts to

approximately 025 ICD-10-CM T50.B91A **Poisoning by other viral vaccines**, accidental (unintentional), initial encounter.[732]

Aborted Fetal Tissue Used in Making Vaccines

Vaccines often contain aborted fetal tissue, and those that do not contain aborted fetal tissue are often developed using aborted fetal tissues. The Vaccine Education Center for the Children's Hospital of Philadelphia explains:

> Vaccines for varicella (chickenpox), rubella (the "R" in the MMR vaccine), hepatitis A, rabies (one version, called Imovax®) and COVID-19 (one U.S.-approved version, Johnson & Johnson (J&J)/Janssen) are all made by growing the viruses in fetal cells. All of these, except the COVID-19 vaccine, are made using fibroblast cells. The COVID-19 vaccine (J&J/Janssen) is made using fetal retinal cells.[733]

The CDC states that there are "[n]o tissues such as aborted fetal cells, gelatin, or any materials from any animal"[734] in the COVID-19 vaccines. But that is misleading because the CDC does not reveal that aborted fetal cells are used in the manufacturing of the COVID-19 vaccines. Furthermore, the CDC is basing its statement that there are no materials from any animals or aborted fetal cells on the fact that the process of making vaccines includes a filtering step that is supposed to remove the animal and fetal cells. That filtering step, though, is not 100% successful. There remain in the vaccines trace amounts of human fetal and animal cells. The British Columbia (BC) immunization information website, run by the BC Ministry of Health, the BC Centre for Disease Control (an agency of the BC Provincial Health Services Authority), the BC Pharmacy Association, and other government and industry organizations, explains that vaccines contain trace amounts of animal and human cells used in production.

> Animal and human cell cultures may be used in the process of making mRNA or viral vector COVID-19 vaccines, but the vaccines do not contain animal or human cells or tissue. The purification process removes nearly all of the cell components so that only **trace amounts of DNA and protein may be present in the vaccine.**[735]

Dr. Brianne Barker, associate professor of biology at Drew University, explains that "in order to make the [Johnson and Johnson COVID-19] vaccine, the scientists give PerC6 [fetal] cells DNA so that they can make the parts of the virus and build that molecular machine—basically the PerC6 [fetal] cells are the factories that make the vaccine for us."[736] The PERC6 fetal cells are allegedly later filtered out of the J&J COVID-19 vaccine before it is put into vials for injection.[737] Pfizer/BioNTech and Moderna used the HEK293 fetal cell lines in their testing stages for their COVID-19 vaccines.[738]

The HEK293 fetal line derived from an elective abortion in the 1970s is routinely used to produce proteins and cultivate viruses.[739] HEK is an acronym for human embryonic kidney cells.

The WI-38 fetal line was derived from fetal tissues harvested from an elective abortion in the 1960s to generate attenuated viruses.[740]

The MRC-5 fetal line was derived from fetal lung tissues harvested from an elective abortion in 1966. The abortion records indicate that it was taken from a 14-week male fetus removed for psychiatric reasons from a 27-year-old woman with a genetically normal family history. MRC-5 is used to generate attenuated viruses.[741]

The origin of PERC6 fetal line is documented through direct testimony before the Food and Drug Administration's Vaccines and Related Biological Products Advisory Committee from Dr. Alex Van Der Eb, who stated: "So I isolated retina [cells] from a fetus, from a healthy fetus as far as could be seen, of 18 weeks old. There was nothing special in the family history, or the pregnancy was completely normal up to 18 weeks, and it turned out to be a socially indicated abortus, abortus provocatus, and that was simply because the woman wanted to get rid of the fetus."[742] The PERC6 fetal line is currently used in the research and development of vaccines.

Novavax has publicly proclaimed: "No human fetal-derived cell lines or tissue, including HEK293 cells, are used in the development, manufacture or production of the Novavax COVID-19 vaccine candidate, NVX-CoV2373."[743]

The HEK293 fetal line mentioned by Novavax refers to the human embryonic kidney (HEK) cells of the victim of an elective abortion in the 1970s.[744]

HEK293 is not the only human fetal cell line. It is rather suspicious that Novavax would specifically cite that particular cell line and claim that it was not used in the "development, manufacture or production" of its COVID-19 vaccine when it turns out that Novavax, indeed, used that very cell line when "testing" the efficacy of its vaccine. Is not testing part of the development of the vaccine? Absolutely!

It seems that Novavax has been caught in a subtle deception. It is more properly described as a bald-faced lie. Novavax funded research that studied the efficacy and safety of their COVID-19 vaccine. That study expressly states that it involved the use of "human embryonic kidney (HEK) 293F cells."[745] Novavax cannot distance itself from the testing because researchers who worked on the study were identified as being employed by or affiliated with Novavax, Jing-Hui Tian, Alyse D. Portnoff, Nita Patel, Michael J. Massare, Greg Glenn, and Gale Smith.[746]

When presented with that damning evidence, Novavax claimed that it "did not use HEK293 cells in the testing of NVX-CoV2373."[747] Novavax, apparently, understood that testing was part of the development of its COVID-19 vaccine and decided to deny that it used the aborted fetal cell line of HEK293 in its testing, although the published paper was, in part, a "testing" study. Thus, rendering Novavax's denial untrue.

Furthermore, the statement from Novavax denying that it used aborted fetal cells in testing its COVID-19 vaccine was later impeached by a letter sent by Novavax to the Charlotte Lozier Institute, wherein Novavax officially admitted:

> Testing was conducted to compare the structural integrity of the SARS-CoV-2 spike protein produced in the Sf9 insect cells versus the spike protein produced in the mammalian human embryonic kidney HEK 293F cells. The comparison determined the Sf9 cell technology produced spike proteins were comparable in structural integrity as the spike proteins produced in the HEK 293F cell.[748]

It seems that Novavax is pathological in its deception. In the same letter sent by Novavax to the Charlotte Lozier Institute, where it admitted that its vaccine was tested on aborted fetal tissue, Novavax stated that "fetal-derived cell lines were not used in the manufacture, testing, or production of the Novavax COVID-19 vaccine."[749]

"Oh what a tangled web we weave when first we practice to deceive."

The Inova Hospital System is spreading the Novavax lie. Indeed, the Inova imprimatur of the Novavaz vaccine includes the provably false statement that "the Novavax vaccine has no linkage to cell lines from aborted fetuses." Inova prefaces its conclusion with an official statement from Novavax that "no human fetal-derived cell lines or tissues are contained in the Novavax COVID-19 vaccine, adjuvanted, or used in the development, manufacture, or release testing."

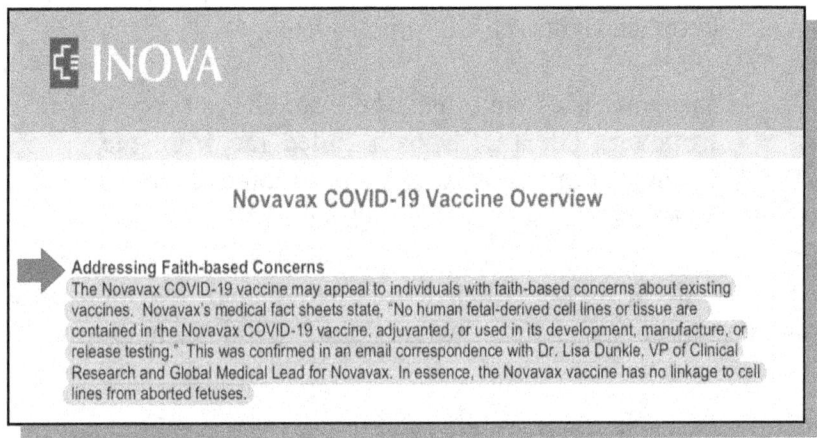

Release testing is something that is done after the release of a product. Apparently, Novavax is now quibbling that they did not test their product on aborted fetal cells after the product was released. I guess they hope that will be enough to pull the wool over the eyes of most who will not realize that Novavax, in fact, tested their COVID-19 vaccine on aborted fetal cells before releasing it. Proof that the equivocation is simply an effort by Novavax to obfuscate their guilt in using aborted fetal tissue is found in the statement by INOVA that "[i]n essence, the Novavax vaccine has no linkage to cell lines from aborted fetuses." Read that again. INOVA interprets Novavax's claim that there was no release testing using fetal tissue, as meaning that the vaccine has no linkage to aborted fetuses. That is what Novavax wants people to believe. But it is a deception; it is not true.

Abortion is the sin of unjustifiable homicide. God states that we are living souls from the moment of conception in the womb.

> For thou hast possessed my reins: thou hast covered me in my mother's womb. I will praise thee; for I am fearfully and wonderfully made: marvellous are thy works; and that my soul knoweth right well. (Psalms 139:13-14)

> Listen, O isles, unto me; and hearken, ye people, from far; The LORD hath called me from the womb; from the bowels of my mother hath he made mention of my name. (Isaiah 49:1)

Indeed, we are ordained to be living souls by God before our conception in our mothers' wombs. God forms us in the womb.

> Before I formed thee in the belly I knew thee; and before thou camest forth out of the womb I sanctified thee, and I ordained thee a prophet unto the nations. (Jeremiah 1:5)

God is the creator of all things, including the creator of each man in his mother's womb.

> As thou knowest not what is the way of the spirit, nor how the bones do grow in the womb of her that is with child: even so thou knowest not the works of God who maketh all. (Ecclesiastes 11:5)

God of the Lord of all, both born and unborn.

> I was cast upon thee from the womb: thou *art* my God from my mother's belly. (Psalms 22:10)

Fetuses in the womb are sentient. We see that in Luke when, Elizabeth was greeted by Mary, who was pregnant with Jesus. John the Babtist, who was unborn and in Elizabeth's womb jumped for joy upon hearing the Mary's greeting.

> And it came to pass, that, when Elisabeth heard the salutation of Mary, the babe leaped in her womb; and Elisabeth was filled with the Holy Ghost: (Luke 1:41)

God hates the shedding of innocent blood.

> These six things doth the LORD hate: yea, seven are an abomination unto him: A proud look, a lying tongue, and **hands that shed innocent blood**, An heart that deviseth wicked imaginations, feet that be swift in running to mischief, A false witness that speaketh lies, and he that soweth discord among brethren. (Proverbs 6:16-19)

The Holy Bible states that God elected Jacob as the heir to the promise. God elected Jacob before he was born.

> That is, They which are the children of the flesh, these are not the children of God: but the children of the promise are counted for the seed. For this is the word of promise, At this time will I come, and Sara shall have a son. And not only this; but when Rebecca also had conceived by one, even by our father Isaac; (For the children being not yet born, neither having done any good or evil, that the purpose of God according to election might stand, not of works, but of him that calleth;) It was said

unto her, The elder shall serve the younger. As it is written, Jacob have I loved, but Esau have I hated. (Romans 9:8-13)

Notice also what God states about Jacob and Esau. God elected Jacob before they were born and before either he or Esau had done any good or evil. That means that children who are aborted have not done any evil. There is no justification for their death; they are innocent. The killers are culpable, and those who encourage and abet them in their deadly scheme are accomplices in that sin. Unless they repent and turn in faith to Jesus Christ, they will be punished by God accordingly. *See* Matthew 25:31-46; Romans 2:3-9; 2 Corinthians 5:10; Revelation 20:11-15.

Abortion is homicide. God has commanded that we shall not kill one another. "Thou shalt not kill." (Exodus 20:13)

27 Vaccines Are Dangerous Medical Quackery

The COVID-19 vaccine is not an anomaly. It is just the most recent vaccine atrocity. Vaccination is medical quackery.[750] But because vaccinations fulfill the perverted ends of Satan and his minions, the practice flourishes. Vaccines are unsafe and ineffective. James Howenstine, M.D., in his book, *A Physicians Guide to Natural Health Products*, revealed that "[a] New Zealand study disclosed that 23% of vaccinated children develop asthma compared to zero in unvaccinated children."[751] One suppressed study proves that "vaccinated children appear to be significantly less healthy than the unvaccinated."[752]

In that study funded by The Institute for Pure and Applied Knowledge (IPAK) and published in the International Journal of Environmental Research and Public Health it was determined that unvaccinated children are significantly healthier than vaccinated children.[753] The conclusion from the study is that vaccinating children causes them to suffer a "significant" increase in asthma, allergies, breathing issues, behavioral issues, ADHD, respiratory infections, otitis media (ear infections), ear pain, infections, conjunctivitis (eye infections), eye disorders, eczema, dermatitis, urticaria (hives), and anemia.

The study made a notable finding. "Remarkably, zero of the 561 unvaccinated patients in the study had attention deficit hyperactivity disorder (ADHD) compared to 0.063% of the (partially and fully) vaccinated."

The chart below shows the "[c]umulative office visits in the vaccinated (orange) vs. unvaccinated (blue) patients born into [Dr. Paul Thomas' pediatric] practice: the clarity of the age-specific differences in the health fates of individuals who are vaccinated (2763) compared to the 561 unvaccinated in patients born into the practice over ten years is most strikingly clear in this comparison of the cumulative numbers of diagnoses in the two patient groups. The number of office visits for the unvaccinated is adjusted by a sample size multiplier factor (4.9) to the expected value as if the number of unvaccinated in the study was the same as the number of vaccinated."[754]

The study reported: "The visual impact of the cumulative office visit plots is striking; more so than other plots, the time element (day of life) provides an index by which to compare the accumulation of human pain and suffering from potential vaccine side effects ... [chart below]. These results are worth studying closely and noticing the variation among the cumulative office visits per condition and the stark differences between the rates of billed office visits in the most and unvaccinated patients born into the practice." Below are charts that graphically illustrate the difference in the number of office visits for various diagnosed ailments between vaccinated children ([upper light gray] orange line) and unvaccinated ([lower dark gray] blue line) children. The stark difference illustrates the significantly better health of unvaccinated children.

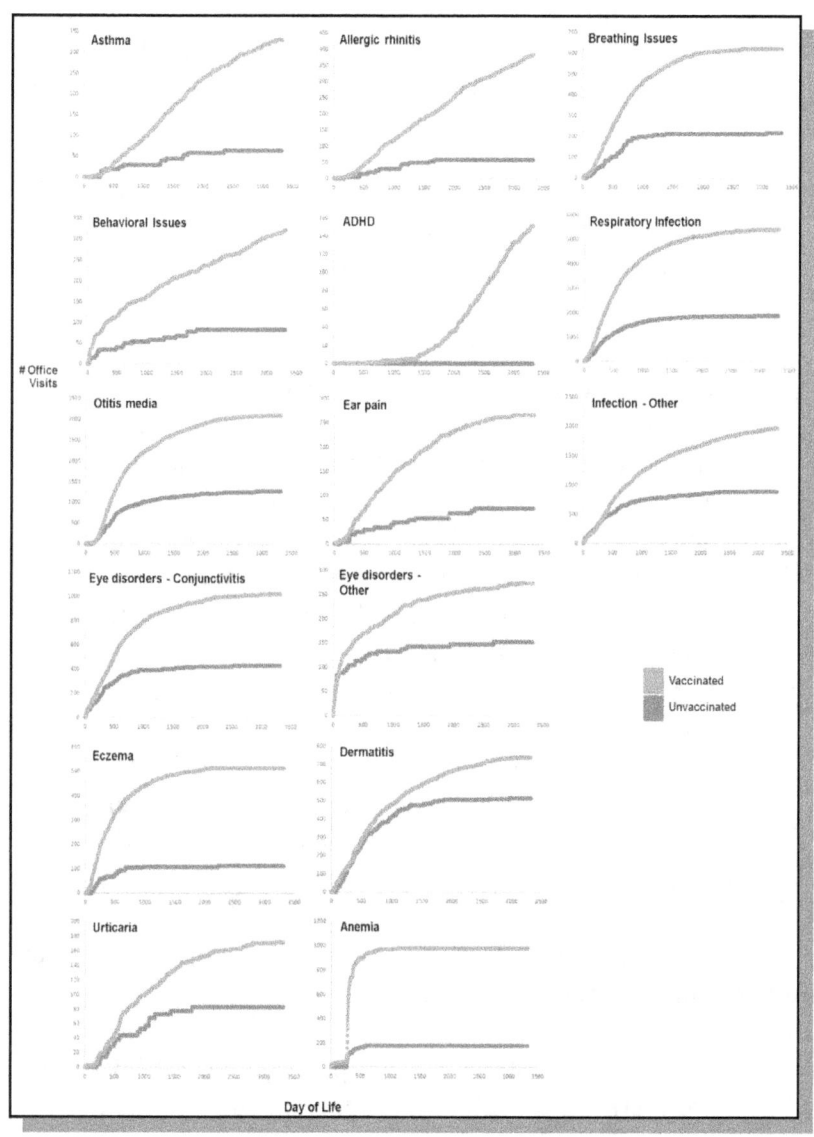

The above study was later retracted based on the unsubstantiated complaint from an anonymous source.[755] The study's authors revisited the data to address the claim by the complainant and found that the complaint was without merit. Their confirmation study was published and has not been refuted or retracted. Their revisit of the study confirmed their initial conclusions that vaccinated children are significantly less healthy than unvaccinated children.

> Studies finding associations between vaccines and adverse conditions have been targeted for retraction. Here, we revisit data from one such study, comparing the increase in office visits for conditions independent of the routine "well-child" visits (hereafter, Health Care Visits; HCVs). The retraction occurred after >1/4 of a million people had read the peer-reviewed study. It was targeted by one anonymous reader who complained he did not believe the published results. His complaint hinged on the supposition —unsupported by any data —that vaccinated children made their scheduled HCVs more regularly than unvaccinated, implying that those unkept appointments led to fewer diagnoses. We show, here, new data from the same practice that the opposite is true. When the data for vaccinated versus unvaccinated children are examined, the critic's claim is exactly reversed.[756]

Steve Kirsch explains the motive behind the skulduggery in retracting Dr. Thomas' study.

> The [Thomas] study was unethically retracted by the journal over the objection of the authors, i.e., the journal didn't follow the COPE guidelines. They said that "the conclusions were not supported by strong scientific data" which is NOT a valid reason to retract a study once it is published. The journal retracted the paper after an anonymous person claimed (without any evidence) that the

results could be due to fewer office visits by the unvaxxed. The author provided evidence that this was not the case, but the journal ignored the evidence. Why? Because the paper got 250,000 views, it had to be retracted because it was counter-narrative and too popular. Later, a new paper showed proof that the reason the journal gave for retracting the paper was clearly false. The journal decided not to admit they were wrong and did not reverse the retraction of the Thomas paper. This is corruption of the highest magnitude.[757]

Please notice the chart below relating to ADHD (Attention-Deficit/Hyperactivity Disorder). ADHD begins to manifest as soon as the vaccinated children begin going to school and their ADHD behavior becomes noticeable relative to their classmates. What the study chart does not break out from ADHD are the children who are also suffering from autism. Autism falls within a spectrum and is often referred to as Autism spectrum disorder (ASD). Children and Adults with Attention-Deficit/Hyperactivity Disorder (CHADD) is an organization that provides support, education and encouragement to parents, educators and professionals regarding ADHD issues on a grassroots level. CHADD explains the relationship between ADHD and ASD:

> More than half of all individuals who have been diagnosed with ASD also have signs of ADHD. In fact, ADHD is the most common coexisting condition in children with ASD. On the flip side, up to a quarter of children with ADHD have low-level signs of ASD, which might include having difficulty with social skills or being very sensitive to clothing textures, for example.
>
> Both ADHD and ASD are neurodevelopmental

disorders (brain development has been affected in some way). That means both conditions/disorders affect the central nervous system, which is responsible for movement, language, memory, and social and focusing skills. A number of scientific studies have shown that the two conditions often coexist, but researchers have not yet figured out why they do.

Objective research has established a direct link between vaccination and ASD. The chart below tells a clear story that vaccines cause ADHD. CHADD says that researchers have not yet figured out why ASD and ADHD often coincide with one another. That is not true. All one need to do is look at the chart below and realize that ADHD and ASD are both neurodevelopmental disorders to understand that they are both caused by vaccine poisoning.

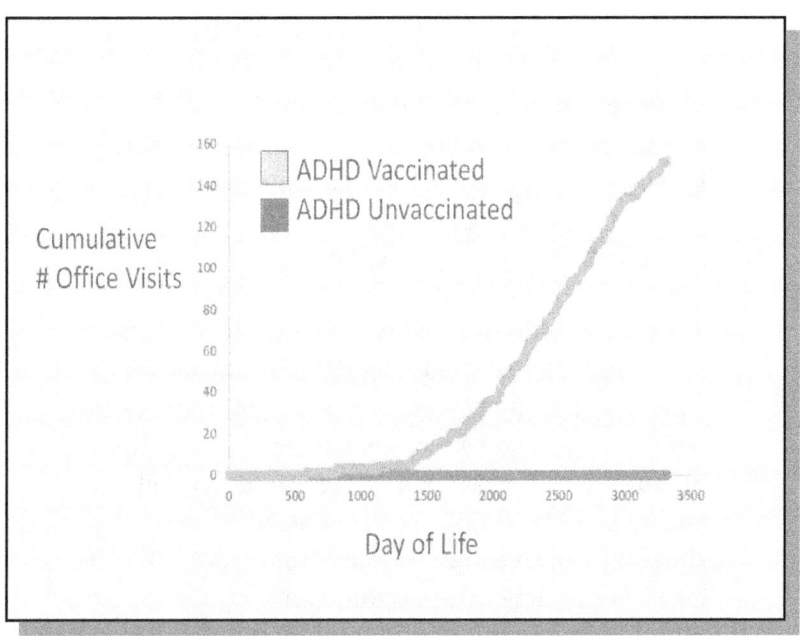

The two researchers who conducted the study, Dr. James Lyons-Weiler and Dr. Paul Thomas are not anti-vaccination doctors. But publishing data that refutes the vaccine paradigm comes with a cost. As a direct result of this study, the state medical board suspended the medical license of one of the researchers, Dr. Paul Thomas, within a week of the publication of the article. The suspension was in retaliation for having published the study showing the harmful effects of childhood vaccinations. The suspension was an unprecedented action because it was done summarily prior to any adversarial hearing. He is being punished as an object lesson for anyone who would have the temerity to publish the truth about vaccinations being harmful to the health of patients. Jeremy Hammond explains:

> On December 3, 2020, the Oregon Medical Board issued an emergency suspension order to prevent renowned pediatrician Paul Thomas, MD, from

seeing his patients by stripping him of his license.

The ostensible reason given by the board for this action against Thomas, who is affectionately known as "Dr. Paul" by his patients and peers, is that his "continued practice constitutes an immediate danger to public health".

Thomas is perhaps most well known as coauthor, along with Dr. Jennifer Margulis, of the book The Vaccine-Friendly Plan, which provides guidance to parents who want to protect their children from infectious diseases but have concerns about vaccines. The book is a bestseller currently showing a five-star rating from over 1,800 customer reviews at Amazon.com.

Since 2008, Thomas has practiced pediatrics out of his clinic, Integrative Pediatrics, which is in Beaverton, Oregon, within the metropolitan area of Portland.

The main accusation leveled at Thomas by the state medical board is that he has "breached the standard of care" in his practice by having many patients who are not vaccinated strictly according to the routine childhood schedule recommended by the Centers for Disease Control and Prevention (CDC).

The story the medical board tells is one of a reckless and "bullying" doctor who coerces his pediatric patients' parents not to follow the CDC's recommendations and whose gross negligence in this regard has caused harm to children and negatively impacted the health of the community.[758]

But that's not the true story.

The *true* story is that parents have flocked to Integrative Pediatrics precisely because they've been bullied, with the state's approval, by pediatricians in other practices who choose to dutifully serve the bureaucrats in government by compelling parents to strictly comply with the CDC's schedule.

Parents who *did* comply and then witnessed their children suffer harm as a result are mocked and derisively labeled "anti-vaxxers" for learning hard lessons from their firstborn children that they then apply to younger siblings by making different parenting choices. (Often, such parents respond to the derogatory label by insisting on being described as "ex-vaxxers", but government officials and the major media institutions refuse to hear them.)

Parents who *do* vaccinate their children, but not strictly according to the CDC's schedule, are also lumped into the group monolithically labeled "the anti-vaccine movement" by apologists for the one-size-fits-all approach of public vaccine policy.

These parents have all been told a million times that vaccines are "safe and effective". They are well aware of the arguments in favor of vaccinations that we all hear incessantly from government officials, medical professionals, and the mainstream media.

They are also perfectly familiar with the tale of how, in 1998, public enemy number one, Dr. Andrew Wakefield, published a fraudulent study in

The Lancet, later retracted, claiming to have found an association between the measles, mumps, and rubella (MMR) vaccine and autism. In my own case, our son's pediatrician told us during an early well-child visit that Wakefield was serving time in prison for what he'd done, which I knew was untrue. This attempt to persuade us into compliance consequently served only to reaffirm our conviction that we shouldn't assume doctors are trustworthy and should rather do our own research, think for ourselves, and trust our own judgment. These parents know that numerous studies have since been published that failed to find an association.

They know that, by choosing to dissent from or criticize public vaccine policy, they are placing a target on their back. They know they will be met with disapproval by other members of their own family, accused of being irresponsible parents, scolded, and scorned. They know that they will be viciously attacked by government officials and policy advocates masquerading as journalists, as well as by doctors and other members of their community. (I, too, have experienced rifts within my family over this issue, and, naturally, as someone who has for years been publicly criticizing public vaccine policy, I have experienced countless personal attacks on my character.) (parenthetical originally in endnote)

And yet, despite the bullying and intimidation, they remain unmoved. There is one simple reason for this: they see it as their duty as responsible parents to act in their children's best interest no matter what societal pressures are placed on them to conform with expected behavior. Consequently, they do their own research, think for themselves, draw their own conclusions, and take a stand to protect their children.

In many cases in Portland, parents who face the scornful intimidation of a routine well-child visit at their pediatrician's office and still insist on exercising their right to make an informed choice not to vaccinate are told that they must either comply with the CDC's recommendations or find another pediatrician. (Just since publishing this article, my family has also experienced this kind of bullying due to a policy change at our son's pediatric practice. On May 5, 2021, we were given an ultimatum by one of the doctors there to either vaccinate him according to the AAP's recommendations (synonymous with the CDC's recommendations) or never come back. We declined the unnecessary and risk-carrying pharmaceutical products and so were expelled. [...]) (parenthetical originally in endnote)

And, so, they go to Dr. Paul.

With respect to the medical board's suspension order, Paul Thomas says that he knew the moment The Vaccine-Friendly Plan was published that this day was coming. He knew at the time that, because he was challenging the CDC's schedule and therefore the "standard of care" of the medical establishment, he would be placing a target on his back and risking his career.

But he did it anyway.

Why?

The Oregon Medical Board wants us to believe it's because he's a villain who demonstrates reckless disregard and poses a danger to public health. The media have run with that story.

But what the results of the study do demonstrate to a reasonable degree of certainty is that his unvaccinated patients are healthier than vaccinated children and place less of a burden on the health care system.

However, what neither the board's order nor the media have disclosed is that the board's suspension order was issued just eleven days after Thomas published a study in a peer-reviewed medical journal showing that, among the children born into his practice, those who remained completely unvaccinated were diagnosed at significantly lower rates than vaccinated children for a broad range of chronic health conditions and developmental disorders.

The difference in health outcomes was even more dramatic when Thomas and his coauthor, research scientist Dr. James Lyons-Weiler, looked at cumulative incidence of office visits for given diagnoses rather than incidence of diagnoses alone. This result strongly suggests that his vaccinated patients not only suffer from a higher rate of chronic health conditions, but also that their conditions are more severe, therefore requiring more frequent visits to his clinic.

The study is titled "Relative Incidence of Office

Visits and Cumulative Rates of Billed Diagnoses Along the Axis of Vaccination." It was published in the International Journal of Environmental Research and Public Health on November 22, 2020.

As Thomas and Lyons-Weiler emphasize in the study, they do not show that vaccinations are the cause of the evidently worse health outcomes among vaccinated children. But what the results of the study do demonstrate to a reasonable degree of certainty is that his unvaccinated patients are healthier than vaccinated children and place less of a burden on the health care system.[759]

Importantly, this was data that the medical board had asked Thomas to produce to support his practice of vaccinating patients according to the principles of his "Vaccine-Friendly Plan".

Yet, when Thomas surmounted this challenge by obtaining Institutional Review Board (IRB) approval and publishing the deidentified data comparing health outcomes between vaccinated and unvaccinated children, the board's emergent response was to suspend his license until further notice "while this case remains under investigation"—and on grounds that are completely belied by the publicly available evidence. (endnote deleted)

The real story here isn't one of a rogue doctor dismissing science and recklessly endangering his pediatric patients by bullying their parents into accepting "alternative" care. The real story is one of a rogue medical board dismissing science and recklessly endangering public health by encouraging pediatricians to bully their parents into strict compliance with the CDC's schedule and selecting Paul Thomas, MD, to set an example to other physicians of what their punishment will be if they instead choose to respect parents' right to informed consent.

But that story doesn't begin in December of 2020. To tell the true story and fully appreciate its significance, we need to go back and review the sequence of events that led Paul Thomas to this pivotal moment in his life's journey.

On 16 July 2021, the MDPI retracted the article with the following cryptic notice. "The journal retracts the article 'Relative Incidence of Office Visits and Cumulative Rates of Billed Diagnoses along the Axis of Vaccination' cited above. Following publication, concerns were brought to the attention of the editorial office regarding the validity of the conclusions of the published research. Adhering to our complaints procedure, an investigation was conducted that raised several methodological issues and confirmed that the conclusions were not supported by strong scientific data. The article is therefore retracted. This retraction is approved by the Editor in Chief of the journal. The authors did not agree to this retraction."[760] The MDPI did not indicate what were the "methodological issues" or specify how the conclusions "were not supported by strong scientific data." That lack of specificity for such an extraordinary action suggests the retraction of the article by the MDPI was not due to methodological issues or that it was not supported by strong scientific data but was rather due to financial and political pressure put on MDPI.

The following report was posted on the Institute for Pure and Applied Knowledge (IPAK) website:

> Independent journalist Jeremy Hammond has authored a definitive and thorough report[761] that reveals that the Oregon Medical Board is guilty of wrong-doing because they tried to coerce Dr. Thomas into changing his lawful pediatric practice into an unlawful medical practice under Oregon's state law.

The IPAK report explains that the real story isn't a negligent doctor dismissing science and recklessly endangering his pediatric patients by hoodwinking parents into not vaccinating their children. The real story is one of a villainous medical board endangering public health by encouraging pediatricians to scare parents into strict compliance with the CDC's schedule. The rogue medical board selected Dr. Thomas, MD, to set an example to other physicians of what would happen to them if they choose to accede to the parents' right to informed consent.

> Under Oregon state law, phyisicians, including pediatricians, must provide for fully informed consent and respect vaccine refusal. The board had tried to sanction Dr. Thomas for allowing patients to use antibody titre-testing as evidence of immunity. It [the Hammond report[762]] found that the board's actions were "ludicrous given the fact that Oregon law only requires one dose of mumps vaccine, and it specifically allows for the use of antibody testing as evidence of immunity in lieu of evidence of vaccination."

The report also completely rebuts all eight of the allegations of medical misconduct alleged by the Oregon Medical Board. Under current Oregon law, The Board answers to the Governor of the State of Oregon.[763]

Rhoda Wilson reveals in the April 11, 2022, edition of The Expose a groundbreaking study comparing the health of a group of 1,482 unvaccinated adults and children to the national statistics on the health of vaccinated adults.[764] The study conducted by an organization called *The Control Group* reveals that unvaccinated adults are significantly healthier than vaccinated adults.[765]

The Control Group filed a complaint in federal court seeking a declaratory judgment and injunctive relief against the federal government alleging its vaccine laws, regulations, and policies are unscientific and violate the constitutional rights of the people.[766] But their complaint was dismissed and "on October 3, 2022, the US Supreme Court denied The Control Group's petition for writ of certiorari. So this health freedom case is now closed."[767]

Despite the failure of the Control Group in court, the facts that they established in their study will have a long-term benefit to all who seek justice in the future. The study is robust and unimpeachable. Dr. Stephen Malthouse states:

> Every so often a study comes along that shakes the bedrock of medicine. The Control Group compared unvaccinated adults to vaccinated adults in the US and what they discovered is incredible. Perhaps one of the most surprising findings is that vit K shots, containing aluminum in most cases (although not always disclosed on the list of ingredients), played a significant role in adult (and childhood) chronic disease. If you get rid of vit K shots and all vaccinations, the incidence of heart disease,

asthma, autism, and other severe disorders goes practically to zero.[768]

Below is a sample of some of the charts that were filed as exhibits in the litigation by the Control Group.

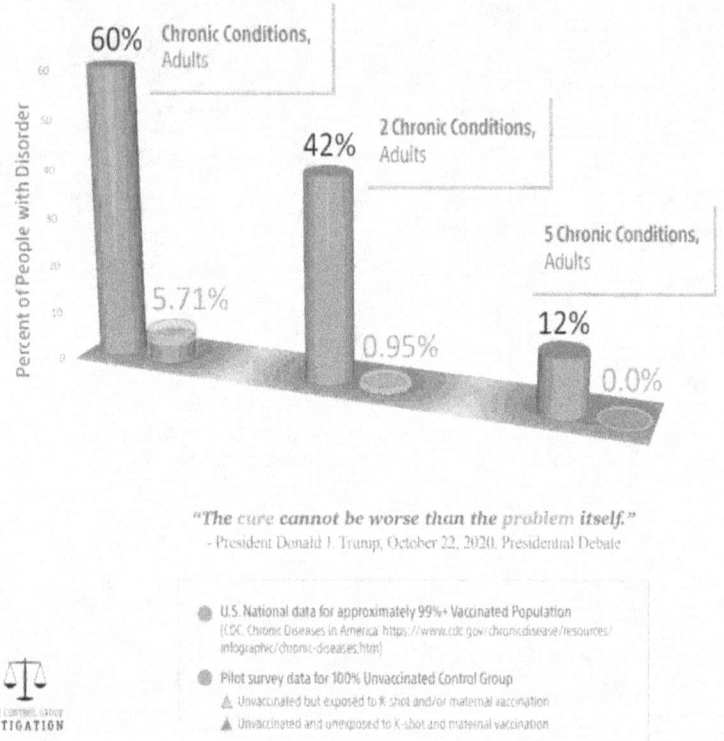

60% of adults in the vaccinated population had chronic health conditions, while **5.71%** of adults in the unvaccinated group had chronic health conditions. **42%** of adults in the vaccinated population had 2 chronic health conditions, while **0.95%%** of adults in the unvaccinated group had 2 chronic health conditions. **12%** of adults in the vaccinated population had 5 chronic health conditions, while **0.0%%** of adults in the unvaccinated group had 5 chronic health conditions.

2020 Pilot Survey Data Comparison
VACCINATED -vs- UNVACCINATED

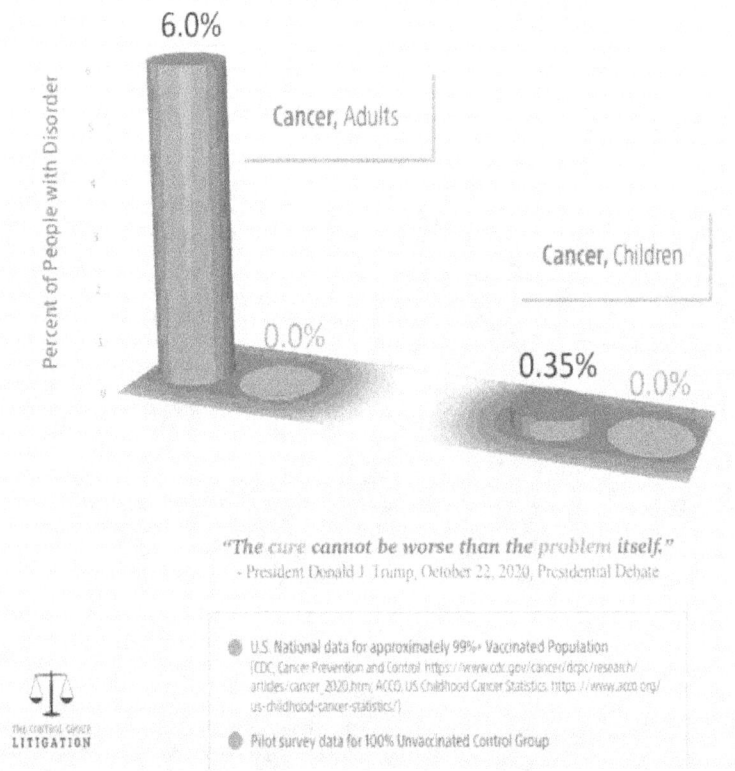

"The cure cannot be worse than the problem itself."
- President Donald J. Trump, October 22, 2020, Presidential Debate

- U.S. National data for approximately 99%+ Vaccinated Population (CDC, Cancer Prevention and Control https://www.cdc.gov/cancer/dcpc/research/articles/cancer_2020.htm; ACCO, US Childhood Cancer Statistics, https://www.acco.org/us-childhood-cancer-statistics/)
- Pilot survey data for 100% Unvaccinated Control Group

6% of adults in the vaccinated population had cancer, while **0%** of adults in the unvaccinated group had cancer. **0.35%** of children in the vaccinated population had cancer, while **0.0%** of children in the unvaccinated group had cancer.

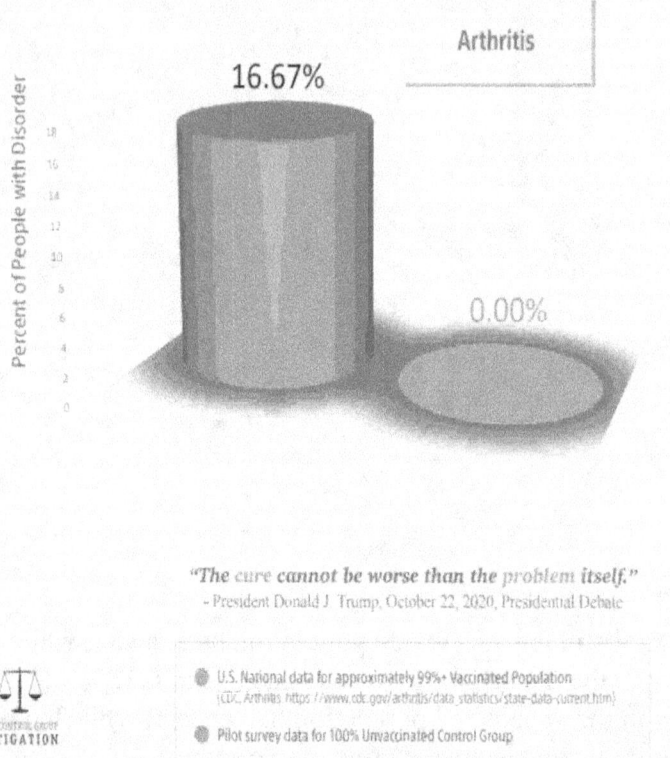

16.67% of adults in the vaccinated population had arthritis, while **0.0%** of adults in the unvaccinated group had arthritis.

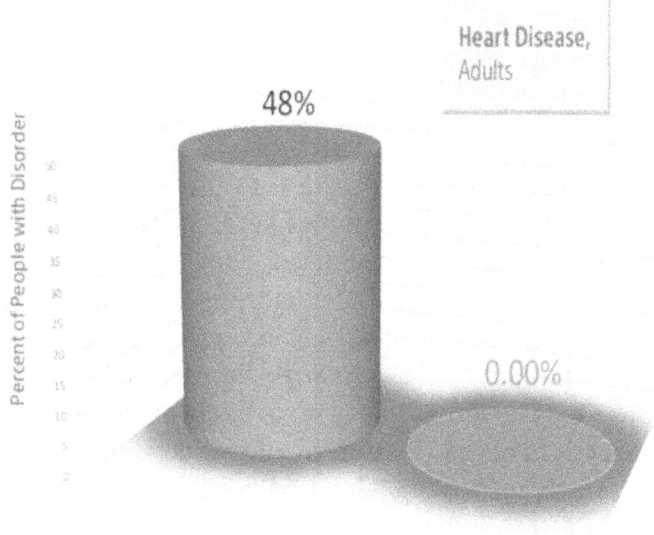

2020 Pilot Survey Data Comparison
VACCINATED -vs- UNVACCINATED

Heart Disease, Adults

"The cure cannot be worse than the problem itself."
- President Donald J. Trump, October 22, 2020, Presidential Debate

LITIGATION

- U.S. National data for approximately 99%+ Vaccinated Population (AHA, Cardiovascular diseases affect nearly half of American adults, statistics show. https://www.heart.org/en/news/2019/01/31/cardiovascular-diseases-affect-nearly-half-of-american-adults-statistics-show)
- Pilot survey data for 100% Unvaccinated Control Group

48% of adults in the vaccinated population had heart disease, while **0%** of adults in the unvaccinated group had heart disease.

Yet another study in 2020 came up with the same results. The study found that vaccinated children were much sicker than unvaccinated children. The researchers concluded:

> In this study, based on a convenience sample of children born into one of three distinct pediatric medical practices, higher ORs [odds ratios] were observed within the vaccinated versus unvaccinated group for developmental delays, asthma and ear infections.[769]

The 2017 Mawson study comparing the health of vaccinated children to the health of unvaccinated children concluded that the vaccinated children were much less healthy than the unvaccinated children.[770] Indeed, the study showed that vaccinated children were 2.4 times more likely to have chronic illnesses, 2.9 times more likely to develop eczema, 3.7 times more likely to incur a neurodevelopmental disorder, 4.2 times more likely to develop autism, 4.2 times more likely to develop ADHD, 5.2 times more likely to develop learning disabilities, and 30.1 times more likely to develop allergic rhinitis.

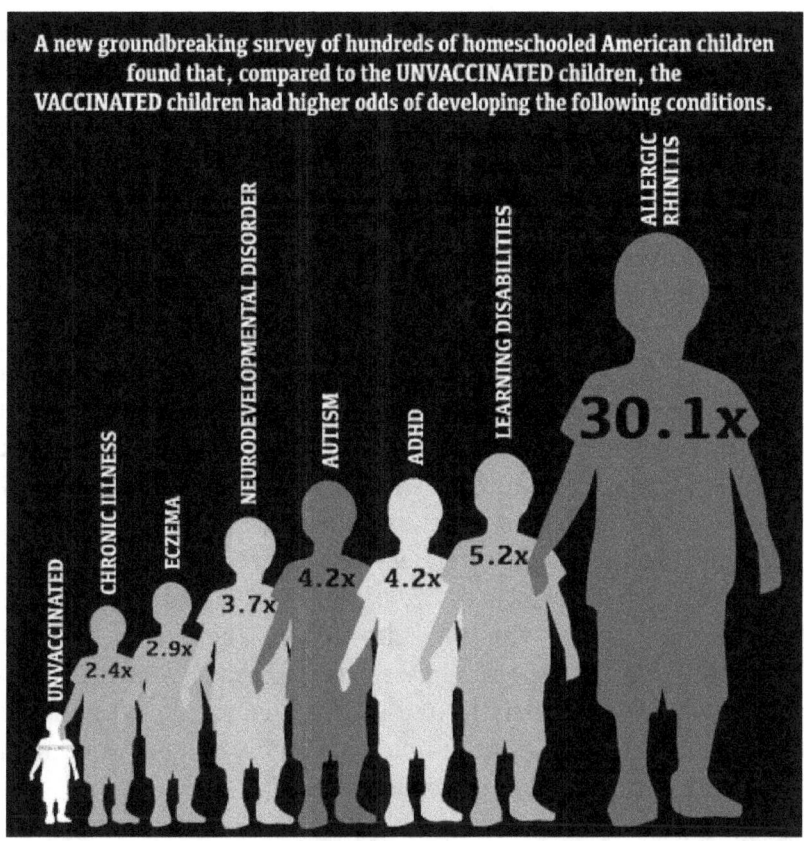

Other studies have confirmed the Mawson results.[771] For example, Steve Kirsch surveyed the parents of 10,000 children and found a 5-fold increase in autism for vaccinated children compared to unvaccinated children.[772] A study of 9,000 boys in California and Oregon found that "vaccinated boys had a 155% greater chance of having a neurological disorder like ADHD or autism than unvaccinated boys."[773] It seems that sinus issues are endemic with vaccines. The Mawson study showed a 30.1-fold greater incidence of allergic rhinitis among the vaccinated children compared to the unvaccinated children; Kirsch found that vaccinated children showed a 33-fold greater incidence in sinusitis compared to the unvaccinated children.

In November 2012, Dr. Coleen Boyle, the CDC's Director of the National Center on Birth Defects and Developmental Disabilities, testified under oath before the House Committee on Oversight and Government Reform that "we have not studied vaccinated versus unvaccinated [children]." Robert F. Kennedy Jr. states, "that was perjury."[774] Kennedy, through Freedom of Information requests, found out that, indeed, the CDC has done vaccinated vs. unvaccinated comparative health studies.

Kennedy discovered that in 1999, the CDC employed an in-house researcher, Thomas Verstraeten, to conduct a vaccinated vs. unvaccinated study using CDC's giant Vaccine Safety Datalink (VSD). The study evaluated whether cumulative ethylmercury exposure from thimerosal-containing vaccines after one month of life increased "the subsequent risk of degenerative and developmental neurologic disorders and renal disorders before the age of six."[775] The study results proved that vaccines were dangerous to the health of children. The study concluded that "high exposure to ethylmercury from thimerosal-containing vaccines in the first month of life increases the risk of subsequent development of neurologic development impairment."[776]

In particular, the study found that the relative risk of autism for vaccinated children was 7.6 times greater than the unvaccinated children. The study also found that the relative risk of sleep disorders for vaccinated children was 5 times greater than unvaccinated children. The study further found that the relative risk of speech disorders for vaccinated children was 2.1 times greater than unvaccinated children. The study found that the relative risk for neurological development disorders for vaccinated children was 1.8 times greater than unvaccinated children.

The CDC could not allow that information to get out. So they instituted a plan to coverup the results of the study. Robert F. Kennedy Jr. explains:

The world's largest vaccine maker GSK whisked Verstraeten off to a sinecure in Brussels and CDC handed his raw data to his CDC boss Frank DeStefano and another researcher, Robert Davis who served as a vaccine industry consultant. Those two men tortured the data for 4 years, removing all unvaccinated children, to bury the autism signal before publishing a sanitized version purporting to exculpate the vaccine. The CDC then cut off public access to the VSD and to this day aggressively blocks any attempts by researchers to study health outcomes in vaccinated vs. unvaccinated populations.[777]

The fraudulently altered study that ended up being published changed the actual conclusion in the original study from showing that "high exposure to ethylmercury from thimerosal-containing vaccines in the first month of life increases the risk of subsequent development of neurologic development impairment"[778] to, instead, say that "[n]o consistent significant associations were found between TCVs [thimerosal-containing vaccines] and neurodevelopmental outcomes."[779]

Kennedy caught government health officials red-handed lying to Congress and engaging in fraud to conceal the dangers of childhood vaccines. This is not merely negligence or dereliction of duty; it is part of a well-funded conspiracy to injure and kill children. This is the behavior of sociopathic criminals. The childhood vaccine scheme constitutes organized crime that is more sophisticated and more dangerous than any mafia syndicate.

The pharmaceutical companies and the governments of the world know that vaccines cause harm. All published vaccine studies funded by pharmaceutical companies and governments are scams. Steve Kirsch explains how pharmaceutical company and government funded researchers accomplish the deception.

When you read the peer-review literature carefully, you'll find that they always consider the "unvaccinated" group to have kids without the particular vaccine under study. So when they compare the MMR vaccine, they compare it to the kids who didn't get the MMR vaccine. So it's like comparing the autism rates of kids who got 28 vaccines with the rates of kids who got 27 vaccines. This is how they hide the signal. They design studies which are designed to fail. Just because they don't find a signal, it doesn't mean that it isn't there. It just means their study design didn't find the signal. They will NEVER compare the chronic disease rates in kids who got all recommended vaccines (well over 50 shots, many with multiple vaccines) vs. completely unvaccinated kids. It simply has never happened. The excuse that unvaccinated kids are too hard to find is ridiculous. The Amish have thousands of such kids and there are hundreds of such kids that can be located in a heartbeat. All they have to do is call me and I'll be happy to help.[780]

Steve Kirsch challenged the seminal government-funded research study from Denmark that allegedly showed no causation between the MMR vaccine and autism.[781] Kirsh alleged that the researchers purposely "chose a study design that was designed to look credible but obscure any signal."[782] In essence, the study was a scam. Kirsch challenged one of the study's principal authors, Professor Anders Hviid, to provide the underlying data and defend his study. Kirsch even offered him $25,000 if Professor Hviid could successfully defend his study. Professor Hviid refused the offer and took steps to block Kirsch. Kirsch sent Professor Hviid an article he wrote detailing his challenge of the research and asked him for comments; Hviid did not respond and instead immediately made his tweets only viewable by followers;

Professor Hviid then did not allow Kirsch to follow him on Twitter. Professor Hviid refuses to address the errors in his study. As Kirsch points out, truth does not mind being questioned; a lie does not like being challenged.

There is convincing evidence that the Denmark autism study was part of a coordinated plan to mislead the public about the dangers of vaccines.[783] Fraud is woven through the warp and woof of the study. Notably, one of the study's co-authors, Dr. Paul Thorsen, is presently a fugitive from justice; he is charged with wire fraud and money laundering for stealing infant disability and autism study grant money.[784]

A randomized study published in 2018 by the highly respected Dr. Peter Aaby found that the Diphtheria–Tetanus–Pertussis (DTP) vaccine caused children to die at a higher rate than unvaccinated children.[785] By the way, Dr. Aaby is not against vaccinations. Indeed, he promotes vaccinations. Yet he concluded that the DTP vaccine is killing children. Aaron Siri explains that Dr. Aaby is a long-time promoter of vaccines:

> Dr. Aaby is renowned for studying and promoting vaccines in Africa with over 300 published studies. ... Among his accolades, in 2000, Dr. Aaby was awarded the Novo Nordisk Prize, the most important Danish award within health research, and in 2009, the Danish Ministry of Foreign Affairs selected Dr. Aaby as a leader in the fight against global poverty.[786]

The conclusion of Dr. Aaby's study was that "[a]lthough having better nutritional status and being protected against three infections, 6–35 months old DTP-vaccinated children tended to have higher mortality than DTP-unvaccinated children. All studies of the introduction of DTP have found increased overall mortality."

Other studies have shown that the mortality rate for DTP-vaccinated children is two (2) times greater than for unvaccinated children. Dr. Aaby explains that "[a]ll studies that documented vaccination status and followed children prospectively indicate that DTP has negative effects; a meta-analysis of the eight studies found 2-fold higher mortality for DTP-vaccinated compared with DTP-unvaccinated."

Doubling the mortality rate is bad enough, but that is not the whole story. The studies referenced by Dr. Aaby were biased in favor of the vaccinated group because the vaccinated groups were healthier babies. Dr. Aaby explains that "the 'unvaccinated' control children in previous studies having been a frail subgroup, too frail to get vaccinated." Thus, the unvaccinated babies did not receive the DTP vaccine because the doctors determined they were too frail and unhealthy to tolerate a vaccination. But when the study measured babies of similar health, the detrimental effect of the DTP vaccine is revealed in all its horror. Dr. Aaby explains that "DTP [vaccination] was associated with 5-fold higher mortality than being unvaccinated."[787]

That is bad enough, but it gets worse. You see, the unvaccinated group cited by Dr. Aaby in his conclusion simply means unvaccinated with DTP. The "unvaccinated" babies in that group had, in fact, been vaccinated with the oral polio vaccine (OPV). When the children that received the OPV are excluded from the unvaccinated group, the mortality rate for children receiving a DTP vaccine skyrockets to ten (10) times that for children receiving no vaccination. That suggests that there is also an increase in mortality due to the OPV.

When isolating only the DTP-vaccinated children and comparing them to the truly unvaccinated children, the simple conclusion is that vaccinating a child with the DTP vaccination increases his chances of dying in the first 6 months of his life by ten (10) fold.

Dr. Aaby concluded that "[a]ll currently available evidence suggests that DTP vaccine may kill more children from other causes than it saves from diphtheria, tetanus or pertussis. Though a vaccine protects children against the target disease, it may simultaneously increase susceptibility to unrelated infections." Many countries, including the U.S., replaced The DTP vaccine with the DTaP vaccine long ago.[788] The 'a' stands for 'acellular' pertussis.

The newer DTaP vaccine is alleged to be somewhat safer than the DTP vaccine, but it is just as ineffective as the DTP vaccine. A 2014 study proved that the DTaP vaccine is ineffective. The study examined the effectiveness of the DTaP vaccine in preventing the 2012 Wisconsin pertussis outbreak.[789] Researchers determined that the efficacy of the vaccine quickly waned. For example, only 11.9% of the children who had received the DTaP vaccine in 2008 and 2009 were protected from getting pertussis during the 2012 Wisconsin pertussis outbreak. Mathematician Igor Chudov reviewed the statistics in the study and concluded that the protection afforded by the DTaP vaccine was effectively zero four years after vaccination.[790] The DTaP vaccine is worthless. Yet, governments and doctors falsely promote the DTaP vaccine as safe and effective.

The DTP vaccine is still being administered in about 40 countries worldwide. What informed parent would agree to vaccinate their child with the DTP vaccine? Indeed, why would any informed parent allow their child to be inoculated with any vaccine?

The above 2018 study by Dr. Aaby confirmed the results of a prior 2017 study he did showing the deadliness of the DTP vaccine. In 2017, the Informed Consent Action Network (ICAN) and the Vaccine Science Foundation (VSF) informed the UN about Dr. Aaby's 2017 study showing the deadliness of the DTP vaccines. Yet, with that knowledge, the UN continued to fund and promote the DTP vaccines. ICAN again implored the UN to stop the DTP program after Dr. Aaby's 2018 study was published. Yet the UN continued to promote and fund DTP vaccinations, knowing that the vaccine was killing children.

Attorney Aaron Siri sent a letter on January 28, 2021, on behalf of the ICAN to the United Nations Special Rapporteur on Torture and Other Cruel, Inhuman or Degrading Treatment or Punishment. In that letter, Siri called out UNICEF for funding and promoting the DTP vaccine while knowing that the vaccine is killing children. It seems that the UNICEF vaccine program killing children is quite profitable. Siri reveals in his letter that "in 2019 alone, UNICEF purchased over $1.656 billions of vaccine products from these companies and spent an equally significant sum paying companies for their distribution, in total amounting to over a third of UNICEF's budget."[791] As shocking as it may sound to read, it is a fact that high officials are knowingly killing children for profit through vaccination. Siri challenged the UN to stop killing children through the DTP vaccine program.

> The seminal study regarding DTP and mortality found that children receiving this product during the first six months of life died at 10 times the rate when compared to children that did not receive this product. Despite this, and many similar studies, the United Nations Children's Fund ("UNICEF"), continues to purchase, promote, and distribute DTP to developing and underdeveloped countries, and pushes its use on every newborn child long after knowing that the clear dangers it poses caused developed nations to stop using DTP decades ago. ... UNICEF has and continues to be instrumental and the central worldwide actor in the purchase,

promotion and distribution of DTP in many developing countries. UNICEF has continued this conduct despite the clear evidence that it increases mortality and despite the fact that DTP has not been subjected to a single randomized placebo-controlled trial to prove its safety.[792]

One thing the medical system has done to conceal that vaccines are causing infant deaths is to label the deaths as being a "syndrome." Hence, we find that what used to be called crib death is now called sudden infant death syndrome (SIDS). Thus, the focus is on the death, leaving the medical community to conjure up some mythical cause to steer the public away from vaccines.

The medical community refuses to acknowledge that vaccines cause SIDS. Instead, they falsely claim that "[r]esearchers do not know exactly what causes SIDS."[793] They claim that they do not know what causes SIDS, but from that alleged position of ignorance, they recommend a way to prevent it by having babies sleep on their backs. A campaign was instituted to do that called "Back To Sleep." When back-sleeping was found not to stop SIDS, the medical community changed the program's name in 2022 to "Safe To Sleep."[794] The medical community maintained the back-sleeping recommendation but added a bunch of other precautions to the mix. It does not matter to the medical community that its recommendations are ineffective. Effectiveness is not the point; concealing vaccines as the cause of SIDS is the goal of "Safe To Sleep."

The Safe To Sleep program is propaganda for the public. Knowledgeable doctors know full well that vaccines cause SIDS. The incidence of SIDS has increased in tandem with rising vaccination rates.[795] The unmistakable correlation cannot be missed. It is being covered up by medical sociopaths who act as protectors of the pharmaceutical companies making the deadly vaccines.

Furthermore, anecdotal proof is abounding. Often anecdotal cases can be dismissed as "idiopathic." But when cases of sudden infant deaths happen to identical twins immediately following vaccination, the inference of causation is compelling. Indeed, one doctor explains that "cases of identical twins developing a condition immediately following an intervention are often considered a gold standard in proving causality.[796] That doctor tracked down 10 cases of twin SIDS, each happening shortly after receiving vaccines, including, but not limited to, DTP, hepatitis B, and oral polio. The vaccines killed the twins. Any other cause is almost impossible. Such evidence is being concealed because it would end the profitable practice of infant vaccinations.

Mathematician Igor Chudov made a significant discovery. He uncovered evidence of a correlation between infant vaccinations and infant deaths.[797] The correlation is that children who do not receive vaccines are less likely to die as infants. Of course, correlation does not necessarily mean causation, but one can make reasonable inferences when there is no other probable cause. Indeed, the correlation of decreased infant deaths with decreased vaccinations without any other causal link establishes probable cause that the vaccines are causing infant deaths.

Chudov looked at Florida statistics reflecting a drop in childhood vaccinations in 2021.[798] He found that the reduction in childhood vaccinations correlated with a concomitant decline in infant deaths.[799] Keep in mind that Chudov was not examining COVID-19 vaccines. The vaccines under consideration were the routine vaccines received in accordance with the childhood vaccine schedule.

Infant vaccination decreased by 14.1% in 2021, which correlated directly with a drop in 2021 in all-cause infant mortality of 8.93% in 2021. Notably, the the decrease in infant mortality happened as deaths of other age groups increased significantly.

That 8.93% drop in infant mortality happened at the same time that there was a 14% drop in childhood vaccinations. Carina Blackmore, the Director of the Division of Disease Control and Health Protection Coverage For the State of Florida, stated that in 2021 there was a decrease in childhood vaccinations in Florida by "an alarming 14.1 percentage points since 2020, from 93.4 to 79.3 percent statewide."[800]

Chudov concluded that the "14 percent decrease in vaccination coverage is associated with 9 percent decrease in infant mortality."[801] That significant finding should be of concern for all parents and doctors. That kind of evidence has been known for years. But governments and social scientists have kept it hidden from the public. The medical community is also aware of the evidence revealing the dangers of vaccines, but doctors and scientists have shown a suspicious lack of curiosity about the damning evidence. There is a good reason the medical community has disregarded this incriminating evidence - "money." For the love of money is the root of all evil." 1 Timothy 6:10. Pharmaceutical companies massively fund virtually every medical school. He who pays the piper calls the tune.

In addition, pediatricians do not want to hear about or explore any evidence about the dangers of vaccines because they make large amounts of money by administering those vaccines. Indeed, most pediatricians refuse to treat unvaccinated children because they are paid a bounty for every fully vaccinated child in their practice above a certain threshold.[802]

Furthermore, in 2021, the American Medical Association (AMA) amended its Code of Medical Ethics Section 8.7 to include an ethical responsibility to encourage patients to get vaccinated.[803] With that, the AMA (being under the thumb of the pharmaceutical industry) has determined that it is an ethical violation for a physician not to encourage patients to accept immunization.[804] A physician cannot be neutral on the issue of vaccination; he must "encourage" vaccination or be subject to license suspension by their state medical board for violating the AMA code of ethics.[805]

Mark Blaxill and Amy Becker studied mortality rates during the COVID-19 lock-downs.[806] They discovered a startling fact. Infant mortality actually went down during the COVID-19 lockdowns. There was a significant decrease in the number of infant deaths. Blaxill and Becker attributed that drop to the inability of parents to do well-baby doctor checkups with the obligatory vaccinations. Fewer vaccines = fewer infant deaths. Blaxill and Becker stated:

> Starting in early March, expected deaths [for children under 18 years old] began a sharp decline, from an expected level of around 700 deaths per week to well under 500 by mid-April and throughout May. The Centers for Disease Control and Prevention. National Center for Health Statistics Mortality Surveillance System.
>
> As untimely deaths spiked among the elderly in Manhattan nursing homes and in similar settings all over the country, something mysterious was saving the lives of children. As springtime in America came along with massive disruptions in family life amid near-universal lockdowns, roughly 30% fewer children died.

***

Was this a protective effect of school closures? Were teenagers getting themselves into risky situations at a lower rate? No. There was very little effect among school age children or adolescents.[807]

Incidentally, since the publication of Blaxill and Becker's

article, the CDC has removed the page that memorialized the fact that almost all of the reduction in childhood deaths came from infants. Blaxill and Becker explain that the CDC statistics showed:

> **Virtually the entire change came from infants.** Somehow, the changing pattern of American life during the lockdowns has been saving the lives of hundreds of infants, over 200 per week.

***

What has changed during this period that might have such an effect?

***

> One very clear change that has received publicity is that public health officials are bemoaning the sharp decline in infant vaccinations as parents are not taking their infants into pediatric offices for their regular well-baby checks. In the May 15 [2020] issue of the CDC Morbidity and Mortality Weekly Report (MMWR), a group of authors from the CDC and Kaiser Permanente reported **a sharp decline in provider orders for vaccines as well as a decline in pediatric vaccine doses administered.** Santoli, Jeanne M et al. Effects of the COVID-19 Pandemic on Routine Pediatric Vaccine Ordering and Administration — United States, 2020. cdc.gov.[808] [Online] May 15, 2020. These declines began in early March, around the time infant deaths began declining.[809]

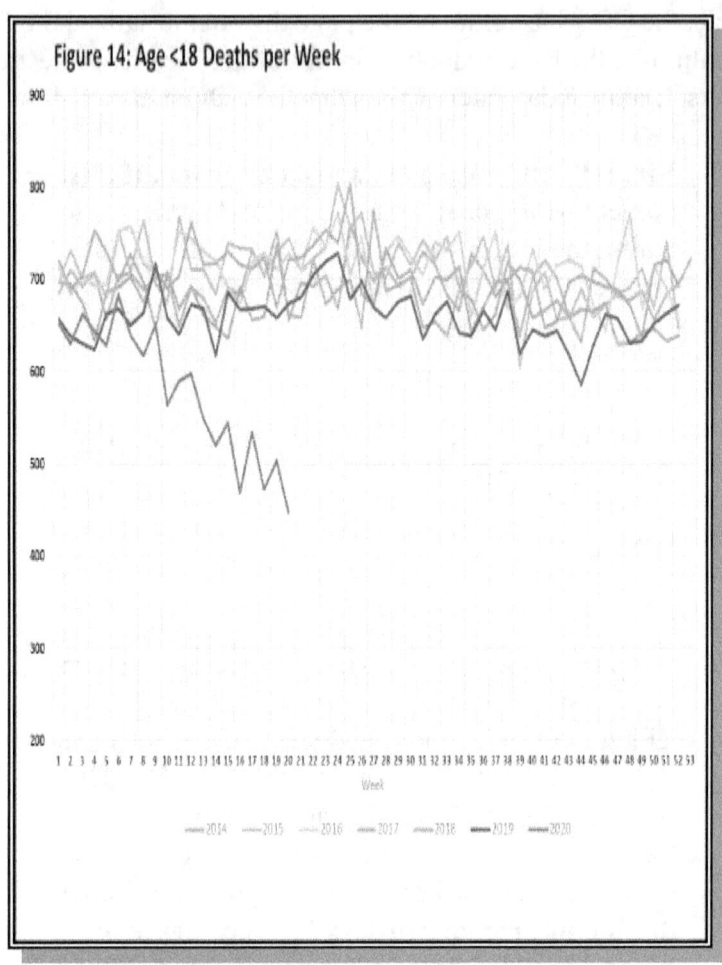

Figure 41: Chart showing a precipitous drop in child deaths early in 2020 that correlated directly with the COVID-19 lookdowns. Virtually the entire drop in deaths among children under 18 years old came from infants. The COVID-19 lockdowns prevented parents from taking infants for well-baby checkups and getting vaccinated. The reduction in infant deaths also correlated directly with a sharp decline in provider orders for vaccines and a decline in pediatric vaccine doses administered.

A 2011 study compared the infant mortality rate (IMR) of 34 countries to the number of vaccines required by their 2009 national vaccine schedule within the first year of infancy.[810] If vaccines were safe and effective, as the pharmaceutical companies and the CDC claim, the greater the number of childhood vaccines would mean a lower infant mortality rate. But the opposite was found. The study revealed a direct correlation between the number of childhood vaccines and the mortality rate. The more vaccines administered to infants, the higher the infant death rate.

In 2009, the U.S. vaccine schedule called for 26 vaccine doses within the first year after birth, and the infant mortality rate in the U.S. was 6.22 per 1,000. The U.S. had the highest number of infant vaccines of all 34 countries in the study. The report also found that the U.S. had the highest infant mortality rate among all 34 countries. The researchers explained:

> Despite the United States spending more per capita on health care than any other country, 33 nations have better IMRs. Some countries have IMRs that are less than half the US rate: Singapore, Sweden, and Japan are below 2.80. According to the Centers for Disease Control and Prevention (CDC), "The relative position of the United States in comparison to countries with the lowest infant mortality rates appears to be worsening."

***

> The infant mortality rate is expressed as the number of infant deaths per 1000 live births. According to the US Central Intelligence Agency (CIA), which keeps accurate, up-to-date infant mortality statistics throughout the world, in 2009 there were 33 nations with better infant mortality rates than the United States. The US infant

mortality rate of 6.22 infant deaths per 1000 live births ranked 34th.

The researchers broke the countries into five categories based on the number of vaccines routinely given to the children in each country. The researchers then charted the number of vaccines in each quintile against the average mortality rate for those countries. The chart revealed a direct correlation between the number of vaccines and the average infant death rate. The more vaccines administered to infants, the higher the infant death rate.

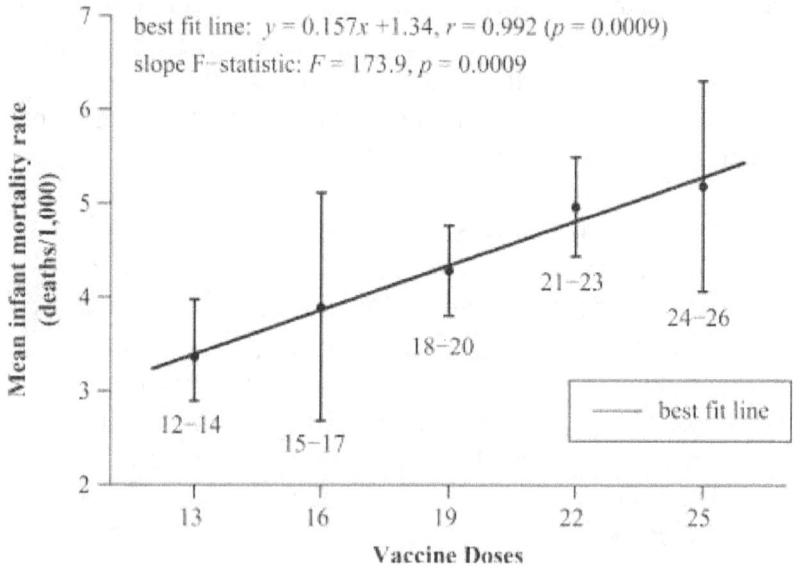

The r-value between the number of infant vaccines and infant deaths was 0.992. The lowest r-value possible is 0.0, and the highest positive r-value is 1.0. An r-value of 1.0 means a perfect one-to-one positive linear correlation between two variables. Generally, an r-value greater than 0.7 indicates a strong correlation between variables. In this case, an r-value of 0.992 indicates a very strong correlation that more infant vaccines will result in more infant deaths. The r^2 for the statistics was 0.983. That means an increase in infant vaccinations explains 98.3% of infant deaths. The *p*-value for the statistics was 0.0009. That means that the probability of the outcome happening by chance was 0.09%. Thus, it can be said with a high degree of scientific certainty that as more vaccines are given to infants, those vaccines will cause more infant deaths. That is scientific proof that vaccines kill infants.

Lest you think that the above quoted doctors and their studies are anomalies, please understand that doctors and scientists through the centuries have witnessed first-hand the injuries caused by vaccines and have been speaking out against that superstitious practice.

Dr. Archie Kalokerinos was a vaccine believer when he first worked as a medical doctor among Australia's aboriginal people in the 1950s. But he soon realized that the children were becoming sick and dying after getting vaccinated. He wrote a book about his experience titled *Every Second Child*. Brett Wilcox explains:

> *Every Second Child* was so named because up to half of the vaccinated Aboriginal infants died following vaccination, which Kalokerinos attributed to an acute vitamin C deficiency. Kalokerinos learned independently what professionals had come to learn in Africa and India and what vaccine manufacturers had known all along: vaccines injure and sometimes kill immunocompromised children.[811]

Dr. Kalokerinos reveals in his book the devastation wrought by the vaccine programs in the aboriginal populations of Australia:

> A health team would sweep into an area, line up all the Aboriginal babies and infants and immunise

them. There would be no examination, no taking of case histories, no checking on dietary deficiencies. Most infants would have colds. No wonder they died. Some would die within hours from acute vitamin C deficiency precipitated by the immunisation. Others would suffer immunological insults and die later from 'pneumonia', 'gastroenteritis' or 'malnutrition'. If some babies and infants survived, they would be lined up again within a month for another immunisation. If some managed to survive even this, they would be lined up again. Then there would be booster shots, shots for measles, polio and even T.B. Little wonder they died. The wonder is that any survived. The excitement of this realisation is difficult to describe. On one hand, I was enthralled by the simplicity of it all, the 'beautiful' way by which the pattern fitted everything I had been doing. On the other hand, I almost shook in horror at the thought of what had been, and still was going on. We were actually killing infants through lack of understanding.[812]

28 Vaccines Cause Autism

Autism has exploded from a rate of 1 in 10,000 children in 1970 to 1 in 54 children by 2020.[813] That explosion in autism has correlated with the increase in childhood vaccinations. The correlation is unmistakable. The conclusion is ineluctable; childhood vaccinations cause autism. With each new vaccine comes an increased incidence of autism. In the United States, children have gone from receiving only the DTP and smallpox vaccines in 1940 to receiving the MMR, polio, and DTP shots in 1980, to now receiving 11 vaccines, involving 29 separate shots before the child reaches the age of 15 months old, according to the 2023 CDC childhood vaccine schedule.[814] The poor children have their immune systems bombarded with 19 shots before they reach six months old.[815]

Synaptogenesis is the formation of synapses in the brain, which are the contact points where information is transmitted between neurons. Intense synaptogenesis occurs in children as they grow during the first 18 months. Vaccines produce immune activation, which disrupts synaptogenesis in a child's brain. There is likely a synergistic effect caused by neurotoxic ingredients in the vaccines, like aluminum or mercury, at the very time the brain is developing. This adverse effect on the child's brain causes autism.

A medical researcher explains:

> The science reviewed here tells a consistent and compelling story: that vaccines may cause autism by stimulating immune activation and elevated cytokines in the brain. Al [aluminum] adjuvants are implicated as a cause of autism because they can be transported into the brain, because they cause microglial activation at vaccine-relevant dosages, and because aluminum induces IL-6 in the brain.[816]

Aluminum is used as an adjuvant in vaccines given to children. Vaccine advocates claim that an aluminum adjuvant dissolves in the blood and is removed by the kidneys. But that claim is based on the assumption that the aluminum is ingested by drinking it. That is not the case when aluminum is contained in a vaccine injected into the body. Research has shown that aluminum travels from the injection site throughout the body to the brain.[817] The aluminum remains in the organs of the body, wreaking havoc. Aluminum causes inflammation in the brain. A single vaccine shot contains more than enough aluminum to inflame an infant's brain.[818]

Researchers using fluorescence microscopy have found high levels of aluminum in the brain tissue of those who have autism.[819] That is significant because, as explained by Dr Chris Shaw, Neuroscientist and aluminum researcher at University of British Columbia, "the existing evidence on the toxicology and pharmacokinetics of Al [aluminum] adjuvants…altogether strongly implicate these compounds as contributors to the rising prevalence of neurobehavioural disorders in children."[820]

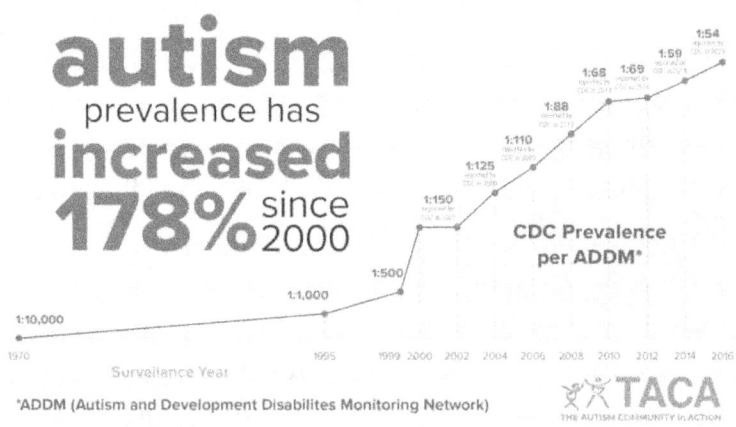

A study of newborn boys showed that those who were vaccinated with Hepatitis B had threefold greater odds for autism compared to boys who were not vaccinated.[821] Another study involving 666 children that compared 405 vaccinated children with 261 unvaccinated children revealed that vaccinated children had 4.7 times greater diagnoses of autism.[822]

That study raised a furor among the powerful pharmaceutical companies and allied interests. They took immediate action to force the Frontiers in Public Health Journal to retract publication of the study. It was republished in the Journal of Translational Science, but similar pressure was brought on that journal and it subsequently also retracted publication of the study. It is interesting to note that those who denigrate that study never discuss the details of the study. They limit their discussion to general allegations of bias, with no specifics. Indeed, they cannot allow the information in the study to be generally known.[823] The study can be downloaded from the link provided at the endnote at the end of this sentence.[824] See also the study by Dr. Andrew Wakefield that linked vaccines to autism that *The Lancet* retracted.[825]

You will never hear of a study alleging no connection between vaccination and autism suddenly withdrawn from publication. Indeed, when you look at the studies closely, they studiously limit their study to only the MMR vaccine. Often they are comparing groups where the unvaccinated group has actually received other vaccines, it is just that they did not receive the MMR vaccine. And so the results are announced that the study shows that the MMR vaccine does not cause autism because the rates of autism are the same as for the non-MMR group.

To keep the vaccine wagon rolling, the pharmaceutical companies and their minions must have some studies to establish the safety of their unsafe vaccines. Since their vaccines are dangerous, and they most certainly cause autism, the only way a study can show they are safe is if they rig the study.

In a 2019 Denmark study, the largest study of its kind, researchers in Denmark compared 625,842 vaccinated children with 31,619 unvaccinated children.[826] The unvaccinated children were those that had not received the MMR vaccination. Whereas the vaccinated children had received the MMR vaccination. They concluded that the MMR vaccine did not cause any appreciable difference in the rate of autism between the groups. That is how it was portrayed to the public. But let us look at that study a little closer.

The Novo Nordisk Foundation funded the study.[827] Furthermore, the two principal researchers both received additional financial grants from the Novo Nordisk Foundation during their work on the autism/MMR research.[828] The Novo Nordisk Foundation is a Danish charitable trust with significant corporate pharmaceutical interests.[829] Its wholly owned subsidiary, Novo Holdings, is the holding company for the pharmaceutical companies Novo Nordisk A/S and Novozymes. Novo Nordisk Foundation's assets were estimated in 2021 to be worth approximately US$93.73 billion, making it one of the largest charitable foundations in the world.[830] They have interlocking interests with other giant philanthropic foundations like the Bill and Malinda Gates Foundation.[831] The Gates and Novo Nordisk foundations use their charitable trusts to push agendas that enhance corporate profits.

Pharmaceutical companies, like Novo Nordisk, have an interest in seeing the vaccines continue to be given to children. That is because they make a lot of money on pharmaceuticals that are subsequently needed to address the injuries caused by the vaccines.

Novo Nordisk also profits directly from vaccine manufacturing. Novo Nordisk makes Cetyl Trimethyl Ammonium Bromide (CTAB), which is a germicide that is a powerful cationic surfactant "used in vaccine downstream processing in both bacterial and viral vaccines."[832] Novo Nordisk explains that "CTAB (Cetrimonium Bromide) is recommended by the WHO in bacterial vaccine manufacturing as a purification agent for polysaccharide vaccines."[833] Notably, "[p]olysaccharide vaccines are commonly found in standard children vaccination programs."[834] If a vaccine (like the MMR vaccine) is shown to be unsafe or ineffective, that will hurt the profits of Novo Nordisk.

The Danish research study was also funded by the Danish Ministry of Health.[835] The Danish Health Authority is interested in seeing a study outcome favorable to childhood vaccines. After all, their official stance is that "All young children are vaccinated against the following diseases: Diphtheria, tetanus, whooping cough, polio, ... Meningitis ... Measles, mumps and German measles [rubella] [a.k.a. MMR]."[836]

He who pays the piper calls the tune. The researchers understood that if their research found that the MMR caused autism, the government and Novo Nordisk would be very unhappy with them. Their research grants from the Novo Nordisk

Foundation and the government would end if they found a causal link between the MMR vaccine and autism. It is no big surprise that the researchers concluded what they were paid to conclude. It is interesting to study how they rigged their study to find that MMR vaccines do not cause autism.

The study is rather suspicious because at the outset it cites to Dr. Wakefield's study that was retracted by *The Lancet* that showed a direct correlation between childhood vaccines and autism. That suggests that their research was designed to rebut Dr. Wakefield's study. Indeed, in an email to NPR, the lead researcher, Anders Hvid suggested that the research was prompted by the fact that "the idea that vaccines cause autism is still around despite our original and other well-conducted studies."[837] Hvid was concerned that "[p]arents still encounter these claims [that vaccines cause autism] on social media, by politicians, by celebrities, etc."[838] Although he did not come out and say so, his comments suggested that his research was to refute the MMR-autism causation argument. He had an agenda.

Hvid states that he was concerned about the argument that "vaccines" cause autism. But that is not what he researched. To answer that question he raised about vaccines causing autism, one must compare vaccinated and unvaccinated children. But Hvid did not do that. He compared two groups of vaccinated children. He compared a group that received a single vaccine against five diseases against another group that received that same vaccine plus another vaccine against three diseases. In Denmark, that single vaccine against five diseases is given four times at intervals of 3 months of age, 5 months of age, 12 months of age, and 5 years of age.[839] The second vaccine is given twice, at 15 months old and again at 4 years old.[840] The single vaccine group received the diphtheria, acellular pertussis, tetanus, inactivated poliovirus, and Haemophilus influenza type b (a.k.a., DtaP-IPV/Hib) vaccine. The double vaccine group received the additional vaccine against measles, mumps, and rubella (MMR).

The researchers were careful to label the unvaccinated group "MMR-unvacciated" and the vaccinated group "MMR-vaccinated." The reason for that nomenclature was that the MMR-unvaccinated group was only not vaccinated with the MMR vaccine. The unvaccinated group was not truly unvaccinated. 26,890 of the 31,619 children in the "MMR-unvaccinated" group received other vaccinations. Thus, more than 85% of the children labeled as "MMR-unvaccinated" received vaccinations. They received diphtheria, acellular pertussis, tetanus, inactivated poliovirus, and Haemophilus influenza type b vaccines (a.k.a., DtaP-IPV/Hib). Any one of those vaccines could cause an increase in autism in the "MMR-unvaccinated" group. And certainly, the cumulative effect of those seriatim vaccinations on a young child could be devastating to a child's undeveloped immune system. The only vaccine missed by the unvaccinated group was the MMR vaccine. The high numbers of autism sufferers in the MMR-unvaccinated group would then be compared to the MMR-vaccinated group and allow the researchers to claim that the MMR vaccine does not cause autism because the rate of autism would be similar. The Denmark study authors concluded:

> The study strongly supports that MMR vaccination does not increase the risk for autism, does not trigger autism in susceptible children, and is not associated with clustering of autism cases after vaccination.[841]

That conclusion in the Denmark study can be likened to a study of the intoxicating properties of rum. In our hypothetical rum study, we will have 10 persons consume a shot of vodka, a shot of whiskey, a shot of gin, a shot of tequila, and a shot of rum, and another 10 persons will consume all of those shots of alcoholic beverages but not the shot of rum. Both groups of persons (all 20) end up drunk. Thus, just as do the vaccine researchers, we can conclude that rum could not have caused the drunkenness because both the 10 persons who drank rum and the 10 persons who did not drink rum got drunk. We can then publicly announce that our study proves that rum is not an intoxicating liquor. Those are the kinds of shenanigans being pulled by "scientists" portraying dangerous vaccines as safe to the public.

And so the non-MMR group, being not truly an unvaccinated group, is presenting a higher autism number than would be the case for a truly unvaccinated group. When looking at a study that truly compares a vaccinated group vs. an unvaccinated group, the results are significant. A recent study that compared truly unvaccinated children with vaccinated children revealed that vaccinated children had 4.7 times greater diagnoses of autism.

Notably, the Danish researchers acknowledged the elephant in the room. "A general criticism of observational vaccine effect studies is that they do not include a completely unvaccinated group of children."

They should have compared a purely unvaccinated group against a vaccinated group. But they did not do that. The mainstream media misinforms the public that "[t]here's strong new evidence that a common childhood vaccine is safe."[842] They trumpet statements of the co-author of the Denmark study, Anders Hviid, stated that he hopes the findings will reassure parents. He further stated, "[p]arents should not avoid vaccinating their children for fear of autism."[843] Does that sound like an objective researcher? He is showing his bias by reassuring parents that they should not be afraid that vaccines cause autism. But how would he know that? His study compared two vaccinated groups. And his study was limited to the MMR vaccine. But he went further in his comment to cover all vaccines. That sounds like a promoter of vaccines, not an objective researcher. And it seems that he had an agenda. Mission accomplished.

Pedro Alcantara of the Asociacion Espanola de Pediatria posted the following public comment alleging that the study came to a misleading conclusion.

> Both the control group and the study have previously received a cocktail of vaccines: DTaP-IPV/Hib by 12 months of age. Obviously, if some or all of the vaccines in the cocktail caused autism in susceptible kids, by the time the MMR is administered all the susceptible kids would already be autistic and the extra MMR wouldn't affect much the incidence in the study group relative to the control group. Therefore the correct conclusion would be that "Later MMR vaccination does not increase the risk in comparison to a cocktail of previously administered vaccines". By omitting this last point from the conclusion the reader is misled into believing that the MMR vaccine has been proven safe in absolute terms, that is, compared to lack of vaccination. By making a grand universal statement that "MMR vaccination does not increase the risk for autism, does not trigger autism in susceptible children, and is not associated with clustering of autism cases after vaccination" the authors unduly extrapolate their observations to unvaccinated subjects. Lawmakers maybe mislead into taking wrong decisions affecting public health.[844]

Anthony R. Mawson, Department of Epidemiology and Biostatistics, School of Public Health, Jackson State University, posted a public comment to the authors of the study that said in pertinent part:

> The effect of these analyses was therefore to compare autism rates in two highly vaccinated groups, thereby obliterating the potential impact of vaccines in general. Comparisons should instead be

between fully vaccinated and completely unvaccinated groups of children, or between MMR-only vaccinated and completely unvaccinated children in terms of autism.[845]

While the authors of the study responded to comments made by other researchers, they did not respond to the remarks of Anthony Mawson or Pedro Alcantara. It seems that they had no good explanation for what they did. The researchers rigged the study to falsely show that MMR vaccines do not cause autism by ensuring that both the MMR-vaccinated and the MMR-unvaccinated groups were vaccinated.

Such fraudulent studies are planned in advance for the purpose of coming out with a predetermined result. Brett Wilcox, in his book, *Jabbed*, explains:

> When research emerges demonstrating the risks associated with vaccines and vaccine ingredients, the government often responds by conducting fraudulent studies to shore up the faith of vaccine believers. Dr. Gordon Douglas, director of strategic planning for vaccine research at the National Institutes of Health, explained as much in a 2001 presentation at Princeton University when he said,

> "Four current studies are taking place to rule out the proposed link between autism and thimerosal. In order to undo the harmful effects of research claiming to link the [measles] vaccine to an elevated risk of autism, we need to conduct and publicize additional studies to assure parents of safety."[846]

The Director of Strategic Planning for the NIH, who is supposed to be a public servant looking out for children's safety, is concerned that the studies linking the measles vaccine to autism might be believed. He does not care that the studies are accurate and the prove a real risk of autism. His only concern is that the study may undermine the security that parents have in the safety of the vaccine. He does not warn the parents based on scientific research that the MMR vaccine is dangerous. Instead, he plans out four studies that he announces before they are concluded will "undo the harmful effects of research" that proves that the vaccine is causing autism. How can he be so sure that the four studies he cites will show that the vaccines do not cause autism? Because the studies are rigged.

Brett Wilcox reveals the entities that are really pulling the strings on the puppet known as Dr. Gordan Douglas.

> Robert F. Kennedy Jr. pointed out that when Douglas spoke at Princeton, he was also employed by Aventis, a company that manufactures thimerosal containing vaccines. In addition, Douglas had formerly served as president of Merck's vaccination program. While serving in that capacity in 1991— the beginning of the thimerosal generation and the autism epidemic.[847]

Dr. Douglas knows full well that the mercury-laden thimerosol is neurotoxic. He knew that using mercury in childhood vaccines would cause brain damage (i.e., autism). Brett Wilcox exlpains:

> Robert F. Kennedy [Jr.] asserts that Dr. Maurice Hilleman, one of the fathers of Merck's vaccination programs, warned Dr. Gordon Douglas … that six-month-old children administered the shots on schedule would suffer mercury exposures 87 times the existing safety standards. He recommended that thimerosal use be discontinued,

"especially where use in infants and young children is anticipated."⁸⁴⁸

Dr. Douglas knew from the beginning that the MMR vaccine from Merck caused autism. Yet, right up until 2001, when thimerosal was finally removed, Dr. Douglas was trying to rig fraudulent studies to prove that the MMR vaccine was safe.

The American Academy of Pediatrics (AAP) "calls for the on-time, routine immunization of all children and adolescents" and further "reminds pediatricians that every visit is an opportunity to vaccinate."⁸⁴⁹ The AAP further recommends "COVID-19 vaccination for all infants, children, and adolescents 6 months of age and older."⁸⁵⁰ That is an appalling recommendation in light of the VAERS data showing that the COVID-19 vaccines are associated with 35,347 deaths, 27,113 cases of myocarditis and pericarditis, and 66,462 permanent disabilities as of June 2, 2023.⁸⁵¹ That dangerous recommendation can be explained by the fact that the AAP receives funds from COVID-19 vaccine maker Pfizer.⁸⁵² Indeed, the AAP is almost entirely funded by pharmaceutical companies. Among its top ten donors are pharmaceutical giants Johnson & Johnson, Merck, and Sanofi, all vaccine makers.⁸⁵³ He who pays the piper calls the tune.

Furthermore, the AAP argues against religious liberties by calling for eliminating religious exemptions to vaccinations. "The AAP views nonmedical exemptions to school-required immunizations as inappropriate for individual, public health, and ethical reasons and advocates for their elimination."⁸⁵⁴

The AAP falsely states that vaccines are not associated with autism.⁸⁵⁵ The AAP makes that statement even though the AAP knows that vaccines cause permanent brain damage. The AAP has posted a 1998 paper written by CDC researchers that showed the measles vaccine causes permanent brain damage.⁸⁵⁶ Autism is brain damage caused by vaccines. That 1998 study does not stand alone. There are 214 peer-reviewed studies linking vaccines and autism.[857] Several studies have shown that a vaccinated child is more than four times more likely to be stricken with autism than an unvaccinated child.[858]

Steve Kirsch reports that a "large clinical pediatric practice I am personally very familiar with has eschewed the use of all vaccines and acetaminophen and achieved a zero autism rate over the past 25 years even though autism rates were skyrocketing in adjacent clinics."[859] Another pediatric clinic, Homefirst Medical Services, which has treated more than 30,000 children over a 47-year period, found not a single case of autism among the unvaccinated children.[860] Compare that to the shockingly high rate of 1 in 54 autistic children (as of 2020) reported by the CDC. Incidently, Steve Kirsch conducted a study and found that the rate of autism is closer to 1 out of 3 children.[861]

Dr. Lyons Weiler, Ph.D., is the Scientific Director of the Bioinformatics Analysis Core and a Senior Research Scientist at the University of Pittsburgh. Dr. Weiler got a call from one of the top autism experts in the world, who told Dr. Weiler: "We [autism experts] all know vaccines cause autism. We just aren't allowed to talk about it."[862] Steve Kirsch explains that if autism researchers publically admitted that vaccines cause autism, "they would lose their funding, their job, their license to practice medicine, their hospital privileges, their board certifications, etc."[863]

29   Dangerous Placebos

The gold standard for a scientific study is a randomized controlled trial (RCT). In an RCT, the study participants are selected from the targeted population and randomly assigned to either a trial or control group. In a vaccine study, the trial group receives the vaccine being tested for efficacy and safety. The control group is supposed to receive a placebo injection, which should be an inert liquid like saline. The study participants and administrators should be kept blind as to which persons are in each group.

The control group is supposed to give the background base for determining adverse events. The adverse events in the trial group are compared to the adverse events in the control group to determine if the vaccine is safe. But pharmaceutical companies have a problem. They know their vaccines are unsafe and could never pass muster as safe and effective in a properly conducted RCT. They could fudge the data, but the problem with doing that is it's a crime and they don't want to go to jail.

The pharmaceutical companies have figured out a way to rig their vaccine studies to conceal the health dangers of their vaccines and, at the same time, avoid jail. Pharmaceutical companies use a trick to make their dangerous vaccines appear safe. They use a bioactive ingredient, which they falsely call a "placebo," to administer to the control group. The bioactive injections cause adverse events in the control group. This raises the background adverse events so that when the vaccine group is compared to the control group receiving the "placebo," the vaccine group's adverse events do not look so bad by comparison.

That is what Merck did when it tested Gardasil. Gardasil® is a quadrivalent human papillomavirus recombinant vaccine (qHPV) made by Merck, The 2006 Gardasil package insert describes two placebos used in its testing.[864] One placebo was a inert saline injection given to 320 members of the control group and another was an injection containing amorphous aluminum hydroxyphosphate sulfate (AAHS) given to another 3,470 members of the control group. The total number of persons in the control group was 3,790 (3,470+320=3,790). When the total control group of 3,790 participants was listed they were described as receiving a "placebo." But AAHS cannot be truly described as a placebo. It is a bioactive ingredient that is formulated to cause the body to have an immune response.

A placebo is an innocuous, inactive substance that does not have a physiological effect on the body.[865] Some prefer to call such inert substances dummies.[866] Indeed, Merck acknowledges that a placebo is supposed to be inert and inactive. "On its website, qHPV vaccine's sponsor [Merck] defines a placebo as 'an inactive pill, liquid, or powder that has no treatment value'. This definition is consistent with the decades old notion of placebos as pharmacologically inert substances used to obtain unbiased assessments in experimental research."[867]

But when Merck sought FDA approval for Gardasil in 2006, it administered AAHS to the control group, while misleadingly calling it a placebo. Furthermore, Merck concealed the independent reporting of the systemic effect of the actual placebo (saline solution) on the control group. This was purposeful because Merck specifically broke out the different localized reactions to the injections site for the ""Aluminum-Containing Placebo" and the saline "placebo." That is because it was expected that there would likely be some reaction to the injection site for anything injected into the body. But systemic reactions, like fever and nausea, are a whole other matter. Merck lumped the AAHS control group and the saline placebo control group together when reporting systemic reactions. This had the effect of elevating the systemic adverse events caused by the "placebo" injections. Merck reported the combined 3,790 members of the AAHS and saline control group as a single "placebo" group. It made it appear that the systemic adverse event rate of approximately 38.6% for the Gardasil test group was not so bad because the combined 3,790 members of the control group had 35.1% systemic adverse events. Merck purposely obscured that 92% of the control group received AAHS.

Even though 92% of the control group received a bioactive AAHS injection, Merck described the control group throughout the 15-page package insert as receiving a "placebo." The first mention of an "Aluminum-Containing Placebo" appeared on page 6. But it was only in a chart heading. AAHS is not mentioned again until pages 10 and 12, where it is again listed as an "Aluminum-Containing Placebo," and only in a chart heading. But there was no explanation.

Interestingly, the insert explains: "Each 0.5-mL dose of the [Gardasil] vaccine contains approximately 225 mcg of aluminum (as amorphous aluminum hydroxyphosphate sulfate adjuvant) [AAHS]" among other ingredients. Thus, the test subjects and 92% of the control group were injected with AAHS. When you realize that the purpose of AAHS is to stimulate the immune response and that immune response is the catalyst for adverse events, you get an idea of the trick Merck was pulling. They wanted the control group's immune system ramped up to have as many adverse events as possible to make the expected adverse events from Gardasil not look so bad by comparison to the "placebo" injected control group.

Once Merck received its 2006 FDA approval for Gardasil it slithered back and rewrote its package insert to explicitly describe the use of AAHS as the "placebo" in the control group.[868] In September 2008, Merck published a new Gardasil package insert that made 68 references to AAHS use in the control group. Suddenly the group of 3,790 people in the control group that was labeled in 2006 as receiving a "Placebo" was now listed as receiving "AAHS control or Saline Placebo." Merck then explains in the package insert that "AAHS Control = Amorphous Aluminum Hydroxyphosphate Sulfate." Once they obtained FDA approval and the coast was clear, Merck decided to go back and tidy up its package insert to reflect what was really happening in the trials.

Peter Doshi, Ph.D., is an Associate Professor of Practice, Sciences, and Health Outcomes Research at the University of Maryland School of Pharmacy. He wrote an article with other scientists exposing the fraud of vaccine researchers using bioactive placebos. In particular, he cited the example of the Merck Gardasil study using AAHS with Merck misleadingly calling it a "placebo." Dr. Doshi correctly identifies that practice as an ethical issue. Dr. Doshi describes the problem:

> [T]he efficacy and safety analyses of these five qHPV [Guaradasil] vaccine trials were conducted as if the trials were controlled with inert placebo when they were not. None of the key publications for these trials, which have been used to inform regulatory and health decision making, appear to discuss how AAHS-containing control could affect the interpretation of results.[869]

Doshi was troubled that Merck lied to the trial participants by telling them they would receive an inactive placebo. When in fact they were receiving a bioactive AAHS injection.

> We also consider that the use of the term 'placebo' to describe an active comparator like AAHS inaccurately describes the formulation that the control arm participants received, and constitutes an important error that requires correction. If trial participants were told they could receive 'placebo' (widely defined as referring to an 'inactive' or 'inert' substance) without being informed of all non-inert contents of the control arm injection, this raises ethical questions about trial conduct as well.[870]

Using a bioactive ingredient that is actually one of the adjuvants used in the Gardasil injection renders the study results almost useless. Dr. Doshi explains:

> With respect to adjuvants in vaccines, the FDA has noted that 'adjuvants have their own pharmacologic activity, which may affect both the immunogenicity and the safety of vaccines. Adverse reactions may include local reactions such as pain, swelling, injection site necrosis, and granulomas. Systemic reactions may include nausea, fever, arthritis, as well as potential immunotoxic reactions. Unexpected, rare events may also occur'.[871]

Dr. Doshi opined that the reasons given by Merck for using AAHS in the control arm were not credible. Merck claimed that it wanted to test only the HPV virus-like particles and therefore used the AAHS in the control group. But that appears to be a deceptive cover story that makes no sense. If that was Merck's objective, it could not accomplish it by only using AAHS. Merck should have included all other excipients that were in the Gardasil vaccine to inject in the control group. Dr. Doshi explains:

> According to qHPV vaccine's prescribing information, each dose of vaccine contains '9.56 mg of sodium chloride, 0.78 mg of L-histidine, 50 mcg of polysorbate 80, 35 mcg of sodium borate, <7 mcg yeast protein/dose and water', in addition to AAHS and HPV virus-like particles. To test HPV virus-like particles, as the manufacturer stated was its intention in using an AAHS control, the control would logically have also included these other ingredients in addition to AAHS.[872]

Finally, Dr. Doshi explains that the study would be irrelevant even if Merck included all other ingredients in the control group injection. To conduct such a study would be scientifically irrational. A vaccine trial aims to assess the safety and efficacy of the vaccine as manufactured and not just one component of the vaccine. That is because there is a synergism between the ingredients in the vaccine, and people are injected with all those ingredients, not just the antigen in the HPV virus-like particles.

> [T]he stated rationale of using AAHS control, to characterise the safety of the HPV virus-like particles, lacks clinical relevance. The clinically relevant question is what are the effects (benefits and harms) of qHPV vaccine—the whole product, not one of its components.[873]

Clearly, the real reason that Merck used AAHS and misleadingly labeled it as a "placebo" in its control group was to ramp up the adverse events in the control group to then show that the Gardasil vaccine was safe compared to the control group receiving a "placebo." Those reading the study will not realize that the "placebo" was not a placebo at all but an injection of a bioactive substance made up of amorphous aluminum hydroxyphosphate sulfate (AAHS).

Merck is not alone. All pharmaceutical companies making childhood vaccines use the same deceptive trick. An author of a book titled *Turtles All the Way Down* needed to remain anonymous to protect himself from backlash in the medical community. The anonymous author explains how the pharmaceutical companies rig the trials while staying out of jail:

> Vaccine trials in general, and childhood vaccine trials specifically, are purposely designed to obscure the true incidence of adverse events of the vaccine being tested. How do they do this? By using a two-step scheme: First, a new vaccine (one which does not have a predecessor), is always tested in a Phase 3 RCT in which the control group receives another vaccine (or a compound very similar to the experimental vaccine, see explanation below). A new pediatric vaccine is never tested during its formal approval process against a neutral solution (placebo). Comparing a trial group to a control group that was given a compound that is likely to cause a similar rate of adverse events facilitates the formation of a false safety profile.[874]

The pharmaceutical companies use the word "placebo" to describe the injection given to the control groups in their studies of childhood vaccines. But the "placebos" always contain bioactive ingredients that cause adverse events. Those adverse events in the control group are then used as the supposed background rate of adverse events to compare the tested vaccine's safety. The tested vaccine may be quite dangerous, but because it is often being compared to an equally dangerous bioactive "placebo" the pharmaceutical companies can announce that the vaccine is safe because it does not significantly increase the rate of adverse events as compared to the control group receiving a "placebo." Shocking as it may sound, it is a historical, scientific fact that no vaccine on the CDC childhood vaccine schedule was ever tested in a randomized controlled trial using an inert placebo for the control group.

The CDC has described the hepatitis A vaccine as "very safe." The CDC recommends that children get a two-shot administration beginning as early as 12 months old.[875] Merck, in 1996, tested its hepatitis A vaccine (VAQTA®) against a control group that was given a "placebo" containing an aluminum diluent. Aluminum is a bioactive ingredient that not only stimulates the immune system but it is also neurotoxic. There are significant side effects to being injected with such a heavy metal. Merck described the placebo as (alum diluent). That means that the aluminum was a diluent. A diluent is a substance used to dilute other ingredients. That suggests the "placebo" carried other unspecified ingredients diluted in the aluminum carrier.

It is not surprising then to find that the 1996 Merck VAQTA® hepatitis A study showed systemic side effects for the control group receiving the 'placebo" that in most instances were equal to or greater than those in the test group getting the VAQTA® vaccine. With that trick, Merck was able to say in their VAQTA® package insert that "[t]here were no significant differences in the rates of any adverse events or adverse reactions between vaccine and placebo recipients after Dose 1."[876]

Another example of the "placebo" scam run by pharmaceutical companies is a 2002 safety trial study for a new DTaP (diphtheria, tetanus, and pertussis) vaccine. The CDC has concluded that "DTaP and Tdap vaccine [sic] are safe and effective at preventing diphtheria, tetanus, and pertussis."[877] The CDC based its conclusion that the DTaP vaccine was safe on a rigged study.

In the DTaP study, the "control group" received the older DTP vaccine.[878] In that study, 1 in every 22 subjects in the experimental group became so ill that they were admitted to the hospital.[879] But a similar rate of hospitalization was also reported in the control group. The study thus reported that the "rates of vomiting, convulsions and hospitalizations ... were not significantly different between the two groups."[880] The study showed that the new DTaP vaccine and the older DTP vaccine both have a high rate of adverse events, which caused many children to be hospitalized. But the point of the study was to measure the safety of the new vaccine against the older vaccine and not to measure the vaccine's safety in absolute terms. With the rigged criteria of relative safety, the FDA and the vaccine maker were able to announce a finding that the new vaccine was just as safe as the older vaccine because the rate of hospitalization was the same for both. But no rational person would ever say that a vaccine is safe that causes 1 out of every 22 children to be hospitalized. The trial showed that both the old and new vaccines were unsafe. But because the vaccine maker did not use an actual placebo there was no comparison to an inert (saline solution) the danger of the new DtaP was obscured.

The scam artists at the Pharmaceutical companies argue that when they have a childhood vaccine that has been proven effective, it is unethical not to administer that established vaccine to the control group. That is their cover story, but it is a provable lie. The testing of Prevnar® proves the lie. Prevnar® is supposed to guard against pneumococcus bacterium. Before Prevnar® there was no established childhood vaccine against pneumococcus bacterium. And so, no ethical claim could be made not to use an inert saline solution for the control study group. Nonetheless, Pfizer chose not to test Prevnar® against a true control group using a saline solution. Instead, Pfizer used a bioactive meningococol bacterium "placebo."

It gets worse; the control "placebo" was an investigational

vaccine. An investigational vaccine is an experimental vaccine that has only been tested in a laboratory and is approved by the FDA for use on persons for testing purposes only.[881] An investigational vaccine has not been shown to be safe or effective. That means the "placebo" vaccine given to the control group was an unproven and possibly unsafe vaccine that could cause unknown adverse events. The testers introduced an unknown variable into their test.

Pfizer went a step further in contaminating the test. Pfizer gave both the control group and the test group the DTaP vaccine. The Pfizer Prevnar® insert states:

> Efficacy was assessed in a randomized, double-blinded clinical trial in a multiethnic population at Northern California Kaiser Permanente (NCKP) from October 1995 through August 20, 1998, in which 37,816 infants were randomized to receive either Prevnar® or a control vaccine (an investigational meningococcal group C conjugate vaccine [MnCC]) at 2, 4, 6, and 12-15 months of age. Prevnar® was administered to 18,906 children and the control vaccine to 18,910 children. Routinely recommended vaccines were also administered which changed during the trial to reflect changing AAP and Advisory Committee on Immunization Practices (ACIP) recommendations.[882]

Pfizer did all it could to obscure the dangerousness of Prevnar. It was as though they knew that Prevnar would be shown in the study to be dangerous to children. The test did not disappoint. Sure enough, the study resulted in about 1,000 infants being hospitalized; that amounted to one out of every 35 infants in the study being hospitalized.[883] One out of every 16 children in the trial needed to be taken to the emergency room within 30 days of being vaccinated.

The study reported 5 cases of sudden infant death syndrome (SIDS) among the Prevnar test group and 8 cases of sudden infant death syndrome among the control group receiving the "placebo." Prevnar was shown to kill children, yet because they rigged the study to ramp up the control group's deaths by giving the control an experimental vaccine, they concluded that Prevnar was safe. Furthermore, the study authors stated: "The number of SIDS deaths in the efficacy study from October 1995 until April 20, 1999, was similar to or lower than the age and season-adjusted expected rate from the California State data from 1995-1997."[884] The study authors compared the SIDS data in the study to the SIDS data from a state that mandates childhood vaccinations and does not allow religious exemptions.

It is interesting that many of the childhood vaccine studies report SIDS data. But when people try to link SIDS to vaccines, they are considered conspiracy theorists or anti-vax wackos.

But Pfizer was not done. They must keep the poisons coming. Prevnar was purported to work against 7 strains of pneumococcus bacteria. In 2010, it updated its Prevnar vaccine to cover 13 pneumococcus bacterial strains. The new vaccine was branded Prevnar 13. How did they study the new vaccine for efficacy and safety? Well, they were not about to use an inert saline solution for the control group. So, they tested Prevnar 13 against the control group receiving the previously approved predecessor Prevnar vaccine.[885] What was the result? The Prevnar 13 package insert reveals:

> **Serious adverse events** reported following vaccination in infants and toddlers occurred in **8.2%** among Prevnar 13 recipients and **7.2%** among Prevnar recipients.[886]

You read that correctly. The FDA approved Prevnar 13 as safe even when **8.2% (one out of every 12 children) suffered a** "**serious adverse event**" from the vaccine. But because Prevnar 13 was compared to an equally dangerous predecessor vaccine, it was deemed by the FDA to be safe. There was a lot of money at stake with Prevnar and its successor vaccine, Prevnar 13. Reuters reported in 2014 that Prevnar and Prevnar 13 combined annual sales of almost $4.5 billion made them Pfizer's second-biggest franchise.[887]

This same scam is being run for adult vaccines. For example, Jeremy Howick revealed that "in the COVID-19 vaccine developed by the University of Oxford, the control group receives a meningitis and septicaemia vaccine as a placebo."[888] The Oxford COVID-19 vaccine is made by AstraZeneca and sold under the brand names Covishield and Vaxzevria.

On April 29, 2020, Pfizer-BioNTech announced the phases 1-2 studies (NCT04368728) of its COVID-19 vaccine.[889] The trial was described as "a Phase 1/2, randomized, **placebo-controlled**, observer-blind, dose-finding, and vaccine candidate-selection study in healthy adults."[890] One would naturally think that Pfizer-BioNTech would conduct the study using an inert saline solution. But you would be wrong.

The Informed Consent Action Network (ICAN) filed a Freedom of Information Act request with the FDA asking for the ingredients of the "placebo" used in the Pfizer-BioNTech studies. The FDA responded by denying the request. The FDA stated in pertinent part that information was a "trade secret" and thus "confidential commercial information."[891]

Dear reader, think about that. The placebo used in the control groups for the Pfizer-BioNTech COVID-19 vaccine trials is considered a confidential trade secret. We know from that alone that the placebo was not an inert substance like saline because saline is not and cannot be a trade secret. Thus, we know that the ingredients for the "placebo" were very likely bioactive.

Pfizer-BioNTech likely used their usual procedure of administering a bioactive ingredient to the control group to set a very high level of adverse events against with which to measure the mRNA COVID-19 vaccine to make the mRNA COVID-19 falsely appear safe. We now know that their scheme worked because the Pfizer-BioNTech COVID-19 vaccine won emergency use authorization and immediately began injuring and killing people.

30   Pediatricians Are Paid Bounties

This author talked to a couple with a newborn baby who had to leave their pediatrician's office because the pediatricians would not allow them to forgo getting their child vaccinated. The pediatricians continually pushed to allow the nurse to vaccinate their newborn baby. When the parents requested that the nurses and doctors please stop continually pestering them to have their child vaccinated, she was told that their office would allow a delay in the vaccination schedule but they would eventually have to get their child fully vaccinated.

The pediatric office has posted on its website a notice that it follows "the national standards of care set forth by the Centers for Disease Control and Prevention (CDC) and the American Academy of Pediatrics (AAP)."[892] According to the CDC vaccination schedule, their child would need to receive more than 47 total doses of vaccines (including boosters) that covered 17 different diseases before the child reached 15 months old. That pediatric practice of 15 doctors stated that if the parents persisted in not allowing them to vaccinate their child they would need to abide by their written policy, which required them to "find another pediatrician who agrees with your beliefs."[893]

The parents called pediatricians to find another doctor for their newborn child. The first four offices that the parents called refused to treat their child unless they agreed to have him vaccinated. A fifth office finally agreed to see their child without him being vaccinated, but only if they submitted a religious exemption.

The American Academy of Pediatrics (AAP) is a corporate and government mouthpiece that touts the wares of drug and vaccine manufacturers. Most Pediatricians mindlessly follow the recommendations of the AAP. The AAP advocates strong-arm tactics to coerce parents to vaccinate their children; it advises pediatricians that it is an "acceptable option to pediatric care clinicians to dismiss families who refuse vaccines."[894]

Moral degenerates run the AAP. For example, the AAP has issued an official policy statement supporting transitioning prepubescent children from male to female and vice versa.[895] The AAP thinks that prepubescent children should be allowed to change their gender despite objections from parents. The AAP approves transgenderism and states that it is outdated thinking to opine that a prepubescent child is not mature enough to change his or her gender. The AAP says that parents and doctors should affirm a child's decision to transition from one gender to another and not try to dissuade the child from that course. The AAP calls efforts to stop a child from identifying as or transitioning to a sex other than his or her biological sex "inappropriate," "deleterious," "unfair," "deceptive," and "outside the mainstream of traditional medical practice." The AAP states that it approves children undergoing cross-sex hormone therapy and irreversible transexual "gender affirming" surgeries. The AAP thinks that Pediatric primary care providers should be "a reliable source of validation, support, and reassurance" to prepubescent children seeking to transition from one gender to another. The AAP undermines the authority of parents over their children. In cases where the family objects to their child transitioning from one sex to another, the

AAP recommends that pediatricians seek legal help to ensure that they do not violate the local consent laws in their efforts to help the child transition over the objection of the parents.

It seems that there is a medical phalanx set up to push parents into vaccinating their children. The Immunization Action Coalition (IAC) provides doctors with a "Sample Vaccine Policy Statement: Ready for you to adapt for your practice."[896] That policy statement template states, in pertinent part that "if you should absolutely refuse to vaccinate your child despite all our efforts, we will ask you to find another healthcare provider who shares your views. We do not keep a list of such providers, nor would we recommend any such physician."[897]

The Immunization Action Coalition is funded "in partnership with the Centers for Disease Control and Prevention (CDC)" which "provided financial support to IAC."[898] The Children's Health Defense revealed that the CDC has acted as a captured government agency that is under the control of the vaccine industry.

> The latest data and science show that specific vaccines are unequivocally not safe. Yet government officials – with well-documented conflicts of interest with the $50 billion vaccine industry – systematically obscure the risks while exaggerating the benefits of vaccines.
>
> The government has quietly admitted culpability by paying out over $4 billion for thousands of injuries and deaths caused by vaccines underscoring that vaccine injuries can and do happen, including autism. And, an HHS-funded study concluded that fewer than 1% of vaccine injuries are even reported.

Big Pharma is exerting influence over WHO, FDA and CDC to fast track and short cut safety studies in order to gain more profits faster. Big Pharma has zero financial risk when children get vaccine injured because the government prevents victims from suing big pharma – resulting in big pharma not being concerned about child vaccine safety.

***

And CDC, frankly, is a vaccine company; it owns 56 vaccine patents and buys and distributes $4.6 billion in vaccines annually through the Vaccines for Children program, which is over 40% of its total budget. Further, Pharma directly funds, populates and controls dozens of CDC programs through the CDC foundation. A British Medical Journal editorial excoriates CDC's sweetheart relationship with pharma quotes UCLA Professor of Medicine Jerome R. Hoffman "most of us were shocked to learn the CDC takes funding from industry… It is outrageous that industry is apparently allowed to punish the CDC if the agency conducts research that has potential to cut into profits."[899]

The parents of the above mentioned child have come up against a massive syndicate funded by vaccine manufacturers. The couple's ordeal in finding a pediatrician who will treat their unvaccinated child is not unusual. Alex Pietroski, a reporter for Waking Times, alleged that "it is now very difficult to find a pediatrician who will accept a family who doesn't vaccinate. Even parents who partially vaccinate or follow a different schedule have a hard time finding a doctor. Here's why: doctors have to vaccinate a certain percentage of their patients or they don't get their bonus. BCBS [Blue Cros Blue Shield] says doctors need to vaccinate 63%

of their patients to get the payout [of $400 per vaccinated child]."⁹⁰⁰

This author researched Pietroski's allegation. Indeed, many pediatricians refuse to see child patients whose parents have decided not to have their children receive vaccines.⁹⁰¹ Doctors are increasingly encouraged to refuse service to the unvaccinated child patients based on a policy published in 2016 by the American Academy of Pediatrics (AAP) that allows pediatricians to dismiss the child patients of parents who refuse vaccines.⁹⁰² The Greenville News reported that "[a] two-month-old baby was recently denied care at a Carolina Forest pediatrician's office due to his parents' stance on vaccines."⁹⁰³ The report reveals:

> That decision stems from a policy adopted by recommendation of the American Academy of Pediatrics, according to Brian Argo, chief financial officer of Conway Medical Center, which operates CPG Pediatrics.⁹⁰⁴

You will notice that the spokesman for the pediatric office was the "chief financial officer." Why would the chief financial officer be the one who is giving the reasons for the policy of refusing service to unvaccinated children? Brian Argo has an MBA⁹⁰⁵, not an MD; he is a financial expert; he is not a medical expert. You would think that there would be a medical reason for the policy. You would think that the pediatrics office would appoint a medical doctor to give a medical reason for the policy. Instead, the pediatric office appoints a financial officer to present the rationale for refusing service to unvaccinated children. But he does not give a financial reason, nor does he give a medical reason; he gives as the reason a recommendation by the AAP. Unsurprisingly, he did not say that the pediatric office makes a lot of money by vaccinating children, and every unvaccinated child in its medical practice threatens that money stream.

Pietroski, however, alleges that there is a financial motive at the core of pediatricians not allowing unvaccinated children in their practice. Pietroski made a fantastic allegation that many pediatricians will not treat unvaccinated children because they need a certain threshold of patients in their medical practice to be vaccinated to be paid a bounty from insurance companies for each vaccinated child. It seems that the stick of medical licensure suspension for violating the AMA and AAP regulations if the pediatrician fails to vaccinate children is matched by the carrot of financial reward for doctors who push vaccines on the uninformed parents of children.

I researched Pietroski's allegation. What I found was surprising. The evidence establishes that his allegation is true. One example of this is under the Blue Cross Blue Shield *Childhood Immunizations- Combo 10* program. Under that program, if a pediatrician can convince 63% of the parents of children in their practice to receive the full schedule of the ten listed vaccines before the child's second birthday, the pediatrician will receive a $400 bounty per vaccinated child from Blue Cross Blue Shield.[906] That program presents a perverse monetary incentive for pediatricians to push for childhood vaccines. By the way, this is only one of the incentive programs being run by one insurance company in Michigan. There are, no doubt, many others. Below is a screenshot from page 15 of the 2016 Blue Cross Blue Shield "Performance Recognition Program, Provider Incentive Program," outlining the details of its *Childhood Immunizations- Combo 10 program.*

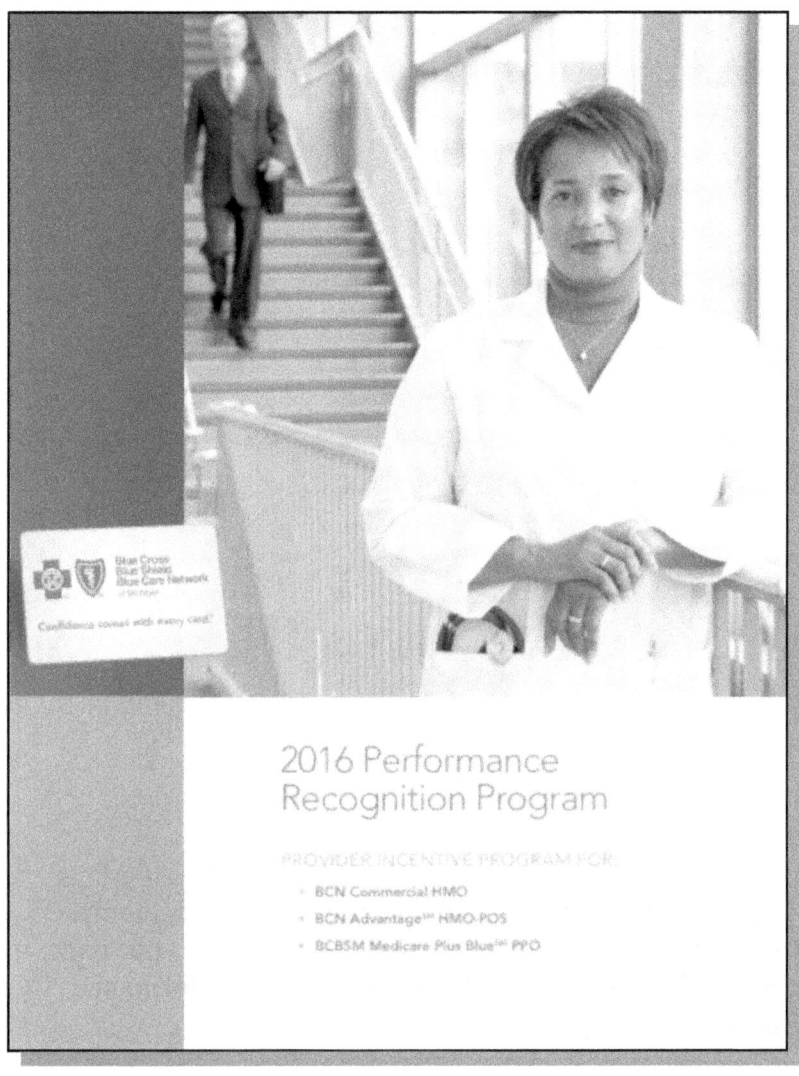

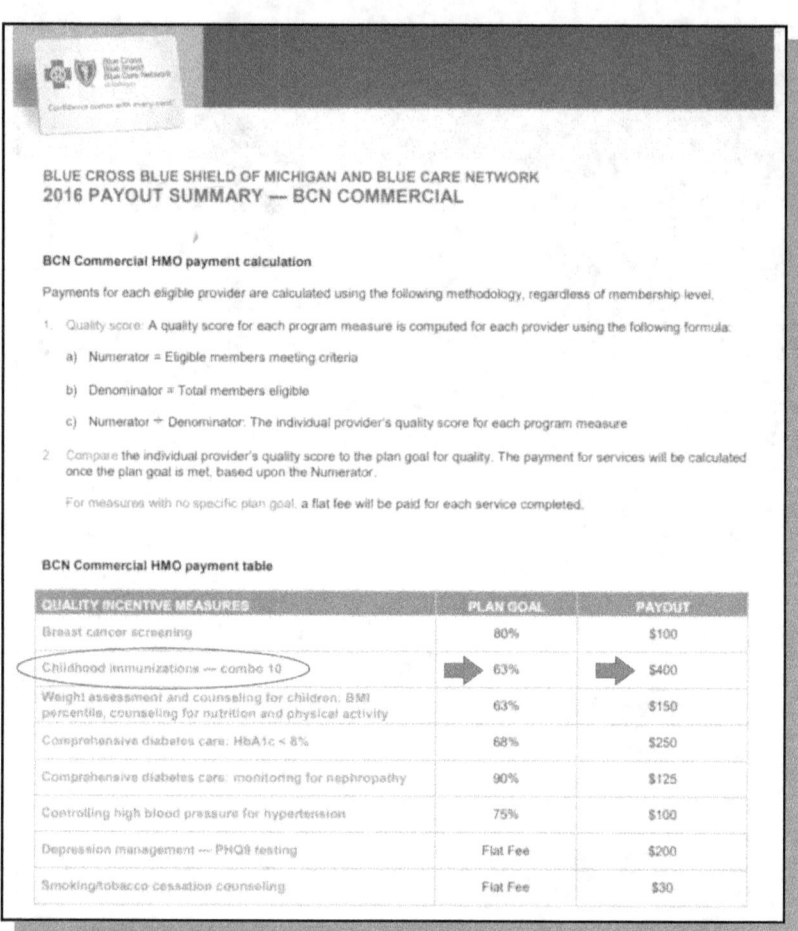

Figure 45: Chart (annotated) with instructions appearing on page 4 of the Blue Cross Blue Shield 2016 Performance Recognition Program.

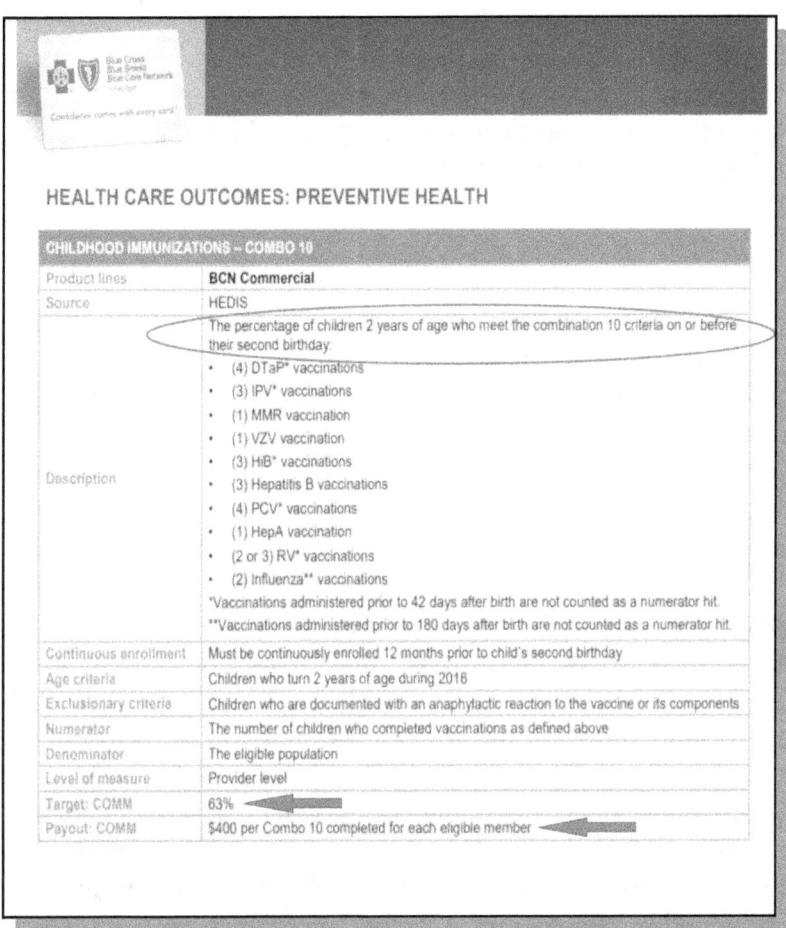

Figure 46: Chart (annotated) appearing on page 15 of the Blue Cross Blue Shield 2016 Performance Recognition Program.

The Blue Cross Blue Shield *Childhood Immunizations-Combo 10* program pays a bounty of $400 per child. But the pediatrician must have at least 63% of his patients vaccinated to receive any money. If the vaccinated population of children in his practice drops below 63%, the pediatrician receives nothing. To meet the plan goal, the eligible children receiving the required ten vaccines (numerator) is divided by the total eligible children in the practice (denominator). If that figure is 63% or more, then the doctor receives his bounty based on the number of children in the numerator. The Blue Cross Provider Incentive Program states: "The payment for services will be calculated once the plan goal is met [63%], based upon the Numerator."[907] If the fraction is less than 63% the doctor receives nothing.

It would not be unusual for a pediatrician to make approximately $53,000 yearly from Blue Cross Blue Shield's childhood vaccine incentive program. In 1999, a research study published in the Journal of the American Medical Association examined eighty-nine pediatric practices in 31 states involving 373 individual pediatric practitioners.[908] The study found that "each practitioner cared for an average of 1546 patients" over a two-year period. That is an average of 773 patients each year. The study was not a measure of office visits; it was a measure of individual patients treated regardless of the number of office visits. Thus, one patient visiting the office three times over the two-year period would be counted as a single patient. The study found that 27.4% of all pediatric patients were 2 years old or younger. On average, each pediatrician treated 211.8 (773 x 0.274 = 211.8) patients that were two years old or younger per year. That means that the average pediatrician can count on a bounty payout of approximately $84,720 per year from the Blue Cross Blue Shield Childhood Immunizations- Combo 10 program.

The $84,720 figure assumes that the doctor is able to convince 100% of his parents to vaccinate their children. If he is only able to convince 63% of parents, which is the bare minimum to qualify for the bounty, he would stand to make $53,374. Thus, the average pediatrician can make between $53,374 and $84,720 per year in vaccine bounty payments. The critical driver for him to push vaccinations on every parent is that if his rate of child vaccinations drops below 63% he will make nothing under that program.

This financial incentive to have a certain threshold (63%) of fully vaccinated children in their practice explains perfectly why some pediatricians will not allow unvaccinated children in their practice. Every child in their practice who is not fully vaccinated will bring them closer to their minimum threshold and threaten their $400 bounty for each vaccinated child. The Pediatrician, who you think should be looking out for your child's best interest, has a monetary incentive to ignore the mountain of evidence that vaccines are both ineffective and dangerous to children. Now you know why there has been no push-back from pediatricians about the acceleration of vaccines being injected into infants. They are financially incentivized to be willfully ignorant doctors.

The avarice of doctors has reached such a level that some will risk the lives of their patients for a buck. In a 2016 post on *Wellness and Equality*, the writer reveals how one pediatrician was willing to inject a vaccine into a child even after the child had a prior severe life-altering vaccine reaction. The pediatrician did not care about the harm the vaccine could cause to the child.

> When my friend's child suffered a life-threatening reaction to a vaccine a week after her first birthday, my friend assumed her pediatrician would write her a medical exemption from future vaccines. Shortly after receiving a routine set of vaccines, the happy, vibrant one-year-old spiked a 106 degree fever, began having seizures, and was hospitalized. When the unexplained "illness" passed after a week in the hospital, the little girl had lost her ability to walk. My friend describes how her daughter, who had learned to walk several months earlier at 9 months, suddenly "stumbled around like a drunk person" for weeks following the vaccines. My friend met with a team of pediatricians, neurologists, and naturopathic doctors, and they agreed: Her daughter had suffered a brain injury caused by a

reaction to one of the vaccines. Hoping the injury would be temporary and that she might recover and ease her brain inflammation if they could help her small body quickly eliminate the vaccine additives that caused the reaction, my friend's daughter underwent an intensive detoxification program overseen by a nutritionalist. Slowly, her daughter relearned to walk.

My friend is a practicing attorney who graduated from a Top 10 college. The evidence was overwhelming that her daughter's reaction had been caused by vaccines, she told me.

But a few months later, when she took her daughter back into the pediatrician for a visit, he wanted to vaccinate her daughter again. She was baffled. Why?

After a reader sent us a link to a PDF file of Blue Cross Blue Shield's Physician Incentive Program available online, *Wellness & Equality* learned that insurance companies pay pediatricians massive bonuses based on the percentage of children who are fully vaccinated by age 2.[909]

Some pediatricians are money-grubbers who care nothing about the well-being of the children they treat.

For the love of money is the root of all evil: which while some coveted after, they have erred from the faith, and pierced themselves through with many sorrows. (1 Timothy 6:10)

Once Blue Cross and Blue Shield realized their scheme was being publicized, it took steps to prevent further revelations.

> After *Wellness & Equality* published [the] article, Blue Cross Blue Shield locked online access to their incentive program and then removed the page altogether.[910]

J.B. Handley, the co-founder of Generation Rescue, revealed the dark secret of how much money pediatricians make by administering vaccines to children.

> [W]henever I meet a pediatrician I ask them a simple question: what percentage of your revenue come from vaccine administration? The number always astounds me. The answers I get are that anywhere from 50-80% of their revenue comes from giving vaccines. Imagine that.[911]

In his book, Jabbed, Brett Wilcox revealed that "a pediatrician told a Minnesota audience in 2016 that he loses $700,000 a year because he doesn't push vaccines according to the U.S. vaccine schedule."[912]

COVID-19 Vaccine Bounties

On April 13, 2023, U.S. Congressman Thomas Massie reported on Twitter that Anthem Medicaid paid a bounty to push COVID-19 vaccines under its "COVID-19 Vaccine Provider Incentive Program."[913] The bounty gave progressively increased payments for each vaccinated patient based on the percentage of Anthem vaccinated members. For example, if the doctor provided at least one dose of a COVID-19 vaccine before September 1, 2021, to a patient, the doctor would receive a $20 bonus per vaccine administered if at least 30% of his Anthem patients were vaccinated. However, the payment increased to $125 per vaccinated patient if 75% of the Anthem members were vaccinated. The amount increased substantially if the patient was vaccinated between September 21, 2021, and December 31, 2021.

If the doctor provided at least one dose of a COVID-19 vaccine to a patient before December 31, 2021, the doctor would receive a $100 bonus per vaccine if at least 30% of his Anthem patients were vaccinated. However, the payment per COVID-19 vaccine increased to $250 per vaccinated patient if 75% of the Anthem members were vaccinated before December 31, 2021. Below is the official schedule of bounties provided to doctors by Anthem, which Rep. Massie obtained. Other insurance companies almost certainly have similar incentive programs. You have reason to question your doctor's objectivity when he recommends you take the COVID-19 vaccine. He likely has a pecuniary interest in convincing you to take the vaccine.

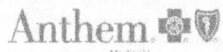

Anthem Blue Cross and Blue Shield Medicaid

COVID-19 Vaccine Provider Incentive program

Getting vaccinated against COVID-19 is one of the best and safest ways people can protect themselves and their families against the virus. As a participating practice in the COVID-19 Provider Vaccine Incentive program, we recognize your hard work by offering incentives for helping patients make the choice to become vaccinated.

Eligibility

The COVID-19 Vaccine Provider Incentive program is open to you if you are a participating Kentucky primary care provider with an Anthem Blue Cross and Blue Shield Medicaid (Anthem) panel size of 25 or more members. All Anthem members identified as receiving COVID-19 vaccination services are included in the methodology. Vaccine results will be determined by a COVID-19 vaccine claim or by confirmation from the Kentucky Vaccine Registry.

The results will be calculated for two time periods:
- September 1, 2021 – Initial incentive payment
- December 31, 2021 – Final incentive payment

How you can qualify for a bonus

If your practice meets the below thresholds for vaccination with at least one dose by September 1, 2021, you will receive the initial incentive payment based on the following rates:
- 30% Anthem members vaccinated – $20 bonus per vaccinated member
- 40% Anthem members vaccinated – $45 bonus per vaccinated member
- 50% Anthem members vaccinated – $70 bonus per vaccinated member
- 60% Anthem members vaccinated – $100 bonus per vaccinated member
- 75% Anthem members vaccinated – $125 bonus per vaccinated member

The final incentive payment is calculated based on members who are newly vaccinated between September 1, 2021 and December 31, 2021 (see the *Appendix* for calculation examples). If your practice meets the below thresholds for vaccination with at least one dose by December 1, 2021, you will receive the final incentive payment based on the following rates:
- 30% Anthem members vaccinated – $100 bonus per newly vaccinated member
- 40% Anthem members vaccinated – $150 bonus per newly vaccinated member
- 50% Anthem members vaccinated – $175 bonus per newly vaccinated member
- 60% Anthem members vaccinated – $200 bonus per newly vaccinated member
- 75% Anthem members vaccinated – $250 bonus per newly vaccinated member

https://providers.anthem.com/ky

Anthem Blue Cross and Blue Shield Medicaid is the trade name of Anthem Kentucky Managed Care Plan, Inc., independent licensee of the Blue Cross and Blue Shield Association. Anthem is a registered trademark of Anthem Insurance Companies, Inc.

31 Buying Influence to Injure and Kill

The strange phenomenon of colleges nationwide issuing vaccine mandates in virtual lockstep is explainable. They were not making independent judgments about the safety and efficacy of the COVID-19 vaccines. They mandated the COVID-19 vaccines because the federal government paid them to do it. The federal government created a financial incentive for universities to mandate COVID-19 vaccines.

College administrators don't care about the well-being of the students; they care about money. The universities are staffed with highly qualified scientific researchers with worldwide data and studies at their fingertips. College administrators know with certainty that the COVID-19 vaccines are unsafe and ineffective. But they have been paid off. The universities mandating the COVID-19 vaccines are run by sociopaths who are perfectly okay with injuring the students and staff because they get money from the federal government to do it.

U.S. colleges and universities are being paid billions of dollars from the federal government Coronavirus Aid, Relief, and Economic Security (CARES) Act to mandate student and staff COVID-19 vaccinations. The precondition for receiving the

CARES money is that the universities comply with COVID-19 vaccine mandates.

The universities do not serve the students. They are more beholden to their paymaster, the federal government. **For example, Yale University made more money from the CARES Act in 2022 ($607 million) than from student tuition ($475 million).**[914] Dr. Michael Nevradakis, Ph.D., and Lynn Comerford, Ph.D., revealed that "since 1998, Yale has received $9 billion from HHS — $1 billion of which has been disbursed since 2020."[915] It is no surprise then to find that Yale's "COVID-19 Vaccination Policy" includes an oppressive COVID-19 vaccine mandate.

> The university requires all students, faculty, staff, and postdoctoral/postgraduate trainees — other than those with approved medical or religious exemptions — to receive a primary COVID-19 vaccine series and to obtain a booster shot within 14 days of eligibility. Additionally, students — other than those with approved medical or religious exemptions —must receive an updated, bivalent booster by the start of the spring semester (in any event, no later than January 31, 2023), regardless of how many previous monovalent boosters they received.[916]

On April 1, 2021, HHS announced that it was establishing a nationwide network of "trusted voices" to encourage people to get COVID-19 vaccinations. The trusted voices were labeled "The COVID-19 Community Corps." Among the founding members of this Orwellian campaign to poison the populace through deceptive marketing were the nation's premier medical and health associations, including, but not limited to, the American Medical Association (AMA), American Academy of Pediatrics (AAP), American College of Obstetricians and Gynecologists (ACOG), American College of Physicians (ACP), and American Association of Nurse Practitioners (AANP).[917]

Why would these medical organizations agree to work with HHS to encourage people to get COVID-19 vaccines? The answer is as old as time; they are being paid very handsomely to prostitute themselves and act as shills and huxters for the government. For example, the ACOG alone received $11 million from HHS.[918] Attorney Maggie Thorp, and her OBGYN husband Jim Thorp, M.D., revealed that receipt of the money was contingent on "ACOG's full compliance with CDC guidance on COVID-19 infection and control."[919] The ACOG is not just a professional organization; it holds great sway over its members. Maggie and Jim Thorp explain:

> Meet the American College of Obstetricians and Gynecologists (ACOG). Founded in 1951, ACOG holds itself out as the "premier professional membership organization for obstetricians and gynecologists" and is the leading organization representing physicians and specialists in obstetrical care. ACOG is entrenched across two continents – it has more than 60,000 members and is composed of 12 geographic districts made up of 98 sections spanning North, South, and Central America.[920]

The ACOG had initially taken the position that "[i]n the interest of patient autonomy, ACOG recommends that pregnant individuals be free to make their own decision regarding COVID-19 vaccination."[921] But after HHS made its $11 million payoff to ACOG, on July 30, 2021, the ACOG changed its position on the COVID-19 vaccine from one of deference to the mother's decision to one of strongly recommending the COVID-19 vaccine for pregnant women. That recommendation was made in the face of no evidence of the vaccines' safety or efficacy for pregnant women; indeed, the COVID-19 vaccine clinical trials failed to include pregnant women. There was no science to support ACOG's change in position, but the payment of $11 million certainly explains it.

Flush with its windfall of $11 million from HHS, ACOG obediently whipped its doctors into line by publishing "key recommendations," including:

> The American College of Obstetricians and Gynecologists (ACOG) strongly recommends that pregnant individuals be vaccinated against COVID-19. Given the potential for severe illness and death during pregnancy, completion of the initial COVID-19 vaccination series is a priority for this population.

***

> ACOG recommends that pregnant and recently pregnant people up to 6 weeks postpartum receive a bivalent mRNA COVID-19 vaccine booster dose following the completion of their last COVID-19 primary vaccine dose or monovalent booster.[922]

All patients who refuse to get the COVID-19 vaccine must have their medical record reflect their refusal. Notably, one of the ACOG "key recommendations" is for the doctor to convince the patient who refused previous vaccination efforts to get vaccinated at the next office visit.

> For patients who do not receive any COVID-19 vaccine, the discussion should be documented in the patient's medical record. During subsequent office visits, obstetrician–gynecologists should address ongoing questions and concerns and offer vaccination again.[923]

This hard-sell strategy clearly deviates from ACOG's previous position that "pregnant individuals be free to make their own decision regarding COVID-19 vaccination." A little known fact is that under the "Cooperative Agreement" between HHS and the ACOG that was part of the arrangement to get the millions of dollars from HHS, "the recipient is expected to provide to CDC copies of and/or access to COVID-19 data collected with these funds."[924] That means the patient's decision whether to get a COVID-19 vaccine will likely be reported to the CDC. The CDC is a component agency of HHS.

The $11 million payoff from the HHS turned the ACOG into liars. One of the "Key Messages" about COVID-19 from the ACOG is the claim that the COVID-19 vaccines do not cause infertility, spontaneous abortion, or fetal defects. That assurance is false. Evidence from Pfizer's studies reported in January 2021 (and publically revealed under an FOIA order on April 28, 2023) showed that rats who had taken the COVID-19 vaccine were twice as likely to suffer pregnancy loss.[925] Furthermore, the Pfizer studies showed a 14-fold increase in birth abnormalities among the COVID-19 vaccinated rats compared to the control group.[926]

On April 29, 2023, it was revealed that in human trials, the Pfizer COVID-19 vaccine was shown to cause spontaneous abortions in 21% of women receiving the COVID-19 vaccine.[927] Babies born to mothers who had been vaccinated suffered damages ranging from pneumothorax to death.[928] Indeed, 19% of the infants exposed to the COVID mRNA vaccine via their mothers' milk suffered from 48 different adverse events ranging from diarrhea to vomiting.[929] Amy Kelly, who is the Program Director of the War Room/DailyClout Pfizer Documents Analysis Project, explains:

> Despite Pfizer and the FDA knowing by April 20, 2021, the extent of damage to fetuses and babies, including the fact that fetuses and newborns had died, on April 23, 2021, inexplicably [CDC

Director] Dr. Rochelle Walensky held a White House press briefing where she recommended pregnant women get vaccinated.[930]

ACOG is as culpable as the CDC. While the ACOG had no scientific or medical reasons, they had eleven million other reasons to "strongly recommend[] that pregnant individuals be vaccinated against COVID-19." The ACOG doctors have literally been given a script to follow to deceive and badger their patients into getting vaccinated. The script did not allow for any consideration of each patient's unique health needs or condition. It is a one size fits all recommendation to get vaccinated. There is no proviso in the script for informed consent. It is a script to push, prod, and cajole compliance. The ACOG script prodding pregnant women to get vaccinated remains unchanged despite the mountain of evidence that the COVID-19 vaccines are ineffective and dangerous. It is a violation of the Hippocratic oath to first do no harm. It is not the practice of medicine; it is more the administration of a superstitious religious sacrament.

You realize who is behind this effort to poison and kill mothers and infants when you follow the money. The "CDC Foundation" was created by Congress.[931] It is a public charity that has been given statutory authority to fund the CDC. The CDC accepts funds from the CDC Foundation. Of course, the CDC Foundation wields tremendous control over the CDC. The funds the CDC Foundation provides are then funneled to medical associations such as the ACOG to push doctors into administering vaccines. Take a wild guess who funds the CDC Foundation? The CDC Foundation is funded by all the usual suspects: pharmaceutical companies that make vaccines like Pfizer, Merck, Johns & Johnson, and organizations that profit from vaccines or are funded by those who so profit, like the Bill & Malinda Gates Foundation, the GAVI Alliance, and the World Health Organization.[932] He who pays the piper calls the tune. The powerful pharmaceutical interests use their funding control over the CDC to, in turn, see that those funds are used to control what the doctor tells his patients about the safety and efficacy of vaccines. This is a new spin on trickle-down economics. Any doctor who kicks against the pricks and does not follow orders soon finds himself out of a job.

32 Jacobson v. Massachusetts

The U.S. Constitution establishes the federal government and its relationship to the states and people. The powers of the federal government are expressly granted and enumerated in the Constitution. The Tenth Amendment provides that all powers not granted to the federal government are reserved to the states and people, respectively. The first ten amendments to the Constitution (The Bill of Rights) expressly limit the powers of the federal government. The Ninth Amendment provides that rights not enumerated in the Bill of Rights are nonetheless retained by the people.

First Amendment

>The First Amendment provides:

>Congress shall make no law respecting an establishment of religion, or prohibiting the free exercise thereof; or abridging the freedom of speech, or of the press; or the right of the people peaceably to assemble, and to petition the Government for a redress of grievances.

>The First Amendment has been interpreted to apply to the

state governments by incorporating it into the 14 Amendment Due Process clause. *See, E.g., Cantwell v. State of Connecticut*,[933] (Connecticut State law requiring Jehovah's Witnesses to obtain a certificate as a condition of soliciting support for their views amounted to a prior restraint on the exercise of their religion in violation of the First Amendment); *Engel v. Vitale*,[934] (outlawing school prayer in New York public schools as a violation of the First Amendment Establishment Clause); *Kennedy v. Bremerton Sch. Dist.*,[935] (Public school football coach's freedom of religion was infringed by school district which fired him for kneeling at midfield after games to offer a quiet prayer of thanks where he was joined by players and parents. The conduct by the public school coach was considered private and thus did not constitute a violation of the Establishment Clause.)

In *Cantwell v. State of Connecticut*,[936] the U.S. Supreme Court explained:

> The constitutional inhibition of legislation on the subject of religion has a double aspect. On the one hand, it forestalls compulsion by law of the acceptance of any creed or the practice of any form of worship. ... On the other hand, it safeguards the free exercise of the chosen form of religion.[937]

Jacobson v. Massachusetts

This is a good point to address the alleged precedent of *Jacobson v. Massachusetts*.[938] In *Jacobson*, the U.S. Supreme Court upheld a Massachusetts statute empowering municipal boards of health to require that smallpox vaccinations be given to all residents. Failure to obtain the vaccine subjected the violator to a civil fine.

Jacobson v. Massachusetts[939] addressed 14th Amendment Due Process and Equal Protection claims. The principal claim was that mandating a smallpox vaccination violated his constitutionally protected liberty interest in his bodily integrity against forced medical treatment. The U.S. Supreme Court upheld the validity of the vaccine mandate statute. The claimant did not allege a Freedom of Religion claim under the First Amendment. Thus, *Jacobson* should not be considered precedent in a First Amendment claim. In *Jacobson*, the claimant made an offer of proof at his trial that vaccination for smallpox was ineffective and unsafe. The trial court rejected the offer of proof, and the Supreme Court agreed that evidence that the smallpox vaccine was unsafe and ineffective was irrelevant.

The U.S. Supreme Court ruled that the trial court properly took judicial notice of the safety and efficacy of the smallpox vaccine. The Court stated that it must assume the Massachusetts legislature already weighed the scientific debate regarding the safety and effectiveness of the smallpox vaccine and chose to side with the majority position and reject the minority position. It was not for the courts to overrule that public policy decision that vaccines were necessary for the health of the population.

> We must assume that, when the statute in question was passed, the legislature of Massachusetts was not unaware of these opposing theories, and was compelled, of necessity, to choose between them. It was not compelled to commit a matter involving the public health and safety to the final decision of a court or jury. It is no part of the function of a court or a jury to determine which one of two modes was likely to be the most effective for the protection of the public against disease. That was for the legislative department to determine in the light of all the information it had or could obtain. It could not properly abdicate its function to guard the public health and safety. The state legislature proceeded upon the theory which recognized

vaccination as at least an effective, if not the best-known, way in which to meet and suppress the *31 evils of a smallpox epidemic that imperiled an entire population. Upon what sound principles as to the relations existing between the different departments of government can the court review this action of the legislature? If there is any such power in the judiciary to review legislative action in respect of a matter affecting the general welfare, it can only be when that which the legislature has done comes within the rule that, if a statute purporting to have been enacted to protect the public health, the public morals, or the public safety, has no real or substantial relation to those objects, or is, beyond all question, a plain, palpable invasion of rights secured by the fundamental law, it is the duty of the courts to so adjudge, and thereby give effect to the Constitution.[940]

In *Health Freedom Def. Fund, Inc. v. Carvalho*,[941] the entire bench of the U.S. Circuit Court of Appeals for the Ninth Circuit cited *Jacobson* in upholding a COVID-19 vaccine mandate in the Los Angeles Unified School District. The plaintiffs did not raise a First Amendment claim in the Health Freedom case. The plaintiffs raised Due Process and Equal Protection claims only. The plaintiffs' principal claim was that the vaccine mandate infringed their liberty interests in bodily integrity against forced medical treatment. The court reviewed the COVID-19 vaccine under the rational basis standard. Under that low standard, if a statute has a rational relationship to a legitimate government interest, it will be upheld. Only in the most egregious cases, where a public health statute has no real or substantial relation to protecting public health, such that it clearly presents a plain and palpable invasion of fundamental rights, will it be ruled unconstitutional.[942]

The rational basis standard is so low that a vaccine mandate will pass muster even though there is evidence that the vaccines do not provide immunity or prevent the spread of disease. The *Health Freedom* court ruled:

> *Jacobson* thus applies to vaccination requirements regardless of whether such vaccines actually provide immunity and prevent the spread of disease or whether they provide no immunity and merely render COVID-19 less dangerous to those who contract it, so long as policymakers could reasonably conclude that the vaccines would protect the public's health and safety.[943]

Thus, the *Health Freedom* court ruled that under *Jacobson*, the constitutionality of a vaccine mandate turns on whether the legislature *could* have rationally decided that vaccines protect the public health, not whether they *actually* provide immunity or prevent transmission of a disease.[944] The Health Freedom court ruled:

> Whether a vaccine protects the public's health and safety is committed to policymakers, not a court or a jury. Further, alleged scientific uncertainty over a vaccine's efficacy is irrelevant under *Jacobson*. *Jacobson* simply does not allow debate in the courts over whether a mandated vaccine prevents the spread of disease. *Jacobson* makes clear that it is up to the political branches, within the parameters of rational basis review, to decide whether a vaccine effectively protects public health and safety.[945]

The *Health Freedom* court had little difficulty finding that "[t]he Policy easily survives such [rational basis] review because (even assuming the truth of Plaintiffs' allegations [that the vaccines were unsafe and ineffective]) it was more than reasonable for the LAUSD to conclude that COVID-19 vaccines would protect the health and safety of its employees and students."[946]

There you have it. Under the *Jacobson* line of Due Process cases, a court will view evidence of the inefficacy and dangers of vaccines as irrelevant. Thus, the only hope for relief is under the First Amendment. A plaintiff should bring his claim under both the Freedom of Religion and the Establishment Clauses of the First Amendment. Arguably, *Jacobson* and its progeny are irrelevant when the claim is under, not Due Process or Equal Protection, but the First Amendment.

That does not mean that one should not also bring a Due Process claim. *Jacobson's* standard seems to be hanging by a thread. It is hard to reconcile *Jacobson* and *Health Freedom* decisions with recent Supreme Court cases involving the scope of Due Process protection. The Supreme Court has ruled that people have a fundamental Due Process right to bodily integrity against forced medical treatment.[947] "A competent person has a liberty interest under the Due Process Clause in refusing unwanted medical treatment."[948] The U.S. Supreme Court stated that "[f]reedom from unwanted medical attention is unquestionably among those principles so rooted in the traditions and conscience of our people as to be ranked as fundamental."[949]

The Supreme Court has ruled that when the government statute "significantly interferes with the exercise of a fundamental right, it cannot be upheld unless it is supported by sufficiently important state interests and is closely tailored to effectuate only those interests."[950] "The [Due Process] Clause also provides heightened protection against government interference with certain fundamental rights and liberty interests. ... We have also assumed, and strongly suggested, that the Due Process Clause protects the traditional right to refuse unwanted lifesaving medical treatment."[951] If a person has a fundamental right to refuse lifesaving medical treatment, he certainly has a right to refuse allegedly beneficial vaccines.

That strict scrutiny standard requires that an infringement of a fundamental right can only pass constitutional muster if it is the least intrusive means to accomplish a compelling state interest.[952] The Supreme Court has repeatedly set forth the principle that "the Fourteenth Amendment forbids the government to infringe fundamental liberty interests at all, no matter what process is provided, unless the infringement is narrowly tailored to serve a compelling state interest."[953]

Under the rational basis test, the government only needs to show that the vaccine could arguably protect public health. But under strict scrutiny, it must establish that the vaccine is the best (indeed, only) way to protect public health. That standard elevates the safety and efficacy of the vaccines from irrelevance under the rational basis test to primacy, to the forefront of the discussion, under the strict scrutiny standard. There is no way an unsafe and ineffective vaccine could ever pass the strict scrutiny test. If a vaccine cannot protect against infection, it is axiomatic that, according to the germ theory, it cannot prevent the spread of a disease. How could any government rationally argue that the only way it can achieve its allegedly compelling interest in protecting the health of the populace is to mandate that all people get vaccinated with an unsafe and ineffective vaccine? It is a ridiculous argument.

With that Supreme Court strict scrutiny precedent firmly in mind, the *Health Freedom* nonetheless used the lower rational basis standard. The *Health Freedom* court disregarded the Supreme Court precedent by dismissively stating that "[w]hatever the reach of these cases, they did not overrule *Jacobson.*"[954] That is not what one would call a deep legal analysis. In light of the Supreme Court's pronouncements, is hard to fathom how the *Health Freedom* and *Jacobson* decisions can form any lasting precedent. In any event, those cases are irrelevant when analyzing the validity of a First Amendment claim.

The Honorable Judge Stickman in *City of Butler v. Wolf* explains the rather tenuous precedent of *Jacobson*:

> *Jacobson* was decided over a century ago. Since that time, there has been substantial development of federal constitutional law in the area of civil liberties. As a general matter, this development has seen a jurisprudential shift whereby federal courts have given greater deference to considerations of individual liberties, as weighed against the exercise of state police powers. That century of development has seen the creation of tiered levels of scrutiny for constitutional claims. They did not exist when *Jacobson* was decided. While Jacobson has been cited by some modern courts as ongoing support for a broad, hands-off deference to state authorities in matters of health and safety, other courts and commentators have questioned whether it remains instructive in light of the intervening jurisprudential developments.[955]

In *Bayley's Campground, Inc. v. Mills*,[956] where the court denied injunctive relief from COVID-19 restrictions, the court nonetheless stated:

> [T]he permissive *Jacobson* rule floats about in the air as a rubber stamp for all but the most absurd and egregious restrictions on constitutional liberties, free from the inconvenience of meaningful judicial review. This may help explain why the Supreme Court established the traditional tiers of scrutiny in the course of the 100 years since *Jacobson* was decided.[957]

Justice Alito's dissent (joined by Justices Thomas and Kavanaugh) to the U.S. Supreme Court's denial of emergency injunctive relief in *Calvary Chapel Dayton Valley v. Sisolak*,[958] calls into question whether *Jacobson* remains valid precedent. *Jacobson* is a phantom from a bygone era. Justice Alito argued that the Supreme Court should have granted the requested injunction: "We have a duty to defend the Constitution, and even a public health emergency does not absolve us of that responsibility."[959] Justice Alito argued that "a public health emergency does not give Governors and other public officials *carte blanche* to disregard the Constitution for as long as the medical problem persists."[960] Justice Alito warned that "it is a mistake to take language in *Jacobson* as the last word on what the Constitution allows public officials to do during the COVID-19 pandemic."[961] Indeed, he viewed it "a considerable stretch to read the [Jacobson] decision as establishing the test to be applied when statewide measures of indefinite duration are challenged under the First Amendment or other provisions not at issue in that case."[962]

Justice Gorsuch's concurrence in *Roman Cath. Diocese of Brooklyn v. Cuomo*[963], questions *Jacobson's* continued viability as the sweeping precedent many ascribe to it. Justice Gorsuch stated that "Jacobson hardly supports cutting the Constitution loose during a pandemic."[964] He had more to say:

> Why have some mistaken this Court's modest decision in *Jacobson* for a towering authority that overshadows the Constitution during a pandemic? In the end, I can only surmise that much of the answer lies in a particular judicial impulse to stay out of the way in times of crisis. But if that impulse may be understandable or even admirable in other circumstances, we may not shelter in place when the Constitution is under attack. Things never go well when we do.[965]

As noted by the U.S. Court of Appeals for the Second Circuit in *Agudath Israel of Am. v. Cuomo*[966]: "'the *Jacobson* Court itself specifically noted that 'even if based on the acknowledged police powers of a state,' a public-health measure 'must always yield in case of conflict with ... any right which [the Constitution] gives or secures.'"[967] (brackets in original).

33 First Amendment Free Exercise Clause

Since its decision in *Jacobson*, the Supreme Court has set forth a test for infringement of Freedom of Religion under the First Amendment. "Under the Free Exercise Clause, a government entity normally must satisfy at least 'strict scrutiny,' showing that its restrictions on the plaintiff's protected rights serve a compelling interest and are narrowly tailored to that end."[968] A federal district court, in *Bosarge v. Edney*,[969] quoted the U.S. Supreme Court when explaining:

> Where strict scrutiny applies, government policy survives only if it advances interests of the highest order and is narrowly tailored to achieve those interests, meaning that so long as the government can achieve its interests in a manner that does not burden religion, it must do so.[970] (quotation marks omitted)

Jacobson hangs by a thread and presents only a smidgen of authority for upholding mandatory vaccinations.

Neutral and Generally Applicable Statutes

In *Employment Division, Department of Human Resources of Oregon v. Smith*,[971] the U.S. Supreme Court ruled that when a statute or practice is neutral and generally applicable on its face and thus only incidentally infringes on a person's freedom of religion, the government does NOT have to show a compelling government interest.

However, a facially neutral statute that when applied allows a secular exemption from vaccination but disallows the same exemption for religious reasons must be assessed under strict scrutiny. The U.S. Supreme Court has repeatedly explained that "[a] law is not generally applicable if it invites the government to consider the particular reasons for a person's conduct by providing a mechanism for individualized exemptions."[972] The U.S. Supreme Court explains the logic behind that rule is the common-sense observation that "[a] law ... lacks general applicability if it prohibits religious conduct while permitting secular conduct that undermines the government's asserted interests in a similar way."[973] No vaccine mandate can ever be considered a generally applicable law because all vaccine mandates allow for medical exemptions.[974]

The U.S. Court of Appeals for the Tenth Circuit explains that "a government policy that grants an exemption for medical reasons but denies the same exemption for religious reasons is not generally applicable, as it devalues religious reasons by judging them to be of lesser import than nonreligious reasons."[975] (ellipse deleted)

All vaccine mandates must be reviewed under the strict scrutiny standard. That means that in order to disallows a religious exemption, the government must establish doing so is the least restrictive means of accomplishing its allegedly compelling government interest. No vaccine mandate that denies a religious exemption could ever pass that test because it is irrational to allow a medical exemption while denying a religious exemption. That is because, as Justices Gorsuch, Thomas, and Alito explained in their dissent to a denial of injunctive relief requested by doctors, "unvaccinated religious objectors and unvaccinated medical objectors are equally at risk for contracting COVID-19 or spreading it to their colleagues."[976] The dissenting Justices explained that "Maine's decision to deny a religious exemption in these circumstances doesn't just fail the least restrictive means test, it borders on the irrational."[977]

On April 17, 2023, the Informed Consent Action Network (ICAN) secured an historic ruling from a federal court.[978] In *Bosarge v. Edney*,[979] the court ruled a Mississippi law unconstitutional. The law disallowed religious exemptions for childhood vaccinations. Children in Mississippi must obtain childhood vaccines before school enrollment. Violation of the vaccine requirement carried criminal penalties. The state statute allowed for medical exemptions but disallowed religious exemptions for the vaccine requirement. The federal district court issued an injunction preventing the enforcement of the law. The State of Mississippi must now afford its residents a religious exemption against having to vaccinate their children as a requirement to attend school.

The State of Mississippi statute made an unconstitutional value judgment that secular (i.e., medical) motivations for opting out of compulsory immunization are permitted but that religious grounds are not.[980] That distinction unconstitutionally discriminated against a citizen's sincerely held religious beliefs. The U.S. Supreme Court has established that discriminating against a person's religious beliefs in that fashion is subject to strict scrutiny. The federal district court in *Bosarge* ruled that the Mississippi statute requiring vaccination was not neutral and generally applicable because the way it was applied discriminated against students based on their religious beliefs. It allowed a secular exemption to vaccination for medical reasons but disallowed religious exemptions. The state must use the least restrictive means to serve a compelling government interest to discriminate against someone based on his religious beliefs. The State of Mississippi could not make that showing because to allow a secular exemption while disallowing a religious exemption is prototypically NOT the least restrictive means. The U.S. Supreme Court has ruled that the government is prohibited from treating "any comparable secular activity more favorably than religious exercise."[981]

The U.S. Supreme Court has issued similar rulings in recent COVID-19 cases. In *Tandon v. Newsom*,[982] the U.S. Supreme Court ruled that it was unconstitutional for the State of California to issue regulations, ostensibly intended to slow the spread of COVID-19, that placed limits on religious gatherings but treated comparable non-religious activities – such as getting haircuts and retail shopping – more favorably. Similarly, the U.S. Supreme Court, in *Roman Catholic Diocese of Brooklyn v. Cuomo*,[983] ruled that New York regulation that prohibited religious gatherings but permitted similar secular gatherings violated the First Amendment where the secular and religious activities in question presented comparable alleged contagion risks.

Please note that the restrictions in the *Newsom* and *Cuomo* cases were based on the unproven, mythical germ theory. The germ theory is a Satanic superstitious belief conjured to enslave the population. Governments will use that folklore to mask, lockdown, separate, and vaccinate its citizens, allegedly to protect the community from each new contrived boogeyman virus.

The State of Mississippi argued that it had a compelling interest in stopping the spread of infectious disease, but the state cannot discriminate against one's religious beliefs to accomplish that goal. The district court pointed out that "[t]he relevant question is not whether the government has a compelling interest in enforcing its policies generally, but whether it has such an interest in denying a religious exemption to a plaintiff."[984]

The state argued that it wanted to prevent the exposure of its vaccinated children to unvaccinated children. But the law does not do that because unvaccinated children with medical exemptions are not excluded from school. Those unvaccinated children would be mingling with the vaccinated children. Furthermore, teachers, administrators, and other adults in the schools are not required to be vaccinated; they have regular contact with the vaccinated children. Only those unvaccinated children with religious objections to vaccination are prohibited from entering the schools. That is unconstitutional religious discrimination.

Finally, the argument that unvaccinated children threaten vaccinated children with infection implicitly acknowledges that the vaccines do not work. If the vaccines worked to protect the vaccinated person, he should not care whether another is vaccinated.

34 The Religious Freedom Restoration Act

In response to the *Smith* decision, Congress enacted the *Religious Freedom Restoration Act of 1993*[985] (RFRA), wherein Congress cited to the U.S. Supreme Court standard set forth in *Sherbert v. Verner*,[986] and *Wisconsin v. Yoder*,[987] and stated the test for protecting a person's Constitutional right to freedom of religion in those cases should be the standard for reviewing whether a statute (regardless of whether it is generally applicable) violates a person's religious rights. Congress required that when a person alleges a facially neutral law "substantially burdens" his right to freely exercise his religion, the government must establish that the law is the least restrictive means to serve a compelling government interest.

The RFRA initially applied to both state and federal governments. However, the U.S. Supreme Court ruled that the statute could only apply to acts by the federal government.[988] Congress subsequently passed the *Religious Land Use and Institutionalized Persons Act of 2000* (RLUIPA). The RLUIPA amended the definition of religious exercise under both the RLUIPA and the RFRA to read: "The term 'religious exercise' includes any exercise of religion, whether or not compelled by, or central to, a system of religious belief."[989]

Under the Religious Freedom Restoration Act (RFRA), the federal government may not substantially burden a person's exercise of religion, "even if the burden results from a rule of general applicability,"[990] unless the government "demonstrates that application of the burden to the person (1) is in furtherance of a compelling governmental interest; and (2) is the least restrictive means of furthering that compelling governmental interest."[991]

In *Burwell v. Hobby Lobby Stores, Inc.*[992] the U.S. Supreme Court ruled that under the RFRA the government may not require a business to provide health care funding for contraceptive methods that included abortifacients because imposing that requirement on a business conflicted with its sincerely held religious beliefs against abortion. One of the several businesses that objected stated that to force them to provide funding was "against their moral conviction to be involved in the termination of human life after conception, which they believe is a sin against God to which they are held accountable.[993] The owners believed that to provide health care that included abortifacients they would be committing sin by facilitating abortions in violation of their sincerely held religious beliefs.[994]

HHS claimed that Hobby Lobby and the other litigants were wrong to think that providing health care to someone with available abortifacients was tantamount to being an accomplice to abortion. But the Court shot down HHS's argument by saying that it was not for the government or the Court to pass judgment on the plausibility or merits of a person's religious beliefs.[995] The *Hobby Lobby* Court cited *Thomas v. Review Bd. of Indiana Employment Security Div.*,[996] where the Court previously held that it was not for the court to judge the reasonableness of the beliefs of a Jehovah's Witness who did not object to making steel that was used in making weapons but objected when he was reassigned to making the weapons themselves. The Court was simply not competent to assess the reasonableness of the beliefs and could only protect them from infringement by the government. The state denial of unemployment compensation when he was fired because of his religious beliefs forbade violated his First Amendment right to free exercise of religion.[997] The *Thomas* Court was unpersuaded by the fact that another Jehovah's Witness had no problem making weapons. The *Thomas* Court stated that it was not equipped to resolve the many doctrinal and behavioral differences between those who share the same faith. The *Hobby Lobby* Court stated "it is not for us to say that their religious beliefs are mistaken or insubstantial. Instead, our narrow function in this context is to determine whether the line drawn reflects an honest conviction."[998] (ellipse and quotation marks deleted)

35 Title VII of the Civil Rights Act of 1964

Title VII of the Civil Rights Act of 1964[999] addresses employment activities. It applies to local, state, and federal governments as well as private employers with 15 or more employees. Title VII prohibits discriminating against an employee based on his religion, race, color, sex, and national origin.religion in employment practices. Title VII also applies to most federal executive employers, and through the Congressional Accountability Act, applies to most federal legislative employers. Supreme Court Justice Alito explained in his concurring opinion in *E.E.O.C. v. Abercrombie & Fitch Stores, Inc.*[1000] that under Title VII[1001] of the Civil Rights Act:

> An employer may not take an adverse employment action against an applicant or employee because of any aspect of that individual's religious observance or practice unless the employer demonstrates that it is unable to reasonably accommodate that observance or practice without undue hardship.[1002]

If an employment practice infringes on a person's sincerely held religious beliefs, the employer must reasonably accommodate that sincerely held religious practice unless doing so would create an "undue hardship" for the employer. An undue hardship means that the employer would need to incur "substantial additional costs" or "substantial expenditures."[1003]

While the First Amendment is a Constitutional provision that protects a person's religious freedom from government infringement, Title VII is a statute that requires employers to reasonably accommodate an employee's religious practices, unless it would create an undue hardship to do so.

The "undue hardship" standard under Title VII is a lower standard than the compelling state interest standard under the First Amendment. Thus, if the government employer violates Title VII it necessarily has also violated the Constitution. In *Brown v. Polk County*[1004] the *en banc* U.S. 8th Circuit Court of Appeals explained:

> [I]n the governmental employment context, the first amendment protects at least as much religious activity as Title VII does. ... [A]ny religious activities of employees that can be accommodated without undue hardship to the governmental employer, see 42 U.S.C. § 2000e(j), are also protected by the first amendment. In other words, if a governmental employer has violated Title VII, it has also violated the guarantees of the first amendment."[1005]

That does not mean that the undue hardship standard is a low standard by any means. The *Brown* court explained in a string of quotes from prior court decisions that

> Any hardship asserted, furthermore, must be "real" rather than "speculative," [or] "merely conceivable," or "hypothetical." ... An employer "stands on weak ground when advancing hypothetical hardships in a factual vacuum." ...

"Undue hardship cannot be proved by assumptions nor by opinions based on hypothetical facts." ... "Undue hardship requires more than proof of some fellow-worker's grumbling.... An employer ... would have to show ... actual imposition on co-workers or disruption of the work routine."[1006] (citations omitted)

The U.S. Equal Employment Opportunity Commission (EEOC) states that "Title VII of the Civil Rights Act of 1964 requires employers to make a reasonable accommodation for an employee's sincerely held religious beliefs as long as doing so does not pose an undue hardship on the employer."[1007] The courts in past cases had taken the view that an accommodation creates an undue hardship on an employer when it imposes "more than a *de minimis* [small or trifling] cost." But in June 2023, the U.S. Supreme Court, in *Groff v. DeJoy*[1008], ruled that to deny a religious accommodation because the accommodation would constitute an "undue hardship," an employer must show that the burden of accommodating the religious beliefs will cause it to incur "substantial additional costs" or "substantial expenditures."

The EEOC has ruled that the standard for protecting religious beliefs under Title VII "forbids employers from rejecting accommodation requests based on their disagreement with an employee's belief; their opinion that the belief is unfounded, illogical, or inconsistent in some way; or their conclusion that an employee's belief is not an official tenet or endorsed teaching of any particular religion or denomination."[1009] That is the same standard courts follow under a Constitutional First Amendment claim.[1010]

Requiring vaccination may also violate one's sincerely held religious beliefs. It is a violation of a person's sincerely held religious beliefs to require that he get a vaccine under penalty of masking, social distancing, testing, travel prohibition, or termination from employment.

In a case involving a $300,000 judgment against a hospital for refusing to grant a religious exemption for an influenza vaccine, the EEOC has stated that "when considering requests for religious accommodation, the Health Center must adhere to the definition of 'religion' established by Title VII and controlling federal court decisions, a definition that **forbids employers from rejecting accommodation requests based on their disagreement with an employee's belief**; their opinion that the belief is unfounded, illogical, or inconsistent in some way; or their conclusion that an employee's belief is not an official tenet or endorsed teaching of any particular religion or denomination."[1011]

Some courts have erroneously accepted arguments by companies that, because they would incur onerous statutory penalties for each unvaccinated employee, they would suffer an undue burden to grant employees' Title VII religious exemption claims.[1012] Courts should not entertain that argument. That is because Title VII provides an exemption to employers from compliance with any "[state] law which purports to require or permit the doing of any act which would be an unlawful employment practice."[1013]

Thus, a company's undue hardship argument based on a statutory penalty lacks merit because the company is immune from any state law penalties that would interfere with the rights of employees protected by Title VII. Under the Supremacy Clause, federal law is supreme over a conflicting state law. One court explained that "[a] discriminatory state law is not a defense to liability under federal law ... Reliance on state statutes to excuse non-compliance with federal laws is simply unacceptable under the Supremacy Clause."[1014]

The typically proposed accommodation for an exemption to the COIVD-19 vaccine is testing, masking and social distancing. The government cannot offer an option that violates federal workers' constitutional rights and then claim that option is a reasonable accommodation. The option of wearing a mask and being medically tested is not a reasonable accommodation because those procedures infringe on the constitutional rights of the workers. The U.S. Supreme Court in *Cruzan by Cruzan v. Missouri Dep't of Health*,[1015] has advised that "the patient generally possesses the right ... to refuse treatment." The FDA has determined that face masks are medical devices, including cloth face coverings and surgical masks worn for COVID-19 medical purposes.[1016] The *Cruzan* Court's ruling establishes a constitutional right to refuse to wear a medical device.[1017] The same reasoning applies to medical tests that require the insertion of a swab deep into the nostrils of a government employee once every three days.[1018] The federal worker has committed no crime, is not under arrest, is not even suspected of being ill. Such tests are a violation of a worker's bodily autonomy.

36 Unconstitutional Accommodations

A little known fact is that the antigen tests that many employers require are also only allowed because they are have been authorized under an EUA.[1019] Because they are authorized under an EUA they come with the same informed consent restrictions as do the EUA vaccines, and the EUA masks. Thus, neither the government nor any other employer can require experimental masking or experimental testing when an employee refuses to take an experimental vaccine.

The masks recommended by the CDC are not approved. They are authorized by an EUA.[1020] The FDA explains: "On August 5, 2020, the FDA issued an umbrella EUA for certain disposable, single-use surgical masks."[1021] The CDC guidance for wearing FDA EUA masks is in accordance with the FDA power to authorize masks under its emergency powers. Such EUA masks are not FDA-approved medical devices. As such, masks cannot be mandated. EUA masks are unapproved experimental medical devices. The CDC references the definition from OSHA for what a facemask is. According to the pertinent part of the OSHA definition, a facemask means a "mask that is FDA-cleared, authorized by an FDA EUA, or offered or distributed as described in an FDA enforcement policy."[1022] The CDC recommendation of FDA EUA masks, come with the right to informed consent. Masks cannot be mandated.

Masks are medical devices.[1023] Any mask mandate is based on the FDA's emergency use authorization (EUA). The mask requirement is to prevent the spread of COVID-19 during the declared emergency. The mask requirement is for the purpose of following the FDA EUA mask guidance. While the FDA authorized masks under its emergency powers, such EUA masks are not FDA-approved medical devices.[1024] Mandating the use of an EUA medical device violates federal law. All EUA medical devices, including masks, come with the inherent legal right to refuse (21 U.S.C. 360bbb-3(e)(1)(A)(ii)(I-III)).

The FDA's blanket EUA mask letter clearly states that manufacturers cannot advertise masks as being safe or effective at diagnosing or preventing COVID-19.[1025] Indeed, the EUA authorizing letter from the FDA states that such mask manufacturers' "advertising and promotional materials, relating to the use of the product shall clearly and conspicuously state that [t]he product has not been FDA cleared or approved."[1026]

21 U.S.C. § 360bbb-3(e)(1)(A) provides that an EUA product can be used only when "[a]ppropriate conditions designed to ensure that individuals to whom the product is administered are informed ... of the significant known and potential benefits and risks of such use, and of the extent to which such benefits and risks are unknown; and ... of **the option to accept or refuse administration of the product**, of the consequences, if any, of refusing administration of the product, and of the alternatives to the product that are available and of their benefits and risks."

The federal government has violated federal law by:

1) not informing persons of the known and potential benefits and risks of wearing a mask,

2) not informing persons that they have **the option to accept or refuse to wear a mask**,

3) not informing persons of the consequences, in any, of not wearing a mask,

4) not informing persons of available alternatives to wearing a mask, and

5) not informing persons of the benefits and risks of the alternatives.

Those are the typical bases for claims brought by plaintiffs seeking court relief against vaccination after having their religious exemption administratively denied. But there are a couple of legal arguments that have not been raised in the courts because they are not generally known.

37 First Amendment Establishment Clause

An issue that should be raised, but is not being raised, is a First Amendment Establishment Clause argument. People should make a First Amendment Establishment Clause argument against compulsory vaccinations, but they are not. The protest should be against government-mandated vaccines because the compulsory vaccine laws require people to take part in a religious ritual in violation of the Establishment Clause.

Raising this issue in a religious exemption case allows for the introduction of evidence of the unscientific religious origins of vaccines. This is the foundation upon which to introduce evidence of vaccine dangers and ineffectiveness. This book sets forth compelling evidence of those facts. In the absence of an Establishment Clause objection, a court could view such evidence as being irrelevant[1027] or easy to disregard.[1028]

Almost all First Amendment claims for vaccine exemption are brought under the Free Exercise Clause. By thus pigeon-holing their claim, litigants allow the opposing party and the court to begin the legal analysis from the point of assuming the safety and efficacy of vaccines. Consequently, when the court compares the risk to the health of the populace by allowing a religious exemption, it is assuming that the vaccines lower the risk that a disease will be transmitted from one person to another.[1029] But an Establishment Clause claim allows the plaintiff to attack the efficacy and safety of the vaccines under the rubric that they are not based on science but are an unsafe and ineffective religious ritual. The government statutes mandating those religious rituals do so in violation of the Establishment Clause of the First Amendment.

Even if a court rejects the Establishment Clause claim, the evidence undermining the safety and efficacy of the vaccines would bleed over into the Free Exercise Clause claim. The court's ruling, with the backdrop of evidence showing that vaccines are ineffective and unsafe, would more likely find that the government does not have a compelling interest in mandating such hazardous and ineffective vaccines.

There is one recent (and rare) case where the plaintiffs raised the efficacy and safety of vaccines, but the plaintiffs did not allege an Establishment Clause violation. There was no attempt to undermine he germ theory foundation of vaccines, thus, the coast was clear for the court to dismiss the inefficacy and danger evidence as being "too underdeveloped to merit further consideration."[1030] The court assumed the validity of the germ theory upon which vaccination is based, and with that assumption firmly implanted, chose to believe "the publically available data"[1031] that vaccines were safe and effective in preventing the spread of a deadly disease.

The presumption of vaccine safety and effectiveness in court litigation puts the petitioner seeking an exemption at a disadvantage. He stands before the court with two strikes against him. Ordinarily, he would be arguing for a religious exemption from a presumptively safe and effective medical treatment. That is quite different from objecting to the state mandating participation in a religious ritual that *ipso facto* is both ineffective and dangerous.

Once the petitioner raises the issue of the religious origins, dangers, and ineffectiveness of vaccines, the playing field is leveled. Evidence of vaccine ineffectiveness and danger becomes front and center in an Establishment of Religion claim. It places the petitioner in a much more advantageous position when he brings the true, and heretofore concealed, nature of vaccines to light. The U.S. Supreme Court has steadfastly held:

> 'The 'establishment of religion' clause of the First Amendment means at least this: Neither a state nor the Federal Government can set up a church. Neither can pass laws which aid one religion, aid all religions, or prefer one religion over another. Neither can force nor influence a person to go to or to remain away from church against his will or force him to profess a belief or disbelief in any religion. No person can be punished for entertaining or professing religious beliefs or disbeliefs, for church attendance or non-attendance. No tax in any amount, large or small, can be levied to support any religious activities or institutions, whatever they may be called, or whatever form they may adopt to teach or practice religion. Neither a state nor the Federal Government can, openly or secretly, participate in the affairs of any religious organizations or groups and vice versa.[1032]

The Supreme Court has stated the long-held maxim that the establishment clause prohibits the government from requiring a person take part in a religious ritual, or indeed, to profess a belief in a religious doctrine or even in a belief in any religion whatsoever. "We repeat and again reaffirm that neither a State nor the Federal Government can constitutionally force a person 'to profess a belief or disbelief in any religion.'"[1033] "To be sure, this

Court has long held that government may not, consistent with a historically sensitive understanding of the Establishment Clause, make a religious observance compulsory."[1034] If a statute has the purpose or effect of advancing or inhibiting religion, it runs afoul of the Establishment Clause of the First Amendment.[1035] In a decision affirmed by an equally divided U.S. Supreme Court, the Oklahoma Supreme Court stated the general guiding principles of the First Amendment:

> Under the Establishment Clause of the First Amendment, made binding upon the States through the Fourteenth Amendment, Oklahoma cannot pass laws "which aid one religion, aid all religions, or prefer one religion over another." ... The Establishment Clause prohibits government spending in direct support of any religious activities or institutions. ... The Establishment Clause also prohibits the government from participating in the same religious exercise that the law protects when performed by a private party.[1036] (citation omitted)

In *Wooley v. Maynard*,[1037] the U.S. Supreme Court ruled that the state could not require a Jehovah's Witness to display on their car license the state motto "Live Free or Die." The claimant stated that the "slogan is directly at odds with my deeply held religious convictions." The Court stated that the state could not restrict nor compel a person's speech.

The U.S. Supreme Court struck down an invocation given by a Jewish rabbi at a public school graduation ceremony as a violation of the Establishment Clause.. The court determined it violated the Establishment Clause because the school principal made the decision that an invocation should be given, and the principal chose the rabbi who was to give the invocation. The Supreme Court stated that the invocation violated the prohibition against government-imposed religious practice. "It is beyond dispute that, at a minimum, the Constitution guarantees that government may not coerce anyone to support or participate in religion or its exercise, or otherwise act in a way which establishes a state religion or religious faith, or tends to do so."[1038]

Vaccination is NOT based on science. This book proves that vaccination is founded on a superstitious religious belief that is falsely portrayed as science. By mandating vaccines in the workplace and schools, the state has taken sides in favor of a religion and is forcing a person to take part in a religious ritual. That violates the establishment clause of the First Amendment. If inviting clergy to give invocations and benedictions at a schools' graduation ceremony[1039] is considered a violation of the establishment clause, certainly requiring a person to receive a vaccine, that is in reality a superstitious religious ritual, must necessarily also be a violation.

The argument that government vaccination mandates constitute a violation of the Establishment Clause is premised on the fact that vaccination is a religious practice. This book sets forth evidence supporting that premise. And for the government to compel vaccination is to compel one to participate in a religious practice.

The U.S. Supreme Court and the courts in general have never addressed the issue of vaccines being a religious ritual imposed on the public in violation of the Establishment Clause. For example, the U.S. Supreme Court in *Smith* cited "compulsory vaccination laws" among the laws that it considered "valid and neutral laws of general applicability" that would be encumbered if they were subjected to the strict scrutiny requirement of being narrowly tailored to serve a compelling state interest. The Court stated that because of the diverse religious views of the U.S. citizenry federal and state governments "cannot afford the luxury of deeming presumptively invalid, as applied to the religious objector, every regulation of conduct that does not protect an interest of the highest order."[1040]

If the courts were presented with evidence that vaccination is not supported by hard science but is instead a superstitious religious practice, then the compulsory vaccine laws would be viewed differently. They would no longer be viewed as valid neutral laws of general application but rather laws that mandate the people to take part in a religious ritual that is neither safe nor effective. The line of defense would shift from arguing for a religious exemption from medical treatment to seeking a religious exemption from a religious practice. Indeed, if vaccines were recognized for what they are, compulsory vaccine laws could never survive a constitutional objection that they constituted a governmental establishment of religion.

In *Dahl v. Bd. of Trs. of W. Michigan Univ.*,[1041] a First Amendment Free Exercise case, the defendant, a university, asserted in an affidavit that the COVID-19 vaccines were the most effective and reasonable way to guard against the SARS-CoV-2 virus. In response to that bare assertion, the court stated: "We do not dispute that assessment."[1042] Notably, the defendant university used the phrase "most effective and reasonable" rather than "most effective and safe." It seems that they knew about the vaccines' danger and were not going to go on record in a sworn affidavit that the vaccines were safe. The court then found that the university could not establish that denying a religious exemption to the COVID-19 vaccine was the least intrusive means for accomplishing it compelling interest. The *Dahl* court found that the university's vaccine mandate violated the Free Exercise Clause of the First Amendment.

While the court in *Dahl* came to the correct decision, it did so under the wrong rubric. It assumed the safety and efficacy of the vaccines. The pattern of courts accepting the safety and effectiveness of vaccines at the outset is a problem. Litigants should force the issue and bring evidence that the government does not have a compelling interest in vaccination because the vaccines are part of an unsafe and ineffective religious ritual. Forcing compliance to the vaccine violated their right to be free of forced participation in a government-promoted religious practice.

Does 1-6 v. Mills[1043] is an example of what can happen when the validity of the germ theory and the safety and efficacy of vaccines are assumed. In *Does 1-6*, the U.S. Court of Appeals for the First Circuit upheld the denial of an injunction from the enforcement of a Maine State statute that prevented religious exemptions for medical workers. The plaintiffs claimed that the Maine statute that mandated COVID-19 vaccines, which allowed medical exemptions but disallowed religious exemptions, was an unconstitutional infringement of their First Amendment Freedom of Religion Rights.

The *Does 1-6* Circuit Court cited the threat of death from COVID-19 as justification for vaccination.[1044] The *Does 1-6* district court reported that "[a]s of September 14, 2021, Maine had 81,177 total cases of COVID-19, with 969 deaths."[1045] But the court got it wrong. The Maine CDC did not actually report deaths caused by COVID-19. The Maine CDC only reports "COVID-associated deaths."[1046] That is not the same thing as people who died "from" COVID-19. Maine is reporting deaths of people who died "with" COVID-19, not people who died "from" COVID-19.

The Maine CDC reported that a "COVID-associated death" included, but was not limted to, a death in which COVID-19 was included on the death certificate. Under that criterion, there is no requirement that COVID-19 cause death. It only has to be listed on the death certificate as accompanying death. That is because the "COVID-associated" deaths are not deaths *from* COVID-19, they are only "COVID-associated" deaths. The U.S. CDC and the Council of State and Territorial Epidemiologists (CSTE) were pulling a statistical fast one by using death certificates to inflate the death statistics to make the alleged COVID-19 disease seem much worse than it was, which served to deceive the public and the courts.

The CSTE guidelines were driven by the U.S. CDC. Dr. Kristin Held revealed a little-known fact that under CSTE's definitions of COVID-19 cases and COVID-related deaths listed on a death certificate, COVID-19 doesn't have to be the first or second cause, and no COVID-19 testing was required.[1047] Indeed, COVID-19 does not have to be the proximate cause of death; it only has to accompany death. The new standard was used to artificially inflate the COVID-19 death statistics. In May 2020 the U.S. CDC implemented new criteria for reporting a COVID-19 death by advising that COVID-19 could be listed on the death certificate without testing or diagnosis that COVID-19 was the cause of death. The U.S. CDC advised that COVID-19 could be listed on the death certificate if it is "suspected or likely." The CDC was asking health officials and doctors to put on the death certificate "probable" or "presumed" death from COVID-19 based upon a clinical judgment (i.e., a guess) without any actual scientific test or diagnosis.[1048] Dr. (and Minnesota State Senator) Scott Jensen concluded that COVID-19 death statistics are being gamed to inflate the death rate.

It gets worse. The Maine CDC decided to fudge the statistics further. On January 2, 2022, the Maine CDC changed its definition of "COVID-associated deaths to match new standards set by the Council of State and Territorial Epidemiologists (CSTE) and US CDC."[1049] After January 2, 2022, according to the Maine CDC, "a COVID-associated death is defined as a death in which: COVID-19 was determined to be the cause of death or contributed to the death OR a death in which COVID-19 was included on the death certificate OR a death due to natural causes that has occurred within 30 days of specimen collection or symptom onset."[1050] You read that correctly, the Maine CDC reported all persons who died of natural causes within 30 days of having tested positive for

COVID-19 or had alleged symptoms of COVID-19 within 30 days prior to death were considered "COVID-associated" deaths. Thus, a person could be included in the list of those with a "COVID-associated" death without any menation of COVID-19 on his death certificate. That can do nothing but further inflate the already inflated COVID-19 reported deaths and make COVID-19 appear to be much worse than it is. If the germ theory were real and disease is spread from one person to the next through viruses, why was it necessary to artificially goose the data to create a statistical phantom epidemic?

The *Does 1-6* court unwittingly based its decision on manipulated statistics that falsely portrayed COVID-19 as a deadly disease. Once the court established that premise, it was off to the races, denying relief to those seeking religious exemptions that the court mistakenly thought would increase the danger of death to the entire populace. The court then built on that false premise another false premise that the vaccines were safe and effective means to save lives.

The *Does 1-6* court ruled that the statute was neutral and generally applicable and did not violate the First Amendment Free Exercise rights of the medical professionals. In *dicta*, the court stated that the statute also passed the strict scrutiny test; that it was narrowly tailored to address a compelling state interest. The court's opinion was premised on the fact that the "COVID-19 vaccines protect against infection and lower the risk of adverse health consequences, including death, should a vaccinated person become infected. Vaccination also reduces a person's risk of transmitting COVID-19 to others."[1051] Read that carefully because within that statement, the court acknowledged that a vaccinated person can nonetheless become infected. And after saying that, the court stated that there was no alternative to vaccination "[b]ecause those treatments do not prevent infections."[1052] But, as the court pointed out, neither do vaccines prevent infections. But when you are dealing with religious superstition masquerading as science, such contradictions can be expected.

Things turned against the plaintiffs from the beginning. The court record reflects that at a district court hearing apparently uncontested evidence was introduced by the Maine CDC that "unvaccinated persons are substantially more likely to contract COVID-19 and suffer serious medical consequences."[1053] All it took was a custodian of the records to testify that COVID-19 data records were routinely kept in the ordinary course of business, and presto-chango, it became a matter of record that the COVID-19 vaccines were effective in stopping contraction of COVID-19. There was likely no thorough analysis of how the data was collected or how the data categories were defined.

For example, being unvaccinated was a term of art applied by state and federal CDCs. Thus, if a person was vaccinated but allegedly contracted COVID-19 within 14 days of vaccination, they were considered to be unvaccinated. The U.S. CDC classified COVID-19 hospitalizations and deaths of fully vaccinated persons only if those persons are hospitalized or die 14 days or more after the final dose of a COVID-19 vaccine.[1054]

Furthermore, the *Does 1-6* court was not informed that the SARS-CoV-2 virus had never been isolated.[1055] Indeed, Biostatistician Christine Massey reported that the U.S. CDC admitted that it has never isolated any virus.[1056] A little-known fact is that the alleged SARS-CoV-2 virus was identified *in silico*, meaning that it originated from a computer simulation. The SARS-CoV-2 virus is a computer-generated theoretical virus that contains DNA strings all humans have (chromosome 8).

Often, those who were ill with flu symptoms tested positive in a PCR test for SARS-CoV-2. That is because the PCR test is detecting the slightest remnant of the *in silico* DNA string, a string constructed by computer to include DNA found in all humans.[1057] That is why there were so many (97%) false positive PCR tests.

Once persons tested positive for SARS-CoV-2, they were tallied up as COVID-19 patients. The court was not informed that the flu disappeared during the 2020-2021 flu season.[1058] With those false positive tests in hand, it was just a matter of recategorizing persons with flu symptoms from flu cases to COVID-19 cases.[1059] That explains the disappearance of the flu. It was a statistical sleight of hand.

The COVID-19 pandemic was overblown and based on deception. The actual evidence would have shown that the germ theory is based on superstition, the statistics were massaged to give credence to that superstition, and the COVID-19 vaccines are unsafe and ineffective. But the court was not presented with that evidence, and so it was left to conclude that the COVID-19 vaccines were safe and effective as a starting point to deciding whether to allow a religious exemption.

Once the court firmly established its position on the safety and efficacy of the COVID-19 vaccines, it was merely a matter of navigating the legal standards to arrive at an outcome that aligned with the court's preconceived notion. The court opinion is chock-full of incongruities and illogic. For example, the court stated that because the statute disallowed both religious and philosophical exemptions from mandatory vaccination requirements, it did not discriminate against religion in particular. To suggest that disallowing a philosophical objection to vaccines is somehow materially different from disallowing a religious exemption misunderstands what philosophy and religion are. The court is making a distinction without a difference.

The freedom of religion protected under the First Amendment also applies to freedom of belief in a particular philosophy or moral code. A court reviewing a denial of a religious exemption is limited to determining if the exemption request is based on a religious belief and if that religious belief is sincerely held.[1060] A court cannot examine the verity of a plaintiff's belief.

Only in the rarest cases will a court adjudge a belief to not be a sincerely held religious belief. One example is *Friedman v. Clarkstown Cent. Sch. Dist.*,[1061] wherein the court found that the plaintiff was not forthright in answering questions about the basis for her objection to having her son vaccinated and never described her religious beliefs as the reason for her refusing to allow her son to be vaccinated.[1062]

Philosophy cannot be disconnected from religion. Philosophy means "Literally, the love of wisdom."[1063] Getting wisdom is a Christian principle. All search for knowledge leads to God. We are thus commanded by God to "get wisdom" and "get understanding." According to Christian doctrine, one begins to gain knowledge after loving and fearing the Lord.

> He taught me also, and said unto me, Let thine heart retain my words: keep my commandments, and live. Get wisdom, get understanding: forget it not; neither decline from the words of my mouth. Forsake her not, and she shall preserve thee: love her, and she shall keep thee. Wisdom is the principal thing; therefore get wisdom: and with all thy getting get understanding. Exalt her, and she shall promote thee: she shall bring thee to honour, when thou dost embrace her. She shall give to thine head an ornament of grace: a crown of glory shall she deliver to thee. Proverbs 4:4-9.

> The fear of the LORD is the beginning of knowledge: but fools despise wisdom and instruction. Proverbs 1:7.

> My people are destroyed for lack of knowledge. Hosea 4:6-7.

> The heart of him that hath understanding seeketh

> knowledge. Proverbs 15:14.

> Teach me good judgment and knowledge: for I have believed thy commandments. Psalms 119:66.

> A wise man will hear, and will increase learning. Proverbs 1:5.

Noah Webster continues: "But in modern acceptation, philosophy is a general term denoting an explanation of the reasons of things; or an investigation of the causes of all phenomena both of mind and of matter."[1064] If a person seeks answers for the reason things happen, he is immediately met with the sovereign grace of God. All search for knowledge leads ultimately to Jesus Christ. And indeed, Webster explains that religion can be considered a category or branch of philosophy. "[T]that branch of philosophy which treats of God, etc. is called theology."[1065] Theology is "the science which teaches the existence, character and attributes of God."[1066]

When our theology is put into practice, it becomes religion, which Webster states "is godliness or real piety in practice, consisting in the performance of all known duties to God and our fellow men, in obedience to divine command, or from love to God."[1067] The search for knowledge is a continual process. To denigrate one's path to gaining wisdom as only philosophy and not religion is to make a qualitative judgment between worthy and unworthy beliefs. That is improper and not allowed under the First Amendment. Treating others the way you want to be treated is often postulated as a philosphical "golden rule." It is also a command from God.

> Thou shalt love the Lord thy God with all thy heart, and with all thy soul, and with all thy mind. This is the first and great commandment. And the second is like unto it, Thou shalt love thy neighbour as

thyself. On these two commandments hang all the law and the prophets. Matthew 22:37-40.

No one would suggest that a person's belief in the "Golden Rule" is not protected by the First Amendment because it is based in philosophy, while another's belief in that same principle is protected because it is based in religion. All courts are rendered incompetent as a matter of law by the First Amendment to make distinctions between philosophy and religion.

For example, Humanists, who are essentially atheists, follow the Golden Rule not as a religious doctrine, but as a philosophy of life and an ethical guide.[1068] They ignore the loving God part, though. Humanists do not believe in a deity or have any belief in the supernatural. They characterize their belief system as "a rational philosophy informed by science, inspired by art, and motivated by compassion."[1069] Indeed, they believe Humanism is a "joyous alternative to religions that believe in a supernatural god and life in a hereafter."[1070] But that does not mean that a Humanist's belief in the truth of the "Golden Rule" is not valid and protected by the First Amendment.

A Humanist who seeks a religious exemption from vaccination should have as much right to that exemption as any other person who has a philosophy of living, regardless of how wrong others may consider it. Suppose a court understood that vaccines are the imposition of a religious ritual on society. In that case, a Humanist has a valid argument against being mandated to take part in that religious practice.

There are Humanists who consider their Humanism a philosophy and not a religion. There are also Humanists who consider Humanism their religion. A Humanist has a constitutionally protected right to freely have a philosophy, and to consider it a religion, although a non-theistic one. The American Humanist Association explains that "Humanism serves, for many humanists, some of the psychological and social functions of a religion, but without belief in deities, transcendental entities, miracles, life after death, and the supernatural."[1071] The government cannot make a distinction between philosophy and religion whereby philosophy is not worthy of constitutional protection because the government deems it not to be a religion.

If a Humanist says that Humanism is his religion; that is the end of the matter. In that case, the government cannot go further and attempt to distinguish it from religion because Humanism does not involve a deity or an afterlife. The Establishment Clause renders the government incompetent to define what religion is and what it is not. If someone says their belief is a protected religious belief, the government cannot examine the qualitative nature of the beliefs and disqualify them as only an unprotected philosophy.

Buddhism is a philosophy of living whose adherents worship no deity. American Buddhist Monk Thanissaro Bhikkhu (Geoffrey DeGraff) explains that "Buddhism is an ethical system — a way of life — that leads to a very specific goal and that possesses some aspects of both religion and philosophy."[1072] The goal of Buddhism is to overcome suffering through meditation, right thought, and ethical living to ultimately reach nirvana, whereby one is freed from the cycle of reincarnation and suffering.

Buddhism is a philosophy of living that is characterized as a religion. If Buddhists can have their philosophy considered a religion, why can't someone who is not a Buddhist have his philosophy considered a religion? Suppose someone has a philosophy of living that does not align with Buddhism. Does that person not also have the right to freely exercise his philosophy and have it be protected under the Free Exercise of Religion Clause of the First Amendment, the same as a Buddhist?

The Maine legislature's contrast between philosophy and

religion is a distinction without a difference. The *Does 1-6* court erroneously concluded that there was a material difference between a religious and a philosophical objection to vaccination based on the fact that the legislature used those two words in the statute. It then felt clear to say that the statute did not discriminate against religion because it also discriminated against philosophy. If that were the case, all a legislature would need to do to avoid the appearance of religious animus is include philosophy along with religion as a disallowed basis for an exemption. One could imagine a legislature adding all kinds of language to camouflage religious animus. Take, for example, a hypothetical statute passed for the purpose of disallowing religious exemptions but drafted with language that disallows exemptions from vaccines based on moral, ethical, philosophical, spiritual, or religious objections. Based on the *Does 1-6* court's logic, because such a statute does not target religion alone, it does not constitute religious discrimination. But the actual target is religion, just as it is with the Maine statute.

Recall that the statute allowed for medical exemptions. The court put the statutory allowance of a medical exemption on a different plane from the disallowance of the religious exemption. Bizarrely, the court stated with a sweep of its hand "that exempting from vaccination only those whose health would be endangered by vaccination does not undermine Maine's asserted interests"[1073] in maintaining the health and safety of healthcare workers and the public. The court's reasoning was that allowing a medical exemption protected the health of the unvaccinated healthcare worker. Thus, it furthered the state's interest in protecting the health of medical personnel so they could serve the public in need of healthcare.

The standard for review when comparing a secular vaccine exemption against a religious vaccine exemption is by juxtaposing them against the stated objective of the government. The U.S. Supreme Court has stated: "Whether two activities are comparable for purposes of the Free Exercise Clause must be judged against the asserted government interest that justifies the regulation at issue."[1074] However, the *Does 1-6* court pulled a switcheroo, substituting the reason the government gave medical exemptions in place of the government's stated overall health objective. The court used the wrong test. The reason why the government gives a person a medical exemption is not germane to deciding whether the medically exempt person poses the same alleged risk to other persons as a religiously exempt person. Allowing people who are unvaccinated for medical reasons undermines the government's stated health interests in the same way as a religious exemption. The government cannot grant a medical exemption that undermines its stated objective, while, at the same time, deny a religious exemption that does the same thing, even if the medical exemption benefits its recipient by making him healthier.

Furthermore, if the plaintiffs had presented the court with evidence of the vaccine health hazards posed to everyone, the court would have a tough time distinguishing medical exemptions from religious exemptions. The harm posed to all persons from vaccinations would justify both medical and religious exemptions. Thus, making an Establishment Clause argument where the evidence of the ineffectiveness and dangers of vaccines is introduced, cuts off at the pass the health safety argument used by the *Does 1-6* court to allow medical exemptions while disallowing religious exemptions. In the face of evidence that vaccines are dangerous to everyone, the court would not be able to distinguish the unique health threats posed to those who have medical allergies to vaccines from the rest of the population, whom vaccines would also harm. Both a person with an allergy to vaccines and the general populace face health threats from vaccines.

Finally, the court left unresolved the supposed threat that the medically exempt unvaccinated worker poses to the public and other healthcare workers from the supposed virus that they can now allegedly spread. How can one person who is unvaccinated for a medical reason not undermine the state's interest in protecting the public health from the purported spread of the virus, while the person standing next to him, who is unvaccinated for a religious reason does undermine that same interest?

U.S. Supreme Court Justices Alito, Gorsuch, and Thomas, in their dissent to the Supreme Court's denial of injunctive relief in *Does 1-6*, eviscerated the reasoning of the *Does 1-6* court of appeals.

> Now consider the first, second, and fourth of these. No one questions that protecting patients and healthcare workers from contracting COVID–19 is a laudable objective. But Maine does not suggest a worker who is unvaccinated for medical reasons is less likely to spread or contract the virus than someone who is unvaccinated for religious reasons. ... That leaves Maine's third asserted interest: protecting the State's healthcare infrastructure. According to Maine, "[a]n outbreak among healthcare workers requiring them to quarantine, or to be absent ... as a result of illness caused by COVID–19, could cripple the facility's ability to provide care." ... But as we have already seen, Maine does not dispute that unvaccinated religious objectors and unvaccinated medical objectors are equally at risk for contracting COVID–19 or spreading it to their colleagues. Nor is it any answer to say that, if the State required vaccination for medical objectors, they might suffer side effects resulting in fewer medical staff available to treat patients. If the State refuses religious exemptions, religious workers will be fired for refusing to violate their faith, which will also mean fewer healthcare workers available to care for patients. Slice it how you will, medical exemptions and

religious exemptions are on comparable footing when it comes to the State's asserted interests.[1075]

It makes no sense to allow one exemption based on a secular objection while denying the other exemption based on a religious objection. Doing so discriminates against the religious objector's constitutionally protected Freedom of Religion. Indeed, Justices Gorsuch, Thomas, and Alito explained in their dissent to the Supreme Court's refusal to review the denial of injunctive relief in Does 1-6, the court of appeals' ruling upholding Maine's decision to deny the religious exemption requests of the healthcare workers was a "serious error" that "borders on the irrational."[1076]

The plaintiffs in the *Does 1-6* case had an Establishment Clause argument that went unresolved because they did not raise it. If at the outset, the religious origins of the vaccines that reveal their dangers and inefficacy were introduced into evidence under a constitutional Establishment Clause claim, a court would be faced with a very different case. The court would not be able to then begin with the premise that the vaccines are safe and effective. There is no guarantee that the evidence would convince a court, but it would raise the issue and put the court in the position of having to address it. If the court ruled unfavorably, those facts would then be a matter of record for a court on appeal to examine, perhaps rendering a more favorable ruling.

The *Does 1-6* case is typical of litigants challenging vaccine mandates. Plaintiffs usually allow the government to present evidence of the dangers of disease spread without any searching examination or rebuttal. That is a mistake. Litigants should at the outset challenge the germ theory and the validity of the statistics that are presented to support the claim of a pandemic. The case of *Brox v. Woods Hole*[1077] illustrates how a court's assumption of the validity of germ theory and CDC efficacy vaccine statistics at the outset can set the groundwork for an unfavorable court decision. In *Brox*, the judge started his opinion by assuming that the COVID-19 pandemic was the deadliest in history. The court stated:

> The COVID-19 pandemic is among the deadliest pandemics in human history. The disease spread rapidly throughout the world and to date has killed over one million Americans, including 25,000 Massachusetts residents.[1078]

None of what the court stated was true. The court began with a false premise of a dangerous contagion. *Brox* is one of the few cases where the plaintiffs challenged the efficacy of the COVID-19 vaccines and the alleged dangerousness of COVID-19.[1079] Unfortunately, the court did not pay much attention to the plaintiffs' arguments.

The *Brox* court took "judicial notice of information on CDC's website."[1080] Perhaps the court should have explored a little further on the CDC website. If it had done so, it would have found that the CDC COVID-19 death statistics were inflated. About 95% percent of people the CDC reported as having died of COVID-19 in the U.S. were suffering from an average of 4.0 chronic diseases.[1081] That means that the people making up the total the CDC said died from COVID-19 likely died from something else. They died with COVID-19, not from COVID-19. The court did not take judicial notice of those clarifying facts. It is unclear what evidence the plaintiffs introduced to refute the CDC death statistics. What is clear is that the court did not give credence to the plaintiffs' evidence. Thus, the court proceeded on the premise of a perceived danger (that did not exist), which left the plaintiffs fighting the case with one hand behind their backs.

The next chapter in this book, titled, *Inflating COVID-19 Death Statistics*, is excerpted from the book *Vaccine Danger: Quackery and Sin*. It establishes beyond a reasonable doubt that the COVID-19 alleged pandemic was fabricated from fraudulent statistics. The COVID-19 death statistics were artificially inflated to create the appearance of a pandemic, when in reality there was no pandemic. The statistical system for reporting COVID=19 deaths was rigged to capture all persons who have tested positive with COVID-19 as a COVID-19 death if they subsequently died. Persons who died from reasons having nothing to do with COVID-19 were reported as COVID-19 deaths. It got so ridiculous that in one case a man who died from a motorcycle accident was reported as having died of COVID-19.[1082] If the plaintiffs brought that evidence to the court's attention, there is little chance that the court could begin its opinion by assuming that there was a deadly pandemic in need of vaccines.

The *Brox* court followed that false premise with yet another. The court averred that the COVID-19 vaccines were safe and effective in addressing the alleged pandemic.

> To combat the spread of the virus, the United States Food and Drug Administration (FDA) granted emergency use authorizations (EUAs) to COVID-19 vaccines manufactured by Pfizer/BioNTech (Pfizer Vaccine) and Moderna (Moderna Vaccine) in December of 2020 and to a vaccine manufactured by Janssen Biotech, Inc. (Janssen Vaccine) in February of 2021. Before granting full approval of the Pfizer and Moderna Vaccines, the FDA reviewed "hundreds of thousands of pages" of data and conducted independent analyses of the Vaccines' safety and effectiveness. The FDA concluded that the Pfizer and Moderna Vaccines met its "high standards for safety, effectiveness, and manufacturing quality" and gave full approval to the Pfizer Vaccine on August 23, 2021, and to the Moderna Vaccine on January 31, 2022. The Vaccines are extremely effective. But, as is common with vaccines, the

immunity generated by the Vaccines wanes over time. Accordingly, in September of 2021, the FDA approved "booster" doses of the Pfizer and Moderna Vaccines, and it has since approved additional booster doses.[1083]

The court cited CDC and FDA information in support of its statement that the COVID-19 vaccines "are extremely effective." Indeed, the court took judicial notice that the FDA and CDC information and data were accurate.

The court draws much of this background from the websites of the Center for Disease Control and Prevention (CDC) and the United States Food and Drug Administration (FDA). Because the accuracy of this information "cannot reasonably be questioned," the court may take judicial notice of these facts. Fed. R. Evid. 201(b)(2); see also Pietrangelo v. Sununu, 15 F.4th 103, 106 n.1 (1st Cir.2021) (taking judicial notice of "state and federal vaccine distribution data" at preliminary injunction stage); Gent v. CUNA Mut. Ins. Soc'y, 611 F.3d 79, 84 n.5 (1st Cir. 2010) (taking judicial notice of information on CDC's website).[1084]

The *Brox* court got it wrong because the conclusions it took judicial notice of were false. HHS Secretary Robert F. Kennedy Jr., who oversees both the CDC and the FDA, made statements on August 5, 2025, that, in effect, revealed that previously published FDA and CDC claims that the COVID-19 vaccines are safe and effective were misleading.

On August 5, 2025, the Department of Health and Human Services (HHS) announced that it was cancelling 22 mRNA projects worth $500 million.[1085] The HHS cancelled the mRNA projects because "[t]he data show these vaccines fail to protect effectively against upper respiratory infections like COVID and flu."[1086]

Furthermore, HHS Secretary Robert F. Kennedy Jr. admitted the the dangers of the COVID-19 vaccines were not outweighed by the benefits, which was something that previously neither the FDA nor CDC would acknowledge. "After reviewing the science and consulting top experts at NIH [the National Institutes of Health] and FDA [Food and Drug Administration], HHS has determined that mRNA technology poses more risk than benefits for these respiratory viruses."[1087]

The premise of the vaccines was that the benefits would outweigh any health hazards from the vaccines. That is the perverse religious ethic of Molech, where the few who the vaccine would injure must thereby pay the price to protect the many. Robert Kennedy did not refute that ethic; he simply said that the injuries suffered by the few were not worth the purported benefit to the many. We do not need Robert Kennedy to tell us the vaccines were not worth it; ask any of the millions of people suffering lifelong injuries from the vaccines.

The HHS press release contained a link to research backing its assertions. The press release cited 656 peer-reviewed scientific papers establishing that the mRNA vaccines are dangerous to the health of the recipients.[1088] There were an additional 70 peer-reviewed papers cited by HHS that established not only that the mRNA vaccines were ineffective but that they drove vaccine-resistant variants, exacerbating the COVID-19 epidemic. The vaccines were not just ineffective; they prolonged and expanded the pandemic.

The plaintiffs in *Brox* tried to contest the efficacy of the vaccines, but the court rejected their argument. The plaintiffs have appealed the decision of the district court, alleging that the court abused its discretion by taking judicial notice of disputed facts.

The plaintiffs have argued on appeal:

> [J]udicial notice of material facts that are disputed is an abuse of discretion, particularly so where the District Court drew essential support for its ruling from such judicial notice. ... The Authority's vaccine mandate was premised on vaccine efficacy with respect to preventing viral infection and transmission of COVID-19. It is indisputable and clear from the record that COVID-19 vaccines can do no such thing as prevent infection and transmission. Such a policy, in light of the abject failure of COVID-19 vaccines to confer immunity as to the spread of contagion, not only fails to satisfy the rigorous demands of strict scrutiny, but is also arbitrary and capricious.[1089]

The district court based its opinion that the COVID-19 vaccines were effective in preventing the infection and spread of SARS-CoV-2 on data from the CDC website. However, the data cited by the court does not support the claim that the vaccines are effective. The plaintiffs pointed that fact out in their appeal.

> The judicially noticed CDC data included infection prevention figures that ranged from "abysmal (8.4%) to middling (68.9%)." ... [T]he District Court implied that the CDC webpage it referenced established the extreme effectiveness of COVID-19 vaccines with respect to contagion control. Upon even the scantest review, the noticed data demolishes this sweeping and critical conclusion.[1090]

Indeed, the CDC fact-sheet proffered by the government to prove that the COVID-19 vaccines were effective actually reveals that they were ineffective. The plaintiffs explained in their appellate brief:

> The fact-sheet ... stated with respect to the then-dominant Omicron variant of COVID-19, "breakthrough infections in people who are vaccinated are expected". With respect to the then-diminishing Delta variant, "people who are up to date with their vaccines who become infected with the Delta variant can spread the virus to others." For a policy, such as the Authority's, the exclusive purpose of which was to "prevent" infection and transmission, a document, which concedes that the sole means of the policy have no capacity to meet its goal, fails to pass even rational basis muster with respect to appellants' claim under the Free Exercise Clause.[1091]

The court either was not informed or ignored the moves made by the CDC to conceal the ineffectiveness of the COVID-19 vaccines. For example, on May 1, 2021, the CDC took steps to stop the collection and reporting of data regarding breakthrough COVID-19 infections among the vaccinated population if they did not result in hospitalization or death.[1092] The CDC took that action because the ineffectiveness of the COVID-19 vaccines was becoming increasingly apparent and rather embarrassing.

The *Brox* court opinion was issued on December 11, 2023. It involved Massachusetts litigants. It was well known at that time that the COVID-19 vaccines were ineffective. U.S. Senator for Massachusetts, Edward Markey in a letter to the CDC noted that 43.4% of the new COVID-19 infections in Massachusetts were among those who were vaccinated.[1093] How could the COVID-19 vaccines be considered effective when 43.4% of all COVID-19 infections were of people who had been vaccinated? The answer is obvious. The vaccines don't work. They don't work because they are not based on science. They are based on a religious superstition. The COVID-19 vaccines, indeed, all vaccines, are religious rituals being forced on the citizens in violation of the Establishment Clause of the First Amendment. The district court summarily disregarded the plaintiff's vaccine ineffectiveness argument. Perhaps, the court would have shown more deference to the ineffectiveness claim if the plaintiffs brought it under the rubric of an Establishment Clause violation.

The evidence was clear when the court issued its opinion that the COVID-19 vaccines were neither safe nor effective. While the plaintiffs contested the efficacy of the vaccines, it is not clear whether they presented evidence of the vaccine dangers. As described in an earlier chapter of this book, as of July 28, 2022, there have been more adverse event reports in VAERS for the COVID-19 vaccines than all other 70+ vaccines combined during the entire 32-year history of the VAERS database. The World Council for Health concluded that "[t]here is sufficient evidence of adverse events relating to Covid-19 vaccines to indicate that a product recall is immediately necessary."[1094] It is estimated that as of July 15, 2022, the COVID-19 vaccine killed 1,215,000 people. The statistics show that vaccinated persons were dying at more than twice the rate of unvaccinated persons.

The *Brox* court was presided over by U.S. District Court Judge Richard G. Stearns. He is a left-wing democrat appointed to the bench by Bill Clinton, with whom he roomed at Oxford when they both studied there as Rhodes Scholars. Judge Stearns is on record saying that he would not be constrained to follow the rule of law. He reportedly stated: "Rigid insistence on the rule of law as a value that transcends all others, even at the risk of collective suicide is (as Justice Jackson famously warned) simply too high a price to pay."[1095]

With the judge willing to dispense with the rule of law if there is sufficient danger, premising his ruling on the assumption that we were in the midst of "the deadliest pandemics in human history," and "the vaccines are extremely effective," the die was cast. He was prejudiced against allowing a religious exemptions to the COVID-19 vaccines. It was just a matter of justifying his decision. The only way to win in a case like that is to undermine the prejudice of the judge by revealing to him that his assumptions are wrong about viruses, epidemics, and vaccines.

The plaintiffs tried to make the argument that "everyone, whether vaccinated or not, carries an equivalent risk of transmitting COVID-19 given the vaccines' inability to inhibit transmission, and thus it would be irrational, legally indefensible and contrary to the public interest for government to mandate vaccines."[1096] But the judge disregarded that argument by saying that "[t]o the extent that plaintiffs mean to argue that the Authority cannot have acted pursuant to a legitimate or compelling interest because the Vaccines are not effective, this is belied by publicly available data."[1097] The court further stated that "the argument was too underdeveloped to merit further consideration."[1098]

The district court disregarded evidence about the inefficacy of the vaccines, instead relying on the FDA and CDC's efficacy information and data. The court was not going to entertain the inefficacy argument. The court alleged that the inefficacy argument was "underdeveloped." It is not clear what the court meant by that, but the plaintiffs are contesting the ruling on appeal, alleging that the court abused its discretion.[1099]

In the end, the court refused to grant the injunction that would have prevented the enforcement of the COVID-19 vaccine mandate. The court held that the vaccine mandate policy was neutral and generally applicable and therefore subject to only rational basis scrutiny. The court handed the victory to the government on the theory that denying religious exemptions while allowing medical exemptions was rationally related to a legitimate government interest, given that the medical exemptions were of short duration and thus not comparable to permanent religious exemptions.

There are many unfavorable rulings throughout the United States where courts have refused to protect a person's constitutional right to Freedom of Religion under the First Amendment. Such unfavorable rulings would be rarer if the plaintiffs had presented evidence that undermined the scientific premise behind vaccination. If courts, at the outset, were faced with having to consider the legitimacy of vaccines as a medical preventive, many judges would look much more favorably toward the argument for a religious exemption. Plaintiffs should introduce evidence of the dangers and ineffectiveness of vaccines under the rubric that vaccines are not supported by actual science because they are superstitious religious rituals masquerading as science. The religion of vaccinology is being imposed on the citizenry by the government in violation of the Establishment Clause of the First Amendment.

Suppose a court rules against a litigant on the Establishment Clause argument; that does not mean it is a wasted effort. It would be hard for a court faced with evidence of government fraud to then adopt that fraud as a premise for ruling in a case. Thus, a court would be more likely to rule in favor of a plaintiff making a Freedom of Religion argument for a vaccine exemption after the plaintiff has shot holes in the two vaccine bulwarks, safety and efficacy.

In the case of the COVID-19 pandemic scare, once a court accepts that there is a deadly pandemic, the battle lines are drawn unfavorably against the litigants seeking religious exemptions. Another example of this is *Doe v. San Diego Unified Sch. Dist.*[1100] In that case, the U.S. Court of Appeals for the Ninth Circuit assumed that the COVID-9 vaccines were safe and effective in preventing the infection and spread of a deadly virus. It premised its ruling on the validity of the germ theory and the propaganda that there was a deadly COVID-19 pandemic. The court stated that "the public interest weighs strongly in favor of denying Appellants' motion. The COVID-19 pandemic has claimed the lives of over three quarters of a million Americans."[1101] In support of that claim, the court cited the CDC website, COVID Data Tracker.[1102]

But the appellants/plantiffs did not rebut the CDC information. They did not inform the court that the CDC artificially inflated the COVID-19 death statistics. If the court had been informed that the CDC website it relied on misleadingly reported deaths as being from COVID-19 when the deaths could have been from one or more other comorbidities.[1103] Comorbidity is defined as the simultaneous presence of two or more chronic diseases or conditions in a patient. The Court of Appeals was not informed that on the date of its opinion, December 21, 2021, the CDC reported that about 95% percent of people they have reported to have died of COVID-19 in the U.S. were suffering from an average of 4.0 chronic diseases or conditions (comorbidities) in addition to COVID-19.[1104]

Thus, the statistical total COVID-19 deaths cited by the court of "over three quarters of a million Americans" as of December 21, 2021 does not mean that the decedents making up that total actually died from COVID-19. The reported people dying "with" COVID-19 are being misrepresented as people who died "from" COVID-19. This inflated the COVID-19 deaths and created a false sense of danger among the public. It misled the court to begin its review with the premise that "the public interest weighs strongly in favor of denying Appellants' motion."[1105]

Once the field of battle was set firmly on the false assumption of a deadly pandemic, the *Doe* court proceeded to shoot down the plaintiffs' argument for a religious exemption with the double-barreled presumption that "the public interest weighs strongly in favor of denying Appellants' motion" because COVID-19 vaccines are safe and effective.

> The record indicates that vaccines are safe and effective at preventing the spread of COVID-19, and that SDUSD's vaccination mandate is therefore likely to promote the health and safety of SDUSD's students and staff, as well as the broader community.[1106]

Nothing could be further from the truth. This book presents abundant admissible evidence proving that the COVID-19 vaccines are neither safe nor effective. You will read how Dr. Denis Rancourt, Ph.D., in a February 9, 2023, report, took the all-cause mortality increases by country and correlated them to the vaccine rollouts in each country. He extrapolated from that data a death rate for the COVID-19 vaccines of approximately 13 million people.[1107] A vaccine with that kind of record could hardly be considered safe. Furthermore, on February 15, 2023, the Florida Department of Health issued a health alert to doctors and the public regarding the dangers of the COVID-19 vaccines. The Florida Department of Health recorded a troubling 1,700% spike in vaccine adverse events during the 2021 COVID-19 vaccine campaign. In addition, the life-threatening adverse events exploded to an increase of 4,400% during the COVID-19 vaccine program. That means the COVID-19 vaccines are four (4) times more harmful and eleven (11) times more life-threatening than any other vaccine.[1108]

Regarding effectiveness, according to the CDC published statistics, 44.1% of those hospitalized between June 20, 2021 and May 31, 2022, for COVID-19 had been fully vaccinated and received at least one COVID-19 booster shot.[1109] How could such a vaccine be considered effective?

The Plaintiffs only presented the *Doe* court with a Free Exercise of Religion claim. The plaintiffs did not raise an Establishment of Religion claim. The coast was then clear for the court to run roughshod over the rights of the plaintiffs. The court reviewed the case assuming that the school vaccine mandate was neutral and generally applicable. It did not use the strict scrutiny standard as required by Supreme Court precedent. The court misapplied the law and denied the injunction requested by the students.

In the *Doe* case, the plaintiffs were a 16-year-old, Jill Doe, and her parents. Jill *Doe* was a student athlete who played multiple sports. She hoped to obtain a college sports scholarship. She had already developed natural immunity to COVID-19 from a prior infection. She thus should not have needed a COVID-19 vaccine if the germ theory were truly applied. She objected to the vaccine based on her religious beliefs. But the San Diego Unified School District COVID-19 vaccine mandate required all students over the age of 16 to be vaccinated or be banned from attending school in person. Significantly, the vaccine mandate has many secular exemptions, but it expressly prohibits religious exemptions.[1110]

The *Doe* court correctly stated the standard for comparing the secular and religious exemptions."Whether two activities are comparable for purposes of the Free Exercise Clause must be judged against the asserted government interest that justifies the regulation at issue."[1111] But then the court pulled a sleight of hand to enhance the need for a secular (medical) exemption to make the erroneous case that a religious exemption is not comparable to a medical exemption. The court justified the medical exemption on the grounds that it allegedly protected the health of the student by preventing an allergic reaction to the vaccine. The court argued that the school system had a greater interest in allowing a medical exemption. The dissenting judge correctly pointed out that "[t]his argument incorrectly focuses on the reasons for the exemption rather than the asserted interest that justifies the mandate."[1112] The dissenting judge explained:

> But "the reasons why" the School District allows in-person attendance for some unvaccinated

students are irrelevant. *Tandon*, 141 S. Ct. at 1296 (citation omitted). Instead, "[c]omparability is concerned with the risks" in-person attendance by an unvaccinated student poses to the "asserted government interest." Id. (citation omitted). Here, the School District's asserted interest for imposing the vaccine mandate in the first place is to ensure "the safest environment possible for all students and employees" by preventing the transmission and spread of COVID-19. Allowing students who are unvaccinated for medical reasons to attend school in person undermines this interest. Thus, the majority errs at the first step in the framework by focusing on the School District's reasons for offering an exemption, rather than the interest that the School District actually asserts to justify the mandate.[1113]

The medical exemption undermines the school system's stated interest in vaccination in the same way as the religious exemption. The reason for the medical exemption is not relevant. The point is that if the school system allows a secular exemption, it cannot deny a religious exemption, unless it passes the strict scrutiny test, which it cannot do.

The *Doe* court panel misapplied the law when it denied the injunction. And this has been a pattern in the U.S. Ninth Circuit court cases involving its review of First Amendment Religious Rights claims. Don't take my word for it, read what seven judges from the Ninth Circuit said in their dissent from the denial of *en banc* review of the case.

Here we go again. When it comes to dealing with the COVID-19 crisis, the "Supreme Court's instructions have been clear, repeated, and insistent: no COVID-19 restriction can disfavor religious practice." *Tandon v. Newsom*, 992 F.3d 916, 939 (9th Cir. 2021) (Bumatay, J., dissenting in part and concurring in part). The Supreme Court has again and again admonished this court for failing to follow its guidance. Indeed, almost a year ago, the Court expressed frustration that, for the "fifth time," it had to "summarily reject the Ninth Circuit's analysis of California's COVID restrictions on religious exercise." *Tandon v. Newsom*, 141 S. Ct. 1294, 1297 (2021) (per curiam) (emphasis added). With this case, our court is gunning for a sixth.[1114]

The seven dissenting judges continue with an illustration of the injustice the school system's COVID-19 mandate scheme works.

Assume Betty and Bea are 16-year-old twin sisters attending another San Diego high school. Betty has always been more devoted to her faith. She sincerely believes that receiving the COVID-19 vaccine would violate her religion. On the other hand, Bea once had a mild allergy to one of the components of the vaccine and qualifies for the District's medical exemption.8 Of course, Betty and Bea share the same home. Both spent time over the holidays mingling with friends and family. Both are unvaccinated. But starting on January 24, Betty will be banned from campus, while Bea will continue her in-person education. Each day after school ends, Bea goes back to the same home as Betty, they eat the same meal, and interact with the same parents. But every morning, Betty watches her sister go back to school, while she must remain confined at home indefinitely.

> It is abundantly clear that Betty and Bea, both unvaccinated, present the exact same risk of infecting their fellow students. After all, even beyond their vaccination status, they are both in constant interaction with the same group of people. But under the District's vaccination scheme, Bea's medical exemption permits her to enjoy the benefits of an in-person education, while her sister Betty is expelled from campus and condemned to online schooling—all for the crime of adhering to her religious beliefs.[1115]

The vaccine mandate disallowed religious exemptions for students, but it allowed religious exemptions for employees. The seven dissenting judges explained:

> That means that unvaccinated teachers, librarians, custodians, coaches, and staff may appear in person if they are religious, while unvaccinated religious students cannot. No one can seriously deny that unvaccinated religious staff and unvaccinated religious students pose similar health and safety risks of spreading COVID-19 on school grounds. If the staff exemption is consistent with the District's interest in the health and safety of its campuses, it strains credulity to believe that the District could not offer the same for its students.[1116]

Yet another case where the court assumed the deadliness of COVID-19 under the germ theory and the supposed safety and efficacy of vaccines is the U.S. Court of Appeals for the Second Circuit decision in *Miller v. McDonald*.[1117] Those assumptions cleared the way for the *Miller* court to ignore the rule of law and decide not to protect the plaintiffs' right to freedom of religion. But if the plaintiffs had attacked the germ theory and the safety and efficacy of the vaccines under a claim that vaccines are religious rituals being imposed on them in violation of the Establishment Clause, their chances of victory would have been much enhanced.

In *Miller*, the Amish sought religious exemptions to New York mandated vaccination for school students. The vaccine requirement applies to all public and private schools. It only applied to students and not to teachers, administrators, or other employees of the schools. Under the statute, there were medical exemptions allowed, but no religious exemptions. Each day a student went unvaccinated, the school incurred a fine of up to $2,000 per student for each day that student remained unvaccinated. The draconian requirement would effectively shut down all Amish schools. Thus far, the state has imposed a total of $118,000 in fines against three schools. That fine was based on 49 students who were unvaccinated for one day each and one student who was unvaccinated for 10 days.[1118] Presumably the fines would continue to mount.

The stated reason New York repealed the religious exemption to vaccination was that New York had fallen below the CDC's goal of at least a 95% vaccination rate to maintain herd immunity. Eliminating religious exemption was a way to increase the vaccination rates among students in New York. The *Miller* court defined herd immunity as "the percentage of individuals in a community who must be vaccinated to reduce the likelihood of a vaccine-preventable disease's transmission."[1119]

In *Miller*, "[p]laintiffs concede that New York Public Health Law § 2164 satisfies rational basis review—immunization programs reduce disease."[1120] That was a mistake. They allowed the proceedings to begin despite having a distinct disadvantage. They were arguing for a religious exemption from what they acknowledged was an effective medical treatment rather than arguing for a religious exemption from an ineffective state-imposed religious ritual. A statute that mandates participation in a religious ritual could not survive even the low standard of rational basis review. It would be deemed *per se* unconstitutional. The state cannot require citizens to engage in a religious ritual.

The plaintiffs argued (quite correctly) that the statute should be subjected to strict scrutiny because it allowed medical exemptions but disallowed religious exemptions, and school officials had discretion whether to grant any particular medical exemption. The U.S. Supreme Court has made it clear that a law is not generally applicable and thus subject to strict scrutiny if there are discretionary exemptions granted. "The creation of a formal mechanism for granting exceptions renders a policy not generally applicable, regardless whether any exceptions have been given, because it invites the government to decide which reasons for not complying with the policy are worthy of solicitude."[1121]

The *Miller* court ruled that school officials lack discretion to grant or deny medical exemptions; therefore, the vaccine requirement is generally applicable and subject to only rational basis review. The problem is that the court made that statement in the face of an averment that "up to 50% of students had medical exemptions in one school while zero students had a medical exemption in another school in the same community and that medical exemptions are granted inconsistently year to year."[1122] That indicates that school officials are exercising discretion. In any event, the fact that it is the school officials who review and approve the exemption renders the statute not of general application.

In response to that rather compelling averment, the court said that it did not change its conclusion because it could not infer a discretionary element without information about the student population and medical needs. That is not an honest response. The statistics themselves speak loudly. A reasonable inference is that the school administration at each of the schools was exercising discretion. There is otherwise no way that there could be a 50% medical exemption rate in one school with zero in the other.

Suppose 100 persons consumed drink "A" at a sports event and 50% of them died within an hour. At the same event, drink "B" was served to a separate group of 100 people at the sports event, and zero of them died.. You could reasonably infer from that information that drink "A" is deadly. You do not need to know anything about the pre-existing health of the people consuming the two products. The statistics speak for themselves.

When presented with an averment that there were 50% medical exemptions in one school and zero medical exemptions in another school, one can reasonably infer that the officials at each school are exercising discretion whether to grant medical exemptions. But in the face of that compelling averment, the court effectively stopped its ears and babbled "la-la-la, I can't hear you!" The court's argument that it needed to know about the student population's medical needs before it could give credence to those facts was an unconvincing excuse to ignore facts that undermine the gravamen of the court's ruling.

The court then stated that "the statute does not create a system in which school officials are given improper discretion to evaluate the reasons given for a requested medical exemption."[1123] The court moved the goal posts. The issue is not whether the school officials exercised *improper* discretion. The issue is whether the school officials had discretion at all. If the school officials had discretion whether to grant a medical exemption, then the statute is not generally applicable and it must be narrowly tailored to achieve a compelling state interest. The court knew that the statute could not pass that test, and so it bent over backwards to find that the school officials did not have discretion whether to grant medical exemptions.

It matters not if all medical exemptions are granted or if none are granted. The Supreme Court has stated that the issue is whether there is "a formal mechanism for granting exceptions... regardless whether any exceptions have been given."[1124] There was such a formal mechanism in *Miller*. Thus, the exemption scheme should have been subjected to strict scrutiny. A scrutiny it could not have passed because it allowed medical (secular) exemptions, while prohibiting all religious exemptions. The plaintiffs have petitioned the U.S. Supreme Court for a writ of certiorari, asking it to overrule the court of appeals.[1125]

Such injustices will continue as long as judges feel emboldened by the danger posed by supposed viral epidemics and assume that a vaccine mandate is a safe and effective means of saving lives. Litigants should present evidence at the outset establishing that the emperor has no clothes. The proofs should start with evidence that vaccination is not based on actual science, it is based on religious superstition. Plaintiffs should expose the scam germ theory and strip the legitimacy from the false science of virology. From that foundation, the litigant can then knock down the claimed vaccine safety and effectiveness house of cards. A court faced with the objective evidence of the dangers and ineffectiveness of vaccines will have no choice but to rule that vaccinology has as muc health benefit and safety as bleeding. This should all be done under the legal claim that vaccination is a religious ritual being mandated by the government in violation of the Establishment Clause of the First Amendment.

38 Inflating COVID-19 Death Statistics

America's Frontline Doctors (AFLD) is a group of doctors who have joined to fight the government's medical oppression. AFLD has sued the U.S. Government, alleging that the COVID-19 emergency is a scam based upon inflated statistics of death and illness designed to bring about a medical tyranny to take away the freedoms of all Americans. The complaint states in pertinent part:

> [T]he Emergency Declaration upon which they are all based was unjustified. As Plaintiffs allege in detail and will show at trial with expert medical and scientific evidence, including the Defendants' own data and studies, **there is not now, and there never has been, a bona fide "public health emergency" due to the SARS-Cov-2 virus or the disease COVID-19.** Virtually all of the PCR tests were calibrated to produce false positive results, which has enabled the Defendants and their counterparts in state governments to publish daily reports containing seriously inflated COVID-19 "case" and "death" counts that grossly exaggerate the public health threat.[1126]

The false positive COVID-19 tests laid the foundation for creating a pandemic where there was none. Deborah Birx, M.D. revealed how the scheme worked. Dr. Birx was the U.S. Global Aids Coordinator & U.S. Special Representative for Global Health Diplomacy and Physician-Ambassador to the office of the Vice President and the U.S. Government Coronavirus Response Coordinator. During an April 7, 2020, task force press briefing, Dr. Birx was asked by a reporter about the allegations by many that the coronavirus deaths have been artificially inflated. The reporter asked: "Can you talk about your concerns about deaths being misreported by coronavirus because of either testing or standards for how they're characterized?"[1127] Dr. Birx then admitted that, in fact, that the COVID-19 deaths were being inflated. Dr. Birx explained that the United States has taken a "liberal approach" to reporting COVID-19 deaths. She stated that it is "straightforward." That "straightforward" approach is to report someone who dies "with" COVID-19 as a COVID-19 death. Implied in her statement is that any deceased person who tests positive for COVID-19 is recorded as dying "of" COVID-19, regardless of the actual cause of death. To put it more succinctly, every person who dies "with" COVID-19 is recorded as dying "of" COVID-19.

Dr. Birx distinguished the U.S. approach from other countries where, for example, if someone died of heart failure or kidney failure and they test positive for COVID-19, some other countries might report that as a kidney failure or heart failure death and not a COVID-19 death. Not so in the United States. The "liberal approach" taken in the U.S. is that if someone dies with COVID-19 they are added to the COVID-19 death total even though they actually died of kidney failure or heart failure. Dr. Birx answered the reporter's question as follows:

> So, I think, in this country, we've taken a very liberal approach to mortality, and I think the reporting here has been pretty straightforward over the last five to six weeks. Prior to that, when there

wasn't testing in January and February, that's a very different situation and unknown.

There are other countries that if you had a pre-existing condition and let's say the virus caused you to go to the ICU and then have a heart or kidney problem — some countries are recording that as a heart issue or a kidney issue and not a COVID-19 death.

Right now, we're still recording it, and we'll — I mean, the great thing about having forms that come in and a form that has the ability to mark it as COVID-19 infection — the intent is, right now, that those — **if someone dies with COVID-19, we are counting that as a COVID-19 death.**[1128] (emphasis added)

Illinois Department of Public Health Director Dr. Ngozi Ezike followed the guidance from the CDC and admitted that the State of Illinois was recording persons who died with COVID-19 as having died from COVID-19, regardless of whether COVID-19 was the actual cause of the deaths. Health Director Ezike stated:

I just want to be clear in terms of the definition of people dying of COVID. The case definition is very simplistic. It means at the time of death it was a COVID positive diagnosis. ... It means, technically, even if you died from a clear alternate cause, but you had COVID at the same time, it is still listed as a COVID death. So. everyone who is listed as a COVID death, doesn't mean that was the cause of the death, but they had COVID at the time of death.[1129]

That reporting scheme of the State of Illinois was per the

guidance given by the CDC. The CDC was beating the bushes, so to speak, to generate the inflated COVID-19 statistics. The CDC issued guidance to the state health commissioners to alter how they report COVID-19 deaths in order to artificially inflate the deaths from COVID-19.

The CDC data manipulation was planned. And it had a purpose. To create a COVID-19 pandemic where none really existed. It was a massive statistical lie campaign. And it constituted a federal crime. Oregon State Senators Kim Thatcher and Dennis Linthicum petitioned U.S. Attorney Scott Asphaug to approve a grand jury investigation into the criminality of the CDC and FDA.[1130] They based their allegations on information and data from a large team of world-renowned doctors, epidemiologists, virologists, and attorneys.[1131] The Senators averred that in the March 2020 alert, the CDC illegally changed the National Vital Statistics System so that mortality data compilers could massage data to falsely report COVID-19 as the "cause" of death. This new set of rules, which only applied to COVID-19, departed from the standard procedures that had been in effect for the prior 17 years.

The CDC statistics reported deaths as being from COVID-19 when the deaths were actually from something else. Comorbidity is defined as the simultaneous presence of two or more chronic diseases or conditions in a patient. The CDC has reported that 94% percent of people they have reported who have died of COVID-19 in the U.S. (as of August 22, 2020) were suffering from an average of 2.6 chronic diseases or conditions in addition to COVID-19.[1132] Thus, the statistical total of 161,392 deaths (as of August 22, 2020) from COVID-19 reported by the CDC does not mean that the decedents making up that total actually died from COVID-19.

On September 27, 2023, the CDC archived the comorbidities section, indicating that about 5% of the listed COVID-19 deaths were solely from COVID-19. The remaining

95% of the listed COVID-19 deaths involved potentially four (4) causes other than COVID-19. The archived section states:

> For over 5% of these deaths, COVID-19 was the only cause mentioned on the death certificate. For deaths with conditions or causes in addition to COVID-19, on average, there were 4.0 additional conditions or causes per death.[1133]

While the CDC webpage is subtitled, *Provisional Death Counts for Coronavirus Disease 2019 (COVID-19)*, which suggests it is reporting those who have died from COVID-19, the data charts state that it is reporting data of "Deaths **Involving** coronavirus disease 2019 (COVID-19)." By this nuanced equivocation, the CDC misrepresented people dying "with" COVID-19 as people who died "from" COVID-19. This inflated the COVID-19 deaths that were being reported and created a false sense of danger among the public.

The CDC reported that as of August 22, 2020, only 6% of the 161,392 reported COVID-19 deaths were from COVID-19 alone. The remaining 151,708 of persons who died while testing positive for COVID-19 died from some cause (i.e., a comorbidity) in addition to COVID-19. The astounding thing is that each of those 151,708 persons who died had 2.6 comorbidities in addition to COVID-19. That means that 94% of the persons reported dying of COVID-19 actually died from a combination of diseases and injuries, which may or may not be COVID-19.

With this surreal definition of what is a COVID-19 death being pushed by the CDC, the local health officials are only limited by their creativity when deciding that a death is from COVID-19. The Orange County (Florida) Health Officer Dr. Raul Pino did not seem to think it was unusual that a man who died from a motorcycle accident was misrepresented as having died of COVID-19. Dr. Raul Pino even tried to make the irrational argument that it is okay to report a person who died in a motorcycle accident as having died from COVID-19 because "it could have been the COVID-19 that caused him to crash."[1134]

Daniella Lama reporting for Fox 35 News in Orlando discovered that the Florida Department of Health has decided that all persons who test positive for COVID-19 in Florida are automatically listed as COVID-19 deaths if they subsequently die unless there is an extra step taken by the reporting agency to exclude them from the COVID-19 death statistics.[1135] That extra step to exclude the motorcycle decedent was not done, which is why he was listed automatically as a COVID-19 death. Obviously, the statistical system is rigged to capture all persons who have ever tested positive with COVID-19 as a COVID-19 death if they subsequently die. If the extra step is not taken to exclude them from the statistical count then they will be listed as a COVID-19 death. With the fear of the disease ramped up by these artificially inflated COVID-19 death statistics, the public was primed to accept the emergency use authorized COVID-19 vaccines.

Why would county health officials and hospitals go along with this scam? Because there is money in it. "For the love of money is the root of all evil." 1 Timothy 6:19. Minnesota State Senator Dr. Scott Jensen, M.D., revealed that hospital administrations are incentivized to diagnose and treat a person for COVID-19.[1136] The system is financially skewed toward diagnosing and treating COVID-19 even though the patient may not actually be ill from COVID-19. The patients may be in the hospital for an entirely different reason, but if they test positive for COVID-19 or they are diagnosed as having COVID-19, then the hospital hits the financial jackpot and can begin raking in the financial windfall from the federal government through the Coronavirus Aid, Relief and Economic Security Act (CARES Act).

The CDC and NIH are fanning the hysteria of a health

emergency that does not really exist. It is doing so by artificially inflating the COVID-19 numbers in order to portray a false sense of emergency to justify its own draconian COVID-19 orders.

Dr. Kristin Held is the President of the Association of American Physicians and Surgeons (AAPS). On July 20, 2020, she explained in a post the trickery used by the CDC and the State Boards of Health to inflate the COVID-19 infection and death rates.

Dr. Held revealed a little-known fact that "[t]he Council of State and Territorial Epidemiologists (CSTE) adopted new definitions of COVID-19 cases and COVID-related deaths in April [2020] that were adopted by the Centers for Disease Control and Prevention (CDC) in May. The states were then encouraged to adopt the new definitions."

These new definitions had the direct effect of artificially inflating the COVID-19 case and death statistics. Dr. Held reveals that under the new criteria "COVID-related deaths can include anyone who has COVID-19 listed on their death certificate as one of the causes of death- it doesn't have to be the first or second cause, and no COVID-19 testing is required."[1137]

There is a political motivation to increase COVID-19 case and death statistics. Dr. Held reveals that the Federal Government is handsomely compensating the hospitals that go along with that political program. She explains:

> Why would someone want to inflate case counts, and what are the risks and benefits of doing so? As reported in Modern Healthcare, July 17, 2020, "HHS to send $10 billion in round two of relief grants to COVID-19 hot spots." Modern Healthcare reports, "Hospitals that had more than 161 COVID-19 admissions between January 1 and

June 10 will be paid $50,000 for each COVID-19 admission. HHS asked hospitals to start submitting COVID-19 admission data on June 8."

Hospitals that use the new CDC definition stand to make millions of dollars. The first round of HHS grants was $12 billion and paid $76,975 per admission to hospitals that had more than 100 COVID-19 admissions from January 1 through April 1. Clearly, states hit early got tons of money- Illinois got $740 M, New York got $684 M, and Pennsylvania got $655 M alone. Additionally, Medicaid will pay out $15 billion in relief funds- hospitals must apply by August, so the more cases the better the return.

***

Remember, this is on top of the extra money commercial insurers and the extra 20% Medicare pay the hospitals for patients hospitalized "with COVID-19." The hospitals reporting the most cases get the most money. In addition to expanding the definition of a New COVID-19 case to include exposure to a COVID-19 positive patient and a self-reported fever, lowering admission thresholds, and requiring testing on every admission, the ability to code a hospital admission as "with-COVID" is easy and becomes a very lucrative business model.

Dr. Held concludes:

Clearly, hospitals are financially incentivized to code more COVID cases and deaths. Definitions matter. Another sad consequence is that we are losing freedoms and destroying our state and country based on the inflated numbers. Our reopenings are based on these numbers –we have lost our ability to congregate in groups of 10 or more, go to church, school, weddings, funerals, sporting events, concerts, or go anywhere without a mask, or hug our parents, grandparents, children, grandchildren, and the lonely.[1138]

It took time for the states to implement the CDC's new definition for COVID-19. But eventually, that new definition bore the sour fruit planned by the CDC. As the states began implementing the new CDC guidance, we found a spike in COVID-19 cases. In the middle of June 2020, the U.S. COVID-19 cases steadily increased from approximately 20,000 reported cases per day to 300,000 reported cases per day by the beginning of January 2021.[1139] That suspicious spike in numbers came on the heels of the new reporting criteria for cases instituted by the CDC. Dr. Held wonders about that spike.

We must answer the question, what happened June 14-16, because something did when you look at the stats. (Did redefining what constitutes a COVID-19 case, hospitalization, or death change the numbers? Did federal financial aid to hospitals change admitting thresholds and practices? Did the FDA withdrawing its Emergency Use Authorization (EUA) for Hydroxychloroquine (HCQ) alter outpatient treatment resulting in COVID-surging? Was it the Riots? Or what?)[1140]

Dr. Held was writing her suspicions on July 20, 2020, when the spike had only reached approximately 75,000 cases per day. Dr. Held thought that was somewhat suspicious. But the daily increase in COVID-19 cases continued until it reached 300,000 cases per day by January 2021. It seems that the "second wave" predicted by Dr. Fauci and others was something they planned to happen by rigging the COVID-19 numbers. It coincided perfectly with the flu season. Interesting that influenza all but disappeared in the fall and winter of 2020. They just redefined all influenza cases as COVID-19 cases.

Dr. (and Minnesota State Senator) Scott Jensen reveals that the guidance by the CDC is to put COVID-19 down as the cause of death even though the death actually resulted from something else. Indeed, the CDC is advising that COVID-19 is to be considered not on testing and a diagnosis that COVID-19 is the cause of death but rather based upon it being "suspected or likely." Health officials and doctors are being asked to put on the death certificate "probable" or "presumed" death from COVID-19 based upon a clinical judgment (i.e., a guess) without any actual scientific test or diagnosis.[1141] In his expert opinion, Dr. Jensen concluded that COVID-19 death statistics are being gamed to inflate the death rate.

Dr. Scott Jensen was named Minnesota Family Doctor of the Year seven years ago. Now he finds himself and his pristine record and reputation under attack after he exposed the dirty secret that the threat from COVID-19 is not real and the states are deceptively inflating the COVID-19 deaths. The Minnesota Board of Medical Practice has now notified Dr. Jensen that they are investigating him on alleged charges of improper medical practice. Among the charges are that he spread disinformation by "advising against vaccines and masks."[1142] Further, the medical board alleged that Dr. Jensen "promoted conspiracy theories that the Minnesota Department of Health instructed providers to falsify death certificates to list COVID-19."[1143] The Orwellian medical board characterizes good medical advice as "disinformation" and true statements as "conspiracy theories." The pharmaceutical cartel is moving against Dr. Jensen as an object lesson to frighten any doctor who would dare to speak up against their medical tyranny and quackery.

The CDC guidance referenced by Dr. Jensen states in pertinent part:

> In cases where a definite diagnosis of COVID–19 cannot be made, but it is suspected or likely (e.g., the circumstances are compelling within a reasonable degree of certainty), it is acceptable to report COVID–19 on a death certificate as "probable" or "presumed." In these instances, certifiers should use their best clinical judgement in determining if a COVID–19 infection was likely. However, please note that testing for COVID–19 should be conducted whenever possible.[1144]

The CDC states that testing for COVID-19 is ideal but not necessary in order to categorize a death as being COVID-19 as long as the "circumstances are compelling within a reasonable degree of certainty." Basically, that means whatever a particular doctor wants it to mean. The CDC instructions for filling out death certificates are contrary to the traditional method of only putting down the scientific finding for a "cause of death." The CDC guidance opens the door for a doctor to opine under a "reasonable degree of certainty" standard that virtually any death is a COVID-19 death. And that is precisely what the CDC wants. The CDC guidance states:

> Ideally, testing for COVID–19 should be conducted, but it is acceptable to report COVID–19 on a death certificate without this confirmation if the circumstances are compelling within a reasonable degree of certainty.[1145]

Below is the scenario on page 6 of the CDC Guidance for Certifying Deaths Due to COVID-19. Please read it carefully. You do not need to be a doctor to understand that the CDC instructs doctors to lie on death certificates. They are trying to inflate the death statistics. Why else would the CDC give specific instructions in filling out death certificates regarding how to characterize a decedent as having died from COVID-19?

The CDC is interested in ensuring that every possible COVID-19 death is caught. And they have an interest in turning deaths with only inferential COVID-19 evidence into COVID-19 deaths. Why are the instructions contrary to all standard medical procedures for filling out death certificates?

The CDC is instructing Doctors to mark down that a patient died of COVID-19 even without any scientific tests to indicate that the patient had COVID-19 at the time of death. The new standard is now simply an inference that it was "likely" that the patient died of COVID-19. In the scenario presented by the CDC, that likelihood is based on the decedent being exposed five days before her death to a person subsequently diagnosed with COVID-19. The CDC scenario presented on page 6 of the CDC death certificate guidance is as follows:

> An 86-year-old female passed away at home. Her husband reported that she was nonambulatory after suffering an ischemic stroke 3 years ago. He stated that 5 days prior, she developed a high fever and severe cough after being exposed to an ill family member who subsequently was diagnosed with COVID–19. Despite his urging, she refused to go to the hospital, even when her breathing became more labored and temperature escalated. She was unresponsive that morning and her husband phoned emergency medical services (EMS). Upon EMS arrival, the patient was pulseless and apneic. Her husband stated that he and his wife had advanced directives and that she was not to be resuscitated. After consulting with medical command, she was pronounced dead and the coroner was notified.

Comment: Although no testing was done, the coroner determined that the likely UCOD [Underlying Cause of Death] was COVID–19 given the patient's symptoms and exposure to an infected individual. Therefore, COVID–19 was reported on the lowest line used in Part I. Her ischemic stroke was considered a factor that contributed to her death but was not a part of the direct causal sequence in Part I, so it was reported in Part II.[1146]

With those standards in mind, state health officials have been able to classify virtually any death where a person tests positive for COVID-19 as a COVID-19 death, regardless of the actual cause of death, and they are doing so. The vast majority of the deaths being counted as "probable cases" are actually of people who may have had COVID-19 but died from something else. For example, on July 23, 2020, Danielle Waugh from CBS 12 News investigated evidence that only 169 of the 581 reported deaths in Palm Beach County were of persons who allegedly had COVID-19 without any contributing illness.[1147] That calls into question the legitimacy of more than 70% of the reported deaths from COVID-19.

Early on, the states adopted the new CDC guidelines. For example, Virginia Department of Health (VDH) states that "VDH adopted the updated CDC confirmed and probable surveillance case definitions on August 27, 2020."[1148] Indeed, the VDH provided a link directly to the CDC website defining confirmed and probable cases.[1149]

The VDH is like most state health departments who follow the new guidance for reporting COVID-19 cases and deaths. The VDH acknowledges that when it reports COVID-19 cases they are not based on a medical diagnosis of COVID-19. Thus, a person does not need to actually have COVID-19 to be included in the

Virginia COVID-19 statistics. The VDH explains:

> Public health uses standardized case definitions to count cases. These case definitions make it easier to compare data over time, across states, or even between different counties. A case definition is different from a diagnosis, and is used for a different purpose. A diagnosis is helpful for treatment and medical billing while a case definition is used for public health surveillance. For COVID-19, Virginia uses the CDC COVID-19 confirmed and probable case definitions. These definitions suggests [*sic*] that we report two case statuses:
>
> Confirmed cases – Confirmed cases include anyone who tests positive for SARS-CoV-2 RNA in a clinical or autopsy specimen using a molecular amplification test.
>
> Probable cases – There are a few ways to identify a probable case. In Virginia, anyone who is positive using an approved antigen test or anyone who displays a specific set of symptoms and has an epidemiologic linkage (contact with another confirmed or probable case or part of a risk cohort), or anyone whose death certificate mentions COVID-19 or SARS-CoV-2 without a positive lab result counts as a probable case.[1150]

The VDH further acknowledges that the COVID-19 statistics received from hospitals overstate the COVID-19 risk. The hospitalization statistics include "those who have [COVID-19] tests pending" but who have not actually tested positive for COVID-19. The VIDH explains that "[t]hese data do not have the same kind of rigorous case definition that epidemiologic case data do because they are not intended for the same purpose. For healthcare system preparation, an overestimation is better than an underestimation."[1151]

The VDH explains that in order to be consistent, it must use that same overstatement across the board when reporting COVID-19 statistics. "For our purposes, it's important that the same case definition be applied to the numerator (the number of cases that result in hospitalization) and the denominator (the total number of cases)."[1152]

Virginia went beyond the CDC guidance and artificially goosed up its COVID-19 case statistics even more. On or before June 19, 2020, NBC News reported that the State of Virginia would start reporting the number of positive COVID-19 tests as COVID-19 cases rather than the number of persons who tested positive. Thus, a person who receives a positive COVID-19 test result one day and two days later tests positive again would be counted as two confirmed COVID-19 cases rather than one case. Since almost all who tested positive for COVID-19 would repeatedly get tested to determine if they were no longer infected, there could be several positive COVID-19 tests per patient before they tested negative. This inevitably would artificially inflate the COVID-19 cases in Virginia. That is the only thing that such a contrivance would achieve. NBC reported:

> The Virginia Department of Health announced it will now count the number of positive virus tests instead of the number of people who test positive.
>
> That means if one person is tested three-times and all three tests come back positive, it counts as three instead of how the numbers were being counted before, which would have only been one because it was a single patient.[1153]

The only reason to count the number of tests is to deceptively inflate the number of COVID-19 cases in Virginia. There is no way around it. That is out-and-out chicanery.

The inflated COVID-19 numbers can be explained in part by the built-in financial incentive for medical professionals to diagnose a patient with COVID-19. USA TODAY revealed that "[t]he coronavirus relief legislation created a 20% premium, or add-on, for COVID-19 Medicare patients."[1154] There are financial incentives in addition to the 20% premium. Dr. Jensen explained the additional financial incentive for hospitals to make a diagnosis of COVID-19:

> Hospital administrators might well want to see COVID-19 attached to a discharge summary or a death certificate. Why? Because if it's a straightforward, garden-variety pneumonia that a person is admitted to the hospital for – if they're Medicare – typically, the diagnosis-related group lump sum payment would be $5,000. But if it's COVID-19 pneumonia, then it's $13,000, and if that COVID-19 pneumonia patient ends up on a ventilator, it goes up to $39,000.[1155]

USA TODAY checked out the claim by Dr. Jensen. "USA TODAY reached out to Marty Makary, a surgeon and professor of health policy and management at Johns Hopkins Bloomberg School of Public Health, about the claim. Makary said in an email April 21 that 'what Scott Jensen said sounds right to me.'"[1156] USA TODAY determined that Dr. Jensen's claim was accurate.[1157]

Andrew Mark Miller, reporting for the Washington Examiner, revealed that because U.S. hospitals are reimbursed 13,000 for every COVID-19 diagnosis and 39,000 for every COVID-19 patient put on a ventilator, "U.S. Centers for Disease Control and Prevention Director Robert Redfield agreed that some hospitals have a monetary incentive to overcount coronavirus deaths."[1158] Dr. Redfield expressed that opinion while testifying before a U.S. House of Representatives Panel. Dr. Redfield acknowledged that the federal reimbursement scheme creates a perverse monetary incentive for U.S. hospitals to inflate the COVID-19 infection rate. Dr. Redfield explained that "when it comes to hospital reimbursement issues or individuals that get discharged, there could be some play in that for sure."[1159]

Edwin Mora, reported for *Breitbart* that "[a]ccording to Congressman [Blaine] Luetkemeyer, Adm. Brett Giroir from the U.S. Health and Human Services (HHS) Department has conceded that there is an economic incentive for hospitals to inflate their coronavirus fatalities. Giroir 'acknowledged that the statistics he is getting from the states are over-inflated,' the Republican lawmakers said."[1160]

According to Becker's Healthcare, as of April 2020, Virginia hospitals received from HHS $201,000 reimbursement per COVID-19 case. That figure was obtained from Kaiser Health News, which "used a state breakdown provided to the House Ways and Means Committee by HHS along with COVID-19 cases tabulated by The New York Times for its analysis."[1161]

Despite the over reporting, the VDH nonetheless claims that the "the number of cases we have on record is an underrepresentation of the true burden."[1162] That nonsensical statement is based in part on the premise that there are people walking around with COVID-19 who show no symptoms. But that statement is based on the disproven premise of asymptomatic spread of SARS-CoV-2. The asymptomatic carrier theory was born from the fact that the PCR test for SARS-CoV-2 has potentially up to a 97% false positive rate. The medical authorities came up with a way to explain how people who are not sick with COVID-19 nonetheless test positive for the disease. They argue that the well-person tests positive for the disease because he is an "asymptomatic" carrier of SARS-CoV-2. Thus, the false-positive test problem is solved.

The asymptomatic spread theory is a fantastical fraud. That foundational lie underlies the government strategy against the mythical COVID-19 pandemic. In a court action for a preliminary injunction, America's Frontline Doctors (AFLD) averred that the government floated the false asymptomatic spread theory to justify lockdowns, masking, and social distancing measures designed to take away our liberties. The AFLD court filing states in pertinent part:

> **[I]t appears that these Defendants either did lie about asymptomatic spread, or were simply wrong about the science.** The theory of asymptomatic transmission – used as the justification for the lockdown and masking of the healthy – was based solely upon mathematical modeling. This theory had no actual study participants, and no peer review. The authors made the unfounded assumption that asymptomatic persons were "75% as infectious" as symptomatic persons. But in the real world, healthy false positives turned out to be merely healthy, and were never shown to be "asymptomatic" carriers of anything. Studies have shown that PCR test-positive asymptomatic individuals do not induce clinical COVID-19 disease, not even in a family member with whom they share a home and extended proximity. An enormous study of nearly ten million people in Wuhan, China showed that asymptomatic individuals testing positive for COVID-19 never infected others. Since asymptomatic individuals do not spread COVID-19, they do not need to be vaccinated.[1163]

Researchers Torsten Engelbrecht and Konstantin Demeter concluded:

> Lockdowns and hygienic measures around the world are based on numbers of cases and mortality rates created by the so-called SARS-CoV-2 RT-PCR tests used to identify "positive" patients, whereby "positive" is usually equated with "infected."
>
> But looking closely at the facts, the conclusion is that these PCR tests are meaningless as a diagnostic tool to determine an alleged infection by a supposedly new virus called SARS-CoV-2.[1164]

The researchers concluded that the RT-PCR test used to detect COVID-19 is so inaccurate that there may be between 22% and 78% false positives. But there is no way to be sure because there is no gold standard against which to verify the accuracy of the tests.

One study gives an example of the test's inaccuracy. "[A] study from Singapore in which tests were carried out almost daily on 18 patients and the majority went from 'positive' to 'negative' back to 'positive' at least once, and up to five times in one patient."[1165]

The apparent preponderance of false positives for asymptomatic subjects means that the people are asymptomatic because they do not have COVID-19. The asymptomatic carrier model that is being sold to the public is a myth. The positive tests are bogus results. The COVID-19 "outbreaks" and "hotspots" are really not "outbreaks" or "hotspots" at all.

Word has gotten out about the inaccuracies of the PCR test, and so the CDC's hand was forced to stop using it. On July 21,

2021, the CDC announced that laboratories should cease using the PCR to test for COVID-19 beginning on December 31, 2021.[1166] If the PCR test is so inaccurate as to cause the CDC to recommend against using it, why is the CDC waiting until December 31, 2021, to transition to a more accurate test? It seems that the CDC is not at all concerned about the accuracy of its COVID-19 testing. The PCR test will be replaced with the antigen test, which the FDA acknowledges is also inaccurate.

It must be understood that most states report Total COVID-19 Deaths as being the number of confirmed and probable COVID-19 deaths. Virginia is one example. The Total Deaths number for Virginia from COVID-19 is a scam on two levels. First, a probable case does not require that the person test positive for COVID-19. In the written guidance, the CDC has told local officials to put on the death certificate "probable" or "presumed" death from COVID-19 based upon a clinical judgment (i.e., a guess) without any actual scientific test or diagnosis.

It does not take much to be a probable case of COVID-19. One could have a headache and have recently been within 6 feet for at least 15 minutes of someone who is himself a probable case of COVID-19 or a member of a risk cohort for COVID-19 as defined by public health authorities during an outbreak. Thus, neither the person who is supposed to be the spreader of the disease nor the person supposed to have gotten COVID-19 needs to have COVID-19 to be included in the statistics for COVID-19 Total Cases or Total Deaths.

It gets worse. The confirmed cases of deaths from COVID-19 are not what you would think they are. A confirmed COVID-19 death does not mean that the person died *from* COVID-19. It means that the person died *with* COVID-19.

A close reading of the Virginia Department of Health (VDH) rules for reported deaths reveals that the "VDH is counting any death that occurs in a person who was reported to the health department as having COVID-19."[1167]

Thus, the VDH is not reporting only those people who died *from* COVID-19. They are artificially inflating the numbers by including the numbers of people who died from some other cause and tested positive for COVID-19 prior to their death. The VDH death statistics include both those who died *from* COVID-19 and those who died *with* COVID-19, even though those who died *with* COVID-19 actually died from some cause other than COVID-19. The department of health states that it will not include those who died from "an injury or accident" among the COVID-19 deaths. But that is the only exclusion. All other people who die *with* COVID-19 from some cause other than injury or accident are listed by the VDH as a COVID-19 death.

The VDH exclusion criteria only excludes from the COVID-19 statistics deaths due to "injury or accident." What about non-traumatic causes of death like cancer, diabetes, emphysema, heart disease, or stroke? Is someone who dies of any of those illnesses listed, nonetheless, as a COVId-19 death? Apparently so. Thus, if someone dies of cancer but tests positive for COVID-19 he will be listed as a COVID-19 death.

How inflated are the death statistics? The CDC offers an answer. That answer is that only 6% of reported COVID-19 deaths died only from COVID-19. All other reported deaths are people who had comorbidities. The CDC explains that its reported statistics show "health conditions and contributing causes mentioned in conjunction with deaths involving coronavirus disease 2019 (COVID-19). For 6% of the deaths, COVID-19 was the only cause mentioned. For deaths with conditions or causes in addition to COVID-19, on average, there were 2.6 additional conditions or causes per death."[1168]

Some of the comorbidities listed by the CDC include

cardiac arrest, diabetes, Alzheimer disease, renal failure, injury (intentional, unintentional, poisoning, and other adverse events), malignant neoplasms (a.k.a. cancerous tumors). In that partial list, the only comorbidity that is not reported as a COVID-19 death in Virginia by the VDH are those who die from "an injury or accident."

The Colorado Department of Public Health and Environment (CDPHE) has also followed CDC guidelines to inflate COVID-19 numbers. The CDPHE told NBC News 9 Denver that "[w]e classify a death as confirmed when there was a case who had a positive SARS-CoV-2 (COVID-19) laboratory test and then died."[1169] Thus, if a person dies from some cause other than COVID-19, he would still be listed as a COVID-19 death if he tests positive for COVID-19. The CDPHE further explained that simply because there is no test does not mean a person will not be listed as a COVID-19 death. The CDPHE stated: "We also classify some deaths as probable."[1170]

With those standards in mind, they are able to classify virtually any death where a person tests positive for COVID-19 as a COVID-19 death, regardless of the actual cause of death, and they are doing so. A case in Montezuma County in Colorado illustrates that point.

> The coroner of Montezuma County in southwestern Colorado couldn't believe it when the state's health department concluded a May 4 death in his county was the result of COVID-19.
>
> "I know it's not correct," George Deavers told 9Wants to Know Thursday. "Nowhere on the death certificate is COVID even listed. It had nothing to do with his death."
>
> Deavers ought to know. The death certificate he

signed just this week lists the official cause of death for the 35-year old man as "ethanol toxicity."

In other words, Deavers said, he died because he drank too much alcohol.

"We did blood work. The blood work came back at 550 [mg/dL]. Anything over 300 is lethal," he said. To be clear, Deavers did test the body for COVID after he received word that the man might have had recent contact with someone with the virus. That test showed the man did, in fact, have COVID-19, but Deavers said he's "99.9% certain" the virus did not cause the man's death.[1171]

The death certificate indicated the cause of death as ethanol toxicity. There was no mention of COVID-19 as even a contributing factor, yet the state of Colorado reported the man as having died of COVID-19 simply because he had tested positive for COVID-19.

The Colorado Department of Public Health and Environment (CDPHE) disagreed with the coroner who filled out the death certificate. The CDPHE continued to list the death from alcohol poisoning as a COVID-19 death despite the coroner's objection. Indeed, the CDPHE refused to even return the coroner's calls.

Why would they do that? Because the state did not want to give Montezuma County a variance from the state COVID-19 emergency business closure restrictions. The state wanted to artificially pump up the death rate in the county from COVID-19 as an excuse to continue with the business closures in that county. NBC News 9 Denver reported:

In a letter sent Monday to the Montezuma County

Administrator, CDPHE's Executive Director Jill Hunsaker Ryan said, "Our reviewers have some concerns about vulnerabilities in Montezuma County and want to monitor the situation further before considering a variance."[1172]

Indeed, the fraud has gotten so bad in Colorado that State Representative Mark Baisley has sent a formal letter requesting 18th Judicial District Attorney George Brauchler to investigate and criminally prosecute the Executive Director of the Colorado Department of Public Health and Environment (CDPHE), Jill Hunsaker Ryan. Baisley, in the letter, accused Ryan of fraudulently overruling death findings by attending physicians in cases where patients also tested positive for COVID-19 in order to artificially inflate the number of COVID-19-related deaths.[1173]

The Colorado Governor has dismissed any notion of a criminal investigation of the Director of the CDPHE. Of course he would; the director is his subordinate and is acting at his direction. So, how has Colorado Governor Jared Polis addressed the issue? "In a conference call with reporters Friday afternoon, CDPHE officials revealed they would be announcing two numbers concerning deaths among COVID-19 patients going forward. One number would show the total number of people who died while sick with COVID-19. The other number would be how many people had died as a result of COVID-19."

You read that correctly, the State of Colorado has decided to keep two books, just like all crooked businesses do. One book will report the actual deaths allegedly caused by COVID-19. The other book will register the phony "total" number of people who died with COVID-19, which means they only tested positive for COVID-19 and have died from some other cause.

So when you hear the total number of deaths from COVID-19 in Colorado, you cannot be sure you are not hearing the inflated number. The public will not know that the "total" number being reported may only mean the decedent had COVID-19 and could have died from something else. The only reason the governor went from out-and-out lying by reporting all persons dying with COVID-19 as "COVID-19 deaths" to now keeping two sets of books is that he was embarrassed when he got caught fraudulently reporting a death from alcohol poisoning as a COVID-19 death only because the decedent also tested positive for COVID-19.

The CDC scheme made no sense to the electorate, so the governor changed course to cover the fraud. But he still wants to have his cake and eat it too. He wants to keep getting federal money by adding in those who die with COVID-19 to those who allegedly die from COVID-19. That way, the state can get more federal money. The federal government is paying the states a lot to play this deceptive game of hyping the COVID-19 scare, locking us down, masking us, and forcibly vaccinating us. It is what the federal government asked for, and it is paying the states a lot of money to do it. COVID-19 is not a threat to public health but a phantom virus to scare citizens into slavery. It is about tyranny.

Indeed, the State of Colorado brought in more than $360 million from the first $30 billion installment sent from the federal government's CARES Act Public Health and Social Services Emergency Fund to the states.[1174] Those funds were sent to the states to encourage the states to enforce the draconian measures necessary to investigate and inflate case statistics, engage in contact tracing, testing services, personal protective equipment, and emergency preparedness and response.[1175] More COVID-19 cases extended the emergency and ensured federal money would flow. The more tyranny imposed by the states meant more money was sent to the states.

Dr. Anthony Fauci is the Director of the National Institute of Allergy and Infectious Diseases (NIAID), an agency in the

National Institute of Health (NIH). The CDC and the NIH are both operational agencies in the Department of Health and Human Services. Anthony Fauci is portrayed as the nation's top infectious disease expert. He is a member of the White House coronavirus task force. Dr. Fauci does not realize it, but he has confirmed that the fraud by the CDC is knowing and intentional. He did this by trying to explain the acknowledged fact that 94% of COVID-19 decedents had on average 2.5 comorbidities. Dr. Fauci did not dispute that fact. He accepted that fact as true. But how he characterized that fact was breathtaking in its incredulity. Dr. Fauci told an ABC News interviewer on September 1, 2020, that it "does not mean that someone who has hypertension or diabetes who dies of COVID didn't die of COVID-19. They did." Dr. Fauci further stated that "it's not 9,000 deaths from COVID-19, it's 180-plus-thousand deaths."[1176]

That statement by Dr. Fauci is telling. Dr. Fauci is stating a hypothetical case, but he is perfectly comfortable to say that someone (anyone) who is listed in the CDC COVID-19 death list who died with 1) hypertension (i.e., high blood pressure), or 2) diabetes, and 3) COVID-19 most definitely died of COVID-19. Dr. Fauci picks one of the three illnesses (COVID-19), and without even knowing the facts or the patient, he is able to divine that every decedent with those simultaneous illnesses always dies from COVID-19.

Dr. Fauci did not equivocate. He emphatically stated that all the diabetics and people with high blood pressure listed by the CDC as having died of COVID-19, in fact died of COVID-19 regardless of the seriousness of their hypertension or diabetes. No, ifs, ands, or buts about it. He stated emphatically that every person listed by the CDC as a COVID-19 death actually died "from" COVID-19 regardless of the comorbidity. Dr. Fauci was forcible and clear: "So the numbers you've been hearing — there are 180,000-plus deaths [as of September 1, 2020]— are real deaths from COVID-19. Let (there) not be any confusion about that."[1177]

Not only is Dr. Fauci's statement incredible on its face. It is contrary to the known facts. States are reporting persons *with* COVID-19 as being COVID-19 deaths, regardless of their comorbidities that could be the real cause of the deaths. The states are doing that under the specific guidance from the CDC. The CDC is receiving that data from the states that they requested the states to send them. Indeed, an Illinois State Health Official announced during a press conference: "Technically, even if you died from a clear alternate cause but you had COVID at the same time, it is still listed as a COVID death."[1178]

In a Johns Hopkins News-Letter dated November 22, 2020, (later retracted) "Genevieve Briand, assistant program director of the Applied Economics master's degree program at Hopkins, critically analyzed the effect of COVID-19 on U.S. deaths using data from the Centers for Disease Control and Prevention (CDC)."[1179] She found that there was zero increase in deaths across the United States between 2018 and 2020. She determined that "the percentages of deaths among all age groups remain relatively the same." She thus concluded that COVID-19 "has relatively no effect on deaths in the United States."[1180] Briand was puzzled because the CDC had reported a sudden increase in deaths due to COVID-19. There should have been an increase in total deaths reported to the CDC by approximately 267,000. But there was no such increase. When Briand examined the death statistics from the CDC, she made the disturbing discovery that deaths from heart disease, respiratory disease, influenza, and pneumonia dropped during the COVID-19 outbreak. She saw in the statistics that deaths were being shifted from those other categories to COVID-19. "Briand believes that deaths due to heart diseases, respiratory diseases, influenza and pneumonia may instead be recategorized as being due to COVID-19."[1181]

The Briand article was retracted for the reason that Johns Hopkins was concerned that the article "has been used to support dangerous inaccuracies that minimize the impact of the pandemic."*1182* But in the retraction notice, Johns Hopkins actually acknowledged the principal finding made by Briand that the number of deaths due to heart diseases, respiratory diseases, influenza and pneumonia had been shifted to the COVID-19 list of deaths. The retraction states that "Briand also claimed in her analysis that deaths due to heart diseases, respiratory diseases, influenza and pneumonia may be incorrectly categorized as COVID-19-related deaths. However, COVID-19 disproportionately affects those with preexisting conditions, so those with those underlying conditions are statistically more likely to be severely affected and die from the virus."[1183] Notice that the retraction does not dispute Briand's finding, but rather tries to explain it as being caused by the fact that "those with those underlying conditions are statistically more likely to be severely affected and die from the virus."*1184* The retraction notice did not contradict the conclusion of Briand's study that the COVID-19 death statistic is a statistic that lists those who die "with" COVID-19 and not necessarily those who die "from" COVID-19.[1185]

The artificial inflation of COVID-19 deaths is a worldwide phenomenon. On July 16, 2020, Dr. Yoon K Loke and Dr. Carl Heneghan studied the death statistics in England and discovered that they were being artificially inflated.[1186] Dr. Yoon K Loke is Professor of Medicine and Pharmacology, Norwich Medical School, University of East Anglia, UK. Dr. Carl Heneghan is Professor of Evidence-Based Medicine and Director of Studies for the Evidence-Based Health Care Programmes at the University of Oxford. Dr. Heneghan set up and directs the Oxford COVID Evidence Service.

According to the definitions used by the National Health Service (NHS) and Public Health England (PHE) for a COVID-19 death, nobody who tests positive for COVID-19 could ever recover from that disease. Drs. Loke and Heneghan reported that "[a] patient who has tested positive, but successfully treated and discharged from hospital, will still be counted as a COVID death even if they had a heart attack or were run over by a bus three months later."[1187]

The Department of Health uses the PHE statistics to announce COVID-19 deaths. As of July 3, 2020, the PHE has reported 45,199 COVID-19 deaths.[1188] The recent study by Drs. Loke and Heneghan calls into question the accuracy of that death tally. Now, it is not clear how many of those people actually died of COVID-19. "It turns out you could have been tested positive in February, recovered, then hit by a bus in July and you'd be recorded as a Covid death."[1189]

The doctors who did the study calculated that "if the counting method is not changed it would mean all 290,000 people who have tested positive for coronavirus would eventually be added to the death toll, regardless of when and how they died."[1190] That is a real problem because most of the people who are hospitalized for COVID-19 are elderly people who have many comorbidities. When they recover from COVID-19 and are released from the hospital, they are more likely to die in the ordinary course of old age from one of their many comorbidities. And so, the elderly who die from some other illness will be counted as COVID-19 deaths, although they did not actually die from COVID-19.

What is the danger from COVID-19? Anthony S. Fauci is the Director of the National Institute of Allergy and Infectious Diseases (NIAID). He is in charge of the federal response to the COVID-19 threat. On March 4, 2020, Dr. Anthony Fauci testified in a public hearing before the U.S. Congress. During his testimony, Dr. Fauci stated ominously that "the mortality for seasonal flu is point one percent (0.1%). So even if it [the mortality rate for COVID-19] goes down to one percent, it's still 10 times more fatal [than the seasonal flu]."[1191] On March 11, 2020, Dr. Fauci repeated that statistic in testimony before the U.S. Congress. "I think if you count all the cases of minimally symptomatic or asymptomatic infection, that probably brings the mortality rate down to somewhere around one percent, which means it is 10 times more lethal than the seasonal flu."*1192*

Yet, when Dr. Fauci is talking to doctors, he changes his tune. The New England Journal of Medicine is typically only read by doctors and scientific researchers. And so, what did Dr. Fauci say about the COVID-19 virus when writing to doctors? In a March 26, 2020 article in the New England Journal of Medicine, Dr. Fauci stated that "the overall clinical consequences of COVID-19 may ultimately be more akin to those of a severe seasonal influenza (which has a case fatality rate of approximately 0.1%)."[1193]

Keep in mind that statement in the New England Journal of Medicine by Dr. Fauci was made in the midst of medical emergencies being announced in many states that included school and business closures, recommendations of social distancing, and state government-mandated limits on public gatherings. All of these measures were recommended by Dr. Fauci, who had fanned the flames of hysteria over the medical danger of COVID-19 among the public. But while Dr. Fauci was telling the public that COVID-19 was ten (10) times more deadly than the flu, he was telling doctors and scientists that "the overall clinical consequences of COVID-19 may ultimately be more akin to those of a severe seasonal influenza (which has a case fatality rate of approximately 0.1%)."

By the way, Dr. Fauci was joined in that article by his co-author, Robert R. Redfield, who is the Director of the U.S. Center for Disease Control (CDC). Basically, the U.S. health czars are on record admitting that what they continue to tell the public is a deadly virus is not really deadly at all. The COVID-19 scare is a scam. Fauci and Redfield confessed that COVID-19 is no more deadly than the ordinary flu in the middle of the hysteria they created.

In early March, 2020, Dr. Fauci told the public that the COVID-19 is ten (10) times more deadly than the ordinary flu. After that, on March 26, 2020, Dr. Fauci writes to doctors in the New England Journal of Medicine that "the overall clinical consequences of Covid-19 may ultimately be more akin to those of a severe seasonal influenza (which has a case fatality rate of approximately 0.1%)." Then after he writes that statement, he continues to tell the public that COVID-19 is one of the worst pandemics in history and warns against lifting the draconian restrictions on social gathering and mask-wearing.

How was Dr. Fauci able to pull off that statistical sleight of hand, trick Congress, and bring about the hysteria that COVID-19 was ten times more deadly than the common flu? Dr. Ronald B. Brown of the School of Public Health and Health Systems at the University of Waterloo explains that when Dr. Fauci testified before Congress, he compared apples with oranges. Dr. Brown reveals that Dr. Fauci misleadingly compared the Infection Fatality Rate (IFR) for the seasonal flu with the Case Fatality Rate (CFR) for COVID-19.[1194] That resulted in the incorrect conclusion that the novel coronavirus was ten times deadlier than the average flu.

Both the CFR and IFR report in the numerator those who die from the disease. But they each have different denominators. The difference is that a Case Fatality Rate (CFR) only includes in the denominator those who actually are diagnosed with and have symptoms of the disease, whereas the Infection Fatality Rate (IFR) includes in the denominator cases and undiagnosed, asymptomatic, and mild infections. CFR is a subset of IFR. All cases are infections, but not all infections are cases. Thus, there is a greater population of infections than cases. That means that the CFR ratio will always be a larger percentage than the IFR ratio. The graphic below is from Brown's report and illustrates the difference between the CFR and the IFR.

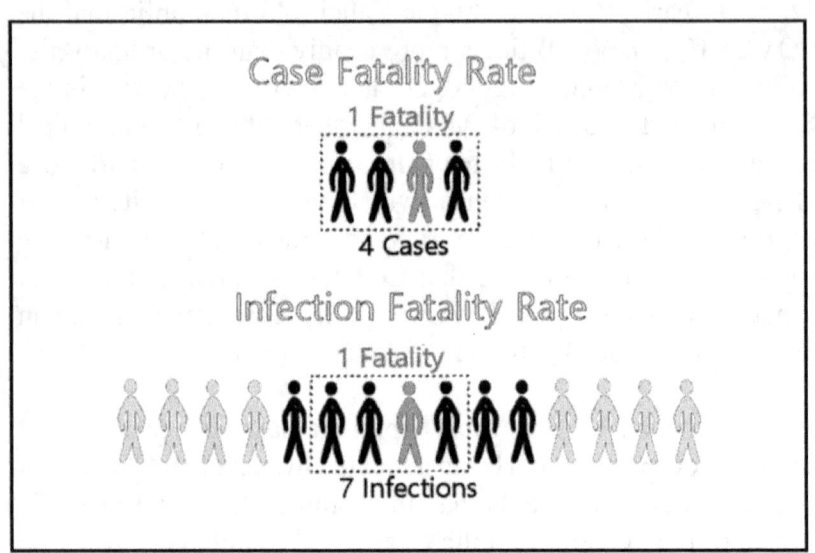

Four (4) cases with one (1) fatality = 25% CFR. Seven (7) infections with one (1) fatality = 14.28% IFR.

Dr. Fauci erroneously reported the CFR for the seasonal flu as being 0.1%. He then stated that the CFR for COVID-19 was 1%. He ominously testified before Congress that simple math reveals that COVID-19 is ten (10) times deadlier than the flu. It turns out that Dr. Fauci was reporting the IFR for the seasonal flu and misrepresenting it as the CFR for the seasonal flu. The actual CFR for the seasonal flu is 1%. That is virtually the same as the CFR for COVID-19. Thus, the lethality of COVID-19 is about the same as the seasonal flu. Dr. Fauci's testimony that COVID-19 is ten (10) times more deadly than the flu was wrong.

When Dr. Anthony Fauci testified in a public hearing before the U.S. Congress on March 4, 2020, and ominously said that "the mortality for seasonal flu is point one percent (0.1%). So even if it [the mortality rate for COVID-19] goes down to one percent, it's still 10 times more fatal [than the seasonal flu],"[1195] he knew that was not true because in a March 26, 2020 article in the

New England Journal of Medicine, Dr. Fauci stated that "the overall clinical consequences of Covid-19 may ultimately be more akin to those of a severe seasonal influenza (which has a case fatality rate of approximately 0.1%)."[1196]

At no time did Dr. Fauci ever retract his misleading public pronouncement that COVID-19 is ten-times more deadly than the flu. Indeed, he doubled down. On July 29, 2020, ABC News reported that Dr. Fauci upped the hysteria another notch when Dr. Fauci "suggested Wednesday that Americans should consider wearing goggles or a face shield in order to prevent spreading or catching COVID-19."[1197] On that same day (July 29, 2020) in an interview with ABC News commentator Dr. Jen Ashton, Dr. Fauci ominously states: "Look at the number of deaths—that's the worst we've had in respiratory outbreak in over 100 years, since the 1918 outbreak of the Spanish Flu. And we still have a ways to go."[1198]

It turns out that the evidence is beginning to show that the actual mortality rate for COVID-19 is indeed more akin to the seasonal flu, just as Dr. Fauci admitted in his New England Journal of Medicine article. Dr. John Ioannidis, who is a professor of medicine and epidemiology at Stanford University, has looked at the worldwide COVID-19 mortality data and concluded that "[a]t a very broad, bird's eye view level, worldwide the IFR [infection fatality rate] of COVID-19 this season may be in the same ballpark as the IFR of influenza."[1199]

Deborah Birx, M.D. is U.S. Global Aids Coordinator & U.S. Special Representative for Global Health Diplomacy and Physician-Ambassador to the office of the Vice President and the U.S. Government Coronavirus Response Coordinator. She stated during a March 23, 2020, White House press conference: "99% of all the mortality coming out of Europe in general is over 50 and pre-existing conditions. The pre-existing condition piece still holds in Italy, with the majority of the mortality having three or more pre-existing conditions. ... Death rates escalate with age and pre-existing conditions. So I really want to be clear that although it may be very low if you're under 40 or very low if you're under 50 or very low if you're under 70, there is an inflection curve. The average age of the person is dying in Italy is in the mid-80s. So there is really a significant issue in our older generation."[1200]

Recall that early in the alleged COVID-19 pandemic, Italy was in the news as being struck by the disease. That was the function of the very large elderly population in Italy. Thus, they had more people dying because they had more older people. "The average life expectancy in Western Europe was 79 years for males and 84 years for females in 2019."[1201] So we know that, in Italy, the people allegedly dying from COVID-19 were dying at the age of the average mortality rate for older people. Furthermore, Italian authorities revealed in March 2020 that 99% of all coronavirus deaths were from people with pre-existing conditions.[1202]

So the people that were trumpeted as dying from COVID-19 early in the purported pandemic were the older sick people. That is the group of people one would expect to die daily. Putting those statistics together, we find the COVID-19 virus is no more deadly than the ordinary flu. And the people threatened by COVID-19 are the same as those threatened by the seasonal flu: older people with pre-existing health infirmities. But the media publicized those deaths as though they were something unusual. The COVID-19 pandemic was just theater. It was false propaganda.

Dr. Ionnidis stated that the fatality rate for COVID-19 could be as low as 0.2%, but no higher than 0.4%. That higher number (0.4%) was gathered from infections among elderly patients and healthcare workers. The more likely 0.2% rate is much lower than the 1-3% range of figures often bandied about by the government fear-mongers. Keep in mind that Dr. Ionnidis is using government-reported figures, which have been proven to be inflated anyway.[1203] Incidentally, the mortality rate in the United

States from all causes is approximately 1%.[1204]

Please recall, as explained above, that the statistics include all deaths "involving" COVID-19 not deaths "from" COVID-19. That means that the persons could have died from some other cause, but the decedent was determined to have COVID-19 at the time of death. Thus they are reported as a death "involving" COVID-19.[1205]

The CDC admits that they double count deaths. "Deaths involving more than one condition (e.g., deaths involving both diabetes and respiratory arrest) were counted in both totals."[1206] That means that a person who is murdered but tests positive for COVID-19 is tallied as both a murder death and a COVID-19 death. It is for that reason that the CDC advises: "To avoid counting the same death multiple times, the numbers for different conditions should not be summated."[1207]

Furthermore, the CDC admits that its statistics of COVID-19 deaths are not confirmed to have COVID-19. The COVID-19 statistics include both "[d]eaths with confirmed or presumed COVID-19."

On February 1, 2021, Patrick Howley, writing for National File, reported that an investigation by the Public Health Policy Initiative uncovered evidence that the Centers for Disease Control and Prevention (CDC) violated federal law by fraudulently inflating COVID-19 fatality numbers.[1208] Howley reported that the investigation revealed that the "CDC illegally inflated the COVID fatality number by at least 1,600 percent."[1209] Howley explained how that was done:

> On March 24th the CDC published the NVSS COVID-19 Alert No. 2 document instructing medical examiners, coroners and physicians to deemphasize underlying causes of death, also

referred to as pre-existing conditions or comorbidities, by recording them in Part II rather than Part I of death certificates as "...the underlying cause of death are expected to result in COVID-19 being the underlying cause of death more often than not." This was a major rule change for death certificate reporting from the CDC's 2003 Coroners' Handbook on Death Registration and Fetal Death Reporting and Physicians' Handbook on Medical Certification of Death, which have instructed death reporting professionals nationwide to report underlying conditions in Part I for the previous 17 years. This single change resulted in a significant inflation of COVID-19 fatalities by instructing that COVID-19 be listed in Part I of death certificates as a definitive cause of death regardless of confirmatory evidence, rather than listed in Part II as a contributor to death in the presence of pre-existing conditions, as would have been done using the 2003 guidelines. The research draws attention to this key distinction as it has led to a significant inflation in COVID fatality totals. By the researcher's estimates, COVID-19 recorded fatalities are inflated nationwide by as much as 1600% above what they would be had the CDC used the 2003 handbooks.[1210]

The graph below is from the Public Health Policy Initiative report and represents the actual deaths due to COVID-19 if those deaths had been reported according to the traditional CDC rules that were listed in the 2003 CDC Medical Examiner's and Coroner's Handbook on Death Registration,[1211] which were in effect until the CDC issued the new COVID-19 reporting rules on March 24, 2020. The new reporting rules only apply to COVID-19. All other causes of death still follow the traditional rules set forth in the 2003 CDC Handbook.[1212] Notice how the new CDC guidance for reporting COVID-19 deaths initiated in the March 24, 2020 COVID-19 Alert No. 2[1213] artificially inflated the number of deaths from COVID-19 1600%.

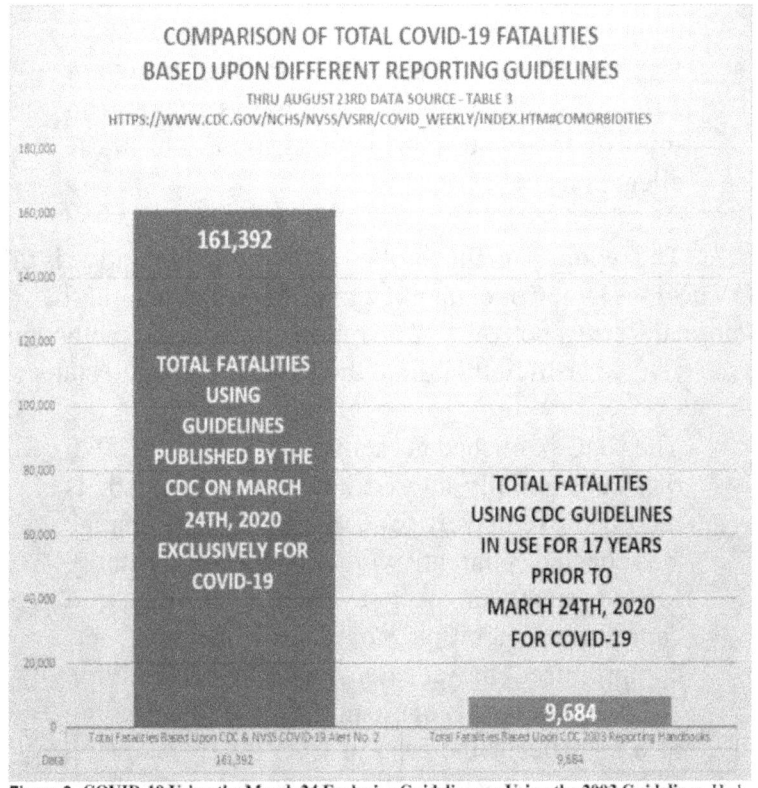

Figure 9. COVID-19 Using the March 24 Exclusive Guidelines vs Using the 2003 Guidelines. Had the CDC used the 2003 guidelines, the total COVID-19 be approximately 16.7 times lower than is currently being reported. [1][30][State & Territory Health Departments]

Howley explains the effect of the CDC fraud and what should be done about it:

By enacting these new rules exclusively for COVID-19 in violation of federal law, the research alleges that the CDC significantly inflated data that has been used by elected officials and public health officials, in conjunction with unproven projection models from the Institute for Health Metrics and Evaluation (IHME), to justify extended closures for schools, places of worship, entertainment, and small businesses leading to unprecedented emotional and economic hardships nationwide. A formal petition has been sent to the Department of Justice as well as all US Attorneys seeking an immediate grand jury investigation into these allegations.[1214]

The report from the Public Health Policy Initiative is titled COVID-19 Data Collection, Comorbidity & Federal Law: A Historical Retrospective.[1215] The report explains the method used by the CDC to artificially inflate the COVID-19 death statistics.

The CDC published guidelines on March 24, 2020 that substantially altered how cause of death is recorded exclusively for COVID-19. This change was enacted apparently without public opportunity for comment or peer-review. As a result, a capricious alteration to data collection has compromised the accuracy, quality, objectivity, utility, and integrity of their published data, leading to a significant increase in COVID-19 fatalities. This decision by the CDC may have subverted the legal oversight of the OMB as Congressionally authorized by the PRA & IQA as well.[1216]

The Public Health Policy Initiative report explains that under this newly adopted CDC reporting scheme, "COVID-19 became emphasized as a cause of death as frequently as possible, while comorbidity was simultaneously deemphasized as causes of death."[1217] The CDC's new rules for reporting COVID-19 deaths had the effect of inflating the reported COVID-19 deaths.

The March 24, 2020 COVID-19 Alert No. 2[1218] from the CDC referred to additional documents providing further guidance, which seemed to be a reference to a March 4, 2020 CDC document titled Guidance for Certifying COVID-19 Deaths,[1219] which explained how to list COVID-19 in Part I of the Death Certificate to show how to list COVID-19 as the "underlying cause" of death. Since the new rules were such a clear departure from the prior practice, it was necessary for the CDC to elaborate with further guidance in April 2020.[1220] But that further guidance did not change the original March 24, 2020, Alert No. 2, which explicitly stated that **"the [new] rules for coding and selection of the underlying cause of death are expected to result in COVID-19 being the underlying cause more often than not."**[1221]

State officials have used the CDC guidance as a license to commit fraud. Officials put on a public facade that they are honestly portraying the death figures as they follow the lead of the CDC in its waltz of deception. But some state officials don't just go along with the flow; they jump on board, give it their all and enthusiastically jimmy up the numbers. For example, Washington State officials have been caught red-handed lying about the COVID-19 deaths in their state. They are engaging in outright fraud to inflate their COVID-19 fatality numbers. Below is a December 16, 2020, press release from the Freedom Foundation:[1222]

> (OLYMPIA, Wash.) — Seven months after a Freedom Foundation investigation showed [the State of Washington government] was inflating the number of COVID-19 fatalities in Washington state and promising to fix its flawed reporting procedures, further research[1223] indicates the state's

Department of Health (DOH) is still over-reporting the totals by potentially hundreds of deaths.

The Freedom Foundation found that the government of Washington State was artificially inflating the reported COVID-19 deaths. The Freedom Foundation began investigating the state's shenanigans in May 2020. The Freedom Foundation found at that time that the Washington "DOH was attributing to COVID-19 every death in which the deceased previously tested positive for the virus." That means that if someone had ever tested positive for COVID-19 at any time in his life and subsequently died, the State of Washington would count that person as having died from COVID-19, regardless of the actual cause of death. That is fraud. The Freedom Foundation determined:

> Washington's data was riddled with cases — as much as 13 percent of the total — in which the death certificate made no reference to COVID-19 as a cause of death. In several cases, even gunshot deaths were chalked up to the virus.[1224]

Governor Jay Inslee dismissed the May 21, 2020 findings of the Freedom Foundation as "dangerous," "disgusting" and "malarkey." He further accused the Freedom Foundation of "fanning these conspiracy claims from the planet Pluto" and not caring about the lives lost to COVID-19.[1225] But his subordinates undermined his claims by acknowledging that the Freedom Foundation was correct. A DOH health statistics manager admitted that the Washington DOH COVID-19 death statistics include deaths of all persons who tested positive for COVID-19 in its totals, even if the victims died from other causes, such as gunshot wounds. She explained that "[o]ur (DOH COVID-19) dashboard numbers do include any deaths to a person that has tested positive to COVID-19."[1226]

Since the Freedom Foundation has been proven correct,

Governor Inslee's opinion, in his official capacity as Governor of Washington, is that the way Washington State was reporting COVID-19 deaths before May 21, 2020, was "dangerous, disgusting, malarkey" and "from the planet Pluto." And since it has been proven that they are still doing it. That makes the Washington officials providing those phony death statistics dangerous, disgusting, and full of malarkey. Those are Governor Inslee's words, not mine.

After having been caught, state officials promised to correct the misreporting. But the Freedom Foundation determined that Washington State officials did not fix anything and continued with the fraud.

> "Make no mistake. This isn't an innocent accounting error we're talking about", said Aaron Withe, Freedom Foundation National Director. "This is a state agency under the authority of Gov. Jay Inslee that continues to misrepresent the number of people who have died of COVID even after it was already caught doing the same thing."
>
> Withe continued, "It's a nakedly political act intended to scare the public into letting him continue to abuse the almost unlimited "emergency powers" that have needlessly bankrupted thousands of Washington businesses and thrown tens of thousands of its residents out of work."[1227]

The follow-up December 2020 probe[1228] by the Freedom Foundation found that "170 death certificates contained no reference whatsoever to COVID-19. Another 171 only referenced COVID-19 as a 'contributing factor' and not part of the causal chain of events leading to death."[1229] Now, that is dangerous, disgusting, malarkey by state officials.

The deceptive practice of artificially inflating the COVID-19 death statistics was worldwide. For example, a UK National Health Service (NHS) Director revealed in a Twitter thread how UK hospitals lied about COVID-19 being the cause of death to create the false illusion of a COVID-19 pandemic. Unsurprisingly, that Twitter thread has since been censored by redacting the most damning information.[1230] But *The Expose* has preserved the original thread.[1231]

The NHS Director explained how in 2016 a strange change began to be instituted that changed how deaths were certified across the UK. Instead of a death being certified by medical professionals who treated the decedent, the certification was to be assigned to a single Medical Examiner at the hospital. Once the NHS Director saw how people who died from causes other than COVID-19 were being classified as COVID-19 deaths, he realized that the 2016 change was part of a plan to create the false impression of a COVID-19 pandemic where there was none. He concluded:

> I have no doubt in my mind, that the Government has planned the entire pandemic since 2016 when they first proposed the change to medical death certification.[1232]

Once the death certification was centralized in a single officer in the hospital, it was not hard to falsify the deaths as COVID-19 deaths with the simple trick of false-positive PCR tests. The NHS Director explained:

> If a patient tests positive for COVID-19 with a PCR Test, this doesn't mean they are infected. If tested again, they may well turn out with a negative test. However, in the NHS, patients are only tested once and this stays on their record throughout their admission. Hospital policies were changed

alongside the implementation of the Medical Examiner System, to ensure that any patient who died within 30 days of a positive test, would have to have COVID-19 as their primary cause of death. This was regulated by the Medical Examiner.[1233]

Persons who died from a myriad of causes were suddenly deemed COVID-19 deaths with a stroke of the pen by the hospital assigned Medical Examiner. The NHS Director explains:

The highest cause of death at every hospital per annum pre COVID-19 is Pneumonia. Pneumonia is a respiratory disease like COVID-19. Pneumonia can be broken down into 4 different causes of death: Bronchopneumonia, spiration Pneumonia, Community-Acquired Pneumonia and Hospital Acquired Pneumonia. These four causes when added together kill the largest number of people on an annual basis prior to the pandemic. The Medical Examiner (one individual in each hospital), was certifying all these pneumonia deaths as COVID-19 deaths. When four different diseases [are] grouped and now being called COVID-19, you will inevitably see COVID-19 with a huge death rate. The mainstream media was reporting on this huge increase in COVID-19 deaths due to the Medical Examiner System being in place.. Patients being admitted and dying with very common conditions such as old age, myocardial infarctions, end-stage kidney failure, haemorrhages, strokes, COPD and cancer etc. were all now being certified as COVID-19 via the Medical Examiner System.[1234]

The entire system was incentivized by money. The NHS Director stated that "[h]ospitals were incentivised to report

COVID-19 deaths over normal deaths, as the government was paying hospitals additional money for every COVID-19 death that was being reported. The Medical Examiner system ensured that COVID-19 was being put down as the cause of death."[1235] Doctors who knew what was going on dared not say anything because they knew it would mean an end to their medical careers.

> Any doctor who argued against COVID-19 as a cause of death was bullied and vilified. The General Medical Council ("GMC") maintains a register of all doctors within the UK. This ensures that there is a fear of being struck off for speaking out against an agenda. The GMC effectively controls all doctors in the UK. Even if a doctor realises what is going on and wants to speak out. They will think twice about talking, as they would be risking their entire career and everything that they've worked so hard for. Doctors essentially have their hands tied, many have families, kids, mortgages and mouths to feed. If I was in their situation, I would think twice about speaking out, for fear of being struck off by the GMC and losing everything.[1236]

The NHS Directors saw clinical decisions in treating patients designed to hasten death.

> The NHS treatment pathway [for CIVD-19] involved patients being placed onto ventilators. There is a 50% chance of death from this clinical decision alone. How many innocent people have died from the clinical decision to place them on a ventilator.[1237]

The NHS Director also saw the strange behavior of doctors promoting the experimental COVID-19 vaccines, which seemed to be the objective of the pandemic hoax.

> In my 12 years of NHS service, never has a doctor pushed or influenced the public to take a vaccine. Yet on social media, I was seeing close friends who were doctors, starting to post on social media that they have taken the vaccine and that the public should. I wouldn't be surprised if doctors were being forced to promote the vaccine by their superiors or if they were receiving monetary gain in doing so.[1238]

The HHS Director saw first-hand the devastation caused by the COVID-19 vaccines.

> During board rounds (where every admitted patient is discussed), we were seeing patients on a daily basis being admitted due to suffering from adverse effects of taking the vaccine. Patients were blacking out after taking the vaccine or suffering from clots or strokes.[1239]

39   5G Radiation Sickness

If the planners of Event 201 were the planners of the COVID-19 pandemic, how could they have such control of events as to ensure the spread of a virus throughout the world to justify their draconian response? The answer is simple; they did not spread anything. The SARS-CoV-2 virus that allegedly causes COVID-19 does not exist. It was a scam from the beginning. They kicked off the scam-demic by using the trick of 5G microwave radiation. When subjects are exposed to 5G radiation, they suffer an illness strikingly similar to a bad flu (i.e., COVID-19). Extreme exposure causes persons to pass out and need hospitalization. They followed up the 5G trick by padding the COVID-19 statistics with influenza cases.

Notably, YouTube considers it disinformation to post "[c]laims that COVID-19 is caused by radiation from 5G networks."[1240] It is simply not something that the social media giants will tolerate. They are doing precisely what the planners of Event 201 suggested should be done. They are censoring information. Why? Because 5G radiation reveals, in part, what is really happening.

Exposure to electrical fields and radio frequency has a detrimental effect on health. Arthur Firstenberg explains:

"Anxiety disorder," afflicting one-sixth of humanity, did not exist before the 1860's, when telegraph wires first encircled the earth. No hint of it appears in the medical literature before 1866. Influenza, in its present form, was invented in 1889, along with alternating current.[1241]

We see a similar pattern today with advances in radio frequency communications.

2002-2003: 3G introduced to the world[1242]
2002-2003: SARS-CoV-1 (SARS) outbreak[1243]

2009: 4G introduced to the world[1244]
2009: H1N1 flu (Swine Flu) outbreak[1245]

2019-2020: 5G introduced to the world[1246]
2019-2020: SARS-CoV-2 (COVID-19) outbreak[1247]

Indeed, research has shown a correlation between 5G radiation and disease suffered by lab animals.

> The health studies conducted in animals revealed that millimeter waves which are used in 5G system, caused change in the body, manifested in structural alteration, suppression of all functions of the organism, the nervous, cardiovascular, immune, blood and other systems with the development complex symptoms. Based on evidence from studied carried out up to today by USA National Toxicology program, Italian Ramazzini study EU Reflex study and a growing number of several scientists say EMW is a "human carcinogen."[1248]

That study is not alone. Many studies show the detrimental

effects of radio frequencies on health. "In May, 2011 the International Agency for Research on Cancer (IARC) concluded that radiofrequency (RF) radiation in the frequency range 30 kHz-300 GHz is a 'possible' human carcinogen."[1249] The 30 kHz-300 GHz range encompasses the frequency range for both 4G and 5G cellular phones.

Dr. Tom Cowan explains that when one is exposed to 5G background radio frequencies, the millimeter waves degrade the oxygen in the atmosphere.[1250] It is as though the person is in a low-oxygen environment at the top of a mountain. Oxygen starvation interferes with certain pathways in your mitochondria, which are organelles in your tissues that use oxygen to make fuel.[1251] The person will suffer hypoxia and come down with all of the symptoms consistent with altitude sickness.

Dr. Cowan explains that "this causes "a hyper-inflammatory response, otherwise known as a cytokine storm, which is the body's way of getting rid of diseased tissue."[1252] That is precisely what we see with the sudden onset of COVID-19 illnesses in areas blanketed with 5G. Dr. Cowan opines that people are dying from hypoxia and an over-enthusiastic inflammatory response, which fits with the misdiagnosis of COVID-19; it is actually sickness from 5G millimeter waves.

On February 5, 2020. Japanese health officials boarded the Diamond Princess at port Yokohama in Tokyo Bay. Those health officials pronounced that 10 persons on board were diagnosed as having coronavirus, later known as SARS-CoV-2 (alleged to cause COVID-19). The ship was ordered quarantined for 14 days. Nobody could leave the ship during the quarantine period. Within three days, another 125 passengers were diagnosed with COVID-19. By February 13, 2020, a total of 218 people were diagnosed with COVID-19.[1253]

A little-known fact is that the Diamond Princess was

sporting some new high-tech 5G towers. An earlier news release explained that "Princess Cruises has announced a new dimension in its connectivity partnership with SES and will become the first global cruise ship fleet with early access to SES's O3b mPOWER network augmenting the Princess Medallion Class experience as it scales across the fleet, according to a press release."[1254]

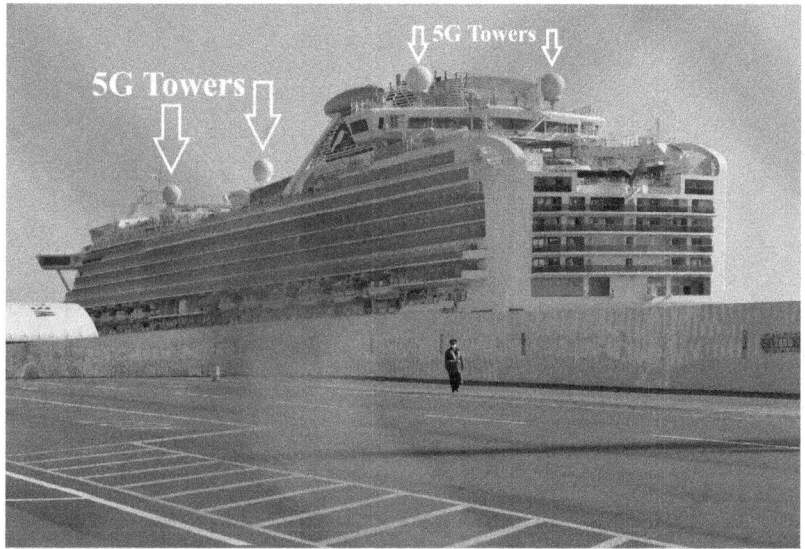

Figure 50: Diamond Princess on or about February 5, 2020, Docked at Tokyo Bay During Its COVID-19 Quarantine (Photograph: Philip Fong/Getty Images)

Is there a connection between the newly installed 5G network on the ship and the passengers being struck ill with coronavirus? It should be noted that only the Princess cruise line that had installed the 5G had outbreaks of COVID-19. In March 2020, the Grand Princess had outbreaks of COVID-19 before docking in San Francisco. The Ruby Princess was reported to have had an outbreak of COVID-19 involving 600 passengers prior to docking on March 19, 2020, in Sydney, Australia. All those ships are Medallion Class ships with the new 5G tower connectivity from SES's O3b mPOWER.

SES explains on its website that the O3b mPOWER is a next-generation 5G satellite signal system.

Together with key stakeholders and technology partners, SES Networks is advancing satellite integration into 5G through standardization, technology development and demonstrations.

***

SES Networks is advancing satellite integration into 5G through standardization, technology development and demonstrations.

***

We've also invested in the revolutionary O3b mPOWER next-generation satellite system, which will augment our existing MEO assets with terabit-scale capabilities.[1255]

Connection Between 5G and COVID-19 Symptoms

What is the effect of 5G on humans? Dr. Magda Havas, Ph.D, sought to answer that question. Dr. Havas "compared the average number of cases, deaths, and tests for COVID-19 per million population in states with and without 5G."[1256]

Dr. Havas found that the standardized testing for states with and without 5G was similar. But he discovered a real difference in COVID-19 cases per million population for those states that deployed 5G. Dr. Havas found that "Covid-19 cases per million are 95% higher and covid-19 deaths per million are 126% higher in states with 5G."[1257]

	Total Cases per 1 million	Total Deaths per 1 million	Total Tests per 1 million	% Cases/Tests	% Deaths/Tests	n
Mean for States with mmWave 5G	2,566	128	14,629	15.64%	0.724%	33
Mean for States without mmWave 5G	1,288	55	14,324	8.82%	0.364%	18
with vs. without mmWave 5G	99%	131%	2%	77%	99%	
p-value for 1 tailed T-test	**0.0199**	**0.0455**	0.8	**0.00345**	**0.0191**	
Correlation to Population Density	0.269	0.169	0.245	0.233	0.154	
Correlation to Pop. Density (excl. outlier Wash DC)	**0.723**	**0.577**	0.496	**0.701**	**0.600**	
Correlation to Air Quality Index	0.110	0.0553	-0.104	0.291	0.187	

A Spanish study proved that countries with 5G had 220% more COVID-19 infections than countries that had not deployed 5G.[1258]

> The results obtained demonstrate a clear and close relationship between the rate of coronavirus infections and 5G antenna location.[1259]

> The case of San Marino is particularly significant. It was the first state in the world to install 5G and therefore, the state whose citizens have been exposed to 5G radiation the longest, and suspiciously, the first state in the world with infections. The probability of this happening is 1 in 37,636.[1260]

Indeed, San Marino is truly a stark indicator of 5G culpability for COVID-19. It was the first European state to adopt 5G technology and had virtually no regulations on its use. Notably, San Marino has the highest incidence per 1,000 population of COVID-19 in Europe. Indeed, its rate is a whopping 27 times greater than the infection rate in Croatia. Why such a stark difference between San Marino and Croatia? The reason is that Croatia does not have 5G.

5G Explains Cruise Ship COVID-19 Outbreak

Does 5G explain the COVID-19 outbreak on the Princess

cruise ships? A researcher has studied the COVID-19 outbreak aboard the Diamond Princess, and he concluded the following:

> When the Diamond Princess data was compared to the controls, it's clear that the death and infection rates of the Diamond Princess significantly surpass the death and infection rates of all the control data. Ongoing use of 5G can result in potential harm to populations. For the above reasons, this paper concludes that 5G wireless technology radiation is a probable factor for causing Covid-19 outbreaks, but still identifies other causes that still need to be tested. Governments are recommended to impose a moratorium on 5G wireless technology until it can be proven that this technology is safe for humans and the environment.[1261]

Wuhan is China's Experimental City For 5G

China has one of the largest 5G networks in the world.[1262] In November 2019, the Chinese government announced plans to blanket China with more than 130,000 5G base stations.

Wuhan, China, which started the entire alleged COVID-19 pandemic, was, interestingly enough, one of the first cities in China to be blanketed with 5G technology.[1263] In April 2018, the Chinese government announced that "[b]y 2020, 5G network will cover every corner of the city."

Sure enough, right on cue, as soon as the 5G network was fired up in Wuhan, the citizens started dropping like flies with symptoms that exactly mirrored the symptoms associated with COVID-19.

Indeed, the same hospital that treated most of the Wuhan COVID-19 patients was bathed in 5G electromagnetic radiation.

CGTN reported:

> In the battle against the novel coronavirus disease (COVID-19), China's leading network service provider, Huawei, built a 5G network at Huoshenshan Hospital in Wuhan, which has played a crucial role in treating coronavirus patients.[1264]

One might wonder why there is not a perpetual illness after an environmental radio frequency innovation. It may be that the exosomes that the body is excreting are in some way also helping to bring equilibrium to the body.[1265] That means the body adapts to the new environment and finds some balance after being exposed to the new technology. But before that point, the initial phase of disruption, there is a spike in death and disease. The world's governments have learned to know what the innovation will do (in this case, 5G) and prepare to use the technology rollout to strip us of some portion of our freedom by characterizing the expected illnesses as a viral pandemic requiring lockdowns, masking, social distancing, relocation camps, and mandatory vaccinations.

40 The Disappearing Flu

5G was good enough to kick-start the fake pandemic. But they knew that they could not irradiate enough people to keep that charade going, so according to plan, they started diagnosing influenza cases as COVID-19. Some who are ill with the flu may test positive for SARS-CoV-12 (alleged to cause COVID-19). That is why the flu disappeared during the 2020-2021 flu season. All persons with the flu were counted not as flu cases but as COVID-19 cases. They then used the COVID-19 scam to push the poisonous COVID-19 vaccines on the population and begin the actual killing. Their objective from the beginning was to force toxic vaccines on the world population.

Statistician John Cullen discovered that the World Health Organization (WHO) influenza data reveals that the COVID-19 statistics are being padded by falsely reporting influenza cases as COVID-19 cases.[1266] But to suggest that influenza cases are being misrepresented as COVID-19 cases is simply not allowed to be mentioned in the mainstream media. The charts below are annotated from the World Health Organization. They reveal that the COVID-19 statistics are being padded by falsely reporting influenza cases as COVID-19 cases.[1267] To suggest that influenza cases are being misrepresented as COVID-19 cases is simply not allowed to be mentioned in the mainstream media.

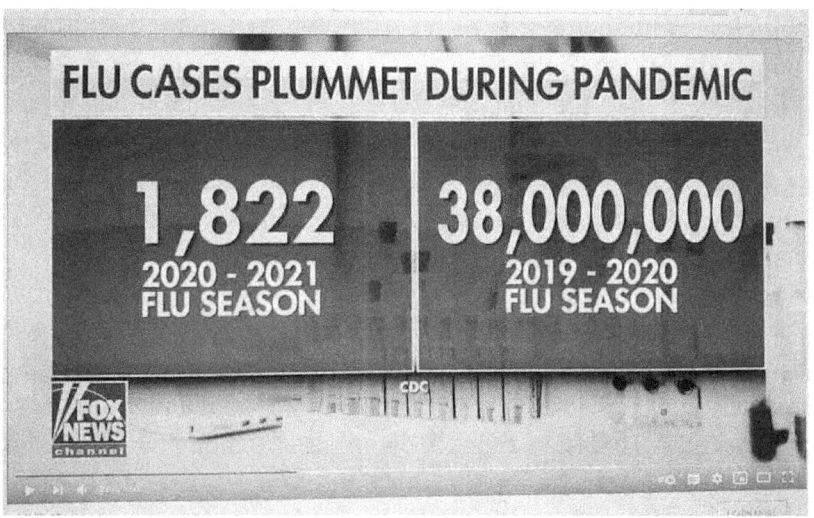

Peter Andrews, writing for Russia Today, reveals that there has been a 98% plummet in flu infections. He then reveals it is impolite within the scientific community to suggest that doctors are misclassifying influenza cases as COVID-19 cases. Andrews explains that "it only seems like the flu has disappeared because doctors and scientists have been wrongly classing other respiratory diseases as Covid. Please note that the boffins are already treating this suggestion as something akin to flat-Earth theory."[1268]

Andrews reveals that "Australia essentially 'skipped' their flu season this year, with not a single case reported since July (their peak). In fact, flu has more or less vanished throughout the Southern Hemisphere." Andrews was writing on October 26, 2020. The Southern Hemisphere had emerged from what should have been their fall and winter flu season. But they had none. And the Northern Hemisphere since followed suit with a collapse in reported flu cases. Jo MacFarlane reporting for The Daily Mail concluded from the WHO data that "flu, it seems, has all but vanished."[1269]

MacFarlane published his article on October 24, 2020, which was the beginning of what is supposed to be the fall and winter flu season in the Northern Hemisphere. MacFarlane could already see from the data that the expected seasonal flu epidemic was not making its appearance. The reported flu cases in the UK were down approximately 90%. He saw the disappearance of the flu revealed by "the figures provide a startling insight into what has become a creeping trend across the world."

Of course, MacFarlane states the obvious. "There are those who claim flu cases haven't vanished at all, but are instead being recorded as Covid-19." But after making that common-sense statement, MacFarlane quickly dismisses the thought. So, what is the explanation he announces for the disappearance of the flu in the midst of the alleged COVID-19 pandemic? It is the theory of … wait for it … "viral interference."

MacFarlane explains that "[w]hen an individual is infected with one virus, they are less likely to be infected by another during that time due to something called 'viral interference'." MacFarlane quotes Dr. Elisabetta Groppelli who claims that "[v]iruses are parasites. Once they enter a cell, they don't want other viruses to compete with. So the virus already in the body will effectively kick the other parasite out." It sounds good, but it is not true. Indeed, when one's immune system is focused on fighting off one particular pathogen, the body's immune resources are focused on that pathogen. With all of the body's immune resources focused on that one pathogen, the person does not have the reserves to fight an unrelated pathogen and is thus is more susceptible to an unrelated pathogen.

That is why the flu vaccine only works for the particular strain of the flu virus that is in the vaccine and no others. Often, persons who receive the flu vaccine end up getting the flu, but it is a different strain of the flu for which they have no protection. Under the theory of 'viral interference' the patient getting a flu shot should be protected from all strains of flu and not just the strain in the vaccine.

The phenomenon of a vaccinated person being more susceptible to an unrelated pathogen is known as pathogenic priming. Vaccines cause pathogenic priming, which injures a person's immune system such that the person is 4.4 times more likely to become ill from some other pathogen. For example, at least six major studies have shown that a person who gets the flu shot has had their immune system pathogenically primed to be more likely to become infected from coronavirus.

The charts below reveal a complete collapse in worldwide cases of influenza after COVID-19 made its appearance in the spring of 2020. Notice the complete disappearance of the flu during the 2020-2021 fall and winter seasonal flu period. That disappearance of flu correlates directly with the reported second-wave of COVID-19 cases and suggests that flu cases are being misreported as COVID-19 second-wave cases.

United States Influenza Cases

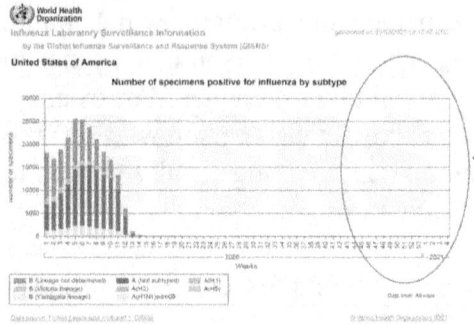

Flu disappears during the 2020-2021 Fall and Winter Flu Season in Direct Correlation with the Alleged COVID-19 Second Wave

The above World Health Organization (WHO) chart shows the number of people infected by influenza in the United States. Each Bar represents the number of infections in the United States for each week of 2020 through week number 4 of 2021. Notice that the influenza infections disappeared in the United States during week 15 of 2020. This correlates very closely with the emergence of COVID-19.

For comparison, below is a WHO chart that shows the number of people infected by influenza in the United States for the entire year of 2019 and the first 4 weeks of 2020. Each Bar represents the number of people infected in the United States for each week of 2019 through week 4 of 2021. Notice the difference from the chart above. This suggests that the disappearance of the influenza in week 15 of 2020 through week 4 of 2021 is because Influenza is being reported as COVID-19 infections. The complete disappearance of the flu during the fall and winter flu season of 2020-2021 suggests that the second wave of COVID-19 cases reported during that period are actually flu cases being falsely reported as COVID-19 cases.

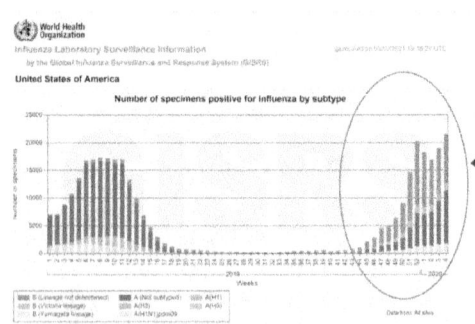

2019-2020 Fall and Winter Flu Season

Worldwide Influenza Cases

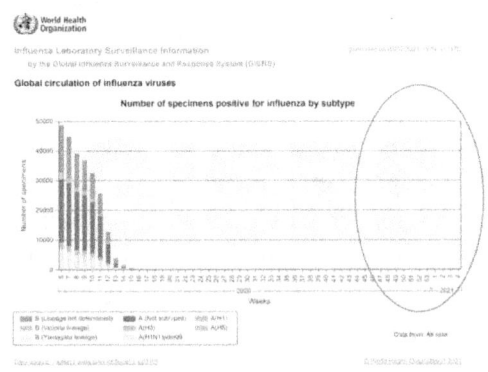

Flu disappears during the 2020-2021 Fall and Winter Flu Season in Direct Correlation with the Alleged COVID-19 Second Wave

The above World Health Organization (WHO) chart shows the number of people infected by influenza in the world. Each Bar represents the number of infections in the world for each week of 2020 through week number 4 of 2021. Notice that the influenza infections disappeared in the world during week 15 of 2020. This correlates very closely with the emergence of COVID-19.

For comparison, below is a WHO chart that shows the number of people infected by influenza in the world for the entire year of 2019 and the first 4 weeks of 2020. Each Bar represents the number of people infected in the world for each week of 2019 through week 4 of 2021. Notice the difference from the chart above. This suggests that the disappearance of the influenza in week 15 of 2020 through week 4 of 2021 is because Influenza is being reported as COVID-19 infections. The complete disappearance of the flu during the fall and winter flu season of 2020-2021 suggests that the second wave of COVID-19 cases reported during that period are actually flu cases

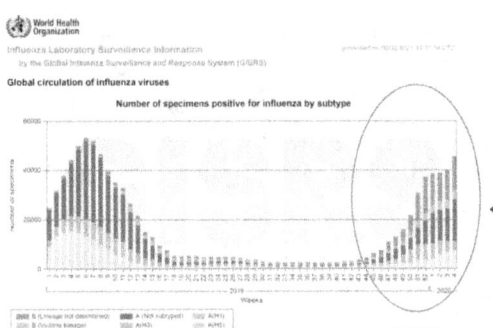

2019-2020 Fall and Winter Flu Season

This author knows someone who was in the ICU with her son at St. Joseph's hospital in Phoenix on August 29, 2020. She spent the day with her son in the ICU and spoke with the nurses. She was told by the nurses that none of the patients in the ICU were COVID-19 patients. Later, she was watching the local news, and it reported that the ICUs in the Phoenix hospitals were filled to 83% capacity with COVID-19 patients. St. Joseph's Hospital is one of the largest hospitals in Phoenix. It is a medical center with more than 500 beds. The local news channel was asked about the discrepancy, and they said they got their information from the local health authorities. The news report was deceptive propaganda. Incidentally, she was with her son in another hospital ICU earlier in the week outside of Phoenix, and there were no COVID-19 patients in that ICU at that time either.

Dr. Vernon Coleman is a general practitioner and a former Professor of Holistic Medical Sciences.[1270] Dr. Coleman is a Sunday Times best-selling author, who has written more than 100 books, selling over 2 million copies in the UK alone. Many of Dr. Coleman's books have been on bestseller lists worldwide. Dr. Coleman summarizes the COVID-19 pandemic scam:

> Covid-19 was, as I have been saying now for three years, nothing more than the rebranded flu. I proved this time and time again. But here, again, are some of the statistics I have used in the past which prove that covid-19 was no more deadly than the flu – because it was the flu. The pandemic myth has been deliberately sustained by the Government, their advisors and the media. But there were no more deaths in 2020 than most other years. Figures from the Office of National Statistics in the UK show that the number of deaths in 2020 was lower than the average for the last 30 years. In 2020 the age-standardised mortality rate per 100,000 people in England and Wales was 1,043.

But the average age-standardised mortality rate for the last 30 years was 1,161 per 100,000. So, there were fewer than average deaths in 2020. Some pandemic, eh? The same is true of every country in the world. Governments and doctors lied. There was no pandemic. It was a gargantuan hoax. And the minute I exposed the hoax I was attacked, vilified and lied about.[1271]

41   State Action by Hospitals

What about a private employer? If the private employer is compelling the employee to get vaccinated in order to comply with a government edict or regulation, then the employer is acting as an agent of the government. The compulsory vaccination would constitute government action in violation of the Constitutional prohibition against the establishment of religion.

The Center for Medicare and Medicaid Services (CMS) working group identified one of the "Strategies that Work" for ensuring medical staff get the flu vaccine: "Make the [flu] vaccinations mandatory for employees. Consequences of non-vaccination may result in termination or suspension of employment."[1272] The CDC explains that "[e]ighteen states establish flu vaccination requirements for hospital healthcare workers, and 16 states establish requirements for hospital patients."[1273] That renders the hospitals virtual arms of the state in implementing state vaccine mandates.

It seems that coercion is the favored approach of CMS. President Biden used CMS as the tool to enforce his COVID-19 vaccine mandate for all healthcare workers. On October 26, 2022, CMS mandated COVID-19 vaccines for all employees of

Medicare and Medicaid-certified facilities. CMS stated that all such facilities "are expected to comply with all applicable regulatory requirements." One of those requirements is that 100% of faculty and staff must be vaccinated, unless they are granted a religious or medical exemption. Failure to reach that level will result in the termination of CMS funding. Facility staff vaccination rates under 100% will trigger an enforcement remedy of termination of CMS for noncompliance for hospitals and certain other acute and continuing care providers.[1274] The threat of CMS funding cut-off hung over hospitals like the Sword of Damocles to coerce compliance with the vaccine requirements. It rendered hospitals virtual arms of the federal government. On June 5, 2023 that interim CMS COVID-19 vaccine requirement expired.[1275] Do not be fooled into complacency. The rule can be resurrected under the next false emergency conjured to require yet another series of vaccines against the next scam pandemic.

The CMS coercion worked like charm with hospitals. For example, Inova Hospital seemed to be acting as an arm of the federal government when it instituted a policy mandating the COVID-19 vaccine for all employees. It seemed to be in lockstep with the edicts and pronouncements of the CDC. For example, on September 1, 2022, the CDC recommended the bivalent COVID-19 boosters manufactured by Moderna and Pfizer-BioNTech with the following statement from CDC Director Rochelle P. Walensky:

> This recommendation followed a comprehensive scientific evaluation and robust scientific discussion.[1276]

Inova Hospital, suspiciously, used virtually identical language in its promotional email recommending the Pfizer BioNTech COVID-19 bivalent boosters to staff:

> *This recommendation followed a comprehensive scientific evaluation and robust scientific*

discussion, both nationally and locally at Inova.

Arguably, Inova was acting as an arm of the government, thus rendering their vaccine mandate government actions constrained by the U.S. Constitution. Incidentally, the "comprehensive scientific evaluation" cited by the CDC and Inova involved eight (8) mice in the case of the Pfizer-BioNTech bivalent booster and ten (10) mice in the case of the Moderna bivalent booster.

In *Lugar v. Emondson* Oil, 457 U.S. 922 (1982), the U.S. Supreme Court ruled that actions of private parties can constitute state actions if (1) the deprivation of a right is caused by the exercise of a rule or conduct is imposed by a private person for whom the government is responsible, and (2) the private person who acts to deprive a right may be fairly said to be a government actor if he acts together with the state or has obtained significant aid from state officials.

In *United States v. Price*,[1277] the U.S. Supreme Court addressed the applicability of 18 U.S.C. § 242 to private actors.

> Private persons, jointly engaged with state officials in the prohibited action, are acting 'under color' of law for purposes of the statute. To act 'under color' of law does not require that the accused be an officer of the State. It is enough that he is a willful participant in joint activity with the State or its agents.[1278]

Price involved the issue of whether a private person can act under color of law for purposes of enforcing 18 U.S.C. § 242. The *Price* court explained that under color of law means the same thing as state action in an 18 U.S.C. § 1983 claim and when bringing a claim for violating the Constitution. The Court stated that "[i]n cases under s 1983, 'under color' of law has consistently been treated as the same thing as the 'state action' required under the Fourteenth Amendment."[1279]

The *Price* Court cited to *Burton v. Wilmington Parking Auth.*,[1280] wherein the U.S. Supreme Court ruled that the plaintiff could bring an action for declaratory judgment and injunctive relief against a private restaurant owner for violating his constitutional right to equal protection of law under the 14th Amendment. The *Burton* Court ruled that because the restaurant owner leased his restaurant from the Wilmington Parking Authority, an agency of the State of Delaware, his discriminatory actions was considered state action. The *Burton* court ruled "that the exclusion of appellant under the circumstances shown to be present here was discriminatory state action in violation of the Equal Protection Clause of the Fourteenth Amendment."[1281] The Burton Court explained:

> By its inaction, the Authority, and through it the State, has not only made itself a party to the refusal of service, but has elected to place its power, property and prestige behind the admitted discrimination. The State has so far insinuated itself into a position of interdependence with Eagle that it must be recognized as a joint participant in the challenged activity, which, on that account, cannot be considered to have been so 'purely private' as to fall without the scope of the Fourteenth Amendment.[1282]

If a state by its inaction in preventing discrimination can be considered to be a party to discrimination by a private person, thus rendering it unconstitutional, a state that mandates a private party vaccinate its employees is certainly a party to the resulting vaccinations. That interdependence between the government and the hospital renders the conduct of the hospitals state action, putting it under the restrictions of the First Amendment to the

Constitution.

Under the PREP Act the government has immunized from liability all health officials who administer COVID-19 vaccines pursuant to federal mandates. The government paid for the vaccines and provided them free of charge to the hospitals. The federal government instructed the hospitals to vaccinate their employees. That federal order to hospitals, with severe financial penalties for failure to abide by it, was to carry out the federal government vaccine mandates. The government is thus responsible for the conduct of the hospitals who required that employees be injected with vaccines paid for by the government pursuant to the government vaccine mandate. Second, the hospitals were acting to impose on their employees a religious practice in violation of the First Amendment Rights of the hospital employees to be free from the government established religious practice of vaccination. The vaccines were paid for by the government, and the hospitals acted as their agents in vaccinating the healthcare employees with the government-purchased vaccines. The hospitals can be fairly said to have been government actors carrying out a government edict. Look for a repeat of this in the future, the next time a scam pandemic is conjured up.

In *Lowe v. Mills*,[1283] the statute imposed onerous penalties on any healthcare provider who allowed a religious exemption for their employees to the statutory COVID-19 mandate. The statute permitted medical exemptions but not religious exemptions. A violation of the COVID-19 vaccine statute by allowing a religious exemption would result in an immediate suspension of the state healthcare license and the imposition of substantial fines of up to 1,0000 per violation per day. The court found that the statutory penalties put an undue burden on the healthcare providers and thus they did not violate Title VII by refusing to provide religious exemptions.[1284]

The *Lowe* court got it backwards. The federal law is

supreme over the state law, not the other way around. The court cannot excuse health care providers' violations of Title VII because to comply with Title VII would result in a state law violation that would cause them an undue hardship. The state law must yield to the federal law. The court in *Barber v. Colorado Dep't of Revenue*[1285] explained:

> Defendant believes that it is compelled to follow the directive from the state, but the Supremacy Clause of the Constitution requires a different order of priority. A discriminatory state law is not a defense to liability under federal law; it is a source of liability under federal law. Reliance on state statutes to excuse non-compliance with federal laws is simply unacceptable under the Supremacy Clause."[1286]

Justice Gorsuch (before his appointment to the U.S. Supreme Court) stated in a concurring opinion in *Barber* that "a state law at odds with a valid Act of Congress is no law at all ... State officials who rely on their compliance with discriminatory state laws as evidence of their reasonableness will normally find themselves proving their own liability, not shielding themselves from it."[1287]

Indeed, Title VII provides an exemption to employers from compliance with any "[state] law which purports to require or permit the doing of any act which would be an unlawful employment practice."[1288] So, the health care providers' undue hardship argument in *Lowe* was without merit. They were immune from enforcement of any penalties under the state statute if they had granted religious exemptions under Title VII.

The court in *Lowe v. Mills* found that the healthcare personnel had a valid claim of a violation of the First Amendment against the government because the statute allowed medical exemptions but did not allow religious exemptions. That being the case, the petitioners, arguably, would also have a First Amendment claim (distinct and separate from their Title VII claim) against the healthcare facilities themselves. The claim would be based on the facilities acting as agents of the government in the enforcement of the vaccine mandate statute. Thus, while their Title VII claim against their employers failed on undue hardship grounds, the employees would have had a remaining First Amendment claim. Under that claim, the employers would be in the shoes of the government, having to argue that denying the religious exemption was the least intrusive means of furthering a compelling government interest. That is a much higher hurdle. Indeed, the *Lowe* court found that the First Amendment claim was still valid against the state statute.

Sin to Do Evil That Good May Come

The second overlooked argument involves freedom of religion. Depending on the status of the claimant, it can be made either under Title VII or the First Amendment or both. The argument is that it is a sin to do evil so that good may come of it. Romans 3:8. That argument is set forth in detail in this book. Often, when employers and governments review a request for a religious exemption from a vaccine program, the entity will disregard any argument about the safety of the vaccine as a basis for the religious exemption. The typical retort is that the safety of the vaccine is only germane to a person seeking a waiver on medical grounds. But that argument can be countered by explaining that the unsafe vaccines cause harm. That harm is evil. It is a doctrine of the Christian faith that it is a sin to do evil so that some good may come of it. In order to lay a foundation for your argument that vaccines are evil requires you to establish that the vaccines are dangerous poisons. Thus, the dangerousness of the vaccines is relevant to your request for a religious exemption.

42 Courts Cannot Question Religious Beliefs

A Bible citation is not necessary, but it is sufficient. Whether the government or a court agrees or disagrees with the Bible passage is irrelevant because the First Amendment prohibits any government entity or court from assessing the legitimacy of religious doctrine. Once a person has set forth a sincerely held religious belief, it is not the province of a government agency or court to further examine the legitimacy of those beliefs. The First Amendment to the Constitution renders all courts incompetent to entertain any objection to the legitimacy of a religious belief.

> "[I]t is not within the judicial ken to question the centrality of particular beliefs or practices to a faith, or the validity of particular litigants' interpretations of those creeds."[1289] Repeatedly and in many different contexts, we have warned that courts must not presume to determine the place of a particular belief in a religion or the plausibility of a religious claim.[1290] (citations placed in endnotes)

It is a long-establish Constitutional principle recognized by the courts that it is "wholly inconsistent with the American concept of the relationship between church and state to permit civil courts to determine ecclesiastical questions."[1291] If a person asserts a sincere religious belief, it is not the function of the courts to further explore that belief. The U.S. Supreme Court, in *Thomas v. Rev. Bd. of Indiana*,[1292] explained that "the resolution of that question is not to turn upon a judicial perception of the particular belief or practice in question; religious beliefs need not be acceptable, logical, consistent, or comprehensible to others in order to merit First Amendment protection."[1293] The courts are not equipped to rule on the legitimacy of religious beliefs.

The government cannot favor one religion over another without violating the Establishment Clause of the First Amendment. In a case where the University of Colorado mandated COVID-19 vaccines and allowed religious exemptions but would "only accept requests for religious exemption that cite to the official doctrine of an organized religion ... as announced by the leaders of that religion."[1294] In applying the exemption standard, the university administration sent emails to each person requesting a religious exemption to provide information about their religious beliefs. The "administration rejected any application for a religious exemption unless an applicant could convince the Administration that [his] religion 'teaches [him] and all other adherents that immunizations are forbidden under all circumstances.'"[1295] That rubric had the effect of denying exemption to all applicants except Christian Scientists and Jehovah's Witnesses. The school administration considered all other requests for exemption to fall under the category of "personal" and not "religious" beliefs. Exemptions were denied for all others, including but not limited to, Roman Catholics, Evangelical Christians, non-denominational Protestants, Buddhists, and members of the Eastern Orthodox Church.

The U.S. Court of Appeals for the Tenth Circuit in *Does 1-11 v. Bd. of Regents of Univ. of Colorado*,[1296] ruled that "a government policy that requires an intrusive inquiry into the validity of religious beliefs violates the Establishment Clause regardless of any purported government interest."[1297] The *Does 1-11* court further ruled that it was unnecessary to decide if the government had a compelling state interest. The court reasoned that "where governmental bodies discriminate out of animus against particular religions, such decisions are plainly unconstitutional, regardless of any compelling interests advanced by the government. ... That is because "government action motivated by religious animus cannot be 'narrowly tailored to advance' 'a compelling governmental interest."[1298] The U.S. Supreme Court has affirmed the principle that "[in] our Establishment Clause cases we have often stated the principle that the First Amendment forbids an official purpose to disapprove of a particular religion or of religion in general."[1299] The U.S. Supreme Court has also stated that such animus toward a particular religion by the government also infringes the freedom clause of the First Amendment.

> The government, consistent with the Constitution's guarantee of free exercise, cannot impose regulations that are hostile to the religious beliefs of affected citizens and cannot act in a manner that passes judgment upon or presupposes the illegitimacy of religious beliefs and practices.[1300]

And that is what the University of Colorado did by rejecting religious exemptions from all people who were not either Jehovah's Witnesses or Christian Scientists. The University of Colorado policy passed judgment on the religious beliefs of students and employees who opposed the COVID-19 vaccine but not necessarily all vaccines. It also discriminated against those whose beliefs were not based on the formal teachings or official doctrines announced by the leaders of a religious organization to which they belonged. The university passed judgment on and presupposed the illegitimacy of religious beliefs that were personal to the applicant. The university was making a ruling based on its assessment of whether a belief was sufficiently organized, sufficiently official, or sufficiently comprehensive. The university simply does not have authority or competence to make those assessments. Such conduct was unconstitutional on its face. The *Does 1-11* court ruled:

> "The clearest command of the Establishment Clause is that one religious denomination cannot be officially preferred over another."[1301] Accordingly, the government may not "pick and choose" religions "on the basis of intrusive judgments regarding contested questions of religious belief or practice."[1302] Such an inquiry violates the Establishment Clause's "prohibition of 'excessive entanglement' between religion and government," and is therefore "unconstitutional without further inquiry."[1303] (citations placed in endnotes)

The school administration could ask "whether" the applicant's sincerely held religious beliefs prevented him from getting the vaccine. It was improper to ask "why" that belief prevents him from getting the vaccine. The school administration deemed that according to Roman Catholic doctrine, it was morally acceptable for a Roman Catholic to be vaccinated and thus a Roman Catholic's decision not to be vaccinated could not be based on a religious objection; it was instead viewed as a personal objection.[1304] The *Does 1-11* court responded:

> That is precisely the sort of religious entanglement the Establishment Clause proscribes. As we have previously admonished the state of Colorado, "[i]t is not for the state to decide what Catholic—or evangelical, or Jewish—'policy' is."[1305] To avoid all doubt: neither is it for the state to decide what "religious beliefs" must be held by Roman

Catholics, or Buddhists, or Orthodox Christians, or anybody. These are "question[s] of religious doctrine on which the State may take no position without entangling itself in an intrafaith dispute. *Id*"[1306] (citation in endnote)

There is no excuse for the school administration to deny an exemption because it thinks that the person's belief is inconsistent with the doctrines of the church denomination to which he identifies. A government institution is simply not allowed to troll through a person's religious beliefs.[1307]

The *Does 1-11* court reviewed an amended policy from the University of Colorado that did not have the restrictive religious doctrine language in the first policy. But the court concluded that the amended policy was also unconstitutional. The court found that the new policy not only continued the establishment and freedom clause violations but also gave preference to those seeking a medical exemption. The court concluded that a "[p]olicy [that] grants secular exemptions on more favorable terms than religious ones, ... is not generally applicable on its face."[1308] That means that such an exemption policy must be reviewed under strict scrutiny, where the government must prove that it is narrowly tailored to achieve a compelling state interest. The University of Colorado could not make that showing. The *Does 1-11* court explained that "a government policy "lacks general applicability if it prohibits religious conduct while permitting secular conduct that undermines the government's asserted interests in a similar way."[1309] (internal quotation marks omitted)

43 Avoid The Sectarian Trap

Often, when people seek an exemption to vaccination, they identify their belief against getting a vaccine with the doctrines of a particular sect. That is a mistake. This author is aware of instances where religious exemptions have been denied because the organization (in this case, a federally chartered non-profit corporation) simply visited the website of the religious sect and found that the sect does not prohibit vaccines. In that case, the sect was Christian Science. The organization told the petitioner that he was not entitled to a religious exemption because the Christian Science doctrine does not prohibit vaccination. Indeed, Christian Science doctrine on vaccination is nuanced, but the organization was correct; Christian Science does not prohibit vaccination. Their official stance on vaccination is as follows:

> For more than a century, our denomination has counseled respect for public health authorities and conscientious obedience to the laws of the land, including those requiring vaccination. Christian Scientists report suspected communicable disease, obey quarantines, and strive to cooperate with measures considered necessary by public health officials. ... As for the issue of exemptions for vaccination in the law ... [i]n the past, many public

officials have been broadly supportive of exemptions when these have not been considered a danger to the wider community. In more recent years, public health concerns relating to vaccinations have risen as exemptions from them have been claimed by larger numbers. Christian Scientists recognize the seriousness of these concerns. ... So we've appreciated vaccination exemptions and sought to use them conscientiously and responsibly, when they have been granted. **On the other hand, our practice isn't a dogmatic thing. Church members are free to make their own choices on all life-decisions, in obedience to the law, including whether or not to vaccinate. These aren't decisions imposed by their church.**[1310]

The organization was wrong to deny the religious exemption based on the official doctrinal announcement from the religious sect. The U.S. Court of Appeals for the Second Circuit explains that "[d]enying an individual a religious accommodation based on someone else's publicly expressed religious views — even the leader of her faith —runs afoul of the Supreme Court's teaching that '[i]t is not within the judicial ken to question the centrality of particular beliefs or practices to a faith, or the validity of particular litigants' interpretations of those creeds.'"[1311] In *Does 1-11 v. Bd. of Regents of Univ. of Colorado*,[1312] the U.S. Court of Appeals for the Tenth Circuit ruled that it was improper for the University of Colorado to deny a Roman Catholic's request for a vaccine exemption because the school administration deemed that according to Roman Catholic doctrine, it was morally acceptable for a Roman Catholic to be vaccinated and thus a Roman Catholic's decision not to be vaccinated could not be based on a religious objection; it was instead viewed as a personal objection.[1313] The *Does 1-11* court stated that it is not for the university to decide what Catholic doctrine or policy is.[1314] While

Doe 1-11 was a Constitutional First Amendment case, that same restriction would apply in a Title VII case.[1315]

Indeed, the Roman Catholic Church has long practiced vaccination as part of its superstitious religious ritual long before it was taken up as part of modern medicine. René F. Najera, who is a doctor of public health (DRPH), in an article published by *The College of Physicians of Philadelphia* explains:

> The Catholic Church's support for vaccination dates back to well before the advent of modern medicine. As early as the 1720s, Jesuits were inoculating indigenous populations in the Amazon against smallpox. (A procedure called variolation involving inoculation with a milder form of smallpox.) A significant milestone occurred in 1757 when Pope Benedict XIV personally received the smallpox inoculation, setting a powerful example for Catholics worldwide. This papal action demonstrated an early understanding of the importance of preventive medicine, particularly remarkable given the limited scientific knowledge of the era.[1316]

Notice that the vaccination began under "limited scientific knowledge." What that means is that the practice of vaccination was based on religious superstition and not science. The Roman Catholic Church was involved in vaccination as a religious practice before Benjamin Jesty's first use of cowpox to inoculate against smallpox in 1774 or Edward Jenner's first cowpox vaccination experiments in 1796. The superstitious practice of vaccination is woven through the web and woof of Catholic religious practice. Najera states:

> In 1822, under Pope Pius VII, the Papal States initiated a comprehensive vaccination campaign

against smallpox. Cardinal Secretary of State Ercole Consalvi issued a detailed decree outlining the vaccination strategy, describing smallpox as a disease that "maliciously robs man of even a minimal life [...] and rages against the human species to destroy it at its infancy." This campaign was revolutionary, as it made the Vatican the first sovereign nation to implement a vaccine mandate. (Massachusetts passed the first law regarding vaccination in 1810.).[1317]

The promotion of vaccination by the Roman Catholic Church is based on religious doctrine. "Pope Francis has repeatedly framed vaccination as a moral obligation, calling it 'an act of love.'"[1318] Devin Watkins summarizes the Vatican doctrine on vaccination:

Pope Francis went on to say that getting a Covid jab that is "authorized by the respective authorities" is an "act of love." Helping other do the same, he said, is also an act of love. "Love for oneself, love for our families and friends, and love for all peoples. Love is also social and political." The Pope noted that social and political love is built up through "small, individual gestures capable of transforming and improving societies." "Getting vaccinated is a simple yet profound way to care for one another, especially the most vulnerable," he said. Pope Francis then prayed to God that "each one of us can make his or her own small gesture of love." "No matter how small, love is always grand," he said. "Small gestures for a better future."[1319]

Notice that there is no discussion of science. There is no discussion of effectiveness. There is no discussion of safety.

Instead, the pope advocated for vaccination on a religous plane. It is a religious obligation. It is the religion of Molech where the few should be sacrificed as "an act of love" for the many. Indeed, the pope has come out against anyone who questions the science, the safety, or the effectiveness of vaccines. He calls all information revealing that vaccines are unsafe and ineffective "fake news" and "disinformation," causing confusion, which must be refuted.[1320] "Pope Francis has repeatedly encouraged Catholics to be vaccinated."[1321]

The Roman Catholic Church's official doctrine regarding the presence of aborted fetal tissue in vaccines is that "it is morally acceptable to receive Covid-19 vaccines that have used cell lines from aborted fetuses in their research and production process."[1322] The Vatican is effectively saying that the few (the aborted children) must be sacrificed for the good of the many. That is the religious ethic of Molech worship.

The U.S. Conference of Catholic Bishops' Ethical and Religious Directives for Catholic Health Care Services has stated that all medical treatment, including vaccination, should, in principle, be voluntary.[1323] "No one should ever be forced to undergo any medical treatment, including vaccination."[1324] But the Catholic Church does not have any official doctrine or teaching against vaccination. Therefore, it will not support any individual's effort to receive a religious exemption from a vaccine mandate.

> A religious exemption, rather than appealing to the judgment of one's individual conscience, appeals explicitly to religious teaching or doctrine. For Catholics, the primacy of one's individual conscience in medical decision-making is also a religious principle in the sense that the Church teaches that one ought to obey his or her informed conscience. However, while there may be good reason for an individual to appeal to his or her own

conscience in refusing COVID-19 vaccination, a Catholic cannot claim that any teaching of the Catholic Church actually prevents him or her from receiving any of the COVID-19 vaccines, since the Church has clearly taught that it is morally acceptable to make use of the available COVID-19 vaccines. Many bishops have asked clergy not to sign religious exemption forms on behalf of Catholics, as such exemptions should be permitted by employers and schools and since it would be erroneous to claim that the Church explicitly teaches that Catholics cannot receive any of the COVID-19 vaccines on doctrinal grounds.[1325]

While the Roman Catholic Church states that, as a matter of ethics, all vaccines should be voluntary, it hypocritically mandates vaccines for Vatican employees and visitors. The Roman Catholic Church not only says it is okay to get a vaccine that was made using aborted fetuses, it mandates those very vaccines. That is not hyperbole. A decree was issued by the Vatican on December 23, 2021, mandated that all visitors and employees who serve the public "will be obliged to provide official documentation proving they have received the full anti-Covid vaccine including the third booster dose."[1326] "According to the decree, staff without a valid 'green pass' proving the state of vaccination or recovery from the virus, will not be able to access the workplace and will be considered a case of unjustified absence, with the consequent suspension of pay."[1327]

The Vatican COVID-19 vaccine mandate applies to all personnel of the Roman Curia, personel of external collaborators and firms, and visitors. Steve Watson, writing for Summit News, explained that "[g]iven that the Pope has given his blessing to the vaccines, religious exemptions are not a thing in this case."[1328] You read that correctly, it seems that the Vatican will not allow a religious exemption for the mandated COVID-19 vaccines.

Indeed, there can be no exemption from the Vatican Vaccine mandate. That is because its edict is part of the *Magisterium* of the Church. According to § 2032 of the Catechism of the Catholic Church:

> To the Church belongs the right always and everywhere to announce moral principles, including those pertaining to the social order, and to make judgments on any human affairs to the extent that they are required by the fundamental rights of the human person or the salvation of souls.[1329]

According to Catholic doctrine, the edicts of the Vatican are imbued with infallibility. Section 2035 of the Catechism of the Catholic Church states:

> The supreme degree of participation in the authority of Christ is ensured by the charism of infallibility. This infallibility extends as far as does the deposit of divine Revelation; it also extends to all those elements of doctrine, including morals, without which the saving truths of the faith cannot be preserved, explained, or observed.[1330]

The Vatican edict on Vaccination follows from Pope Francis' moral judgment that vaccination is an obligatory act of love and a profound way to take care of one another.[1331] According to Catholic doctrine, that pronouncement is imbued with the "charism of infallibility." All Roman Catholics have a duty to obey the edicts of the Catholic Church. Section 2037 of the Catechism states:

> [The faithful] have the duty of observing the constitutions and decrees conveyed by the legitimate authority of the Church. Even if they

concern disciplinary matters, these determinations call for docility in charity.[1332]

The very thing that the U.S. Constitution protects, the Romish Church eschews, freedom of conscience. Section 2039 of the Catechism states that a person should put his conscience aside and bring himself to the blind obedience of Vatican edicts.

> At the same time the conscience of each person should avoid confining itself to individualistic considerations in its moral judgments of the person's own acts. As far as possible conscience should take account of the good of all, as expressed in the moral law, natural and revealed, and consequently in the law of the Church and in the authoritative teaching of the Magisterium on moral questions. Personal conscience and reason should not be set in opposition to the moral law or the Magisterium of the Church.[1333]

The Vatican is an imperial power from which there can be no disagreement because the Roman Catholic Church does not allow freedom of conscience. The Vatican has mandated vaccines. It is an edict from which there can be no exemption. For further information on the Roman Catholic Church and its doctrines, read this author's book, *Solving the Mystery of Babylon the Great*.[1334]

Recall that in *Thomas v. Review Bd. of Indiana Employment Security Div.*,[1335] the Supreme Court was unpersuaded by the fact two Jehovah's Witnesses disagreed on whether it was morally objectionable to make weapons. The *Thomas* Court stated that it was not equipped to resolve the many doctrinal and behavioral differences between those who share the same faith. A person can disagree with the doctrines of his sect and still be able to claim a religious objection to vaccination. The *Hobby Lobby* Supreme Court stated, "it is not for us to say that their religious beliefs are mistaken or insubstantial. Instead, our narrow function in this context is to determine whether the line drawn reflects an honest conviction."[1336] (ellipse and quotation marks deleted)

Having said that, it makes no sense to give an organization a reason to deny a request for a vaccine exemption. It would thus be unwise for any Roman Catholic, Christian Scientist, or anyone else to take the position that they have a religious objection to vaccination based on their adherence to a particular sect's doctrine. A little research might uncover that the sect has no doctrine against vaccination. Then the petitioner would be in the position of arguing that he disagrees with his sect on that issue. That would put the sincerity of the claimed objection to vaccines in question. Why go down that road? The most effective and prudent position is to object based on sincerely held religious beliefs. Stay away from hitching your wagon to a train that may be going in the wrong direction.

It is not necessary to be a member of a recognized religious sect or denomination to assert the religious protection under the First Amendment, the RFRA, or Title VII. For example, in *Lucky v. Landmark Med. of Michigan, P.C.*,[1337] the U.S. Court of Appeals for the Sixth Circuit ruled that the plaintiff raised a valid religious discrimination case under Title VII by averring that she is a Christian who did not belong to any denomination and believed that she "should not have any vaccination enter her body such that her body would be defiled, because her body is a temple." She further stated that "God spoke to her in her prayers and directed her that it would be wrong to receive the COVID-19 vaccine." The court of appeals held that the district court erred when it ruled that she was not entitled to protection under Title VII because she had not established that "her religion has a specific tenet or principle that does not permit her to be vaccinated."[1338]

The Court of appeals stated that the district court was not qualified to render judgment on the validity of her beliefs. Her religious beliefs against vaccination didn't need to be based on some official pronouncement from ecclesiastical hierarchy. The court of appeals stated that no further enhancement was necessary, other than what she had stated. The court stated that the plaintiff's asserted religious beliefs were self-evidently enough to establish that her refusal to receive the COVID-19 vaccine was an aspect of her religious observance or belief. The court of appeals grounded its reasoning on a quote from the U.S. Supreme Court: "It is not within the judicial ken to question the centrality of particular beliefs or practices to a faith, or the validity of particular litigants' interpretations of those creeds."[1339] The court noted that the Supreme Court has "warned, repeatedly and in many different contexts, that courts must not presume to determine the place of a particular belief in a religion or the plausibility of a religious claim."[1340]

And do not be dissuaded by arguments made by institutions that deny religious objections to vaccines by arguing that you must object to all vaccines and not just the vaccine in question. People grow in knowledge and wisdom as they live their lives. It is not unusual to have gotten vaccines and then realize later it was a mistake, a spiritual mistake.

In *Thomas*,[1341] the Supreme Court held that it was not for the court to judge the reasonableness of the beliefs of a Jehovah's Witness who did not object to making steel that was used in making weapons but objected when he was reassigned to making the weapons themselves. The Court was simply not competent to assess the reasonableness of the beliefs and could only protect them from infringement by the government. The U.S. Court of Appeals for the Tenth Circuit in *Does 1-11 v. Bd. of Regents of Univ. of Colorado*,[1342] ruled that it was improper for the University of Colorado to require that the petitioners for an exemption to the COVID-19 vaccine object to all vaccines and not just the COVID-19 vaccine.

44 The Military Vaccine Complex

When all assume that vaccines are safe and effective, the entity from which someone seeks a religious exemption can begin running roughshod over the poor employee. The employee is constrained, as they are unable to argue about the safety and efficacy of the vaccine, because those issues are deemed irrelevant when deciding whether to grant a religious exemption.

The behavior of the U.S. Military during the COVID-19 scam illustrates the problem. In that instance, the military presented the veneer of supposed science that ostensibly established the COVID-19 vaccines were safe and effective. The military was empowered by that framework, built on fraud and deception, to deny 99.75% of all religious exemption requests. The military argued that the safety and effectiveness of the vaccines enhanced the compelling need for military readiness. It was all smoke and mirrors.

On August 24, 2021, "the Secretary of Defense directed the Secretaries of the Military Departments to begin immediate vaccination of all members of the Armed Forces against COVID-19."[1343] On January 10, 2023, the Secretary of Defense rescinded the COVID-19 vaccination mandate. That rescission only happened because Congress passed a law that required the Secretary of Defense to rescind the COVID-19 vaccine mandate.[1344] During the sixteen months when the mandate was in effect, between August 24, 2021, and January 10, 2023, the Department of Defense began a pattern of violating the service members' Constitutional Rights. It routinely denied requests for religious exemptions with letters setting forth boilerplate reasons. "[T]he decision authorities issued their decisions based on determinations of whether or not the vaccination was the least restrictive means of furthering a compelling governmental interest."[1345]

The Department of Defense Inspector General mostly approved the religious discrimination scheme. The Inspector General only criticized the dilatory manner in which the military acted on the religious exemption requests. While the number and percentages of medical exemptions from the COVID-19 vaccine was not revealed in the U.S. Defense Department Inspector General's report, it was reported that there were many medical exemptions allowed.[1346] If even one medical exemption was allowed, according to the Supreme Court standard, denying any religious exemption would not be the least restrictive means to further the government's alleged compelling interest in vaccinating its service members with the COVID-19 vaccine.

The U.S. Defense Department Inspector General's report revealed that as of January 2023, only 339 requests for religious exemptions were approved out of a total of 13,726 (13,387+339) exemption requests. That is an approval rate of 0.25%. That low an approval rate is the smoking gun pointing to Constitutional illegality by the Department of Defense.

Table 13. Number of Religious Accommodation Requests Submitted as of January 2023

Military Service	Requests Approved by Decision Authority	Requests Denied by Decision Authority	Requests In Process	Total Requests by Service
Army	97	1,819	2,512	4,428
Marine Corps	23	3,686	0	3,709
Navy	50	3,256	30	3,336
Air Force*	169	4,626	17	4,812
Total	339	13,387	2,559	16,285

*Air Force numbers include requests from Space Force Service members.
Source: The DoD OIG.

The above statistics may be overstating the approval rates. As of November 29, 2022, the Air Force only allowed religious exemptions to those who qualified (or nearly qualified) for an administrative exemption because they would soon retire.[1347] At that point, there were 135 such exemptions granted. The Air Force revealed during a 2022 litigation that it granted zero requests for religious exemptions to anyone who was not slated to leave within a year.[1348] That means that most (or all) of the 169 exemptions listed in the March 12, 2024, Inspector General Report[1349] were actually administrative retirement exemptions under the guise of religious exemptions.

It further appears that the 339 religious exemptions ultimately granted by the military were part of a hurried window dressing operation. The U.S. Fifth Circuit Court of Appeals revealed that as of February 28, 2022, the Navy had never granted any religious accommodation for any vaccine in the preceding seven years.[1350]

> The Navy has granted hundreds of medical exemptions from vaccination requirements, allowing those service members to seek medical waivers and become deployable. But it has not accommodated any religious objection to any

vaccine in seven years, preventing those seeking such accommodations from even being considered for medical waivers.[1351]

The process for obtaining an exemption was a sham. Notably, there was a standard form for denying a religious exemption, but no standard form existed for granting one. Those seeking a religious exemption were faced with a stacked deck against them. In *U.S. Navy Seals 1-26 v. Biden*, the court revealed the futility of the Navy's religious exemption process.

> Plaintiffs claim their accommodation requests are futile because denial is a predetermined outcome. U.S. Navy SEAL 2's chain of command advised him that "all religious accommodation requests will be denied," because "senior leadership ... has no patience or tolerance for service members who refuse COVID-19 vaccination for religious reasons and want them out of the SEAL community," and that "even if a legal challenge is somehow successful, the senior leadership of Naval Special Warfare will remove [his] special warfare designation." U.S. Navy SEAL 5 averred that "[n]umerous comments from [his] chain of command indicate[d] ... that there [would] be a blanket denial of all religious accommodation requests regarding COVID-19 vaccination." US Navy SEAL 8 averred that his "chain of command ... made it clear that [his] request [would] not be approved and ... provided [him] with information on how to prepared for separation from the U.S. Navy." U.S. Navy SEAL 11 declared that during a chief's meeting, his command master chief told him that "anyone not receiving the COVID-19 vaccine is an 'acceptable loss' to the Naval Special Warfare (NSW) community" and the "legal department

used language such as 'when they get denied,' not 'if they get denied.'"[1352]

In *U.S. Navy Seals 1-26 v. Biden,* the court of appeals denied the government's request for a stay of an injunction issued by a federal district court that prevented the government from enforcing its COVID-19 vaccine mandate against the named plaintiffs. That appellate decision was later reversed in part by the U.S. Supreme Court, insofar as the injunction precluded the Navy from considering vaccination status in making deployment, assignment, and other operational decisions.[1353] The remainder of the injunction preventing the government from taking adverse punitive actions against the plaintiffs continued in force until the COVID-19 vaccine mandate was rescinded on January 10, 2023.

As a result of the denial of religious exemptions, as of February 2023, the military had discharged 7,705 of its finest personnel for refusing to take the COVID-19 vaccine.

Table 15. Service Member Discharge Types as of February 2023

Military Service	Honorable Discharges	General Discharges	Total Service Discharges
Army	281 (15%)	1,622 (85%)	1,903
Marine Corps	1,516 (41%)	2,214 (59%)	3,730
Navy	1,566 (100%)	0 (0%)	1,566
Air Force	34 (7%)	472 (93%)	506
Total	3,397 (44%)	4,308 (56%)	7,705

Source: The DoD OIG.

The 0.25% religious exemption approval rate is pretty close to zero. To get there, the military misapplied the strict scrutiny standard under the *Religious Freedom Restoration Act of 1993*[1354] (RFRA). The U.S. Supreme Court has ruled that the government is prohibited from treating "any comparable secular activity more favorably than religious exercise."[1355]

In *Bosarge v. Edney*,[1356] the federal district court applied the Supreme Court standard and ruled that a Mississippi law was unconstitutional because it allowed medical exemptions but disallowed religious exemptions from vaccinations. The *Bosarge* court stated that it is an unconstitutional value judgment that secular (i.e., medical) motivations for opting out of compulsory vaccinations are permitted but that religious grounds are not. Allowing a secular exemption while disallowing a religious exemption for 99.75% of soldiers is not the least restrictive means.

The only basis the military gave for denying 99.75% of religious exemption requests is the argument that it has a compelling interest in vaccinating the troops. But that is the wrong focus of the strict scrutiny test. The *Bosarge* court explained that "[t]he relevant question is not whether the government has a compelling interest in enforcing its policies generally, but whether it has such an interest in denying a religious exemption to a plaintiff."[1357] That means that if the military allows a single medical exemption, it must allow all exemption requests based on sincerely held religious beliefs.

The review process followed by the military was unlawful. The exemption requests were assessed by review boards that included chaplains. The Inspector General's report reveals that "[o]f the requests we reviewed, we found that chaplain and medical recommendations focused solely on their subject matter expertise. For example, chaplains generally based their recommendations on the sincerity of the Service member's belief."[1358]

That suggests that the religious exemption was being assessed on the merits of the religious claim. That is not allowed. The U.S. Supreme Court has stated, without equivocation, that "it is not for us to say that their religious beliefs are mistaken or insubstantial. Instead, our narrow function in this context is to determine whether the line drawn reflects an honest conviction."¹³⁵⁹ (ellipse and quotation marks deleted)

One court found that the boilerplate language in the rejection letters was legally insufficient and violative of the service members' religious rights under RFRA.¹³⁶⁰ The general boilerplate language claimed that the restriction on religious liberty was the least intrusive means to serve the military's compelling interest. The letters often also questioned the very validity of the religious claims by stating that their religious beliefs were not substantially burdened.¹³⁶¹ In essence, the military determined that many of the religious objections to vaccination either lacked substantive merit or were not sincerely held beliefs.

If the review process were based on the proper standard as announced by the U.S. Supreme Court, to deny 99,75% of claims, the reviewers would be required to determine that 99,75% of the claimants were either not sincere in making their claim, i.e., they were lying, or despite their sincere claim the military had a compelling reason to vaccinate anyway. We now know that the compelling interest was a phantom because the vaccines have been proven to be both unsafe and ineffective. Furthermore, the fact that most of the military personnel who were denied religious exemptions were willing to suffer an involuntary discharge and give up their military careers rather than submit to the COVID-19 vaccine mandate testifies to the sincerity of their religious beliefs. Those two facts leads tot he ineluctable conclusion that the military was wrong all the way around.

The military cannot have it both ways. Religious exemptions are an all-or-nothing proposition. If the military denies even one exemption request that it acknowledges was based on a sincerely held religious belief, it cannot grant any religious exemptions. By the same token, if the military grants even one religious exemption, it must grant all sincerely made requests for a religious exemption.

The compelling interest in vaccination does not go away just because someone holds to a different religious belief. The government is simply not qualified to make qualitative distinctions between religious beliefs. If the government grants a single religious exemption, it cannot deny another religious exemption and claim the denial is the least restrictive means to accomplish its compelling interest in vaccination. It clearly is not the least restrictive means to accomplish a compelling interest because it has allowed 0.25% of religious exemptions and innumerable medical exemptions. You cannot have people walking around unvaccinated and, at the same time, deny a religious exemption to vaccination by saying that there is a compelling need to have everyone vaccinated.

The fact that the military granted 0.25% of religious exemption requests means that in those cases the religious beliefs took precedence over the military's interest in mandatory vaccination. The military cannot then turn around and deny the remainder of the sincere religious exemption requests.

The government is not qualified to say which religious belief is superior to another. If the military's alleged compelling interest must give way to 0.25% of religious beliefs, it must give way to the remaining 97.75% of religious beliefs. Just as the government cannot favor a secular (medical) reason for exemption over a religious reason, it cannot favor one religious reason over another. But that is precisely what the military did. And that is illegal.

Notice that the chaplains were called on to rule on the sincerity of the petitioners' beliefs. But the Inspector General states that the chaplains were in that position due to their subject matter expertise. The Inspector General revealed that "[t]he decision authorities stated that they considered the subject matter expert recommendations."[1362] The government considers its chaplains to be experts on religion. The chaplains are not experts on sincerity. Thus, the only topic where the chaplains could exercise their expertise would be on issues of religious doctrine. But opining on a petitioners doctrinal beliefs is impermissible.

According to Air Force Staff Chaplain Major Matthew J. Streett, when the Air Force reviewed a religious accommodation request, it assessed the merits of the belief. Major Strett testified that the Air Force "reviewed if there is a sincerely held religious belief (as opposed to moral or conscience belief)."[1363] He let the cat out of the bag. A moral belief concerns principles of right and wrong conduct. It is how a person puts his religious beliefs into action. A person's religious beliefs guide his conscience. Major Streett is making a distinction without a difference. His statement reveals that the military assessed whether the person's religious belief was worthy of consideration. If it was not, it was deemed to be only a "moral or conscience belief."

It seems then that the chaplains were actually called on to assess the merits of the petitioners' religious beliefs, under the guise of reviewing their sincerity, since religious doctrine is the only ostensible expertise the chaplains have. The opinion of the chaplain would seem to be important, nah, almost dispositive. Who could ever hope to get a religious exemption in the face of a chaplain who says that your religious belief is not sincere? It would seem that the chaplains had undue influence, the very kind of undue influence prohibited by the Establishment Clause of the First Amendment.

The military chaplain used his unfettered discretion as a purported government expert on religion to examine the merits of a person's relgious beliefs. He then passed judgment on whether the beliefs were truly religious or what the chaplain considers only "moral or conscience beliefs." That is unconstitutional. The U.S. Court of Appeals for the Tenth Circuit in *Does 1-11 v. Bd. of Regents of Univ. of Colorado*,[1364] ruled that "a government policy that requires an intrusive inquiry into the validity of religious beliefs violates the Establishment Clause regardless of any purported government interest."[1365] The court in *Does 1-11* ruled that it did not matter whether the government had a compelling interest because when the government discriminates against a particular religious belief out of animus, such government actions is are plainly unconstitutional.

In *Doe 1-11*, the government considered unapproved religious reasons for a COVID-19 vaccine exemption to be "personal" rather than "religious" beliefs. That is similar to the military's categorization of religious beliefs with which it disagrees as "moral or conscience beliefs." In the *Doe 1-11* case, the government denied all religious exemption requests if they were deemed "personal." Similarly, the military rejected all religious exemption requests that the government chaplain considered to be "moral or conscience beliefs." It does not matter whether the government has a compelling interest when it acts to disfavor one religious belief over another. No action by the government that is based on animus toward one religious belief over another can ever be narrowly tailored to advance a compelling government interest.[1366]

The U.S. Supreme Court has stated that when the government passes judgment on the legitimacy of a religious belief, it infringes the freedom clause of the First Amendment. Indeed, the First Amendment renders the government incompetent to adjudicate the legitimacy of a religious belief. The U.S. Supreme Court in *Masterpiece Cakeshop v. Colorado C.R. Comm'n*[1367] ruled that the government cannot impose regulations or "act in a manner that passes judgment upon or presupposes the illegitimacy of religious beliefs and practices."[1368] The assessment by the chaplain that passes judgment on the legitimacy of religious practices violated the First Amendment.

The chaplains are considered by the government to be subject matter experts in the religious doctrine of their sect. A chaplain is not an expert in determining the sincerity of a person's religious beliefs who is of a different faith. Neither is the chaplain able to assess the sincerity of religious beliefs of someone in his shared faith. In *Thomas v. Review Bd. of Indiana Employment Security Div.*,[1369] the Supreme Court stated that the government is not equipped to resolve the many doctrinal and behavioral differences even between those who share the same faith.

You do not need a religious cleric, especially not a government one, to rule on the sincerity of a person's religious beliefs. Indeed, a government cleric is rendered incompetent by the Establishment Clause of the First Amendment to adjudge any religious issue whatsoever. So what exactly is the function of the chaplain? The chaplain's role in the review process, it seems, is to grease the skids toward denial. And it worked like a charm, with a 99.75% denial rate.

Imagine, for example, a Roman Catholic chaplain assessing the sincerity of a Protestant's religious beliefs. The Catholic and Protestant disagree on almost every point of faith. From the outset, the chaplain disagrees with the Protestant. Indeed, his religious leader, the pope, has issued an edict that vaccination is not a sin but is rather a virtuous act of love. How favorably will that Catholic chaplain look upon the Protestant's petition for a religious exemption? Switch parties' sects and the same issue is presented.

If the chaplain is assessing the sincerely held religious beliefs of someone in his own sect, and he is sure to rule against him. For the chaplain to rule in his favor would impeach the very religious beliefs of the chaplain. He can cloak his opinion as an assessment of the sincerity of his belief, but, in reality he just does not agree with his religious belief. That very real prejudice explains how there was a 99.75% denial rate. Keep in mind that the chaplain has already NOT asked for an exemption, and he has already been vaccinated. A religious cleric who is only in his position because he has been vaccinated and has not himself requested a religious exemption is not an unbiased reviewer. The cards are stacked against the petitioner.

The retort is that the chaplain is not assessing the merits of the religious belief, only his sincerity. But the assessment of sincerity of belief does not call on the chaplain using his expertise of the religious doctrine of his sect. His expertise in his religious sect is his only expertise. You do not need a chaplain to assess the sincerity of a person's religious beliefs. Anyone can do that. A chaplain, who the Inspector General deems to be an expert in religion, might want to assess the merits of a person's religious beliefs. But the Constitution puts such an assessment by the government off limits. Reviewing the merits of a religious exemption claim is precisely what the Supreme Court has said is improper. The government-employed cleric should be the last person to be reviewing a request for a religious exemption. Indeed, the very involvement of government chaplains in reviewing requests for religious exemptions renders the process corrupt. It entangles the government in ecclesiastical matters. The First Amendment renders the government incompetent to rule on religious matters.

The line between reviewing the sincerity of one's belief and the merits of that belief is blurred. In any event, a government inquiry into a person's religious beliefs, for whatever reason, is improper. The First Amendment renders all government officials incompetent in making any judgment about either the sincerity or the merits of one's religious beliefs. The U.S. Tenth Circuit of Appeals, in a COVID-19 vaccine religious exemption case, quoted the U.S. Supreme Court when stating the principle that "inquiries into the sincerity of the Doe's religious beliefs were precisely the sort of trolling through a person's religious beliefs for which this court and the Supreme Court have repeatedly admonished state actors."[1370]

In the rare cases when a chaplain agreed that the military should grant an exemption request from a soldier, sailor, or airman, the command would typically disregard the chaplain and deny the request anyway. For example, a Navy SEAL's chaplain, two Catholic bishops, and commanding officer recommended approval of his COVID-19 vaccine religious exemption, but the Commander of Navy SEAL Special Warfare, without explanation, recommended disapproval. The Deputy Chief of Naval Operations then disapproved his request with boilerplate language that did not refer to any information specific to his request.[1371]

The Inspector General's report indicated that the only reason ever listed for denial was boilerplate language that the vaccine was the least intrusive means of accomplishing the government's compelling interest in vaccination. That is the wrong test. The test should have been whether the person's request for a religious exemption was based on an honest conviction. If so, then the military must decide whether it has a compelling government interest in discriminating against a person based on his religious beliefs and if it can do it in the least intrusive means possible.[1372] That is the real standard, and the military could not ever pass that test.

There is no way that the military can argue that it has a compelling interest in denying a religious exemption to a vaccine to 99.75% of petitioners when it allows a medical exemption from that same vaccine. How is it okey for someone to go unvaccinated for a medical reason while denying 99.75% of soldiers who have a religious objection that same privilege? Both sets of soldiers are theorized to be equally contagious. The only reason for denial of 99.75% of the religious objectors is a value judgment that their religious objection is inferior to the secular medical exemption. That is not allowed. It is unconstitutional religious discrimination to deny 99.75% of vaccine religious exemption requests.

The claimed compelling interest in vaccinating troops

cannot survive scrutiny in court when the military allows administrative and medical exemptions while at the same time denying religious exemptions. In *Doster v. Kendall*,[1373] the U.S. Court of Appeals for the Sixth Circuit cited examples that rendered ridiculous the military's claim of a compelling health interest in vaccinating its troops.

> As for its health interest, the Air Force says that it must reject religious exemptions because those working in "close physical contact" can spread COVID-19. But the Air Force has allowed medical or administrative exemptions even when these exemptions undercut that interest. The Surgeon General, for example, denied Lieutenant Doster a religious exemption because his work as a student "require[d] intermittent to frequent contact with others[.]" But the Air Force granted multiple medical exemptions to pregnant women who worked with him and performed "identical assignments[.]" Likewise, the Surgeon General denied Airman Dills a religious exemption because he had "frequent contact with others" as a passenger representative. Yet Dills worked with "[s]everal" colleagues who obtained other exemptions. The Air Force allowed these members to continue "interacting with people" and "working in close quarters" without change. Perhaps most striking, the Surgeon General denied a religious exemption for Major Corvi (a class member) because her assignment "require[d] intermittent to frequent contact with others." In the same month, she received a medical exemption for her pregnancy. The Air Force does not explain why service members who remain unvaccinated because of their pending retirement or pregnancy pose less of a risk of spreading COVID-19 than those who

remain unvaccinated because of their religion.[1374]

Doster v. Kendall[1375] was later vacated as moot by the U.S. Supreme Court after the Secretary of Defense rescinded the military COVID-19 vaccine mandate. It thus cannot be cited as precedent in any future court cases.

The military's discrimination against religious beliefs in violation of the Constitution was based on subtly twisting the review standard, which facilitated their denial of almost all religious exemption requests. The scheme was successful because the petitioners came to the plate with two strikes against them. Both the petitioners and the government were operating under rules that assumed the vaccine from which the petitioners sought exemptions was a valid, safe, and effective medical treatment. If the petitioners had argued that the vaccine was a superstitious religious ritual, then the evidence of that truth would be admissible in any appeal process to prove that the government was mandating participation in a religious ritual in violation of the Establishment Clause of the First Amendment. That truth would, if accepted, would defeat all vaccine mandates.

Even if in a given case, the Establishment Clause claim failed, the evidence of the religious origins of vaccination would become a matter of record for future review and perhaps a more favorable subsequent decision. Furthermore, the insistence by the petitioner that vaccination is a superstitious religious ritual would establish unimpeachable proof that the request for exemption was based on an "honest conviction"[1376] (a.k.a. sincerely held belief).

Since no medical treatment can be one-size-fits-all, every vaccine mandate must have a medical exemption. Under the U.S. Constitution, if the government grants a medical exemption, it must *ipso facto* also grant a religious exemption that is based on an honest conviction. That is the law.[1377]

The Inspector General of the Defense Department acknowledged that the COVID-19 vaccine mandate must be reviewed under the strict scrutiny standard of the *Religious Freedom Restoration Act of 1993*[1378] (RFRA). The U.S. Supreme Court has long held that under its strict scrutiny standard a rule must be narrowly tailored to address a compelling government interest. A rule is not narrowly tailored "when it leaves appreciable damage to that supposedly vital interest unprohibited."[1379] In the case of vaccine exemption, to allow a person an exemption for a secular medical reason leaves the alleged compelling interest of vaccination unaccomplished with regard to the medically exempt person. If another person is denied his religious exemption, that denial prohibits a religious person from being unvaccinated while leaving a medically exempt person "unprohibited" from being unvaccinated. That is not narrowly tailored and thus an unconstitutional discrimination based on a person's religious beliefs.

The scientific evidence proves that the military does not have a compelling interest in mandating the vaccine. The evidence of the ineffectiveness of the vaccines is important to getting a favorable court ruling regarding a religious exemption. For example, the court in *Navy Seal 1 v. Austin*[1380] granted an injunction against the injection of the military mandated COVID-19 vaccine. The *Navy Seal 1* court called into question the military's conclusion that there were no lesser restrictive means other than vaccination to accomplish its alleged compelling interest, as the court questioned the effectiveness of the COVID-19 vaccines. The military cited data showing the danger of the vaccines to buttress its argument that it had a compelling government interest in vaccinating its personnel. But within that data was evidence that showed the ineffectiveness of the COVID-19 vaccines. The military's argued that that "no lesser restrictive means exists [other than vaccination] because other COVID-19 mitigation efforts, such as masking and social distancing, 'are not 100 percent effective.'"[1381] The court rebutted that claim by pointing out that vaccination is also not 100 percent effective. The court stated:

> For example, Department of Defense data discussed at the hearing and available on the department's website show that between November 24, 2021, and December 22, 2021, the month during which vaccines became mandatory, the military total of new COVID-19 cases rose by 7,515 cases but between December 22, 2021 and February 9, 2021, after vaccination was mandatory and after each branch reported greater than 90% vaccination rates, cases rose by 114,292 cases.[1382]

The court's statement that the vaccines were not 100% effective is the understatement of the year. Indeed, the statistics suggest to any rational reader that the vaccines go beyond ineffectiveness to causing the very disease it is supposed to suppress. There is simply no way that the government could ever prove a compelling government interest in mandating an ineffective vaccine, let alone one that causes the very disease it is purported to prevent. After the Department of Defense rescinded the COVID-19 vaccine mandate, the injunction in *Navy Seal 1 v. Austin*[1383] was dissolved, and the case was dismissed as moot.[1384] A federal district court ruling is not binding precedent in other federal courts. But it can be cited as persuasive authority. However, when a decision is rendered moot, it can no longer be cited even as persuasive authority in subsequent cases.

Navy Seal 1 v. Austin illustrates why the evidence of ineffectiveness is so important. The preferred strategy of the government is to simply state the danger caused by the disease and assume that the court will go along with the allegedly settled science presented through conclusory statements from seemingly authoritative sources that the vaccines are safe and effective. When that pseudo-science, based on fraud and deception, is not rebutted by the opposing party, the outcome is predictable. For example, in *Roth v. Austin*,[1385] the court denied an injunction to stop the mandatory vaccination of service members. The court began its analysis with the premise that the COVID-19 vaccines were safe and effective. The court opened its opinion with the following statement:

> With the evidence provided to the Court in this case, there can be no serious dispute that the available COVID-19 vaccines have dramatically reduced the death toll from COVID-19 in the United States and the world. Further, the data available illustrates that those who have refused to get vaccinated have necessarily had a greater chance to get and spread the virus. Indeed, science shows that those who are unvaccinated have had a dramatically higher likelihood of serious illness or death.[1386]

Every assumption by the court about the effectiveness of the vaccines was erroneous. But when the court begins its decision with a false premise, an unjust ruling will follow. The fate of the service members was sealed after that point.

The plaintiff airmen in *Roth* did their best to rebut the claims of COVID-19 vaccine efficacy. The plaintiffs presented testimony from Dr. Peter A. McCullough, which established the ineffectiveness of the COVID-19 vaccines, thereby refuting the claim that the military had a compelling government interest in the good health of the airmen by mandating vaccination over their religious objections. But the *Roth* court relied on the precedent of another court ruling[1387] and completely disregarded Dr. McCullough's testimony as being "outside the scientific mainstream."[1388] The court was simply not going to go against the "mainstream" so-called science. The following laughably absurd statement by the judge gives us some insight into the prejudice faced by the plaintiffs:

> There is little doubt that if the public had agreed to become vaccinated at the rate [96.8%] that members of the U.S. Air Force had submitted, the pandemic, and indeed the death toll, could have been dramatically different.[1389]

It is hard to win in a court where a judge has a prejudice against evidence that does not align with his pre-conceived notions. Although the strategy of attacking the compelling government interest can be thwarted by a judge who will not consider objective evidence, chances of winning are greatly enhanced in a court with a judge who will listen to reason.

In every case involving a religious exemption, the petitioners should come to court with admissible evidence that the vaccines are unsafe and ineffective, superstitious religious practices. They should present evidence of how the pharmaceutical companies rig the trials to falsely show safety and effectiveness. Otherwise, they will end up in court with judges who will rule on their case, thinking that they are upholding some public good when they deny a religious exemption to vaccination. In most cases, evidence of the religious origins, dangers, and ineffectiveness of vaccines will be a revelation to a judge and you may find a sympathetic ear. But your chances of winning are diminished without presenting such evidence.

The military states it has "a compelling governmental interest in mission accomplishment—including military readiness, unit cohesion, good order and discipline, and health and safety for both the unit and the member."[1390] Who could argue against that? Raising the standard to such a height rendered the religious interests of the service members almost insignificant. The government cannot rely on a compelling interest in the general health of its troops. A pronouncement of an abstract ideal like that is not enough. The government must establish that it has a compelling interest in refusing to exempt from vaccination a particular person who has objected on religious grounds to being vaccinated.[1391]

It is improper to the government to base its disparate treatment of religion when compared to secular activity on a general health concern. The government cannot simply rely on generalities. The RFRA requires the government to prove that its alleged compelling interest requires that it substantially burden the religious liberty of a specific person and that there is no less restrictive way to further that interest.[1392] The U.S. Supreme Court has made it clear that "when judging whether a law treats a religious exercise the same as comparable secular activity, this Court has made plain that only the government's actually asserted interests as applied to the parties before it count—not post-hoc reimaginings of those interests expanded to some society-wide level of generality."[1393] That is because, as the Supreme Court explained, "[a]t some great height, after all, almost any state action might be said to touch on public health and safety and measuring a highly particularized and individual interest in the exercise of a civil right directly against these rarified values inevitably makes the individual interest appear the less significant."[1394]

The real issue is whether mandatory vaccination of religious objectors accomplishes the alleged compelling government interest in preventing infection and spread of COVID-19. Indeed, the *Roth* court restated the compelling interest at issue as "the Air Force's compelling interest is in preventing COVID-19 in the first place."[1395] That is quite a different matter from the general health compelling interest proffered by the military. Objective evidence proves that the COVID-19 vaccines do not prevent COVID-19. The court was misled into believing a false premise which caused an erroneous ruling.

The *Roth* court handed down its ruling on May 18, 2022.

Aproximately seven weeks before that ruling, on or about March 30, 2022, the CDC acknowledged in writing what had long been known in the medical community, that the COVID-19 vaccines do not prevent infection.[1396] The ineffectiveness of the COVID-19 vaccines was an established medical fact when the court ruled that the military had a compelling government interest in vaccinating troops to prevent infection. The court made its ruling on an erroneous premise.

The *Roth* court further stated that "[i]t would be a waste of time and wrong to state that '[s]temming the spread of COVID-19' isn't a compelling interest—the Supreme Court has already decided it is."[1397] The problem with that statement is that from the beginning it was known that the COVID-19 vaccine would not prevent the spread of SARS-Cov-2.

Moderna Chief Medical Officer Tal Zaks admitted that its COVID-19 vaccine may be able to prevent someone from getting sick from COVID-19, but it could not prevent someone from carrying the virus and infecting others.[1398] Indeed, the COVID-19 vaccines so clearly did not prevent the spread of SARS-CoV-2, that the CDC issued a press release on March 8, 2021, saying that fully vaccinated Americans must "continue to take these COVID-19 precautions when in public."[1399] Also on March 8, 2021, the CDC acknowledged the ineffectiveness of the COVID-19 vaccines and advised that residents of non-healthcare congregate settings who had been fully vaccinated against COVID-19 should quarantine themselves for 14 days and be tested for SARS-CoV-2 following an exposure to someone with suspected or confirmed COVID-19. The CDC explained that guidance was "because residential congregate settings may face high turnover of residents [and] a higher risk of transmission."[1400] On July 27, 2021, "CDC Director Rochelle Walensky said recent studies had shown that those vaccinated individuals who do become infected with Covid have just as much viral load as the unvaccinated, making it possible for them to spread the virus to others."[1401]

The statement by the *Roth* court regarding the effectiveness of the COVID-19 vaccines to prevent the spread of the virus is yet another example where the court premised its decision on false information. If the COVID-19 vaccines do not actually prevent the spread of the alleged virus that supposedly causes COVID-19, the government cannot have a compelling interest in manadating those vaccines for the stated purpose of preventing the spread of the alleged virus.

In RFRA vaccine cases, court's focus on whether substantially interfering with a person's religious beliefs is the least restrictive means of achieving the government's compelling interest. But there is no need even to examine whether vaccination is the least restrictive means to accomplishing that goal if vaccination is incapable of furthering the compelling government interest because it is not effective. No government agency could ever show that it has a compelling government interest in mandating an unsafe and ineffective vaccine.

Furthermore, there is no way that the government could survive an Establishment Clause violation in the face of evidence that they are requiring people to participate in a superstitious religious ritual. However, as we saw in *Roth*, victory sometimes depends on the court's receptiveness to the argument. Still, you should present the evidence, make the argument, and allow the court the opportunity to rule on it.

45 Unlawful COVID-19 Mandates

President Joe Biden issued unconstitutional executive orders and executive agency rules requiring federal workers, federal contractors, and the private sector to receive the COVID-19 vaccine.[1402] The problem is that under federal law, no person can be compelled to participate in a medical experiment without informed consent. Indeed, every COVID-19 vaccine manufacturer includes a notice that the recipient of the vaccine should be told that they have the option of accepting or refusing the experimental vaccines. For example, the Moderna fact sheet states: "It is your choice to receive or not receive the Moderna COVID-19 Vaccine. Should you decide not to receive it, it will not change your standard medical care."[1403] They do that because it is a legal requirement.

A person receiving the COVID-19 vaccine must be informed of its dangers and consent to being vaccinated. A person cannot be compelled to take the COVID-19 vaccine. 21 U.S. Code § 360bbb–3, which is the law governing the emergency use authorizations (EUA) of experimental vaccines, requires informed consent that is more limited than in the federal regulations on informed consent for medical experiments. But the statute nonetheless requires certain information be provided to the patient before vaccination, and the patient can withdraw consent and refuse to be vaccinated. The statute, 21 U.S.C. § 360bbb–3(e)(1)(A)(i), requires informed consent for vaccines authorized under an EUA. That code section provides:

> Appropriate conditions designed to ensure that individuals to whom the product is administered are **informed**—
> (I) that the Secretary has authorized the emergency use of the product;
> (II) of **the significant known and potential benefits and risks of such use**, and of the extent to which such benefits and risks are unknown; and
> (III) **of the option to accept or refuse administration of the product,** of the consequences, if any, of refusing administration of the product, and of the alternatives to the product that are available and of their benefits and risks.[1404]

Why is informed consent required for a vaccine under an EUA? Because those vaccines are investigational vaccines (a.k.a., experimental vaccines) whereby the manufacturers of the COVID-19 vaccines authorized under the EUA are under a continuing obligation to report all serious adverse events, including death and hospitalizations that result from the EUA administration of the COVID-19 vaccines. The vaccines are still being studied for safety and effectiveness. A person cannot be compelled to take the vaccine under the threat of any consequences for refusal.

The FDA's guidance on emergency use authorization of medical products requires the FDA to "ensure that recipients are informed to the extent practicable given the applicable circumstances ... That **they have the option to accept or refuse the EUA product ...**"[1405] In the same vein, when Dr. Amanda Cohn, the Executive Secretary of the CDC's Advisory Committee on Immunization Practices, was asked if Covid-19 vaccination can be required, she responded that under an EUA, **"vaccines are not allowed to be mandatory. So, early in this vaccination phase, individuals will have to be consented and they won't be able to be mandatory."**[1406] Cohn later affirmed that this prohibition on requiring the vaccines applies to organizations, including hospitals.[1407] The EUAs for COVID-19 vaccines require fact sheets to be given to vaccination providers and recipients. These fact sheets make clear that getting the vaccine is optional. For example, the fact sheet for recipients states that, "[i]t is your choice to receive or not receive the Covid-19 Vaccine," and if "you decide to not receive it, it will not change your standard of medical care." Attorney Aaron Siri points out that the FDA's position that the COVID-19 vaccines authorized under an EUA cannot be mandated is because informed consent is required by federal statute. Siri explains that "the same section of the Federal Food, Drug, and Cosmetic Act that authorizes the FDA to grant emergency use authorization also requires the secretary of Health and Human Services to **"ensure that individuals to whom the product is administered are informed ... of the option to accept or refuse administration of the product."**[1408]

FDA Interpretation of EUA Medical Experimentation Rules

Other regulatory provisions require informed consent for those participating in medical experiments. The FDA has taken the unofficial position that compliance with the other statutory provisions requiring informed consent are not required for an EUA vaccine. The FDA alleges:

> **Although informed consent as generally required under FDA regulations is not required for administration or use of an EUA product**, section 564 [21 U.S. Code § 360bbb–3] does provide EUA conditions to ensure that recipients are informed about the MCM [Medical Countermeasure] they receive under an EUA.[1409]

The FDA further states:

> FDA must ensure that recipients of the vaccine under an EUA are informed, to the extent practicable given the applicable circumstances, that FDA has authorized the emergency use of the vaccine, of the known and potential benefits and risks, the extent to which such benefits and risks are unknown, that they have the option to accept or refuse the vaccine, and of any available alternatives to the product. Typically, this information is communicated in a patient "fact sheet." The FDA posts these fact sheets on our website.[1410]

The FDA thinks that providing a fact sheet to the recipients of the COVID-19 vaccines is sufficient. "Therefore, FDA recommends that a request for an EUA include a 'Fact Sheet' for recipients that includes essential information about the product."[1411]

The FDA is reading the statutory requirements under Section 564 [21 U.S. Code § 360bbb–3] for administering an unapproved MCM under an EUA as a waiver of the otherwise required informed consent. The FDA's position is presumably based on the following language in subsection (k) of 21 U.S. Code § 360bbb–3:

> If a product is the subject of an authorization under this section, the use of such product within the scope of the authorization shall not be considered to constitute a clinical investigation for purposes of section 355(i), 360b(j), or 360j(g) of this title or any other provision of this chapter or section 351 of the Public Health Service Act [42 U.S.C. 262].

DOJ OLC Opinion

Dawn Johnsen, Acting Assistant Attorney General Office of Legal Counsel, issued an opinion addressed to the Deputy Counsel to the President that public and private entities can legally mandate that employees get injected with the COVID-19 experimental vaccines as a condition of employment.[1412] That opinion seems to be the legal justification for the President's September 9, 2021 decision to mandate COVID-19 vaccinations for the federal workforce.

In the legal opinion, Ms. Johnsen focused on the language found under 21 U.S.C. § 360bbb–3(e)(1)(A)(i) that requires a recipient to be "informed ... of the option to accept or refuse administration of the product, of the consequences, if any, of refusing administration of the product." Ms. Johnsen opines that a person can either "accept or reject" the vaccine, and a company can coerce the employee to make that decision as long as the company informs the employee "of the consequences, if any, of refusing administration of the product."

Ms. Johnsen reads the "option to accept or refuse" condition as merely informational and not conditional. That means the employer only needs to tell the employee the consequences of not taking the vaccine. Then, with that information known, the employee can decide whether to suffer the consequences of accepting or refusing the vaccine.

Ms. Johnsen opines: "These provisions all appear to require only that certain factual information be conveyed to those who might use the product."

DOJ Opines Employment Is Only a "Desirable Activity"

Ms. Johnsen says it is okay that the recipient of the information is faced with a choice at *Morton's Fork*. The worker is between the proverbial rock and a hard place. He is put there by the employer. Ms. Johnsen is okay with that. When someone is at Morton's Fork with two unpleasant choices, his choice cannot be characterized as a free choice. That is because the options are placed before him by the employer who wants him to choose vaccination. So the employer loads up the unpleasantness of not getting a vaccine to coerce him to get one. The employer controls the options. And so the choice is being coerced by the entity presenting the unpleasant options of accepting or refusing the vaccine. The employer wants the employee to take the vaccine and thus sets dire consequences for not doing so. He will be fired if he chooses not to be vaccinated. Thus, according to Ms. Johnsen, the option to accept or refuse the COVID-19 vaccine need not be voluntary.

Ms. Johnsen argues that getting fired or expelled from school is only a secondary consequence of refusal. DOJ characterizes getting fired from your job as simply exclusion from a "desirable activity." Ms. Johnsen thinks that your ability to feed your family is not a necessity, it is only a "desirable activity." Suppose you get fired for refusing to get vaccinated. In that case, DOJ considers you to have exercised your option, and to have chosen, of your own free will, to be excluded from a "desirable activity" of employment over getting vaccinated because you were told ahead of time you would be fired.

On the other hand, if you get vaccinated because you have been threatened with being fired, DOJ considers that exercising your free choice to get vaccinated. The coercive threat of losing your job is perfectly fine to DOJ. Your choice does not have to be voluntary, according to DOJ.

The very language of section 564 of the FDCA (21 U.S. Code § 360bbb-3) assumes that one has the right to refuse. Because it requires the recipient to be informed "of the option to accept or refuse administration of the product." The Congressional

Conference report on the legislation that created both section 564 of the FDCA (21 U.S. Code § 360bbb-3) and section 10 U.S.C. § 1107a interpreted the language in § 360bbb-3 requiring that patients be informed of the option to accept or refuse administration of the product as meaning they had the right to refuse the administration of the EUA product. Section 1107a allows a service member to refuse an EUA unless the President issues an overriding waiver of that right. In the context of explaining the meaning of the presidential waiver under § 1107a the Congressional Conference report states that:

> The amendment would authorize the President to waive **the right of service members to refuse administration of a product** if the President determines, in writing, that affording service members **the right to refuse the product** is not feasible, is contrary to the best interests of the members affected, or is not in the interests of national security.[1413]

Certainly, if the right to refuse found in § 360bbb-3, which applies to all service members and citizens, means that all citizens also have the right to refuse the administration of an EUA vaccine or other product. There is no Presidential waiver provisions for citizens who are not military service members.

The Department of Defense followed the guidance in the Congressional Conference Report. DOD stated in written legal guidance that DOD may not require military service members to take an EUA product because they have a right to refuse the product unless the President exercises the waiver authority contained in 10 U.S.C. § 1107a.[1414]

DOJ agrees with the DOD position because of the consequences that a soldier would suffer if the notice of the option to refuse administration of an EUA vaccine was not interpreted to mean that the soldier had an absolute right to refuse administration. DOJ stated that DOD "understandably does not want to convey inaccurate or confusing information to service members—that is, telling them that they have the 'option' to refuse the COVID-19 vaccine if they effectively lack such an option."[1415] Indeed, that same logic would apply to civilians. What good is it to tell a civilian that he has the option to take a vaccine when exercising that option comes with the consequence of being fired? The civilian, like the soldier, in reality, lacks an option if there are detrimental consequences to exercising that option.

The only distinction between applying the option to refuse the EUA product between a soldier and a civilian is the difference in the consequences to a soldier and the consequences to a civilian. DOJ states that because of the concern that service members, unlike civilian employees, could face imprisonment for refusing an order of a superior officer, it would make no sense for a soldier to be told he has an option to refuse to get vaccinated if he did not have that option. An order that included a proviso that the soldier had the choice of getting a vaccine would be deceptive and confusing if the soldier exercised his right not to get the vaccine and was then punished for exercising the option. DOD and DOJ understand that informing a soldier he has the option to accept or refuse vaccination only to tell him he will be subjected to court-martial, dishonorable discharge, and possibly imprisonment is not a free choice. It is, by its nature, compulsion.

The only difference between a soldier and a civilian is the degree and kind of punishment he will suffer. A soldier could be subject to court martial and a dishonorable discharge from the service. In comparison, a civilian employee could be fired. They are functionally the same. The additional specter of imprisonment that a soldier would face does not change the nature of the right to refuse vaccination. In both civilian and military cases, the option to accept or refuse the administration of the product is meaningless if the person suffers severe consequences for exercising that option. It is nonsense for DOJ to characterize being fired and thus unable to support one's family as simply being excluded from a desirable activity. Only a tyrant thinks like that.

Indeed, even the FDA once understood that being informed of the option to accept or refuse administration of an EUA product in § 360bbb-3 assumes the patient has the right to refuse without compulsion or suffering any consequences. The FDA issued the following regulation in 2005 regarding the EUA Anthrax Vaccine Immunization Program for the Department of Defense:

> With respect to condition (3) [of § 360bbb-3], above, relating to the option to accept or refuse administration of AVA [Anthrax Vaccine Adsorbed], the AVIP [Anthrax Vaccine Immunization Program] will be revised to give personnel the option to refuse vaccination. Individuals who refuse anthrax vaccination will not be punished. Refusal may not be grounds for any disciplinary action under the Uniform Code of Military Justice. **Refusal may not be grounds for any adverse personnel action. Nor would either military or civilian personnel be considered non-deployable or processed for separation based on refusal of anthrax vaccination. There may be no penalty or loss of entitlement for refusing anthrax vaccination.**
>
> This information shall read in the trifold brochure provided to potential vaccine recipients as follows:
>
> You may refuse anthrax vaccination under the EUA, and you will not be punished. No disciplinary action or adverse personnel action will be taken. You will not be processed for separation, and you will still be deployable. There will be no

penalty or loss of entitlement for refusing anthrax vaccination.[1416]

Notice that the FDA interpretation of Section 564 [21 U.S. Code § 360bbb-3] that "[r]efusal may not be grounds for any adverse personnel action" applied to both civilian and military personnel. The FDA reaffirmed that interpretation in its extension of the Anthrax vaccine EUA for DOD personnel on August 3, 2005.[1417]

In its 2007 guidance on EUA products, the FDA made it clear that under 21 U.S. C. § 360bbb–3(e)(1)(A)(i) being informed of the option to accept or refuse administration of the product means that **"[r]ecipients must have an opportunity to accept or refuse the EUA product** and must be informed of any consequences of refusing administration of the product."[1418] Notice that the FDA viewed being informed of the option to accept or refuse the product means that the recipient must have the actual "opportunity to accept or refuse." An opportunity is defined as a convenient means of doing something.[1419] If you suffer for doing something, it is, by definition, inconvenient. If you are punished for doing something, that is the opposite of having an opportunity to do it. The opportunity to refuse is not genuine if the exercise of that opportunity is subjected to a penalty, like being fired or expelled from school.

But when it came to the COVID-19 vaccine, the same statute that the FDA said in 2015 precluded any penalty to service members for exercising the option to refuse vaccination and in 2007 said required an opportunity to accept or refuse a vaccine was suddenly interpreted by the FDA in 2020 to mean that citizens can be fired if they exercise the option to refuse vaccination.

DOJ vs. DOJ

The DOJ under the previous administration opined 14

months earlier, on May 30, 2020, that:

> There is no pandemic exception to the Constitution and its Bill of Rights. Indeed, "individual rights secured by the Constitution do not disappear during a public health crisis." *In re Abbott*, 954 F.3d at 784.[1420]

The above sentiment would preclude any opinion from the DOJ authorizing the coercion of federal workers to be vaccinated with an experimental vaccine under the threat of being subjected to masking, testing, social distancing, and travel prohibitions if they refused. DOJ taking the view that there is no pandemic exception to the Constitution, certainly would not issue an opinion that working to feed your family is simply a "desirable activity" and therefore it would be no great loss if you were fired because you decide not to be injected with an experimental vaccine.

Aaron Siri's Rebuttal

Aaron Siri, attorney for the Informed Consent Action Network, wrote a rebuttal to the DOJ OLC opinion. Mr. Siri wrote a letter of opinion to Dawn Johnsen, Acting Assistant Attorney General Office of Legal Counsel.[1421] Mr. Siri pointed out that the DOJ argument that expulsion from a job, school, and civil society are only "secondary consequences," which does not remove the "option to accept or refuse" defies common sense. He points out that the statutory framework and implementation of 21 U.S. Code § 360bbb-3 "all reflect that 'the option to accept or refuse' was intended to continue the longstanding principle that it is not permissible to coerce anyone to receive an unlicensed medical product."

Mr. Siri points out that the principle of informed consent "was carried forward when Congress included the words 'the right to accept or refuse' in Section 564 [21 U.S. Code § 360bbb-3] is reinforced by the legislative discussions surrounding the passing of Section 564 [21 U.S. Code § 360bbb-3]." He explained:

> On July 16, 2003, in deliberating Section 564, Representative Hays said, without any objection, that:
>
>> [A]ny authority to actually use experimental drugs or medical devices in emergency situations has to be defined and wielded with nothing less than surgical precision. Prior informed consent in connection with the administration of experimental therapy is a basic human right, a right no one should be asked to surrender.
>
> Similarly, on May 19, 2004, Senator Kennedy said while deliberating regarding Section 564 that "[t]he authorization for the emergency use of unapproved products also includes strong provisions on informed consent for patients."[1422]

The statements of Representative Hays and Senator Kennedy indicate that Congress thought that the requirement in Section 564 that the patient be informed of the "significant known and potential benefits and risks of such use" and "of the option to accept or refuse administration of the product" established a requirement of "informed consent." Indeed, Senator Kennedy and Representative Hays were adamant that informed consent be required before anyone was subjected to the administration of an unapproved medical product of any kind when it is authorized for use in an emergency. Senator Kennedy described the language in Section 564 as constituting "strong provisions" requiring informed consent. Informed consent is a higher degree of consent, and all consent must be voluntary to genuinely be consent.

The American Medical Association (AMA) states that "informed consent to medical treatment is fundamental in both ethics and law." The AMA states that when a physician is obtaining a patient's informed consent, he should: "Assess the patient's ability to understand relevant medical information and the implications of treatment alternatives and to make an independent, voluntary decision."

The concept of informed consent for medical experiment subjects is found in every state. For example, in Virginia, the state provides that an agency must obtain the informed consent of anyone taking part in a medical experiment. The Virginia statutes state that the consent must be unconstrained by any coercion: "Informed consent" means the knowing and voluntary agreement, without undue inducement or any element of force, fraud, deceit, duress, or other form of constraint or coercion, of a person who is capable of exercising free power of choice."[1423]

Informed consent in the context of experimental vaccines requires that the patient be fully informed. But regardless of the information provided, his decision to obtain the vaccine must be the product of an unencumbered will that is free of coercion. The litigation regarding the admissibility of confessions offers guidance as to what it means for consent to be voluntary. In *Culombe v. Connecticut*[1424], the U.S. Supreme Court stated that "[t]he ultimate test remains that which has been the only clearly established test in Anglo-American courts for two hundred years: the test of voluntariness. Is the confession the product of an essentially free and unconstrained choice by its maker?"[1425] The *Colombe* Court explained that "The line of distinction is that at which governing self-direction is lost and compulsion, of whatever nature or however infused, propels or helps to propel the confession."[1426] The critical distinction between a voluntary and an involuntary confession is whether the confessor was compelled to confess. For example, threatening to inform the prosecutor of a suspect's refusal to cooperate is viewed by courts to be coercive and render the resulting confession involuntary and inadmissible.[1427] That same concept is found in family law statutes. In Kentucky, voluntary, informed consent is defined by statute, in pertinent part, as:

> "Voluntary and informed consent" means that at the time of the execution of the consent, the consenting person was fully informed of the legal effect of the consent, that the consenting person was not given or promised anything of value except those expenses allowable under KRS 199.590(6), that the consenting person was not coerced in any way to execute the consent, and that the consent was voluntarily and knowingly given.[1428]

Coerced Vaccinations

Under no circumstances can the decision by a federal worker or anyone else to be vaccinated with a COVID-19 vaccine be considered voluntary when it is given under the threat that refusal to do so will result in them being "required to mask no matter where they work; test one or two times a week to see if they have ... acquired COVID; socially distance; and generally will not be allowed to travel for work,"[1429] as stated by President Biden.

Aaron Siri further explains:

The FDA likewise viewed Section 564 as providing a substantive right to refuse when it explained the military exception:

> [A]s a general rule, persons must be made aware of their right to refuse the product (or to refuse it for their

children or others without the capacity to consent) and of the potential consequences, if any, of this choice. An exception to this rule is that the president, as commander in chief, can waive military personnel's right to refuse this product. If the right is not specifically waived by the president for a particular product given under EUA, military personnel have the same right to refuse as civilians.[1430]

The FDA thus makes clear that Section 564 provides a substantive right to refuse, and this right does not exist in the presence of a requirement that imposes negative consequences for refusing.

Similarly, the CDC's Advisory Committee on Immunization Practices ("ACIP") has interpreted Section 564 as a consent provision and not merely a requirement to inform. When responding to an inquiry regarding whether the COVID-19 vaccines can be required, the Executive Secretary of ACIP publicly stated that "under an EUA, vaccines are not allowed to be mandatory. Therefore, early in the vaccination phase individuals will have to be consented and cannot be mandated to be vaccinated."

ACIP's Executive Secretary then reaffirmed to the FDA's Vaccine and Related Biological Products Advisory Committee that no organization, public or private – including hospitals – can mandate the EUA COVID-19 Vaccines:

> Organizations, such as hospitals, with licensed products do have [the] capability of asking their workers to get the vaccine. But in the setting of an EUA, patients and individuals will have the right to refuse the vaccine.

Consistent with the foregoing, the U.S. General Services Administration's ("GSA") Safer Federal Workforce website, applicable to all federal employees and contractors, expressly provided that the EUA COVID-19 vaccines cannot be mandatory.[1431]

The GSA's official position was that "COVID-19 vaccination should generally not be a pre-condition for employees or contractors at executive departments and agencies ... to work in-person in Federal buildings, on Federal lands, and in other settings as required by their job duties."[1432]

Siri reveals that the GSA changed its interpretation of the statute after DOJ released its slip opinion. Now, GSA states that an unvaccinated person can be required to wear a mask, physical distance, be tested, restricted from travel, and even be quarantined.

The DOJ interpretation of Section 564 (21 U.S. Code § 360bbb-3) gives short shrift to the concept of freedom of choice. Section 564 (21 U.S. Code § 360bbb-3) allows "the **option** to accept or refuse administration of the product." "**Option**" is defined in the dictionary as "an act of choosing; the power or right to choose: freedom of choice."[1433] The DOJ opinion eliminates the "freedom of choice" by allowing the choice to be coerced by a threat of being fired, having to wear a mask, being tested, physical distance, etc.

Aaron Siri makes the common-sense observation that "[i]t is illogical that Congress would require that individuals be informed of a freedom of choice if that choice is illusory at the whim of any public or private entity."

National Research Act

Subsection (k) of 21 U.S. Code § 360bbb–3 indicates that an EUA is not to be considered a clinical investigation for purposes of section 355(i), 360b(j), or 360j(g) of this title or any other provision of this chapter or section 351 of the Public Health Service Act [42 U.S.C. 262]. But that language does affect other regulations that remain operative regarding an investigative vaccine under an EUA.

Aside from the misinterpretation of Section 564 (21 U.S. Code § 360bbb-3), coercing employees to get an experimental COVID-19 vaccine by the threat of masking, social distancing, medical testing, and travel prohibitions is a violation of the federal regulations and rulings passed under the authority of the National Research Act.[1434]

In the wake of the infamous Tuskegee Syphilis Study, which was terminated on November 14, 1972, Congress enacted The National Research Act.[1435] That law established a National Commission for the Protection of Human Subjects of Biomedical and Behavioral Research.

The commission was tasked with, among other things, conducting "a comprehensive investigation and study to identify the basic ethical principles which should underlie the conduct of biomedical and behavioral research involving human subjects."[1436] In carrying out that task the commission was ordered to "consider at least ... the nature and definition of informed consent in various research Settings."[1437]

The Belmont Report

The National Commission for the Protection of Human Subjects of Biomedical and Behavioral Research issued an authoritative report known as the Belmont Report.[1438] That report summarized the basic ethical principles identified by the Commission that were to be followed by researchers using human subjects in biomedical research.

The pertinent section of the Belmont Report is the section that addresses informed consent. The Belmont Report expressly states that any research subject must be informed of the risks and alternative treatments prior to entering a research study involving an experimental medical treatment. Notably, that informed consent is defined in the Belmont Report as voluntary consent that is free from coercion and undue influence. The report notes explicitly that consent from unjustifiable pressure is not valid consent. "Unjustifiable pressures usually occur when persons in positions of authority or commanding influence -- especially where possible sanctions are involved -- urge a course of action for a subject." The Pertinent language in the Belmont Report explaining informed consent is as follows:

> **Informed Consent.** -- Respect for persons requires that subjects, to the degree that they are capable, be given the **opportunity to choose** what shall or shall not happen to them. This opportunity is provided when adequate standards for **informed consent** are satisfied.
>
> While the importance of informed consent is unquestioned, controversy prevails over the nature and possibility of an informed consent. Nonetheless, there is widespread agreement that the consent process can be analyzed as containing three elements: information, comprehension and

voluntariness.

***

Voluntariness. An agreement to participate in research constitutes a **valid consent only if voluntarily given.** This element of informed consent requires conditions **free of coercion and undue influence.** Coercion occurs when an overt threat of harm is intentionally presented by one person to another in order to obtain compliance. Undue influence, by contrast, occurs through an offer of an excessive, unwarranted, inappropriate or improper reward or other overture in order to obtain compliance. Also, inducements that would ordinarily be acceptable may become undue influences if the subject is especially vulnerable.

Unjustifiable pressures usually occur when persons in positions of authority or commanding influence -- especially where possible sanctions are involved -- urge a course of action for a subject. A continuum of such influencing factors exists, however, and it is impossible to state precisely where justifiable persuasion ends and undue influence begins. But undue influence would include actions such as manipulating a person's choice through the controlling influence of a close relative and threatening to withdraw health services to which an individual would otherwise be entitled.[1439] (emphasis added)

The U.S. Department of Health and Human Services has created a video wherein is explained the meaning and application of the Belmont Report. The video clarifies that "to deny someone autonomy is to deny them respect as an individual. ... Subjects must understand the extent of the risk they are taking. They must know that participation is **voluntary**, that they can withdraw from the research at any point if they choose. ... **Consent must be free of coercion or undue pressure.**"[1440]

The very actions that the President proposed and are being advocated by DOJ and the FDA constitute coercion and undue influence as defined by the Belmont Report. Federal employees are being coerced into being vaccinated under the penalty of being fired. The threat is being made by the employer who controls their job. The employee is under pressure to please his employer who is exercising undue influence over the employees as he decides whether to take part in the experimental COVID-19 vaccine program. Nothing in Section 564 (21 U.S. Code § 360bbb-3) excuses compliance for an EUA with the standards of informed consent in the Belmont Report.

Padma Nambisan explains that the "[t]he Belmont Report has served as an ethical framework for protecting human subjects and its recommendations incorporated into other guidelines. It is an essential reference document for Institutional Review Boards (IRBs) that review and ensure that research proposals involving human subjects conducted or supported by the Human & Health Services (HHS) meet the ethical standards of the regulations."[1441]

The ethical standards memorialized in the Belmont Report have been incorporated into Federal Regulations. The basic HHS Policy for Protecting Human Research Subjects "applies to all research involving human subjects conducted, supported, or otherwise subject to regulation by any Federal department or agency that takes appropriate administrative action to make the policy applicable to such research. This includes research conducted by Federal civilian employees or military personnel." 45 C.F.R. § 46.101(a). The regulations at 45 C.F.R. § 46.101, et seq., were enacted under the legislative authority of 5 U.S. Code

§ 301, 42 U.S.C. 300v-1(b), and 42 U.S. Code § 289.

45 C.F.R. § 46.101(i) provided that "[u]nless otherwise required by law, department or agency heads may waive the applicability of some or all of the provisions of this policy to specific research activities or classes of research activities otherwise covered by this policy, provided the alternative procedures to be followed are consistent with the principles of the **Belmont Report.**"[1442] That means that no agency of the federal government may drop their ethical protections of research subjects below that which is provided in the Belmont Report. Essentially, the Belmont Report sets the minimum standards beneath which no executive branch department may fall. Indeed, § 46.101(c) provides that "[d]epartment or agency heads retain final judgment as to whether a particular activity is covered by this policy and this judgment shall be exercised **consistent with the ethical principles of the Belmont Report.**" Thus no matter what an executive agency does, it must comply with the ethical standard of the Belmont Report, which includes the informed consent provisions. There is no wiggle room. The ethical standards of informed consent apply to all medical research involving human subjects.

45 C.F.R. §46.116 codifies, in part, the informed consent standards of the Belmont Report. That section provides in pertinent part:

> (1) Before involving a human subject in research covered by this policy, an investigator shall obtain the legally effective informed consent of the subject or the subject's legally authorized representative.

> (8) A statement that participation is voluntary, refusal to participate will involve no penalty or loss of benefits to which the subject is otherwise entitled, and the subject may discontinue

> participation at any time without penalty or loss of benefits to which the subject is otherwise entitled;[1443]

45 C.F.R. § 46.111(a)(5) requires that the informed consent must be documented in writing. The written documentation requirement can be waived but there is no allowance for a waiver of the informed consent requirement.

> Informed consent will be appropriately documented or appropriately waived in accordance with §46.117.

Please note that informed consent must be voluntary. If there is a penalty or loss of benefits of any kind, the consent is not voluntary.

Nuremberg Code

It is a well-established principle that non-consensual human medical experimentation violates the Nuremberg Code and customary international law. That principle was considered authoritative and applicable when determining the application of the Alien Tort Statute.[1444] The gravamen of the Nuremberg Code has been adopted in the United States in the *Belmont Report* and under 45 C.F.R. § 46.101, et seq.

The President may try to argue that he is informing the recipients of "the consequences, if any, of refusing the administration of the product." That is a misinterpretation of the statute. It would open the statute up to an interpretation that virtually any penalty is authorized as a punishment for refusing the vaccine as long as the patient is informed. It would turn restrictive statutory language on its head and make it permissive. It is basic that consent must be voluntary. The one obtaining the consent cannot threaten, cajole, or use undue influence. Otherwise, the consent is not voluntary.

21 U.S. Code § 360bbb–3(e)(1)(A)(I) requires informed consent. Such consent must be voluntary to be consent at all. All understand that fact. Indeed, as mentioned earlier, Dr. Amanda Cohn, the Executive Secretary of the CDC's Advisory Committee on Immunization Practices, stated that vaccines authorized under an EUA, "are not allowed to be mandatory. So, early in this vaccination phase, individuals will have to be consented and they won't be able to be mandatory." Informed consent is not informed consent if it is given under compulsion. The President can no more say that all who refuse the vaccine will be jailed until they agree to be vaccinated as he can require all who refuse to be vaccinated to be fired, wear a mask, be tested for COVID, social distance from others, and be prevented from traveling. That all assumes that the codification of the Nuremberg code in the Belmont Report and federal regulations is inapplicable to the EUA vaccines. Since they are applicable, it is clear that President Biden's edict is unlawful. 45 C.F.R. § 46.116(a)(1) explicitly states that "refusal to participate will involve no penalty or loss of benefits to which the subject is otherwise entitled."

No Emergency Exception to Constitutional Rights

The President's order stems from a declared state of emergency. There is no emergency exception to the Constitution. The U.S. Supreme Court has stated the legal maxim that "[t]he Constitution was adopted in a period of grave emergency. Its grants of power to the federal government and its limitations of the power of the States were determined in the light of emergency, and they are not altered by emergency." *Home Building & Loan Ass'n. v. Blaisdell.*[1445]

In the context of unconstitutional COVID-19 restrictions under executive orders issued by the Pennsylvania Governor, the Honorable William S. Stickman explained in *City of Butler v.*

Wolf[1446]:

> [G]ood intentions toward a laudable end are not alone enough to uphold governmental action against a constitutional challenge. Indeed, the greatest threats to our system of constitutional liberties may arise when the ends are laudable, and the intent is good—especially in a time of emergency. In an emergency, even a vigilant public may let down its guard over its constitutional liberties only to find that liberties, once relinquished, are hard to recoup and that restrictions—while expedient in the face of an emergency situation—may persist long after immediate danger has passed.[1447]

Judge Stickman concluded:

> [I]n an emergency, the authority of government is not unfettered. The liberties protected by the Constitution are not fair-weather freedoms—in place when times are good but able to be cast aside in times of trouble. There is no question that this Country has faced, and will face, emergencies of every sort. But the solution to a national crisis can never be permitted to supersede the commitment to individual liberty that stands as the foundation of the American experiment. The Constitution cannot accept the concept of a "new normal" where the basic liberties of the people can be subordinated to open-ended emergency mitigation measures. Rather, the Constitution sets certain lines that may not be crossed, even in an emergency. Actions taken by Defendants crossed those lines. It is the duty of the Court to declare those actions unconstitutional.[1448]

The President lacks any authority to mandate vaccinations of any kind.

First Amendment and RFRA Claims

If a person asserts a sincere religious belief, it is not the function of courts to further explore that belief. In a First Amendment free exercise case, the U.S. Supreme Court, in *Thomas v. Rev. Bd. of Indiana*[1449], explained that "the resolution of that question is not to turn upon a judicial perception of the particular belief or practice in question; religious beliefs need not be acceptable, logical, consistent, or comprehensible to others in order to merit First Amendment protection."[1450] The *Thomas* Court further stated that "it is not within the judicial function and judicial competence to inquire whether the petitioner or his fellow worker more correctly perceived the commands of their common faith. Courts are not arbiters of scriptural interpretation."[1451] The *Thomas* Court required that for the government to intrude on a person's religious liberty requires the government to show that "it is the least restrictive means of achieving some compelling state interest."[1452] That is a very high hurdle indeed.

Furthermore, for the government to allow a medical exemption for the vaccine, which it necessarily must since there are immunocompromised persons who cannot be vaccinated under any circumstances, it must also necessarily allow a religious exemption. The U.S. Supreme Court in Church of the *Lukumi Babalu Aye, Inc. v. City of Hialeah*[1453] explained:

> Neutrality and general applicability are interrelated, and, as becomes apparent in this case, failure to satisfy one requirement is a likely indication that the other has not been satisfied. A law failing to satisfy these requirements must be justified by a compelling governmental interest and must be narrowly tailored to advance that interest.[1454]

That strict scrutiny hurdle is virtually insurmountable, and the *Lukami* Court said so.

> A law that targets religious conduct for distinctive treatment or advances legitimate governmental interests only against conduct with a religious motivation will survive strict scrutiny only in rare cases.[1455]

The two factors, neutrality and generality, are closely related concepts. The vaccine rules of President Biden appear to be neutral on their face, but they are arguably not neutral in application. As the court stated in *Ward v. Polite*,[1456] "[a] double standard is not a neutral standard."[1457] The *Ward* court called for strict scrutiny when a secular exemption to a rule is allowed, but a religious exemption is disallowed. Even if facial neutrality is conceded, that is not enough. As the *Lukumi* Court held, the rule must also be of general application to avoid strict scrutiny. Here, there are medical exemptions allowed. If a medical exemption is allowed, then the rule is, by definition, not of general application. The *Lukumi* Court explained:

> Where government restricts only conduct protected by the First Amendment and fails to enact feasible measures to restrict other conduct producing substantial harm or alleged harm of the same sort, the interest given in justification of the restriction is not compelling. It is established in our strict scrutiny jurisprudence that "a law cannot be regarded as protecting an interest 'of the highest order' ... when it leaves appreciable damage to that supposedly vital interest unprohibited."[1458] (citation omitted)

Judge (now U.S. Supreme Court Justice) Alito applied that standard in a case where police officers were given medical exemptions from a department beard prohibition rule but not religious exemptions. In *Fraternal Ord. of Police Newark Lodge No. 12 v. City of Newark*,[1459] the court ruled that providing medical exemptions while refusing religious exemptions indicates discriminatory intent, which cannot survive even intermediate, let alone strict scrutiny. Allowing a medical exemption while denying a religious exemption puts the vaccine requirement outside the category of general applicability. It would be necessarily discriminatory against religious beliefs, which requires heightened scrutiny. If the government is going to allow an exemption for a secular medical reason, it must also allow an exemption for a religious reason as well, unless there is a compelling government reason to discriminate against a person's freedom of religion in the least intrusive means possible. No such showing has been, nor can be, made here.

Feds for Medical Freedom v. Biden

Recall that on September 9, 2021, President Biden issued Executive Order # 14043.[1460] President Biden mandated that all federal employees get vaccinated against COVID-19 or lose their jobs. A non-profit organization, *Feds for Medical Freedom*, representing more than 6,000 federal workers and contractors, filed for a preliminary injunction. The United States District Court for the Southern District of Texas granted the request and issued a preliminary injunction.[1461] The injunction was based, in pertinent part, on the district court's finding that President Biden did not have the authority to require federal workers to be vaccinated. The *Feds for Medical Freedom* district court found that the President can regulate executive-branch employees' workplace conduct but not their general conduct. The court ruled that since getting vaccinated is not workplace conduct, the President has no authority to require vaccinations.

The *Feds for Medical Freedom* district court ruling was based partly on U.S. Supreme Court precedent in *NFIB v.*

OSHA.[1462] In that case, the U.S. Supreme Court ruled that COVID-19 is not a workplace risk. Rather, it is a "universal risk" that is "no different from the day-to-day dangers that all face from crime, air pollution, or any number of communicable diseases."[1463] Accordingly, the U.S. Supreme Court held that OSHA did not have the authority to require employees to vaccinate against COVID-19.

The *Feds for Medical Freedom* district court noted the curious fact that "even full-time remote federal workers are not exempt from the mandate." If the purpose of the mandate is to stop the spread of COVID-19 in the federal workplace, as alleged by the government, there seems no rational basis to mandate vaccinations for those who stay home.

More importantly, the Texas federal district court had little difficulty in finding that Article II of the Constitution does not grant any power to the President to impose medical procedures on civilian federal employees. The Government appealed the district court injunctive order and the district court ruling was reversed by a Fifth Circuit panel. That panel ruling was subsequently overturned by an *en banc* Fifth Circuit on March 23, 2023. A federal appeals court panel ruling involves three judges. An *en banc* federal appeals court decision involves all the judges for that particular circuit. In this case, nine judges. The *en banc* court affirmed the district court's ruling issuing the preliminary injunction.[1464] On December 11, 2023, the U.S. Supreme Court vacated the *en banc* 5th Circuit judgment, not on its merits, but on the theory that the injunction was moot because in May 2023 the Biden Administration rescinded its executive order mandating COVID-19 vaccines, and thus the injunction was unnecessary.[1465] Mooting the 5th Circuit ruling means that it is no longer considered precedent in future cases.

46 Moral Hazard

The COVID-19 vaccine is killing exponentially more than needed for the regulatory agencies to rise up and take it off the market. But, suspiciously, the COVID-19 vaccines are getting a pass. Why, with the carnage from the COIVD-19 vaccines so clearly apparent, is there still a push to vaccinate the population? The answer is simple. When the Swine Flu vaccine caused death and illness, the vaccine makers were liable for the damages. But now it is different. The drug companies now have immunity from civil liability for the injuries they cause through their vaccines.

The dangers of vaccines are inherent in the practice and cannot be avoided. Vaccines have been acknowledged by the U.S. Supreme Court and the U.S. Congress to be unavoidably unsafe. Congress passed the National Vaccine Injury Act (NVIA) of 1986, granting pharmaceutical companies immunity for injuries caused by the vaccines they manufactured. As explained by the U.S. Supreme Court in *Bruesewitz v. Wyeth*[1466], the reason for that protection is that Congress deemed vaccines to be unavoidably unsafe;[1467] thus no manufacturer would make a vaccine if they had to suffer the liability for injuries they would unavoidably cause.[1468]

Mary S. Holland explains the issue: "The success of the

national vaccine program has come at a cost. Some children are permanently disabled or die from their vaccine exposures. ... Between 1980 and 1986, people who claimed vaccine injury brought over three billion dollars of damages claims to U.S. civil courts against vaccine manufacturers."[1469]

In response to the litigation that held them accountable for the injuries caused by their vaccines, the vaccine manufacturers lobbied Congress, and in 1986 they were able to get the NVIA law passed. That law protected them from civil liability for injuries caused by vaccines that they manufactured.

The underlying legal reasoning of Congress for the 1986 NVIA law was a concept borrowed from the Restatement of Torts law that vaccines were "unavoidably unsafe." Holland explains that "[t]he Restatement describes all vaccines as 'unavoidably unsafe' products and implicitly recommended that manufacturers not be liable for injuries if doctors administered them properly."[1470]

The NVIA set up a system of government compensation for vaccine injuries that has, in practice, served more to prevent compensation than anything else. Robert F. Kennedy explains:

> Parents, legal guardians and legal representatives can file on behalf of children, disabled adults, and individuals who are deceased. According to the vaccine-injured and their loved ones, the program has failed miserably as a litigious, broken system where the injured are up against a government vaccine program, government owned vaccine patents, government health officials who administer the program and government paid attorneys from the Department of Justice. There is no judge, no jury of your peers and no discovery. Claimants feel the system is set up for their claims to fail.[1471]

The U.S. Supreme Court in *Bruesewitz*, supra, ruled that language in the statute categorically preempts even design defect claims against vaccine manufacturers. Holland explains that U.S. Supreme Court ruling "removed incentives for pharmaceutical corporations to conduct the extensive research and development necessary to ensure that FDA-approved vaccines remain as safe and effective as possible after licensure. FDA approval alone has not been a sufficient guarantee of drug safety, owing in part to the FDA's limited authority to compel further safety research after final approval."[1472]

Holland reveals the real-world consequences of the NIVA for vaccine recipients:

> [Gayle] DeLong showed that the proportion of people that reported a serious complication from a vaccine after [enactment of the NVIA in] 1986 is more than double the proportion of people who experienced a serious complication from a disease before a vaccine for it was available. The difference is statistically significant and is likely greater because of underreporting.
>
> DeLong's analysis suggests that the Vaccine Act "gave firms greater incentives to capture the regulator: If consumers cannot sue firms for product liability, the only barrier to sales is regulatory approval."[1473]

The NVIA protects vaccine makers from liability for "unavoidable" injuries caused by vaccines. The NVIA states in pertinent part:

> No vaccine manufacturer shall be liable in a civil action for damages arising from a vaccine-related injury or death associated with the administration

of a vaccine after October 1, 1988, if **the injury or death resulted from side effects that were unavoidable** even though the vaccine was properly prepared and was accompanied by proper directions and warnings.[1474]

In order to make sure the immunity from liability pill goes down easier for the public, the NVIA mandated that the Secretary of HHS "promote the development of childhood vaccines that result in fewer and less serious adverse reactions than those vaccines [presently] on the market."[1475]

That requirement was supposed to be performed by a task force made up of the "Director of the National Institutes of Health [NIH], the Commissioner of the Food and Drug Administration [FDA], and the Director of the Centers for Disease Control [CDC]."[1476]

The NVIA statute required that "within 2 years after December 22, 1987, and periodically thereafter, the Secretary [of HHS] shall prepare and transmit to the Committee on Energy and Commerce of the House of Representatives and the Committee on Labor and Human Resources of the Senate a report describing the actions taken pursuant to subsection (a) during the preceding 2-year period."[1477]

The NIH, FDA, and CDC scoundrels thumbed their noses at Congress. They violated the law by not filing the required reports with the U.S. Congress. Why did they not file the required reports? The only logical reason is that they did not meet as required, and they did not "promote the development of childhood vaccines that result in fewer and less serious adverse reactions than those vaccines [presently] on the market"[1478] as required by the statute.

That is clear evidence that the component agencies of HHS

(CDC, NIH, and FDA) have no interest in the development of safe vaccines for children.

Robert F. Kennedy Jr. discovered the scofflaws at HHS when he filed a Freedom of Information Act request with HHS requesting the reports prepared and transmitted to Congress as required by the NVIA. HHS refused to comply with the request. He sued HHS.[1479] After being served with the lawsuit, HHS admitted that they never filed any required reports with Congress.[1480] That means that the component agencies of HHS (CDC, NIH, and FDA) never formed the required task force and made no effort to see that vaccines were made safer.

The CDC, NIH, and FDA never met to develop a plan for safe vaccines for children. Why? Because CDC, NIH, and FDA know that the pharmaceutical companies have no interest making vaccines safe for children! Vaccines are unavoidably unsafe and the vaccine makers like it that way. Pharmaceutical companies get rich when people are made sick. It is a racket where they cause injury via their vaccines and then make the patent medicines to address the symptoms of the injuries they have caused. There was a fly in their ointment, and that was civil liability for the injuries they caused. The immunity granted by the NVIA solved that problem. Since the NVIA, the pharmaceutical companies have been off to the races creating one ineffective and unsafe vaccine after another.

As explained by Texans for Vaccine Choice, "[t]he [NVIA] removed all liability from vaccine manufacturers when their products injure or kill. Realizing that removing consumer accountability would eliminate any motivation for manufacturers to ensure their products are as safe and effective as they can possibly be, the Mandate for Safer Childhood Vaccines clause was added to the the Act as a check-and-balance." But we now know that there is no check-and-balance. Robert F. Kennedy Jr. explains:

This speaks volumes to the lack of seriousness by which vaccine safety is treated at HHS and heightens the concern that HHS doesn't have a clue as to the actual safety profile of the now 29 doses, and growing, of vaccines given by one year of age.[1481]

The CDC, when asked, was unable to provide any evidence that any childhood vaccine has ever been tested for safety using a placebo control. Indeed, Robert F. Kennedy Jr. points out that "not one of the 72 vaccines on the schedule mandated for our children, have been tested with a placebo." There is a reason. No vaccine could ever survive being tested for safety and effectiveness against a placebo. The pharmaceutical companies know that their vaccines are not only ineffective, they are injurious. Research has shown that childhood vaccines cause injuries.[1482] And that is by design. A design for which the U.S. Supreme Court has ruled the drug companies have immunity from civil liability.

The CDC, NIH, and FDA know it is a fool's errand to try to convince the drug companies to manufacture something safe when to do so would undermine the drug companies' pecuniary interests. The surreptitious goal of the drug companies is to make people sick through vaccines. That is why the CDC, NIH, and FDA had nothing to report to Congress regarding their efforts to develop vaccines with "fewer and less serious adverse reactions." The goal of the vaccine makers is to cause injury. The pharmaceutical companies, CDC, NIH, and FDA all know that vaccines will unavoidably cause injuries. They have no interest in mitigating the damage caused by vaccines because those injuries make the pharmaceutical companies rich through the patent medicines they sell to address the injuries caused by the vaccines.

For example, on December 13, 2021, Pfizer announced:

Pfizer will acquire Arena, a clinical stage company

developing innovative potential therapies for the treatment of **several immuno-inflammatory diseases**. Under the terms of the agreement, Pfizer will acquire all the outstanding shares of Arena for $100 per share in an all-cash transaction for a total equity value of approximately $6.7 billion. The boards of directors of both companies have unanimously approved the transaction.[1483]

Pfizer is acquiring a company that makes drugs that treat the very immuno-inflammatory injuries caused by Pfizer's COVID-19 vaccine. Arena has drugs in the pipeline to treat cardio inflammatory diseases like myocarditis; the Pfizer COVID-19 vaccine has become notorious for causing myocarditis.[1484] Also notable is Arena's development of a drug (Termanogrel) to address microvascular obstructions, which several doctors have identified as the root cause of many illnesses resulting from Pfizer's COVID-19 vaccine.[1485] For example, Dr. Charles Hoffe, MD — who practices in British Columbia, Canada — explained in very simple terms how the mRNA COVID vaccines create the spike proteins which cause widespread microscopic blood clotting that will eventually kill many people within three years of taking the shots.[1486] Pfizer now wants to get in on the action of offering overpriced patent medicines to give to desperate patients suffering from the deadly side-effects of their vaccine. How much more Machiavelian can you get?

Pharmaceutical companies, like Pfizer, act much like a firefighter who is also an arsonist. That sounds strange, but firefighter arson is a real phenomenon. In 1998, Glendale, CA, Fire Department Captain and Arson Investigator John Orr was convicted of four counts of murder and twenty counts of arson for fires he started dating back to 1984.[1487] Orr, like Pfizer, showed no remorse and did not much care who he killed. Orr is not alone. There are many historical accounts of arson fires perpetrated by firefighters. The U.S. Fire Administration reported:

Slowly, the fire service is shedding light on a situation that occurs rarely but which is nevertheless serious: some firefighters intentionally start fires. A very small percentage of otherwise trustworthy firefighters cause the very flames they are dispatched to put out.[1488]

Indeed, the U.S. Fire Administration reported that the South Carolina Forestry Commission (SCFC) said that 47 firefighters had been charged with arson in South Carolina alone. The U.S. Fire Administration report explained that the motives behind firefighter-perpetrated arsons varied. But one of the potential motives is financial. The arsonist firefighter may be seeking increased overtime pay, or he may be fighting fires for a paid-on-call fire service.

Pfizer acts like a firefighter who causes fires for financial gain, but instead of setting a house ablaze, it destroys the health of the vaccinated patient. Like the firefighter who enters the scene to put out the fire he started, Pfizer enters the scene to provide pharmaceutical drugs to treat the ailment caused by its vaccines. Pfizer then profits by supplying the drugs to treat the harm caused by its vaccines.

Pfizer is hell-bent on profiting from the injuries its vaccines cause. On October 5, 2022, Pfizer announced that it acquired Global Blood Therapeutics, Inc. (GBT), a biopharmaceutical company.[1489] The primary money-making drug from GBT is nOxbryta®, which treats sickle-cell anemia. But the company researches and develops drugs for all blood and hemolytic disorders. It is the ideal company for Pfizer to acquire because Pfizer's COVID-19 vaccine causes all manner of blood and hemolytic disorders.[1490]

On March 13, 2023, Pfizer announced that it had acquired one of the world's leading oncology companies, Seagen, for $43 billion. It has now been established that COVID-19 vaccines cause cancer.[1491] Indeed, as Eustace Mullins explains in his book, *Murder by Injection*, all vaccines cause cancer.[1492] Cancer was practically unknown before the scheme of compulsory vaccinations.[1493] Pfizer is "flush with windfall cash from its hugely successful BioNTech-partnered COVID-19 vaccine."[1494] Pfizer is deploying the billions of dollars in profits from its COVID-19 vaccine to acquire companies that address cancer caused by its COVID-19 vaccine. With the acceleration of new vaccines, Pfizer sees cancer treatments to address the cancers caused by vaccines as a growth industry. The acquisition of Seagan is all about making money. Pfizer states that cancer is a growing disease, and they want to profit from it:

> Oncology continues to be the largest growth driver in global medicine, and this acquisition will enhance Pfizer's position in this important space and contribute meaningfully to the achievement of Pfizer's near- and long-term financial goals.[1495]

Believe it or not, the COVID-19 vaccine manufacturers are protected from civil liability beyond the NVIA. The Food and Drug Administration granted emergency use authorization (EAU) for the COVID-19 vaccines. Because the COVID-19 vaccines administered in the U.S. under an EUA are not FDA-approved. The COVID-19 vaccines, being EUA vaccines, fall under the blanket civil liability protection provided by the PREP Act, which is an almost insurmountable barrier to just compensation for injuries caused by EUA vaccines.[1496] While certain of the COVID-19 vaccines have been approved by the FDA (Moderna's SPIKEVAX and Pfizer-BioNTech's Comirnaty), suspiciously, those approved branded vaccines are not available in the United States.[1497]

A "declared public health emergency" as described in the PREP Act is the legal landscape under which the COVID-19 vaccine is being developed. Under the PREP Act, there is a moral hazard where manufactures of the COVID-19 vaccines will be protected from any liability for injuries caused by their COVID-19 vaccines. They have no financial incentive to make a vaccine that is safe or effective. They can sit back and count their billions in profits as they injure the public with impunity. The demand for the product is guaranteed by a marketplace that is rigged by the U.S. and state governments, which will pay for the vaccine and then mandate that the public consume that vaccine. The attitude of the vaccine manufacturers toward the consumer who is injured is "oh well, too bad, so sad, it sucks to be you."

"For the love of money is the root of all evil: which while some coveted after, they have erred from the faith, and pierced themselves through with many sorrows." 1 Timothy 6:10.

The vaccine manufacturers are virtually immune from liability for their negligence in manufacturing vaccines.[1498] This creates a moral hazard where there is no financial incentive for the vaccine manufacturers to make their vaccines safe.

Mary S. Holland has written an excellent law review article in the Emory Law Journal that explains the moral hazard created by Congress in enacting the 1986 U.S. National Childhood Vaccine Injury Act, which established the National Vaccine Injury Compensation Program (NVICP). There is also the subsequent 2005 PREP Act which established the Countermeasure Injury Compensation Program.[1499]

The NVICP had the effect of protecting vaccine manufacturers from civil liability for injuries caused by vaccines that they manufactured. A plaintiff must first pass through the rigorous legal labyrinth of a special vaccine court to obtain compensation from the government. There are a few who push their cases and are able to win in that court.

The vaccine court wears down the plaintiffs. Thus, there are many thousands of vaccine injury victims who suffer in silence. You can expect the same with the COVID-19 vaccine. Indeed it will be even worse. In 2005, Congress passed a tort shield law, the PREP Act, to protect manufacturers of drugs and other "covered countermeasure[s]," including vaccines, from the risk of damages in the event of a declared public health emergency. The standards for recovery for injuries due to the COVID-19 vaccine under the PREP Act are even more onerous than those under the NVICP. "The Countermeasures Injury Compensation Program (CICP) is a Federal government program that administers the compensation Program specified by the Public Readiness and Emergency Preparedness Act (PREP Act)."[1500] There is a strict one year statute of limitations under the PREP Act. Except under rare exceptions, an injured person must file suit within one year of receiving the vaccine alleged to have caused the injury.[1501] Of the thousands of injuries suffered by people from vaccines, the CICP program has only compensated 29 claimants since 2005, paying out a total of $6 million.[1502]

Vaccine Manufacturers have little concern about the safety of the vaccines because when you are injured by their experimental vaccine, they will be immune from liability.

The vaccine manufacturers are cheering on vaccine mandates. That is why the vaccine manufacturers work so closely with the ultimate force, governments. The governments of the world are their real customers. The governments pay for the vaccines. And the governments will then force those overpriced, ineffective, and unsafe vaccines on their people. On July 22, 2020, the Wall Street Journal Editorial Board pointed out that "[l]ife probably won't return to normal until we have a widely distributed Covid-19 vaccine."[1503]

Endnotes

1. Vaccine Danger: Quackery and Sin, ISBN: 978-1-943056-17-0, https://shop.lightningsource.com/b/085?YxrEPNYbLui1eBOXTOxOx7tvWY3tZcjiABZC1MrpkmT.

2. Medicine man Edward Jenner was the father of modern vaccination!, https://www.reformation.org/vaccine.html (last visited on January 6, 2023). See also Charles Ceeithton, M.D., Jenner and Vaccination, 1889, http://www.whale.to/vaccines/creighton_b.html.

3. Eleanor McBean, The Poisoned Needle (1957), http://www.whale.to/a/mcbean.html.

4. Medicine man Edward Jenner, supra.

5. Charles Creighton, M.A., M.D., Encyclopedia Britannica, Ninth Edition, 1875-1889, http://www.whale.to/a/creighton4.html.

6. Id.

7. Id.

8. Eleanor McBean, The Poisoned Needle (1957), http://www.whale.to/a/mcbean.html, quoting Thomas Morgan, Medical Delusions (p. 48-49).

9. Eleanor McBean, supra.

10. Eleanor McBean, supra.

11. Eleanor McBean, supra, quoting Thomas Morgan, Medical Delusions (p. 48-49).

12. Smallpox Vaccination, CDC, https://www.cdc.gov/vaccines/vpd/smallpox/index.html (last visited on January 9, 2013).

13. Smallpox, Mayo Clinic, https://www.mayoclinic.org/diseases-conditions/smallpox/symptoms-causes/syc-20353027 (last visited on January 9, 2023).

14. Smallpox, Mayo Clinic, https://www.mayoclinic.org/diseases-conditions/smallpox/symptoms-causes/syc-20353027 (last visited on January 9, 2023).

15. Kerry Evans, From variolation to vaccination, Labroots, January 1, 2017, https://www.labroots.com/trending/microbiology/4928/variolation-vaccination.

16. R.B. Pearson, The Dream & Lie of Louis Pasteur (1942) (origninally titled: Pasteur, Plagiarist, Imposter), http://www.whale.to/a/b/pearson.html.

17. Burrough Wellcome & Co., Lecture Memoranda, 17th International Congress of Medicine, London, The History of Inoculation and Vaccination for the Prevention of Disease (1913).

18. Burrough Wellcome & Co., supra at 17-18.

19. Ralph W. Nicholas, The Goddess Sitala and Epidemic Smallpox in Bengal, Journal of Asian Studies (1981) 41 (1): 21–44. https://doi.org/10.2307/2055600.

20. Burrough Wellcome & Co., supra at 16.

21. Steve Halbrook, Vaccine Pandemic: Part 1: The Inoculation Controversy of the 1700s, Vaccines and Christianity, January 25, 2019, https://www.vaccinesandchristianity.org/2019/01/25/vaccine-pandemic-part-1-the-inoculation-controversy-of-the-1700s/, quoting James Martin Peebles, Vaccination a Curse and a Menace to Personal Liberty: With Statistics Showing Its Dangers and Criminality (Los Angeles, CA: Peebles Publishing Company, 1913), 14.

22. Steve Halbrook, Vaccine Pandemic: Part 1: The Inoculation Controversy of the 1700s, Vaccines and Christianity, January 25, 2019, https://www.vaccinesandchristianity.org/2019/01/25/vaccine-pandemic-part-1-the-inoculation-controversy-of-the-1700s/, citing William H. York, Health and Wellness in Antiquity Through the Middle Ages (Santa Barbara, CA: ABC-CLIO, 2012), 105, 106.

23. Steve Halbrook, Vaccine Pandemic: Part 1: The Inoculation Controversy of the 1700s, Vaccines and Christianity, January 25, 2019, https://www.vaccinesandchristianity.org/2019/01/25/vaccine-pandemic-part-1-the-inoculation-controversy-of-the-1700s/, quoting James Martin Peebles, Vaccination a Curse and a Menace to Personal Liberty: With Statistics Showing Its Dangers and Criminality (Los Angeles, CA: Peebles Publishing Company, 1913), 14-15.

24. Vaccinia (Smallpox) Vaccines, CDC, https://www.cdc.gov/vaccines/vpd/smallpox/hcp/vaccines.html (last visited on July 30, 2023).

25. Burrough Wellcome & Co., supra at 13-14.

26. Dominik Wujastyk, 'A Pious Fraud': The Indian claims for pre-Jennerian smallpox vaccination, https://www.academia.edu/451964/_A_Pious_Fraud_The_Indian_Claims_for_pre_Jennerian_Smallpox_Vaccination (last visited on July 30, 2023).

27. Dominik Wujastyk, supra.

28. Raymond Obomsawin, Ph.D., Immunity, Infectious Disease, and Vaccination. Video Re-Posted by Edward Hendrie Under Article Heading: The History of Vaccines Proving They Are Ineffective and Dangerous, May 26, 2021, https://greatmountainpublishing.com/2021/05/26/the-history-of-vaccines-proving-they-are-ineffective-and-dangerous/. See also, Ida Honorof and Eleanor McBean, Vaccination, The Silent Killer: A Clear and Present Danger (1977), https://archive.org/details/vaccinationsilen00hono, and Eleanor McBean, The Poisoned Needle (1957), http://www.whale.to/a/mcbean.html.

29. Eleanor McBean, supra.

30. Rene F. Najera, Papal Patronage: A History of Vatican Leadership in Vaccine Science and Public Health, The College of Physicians of Philadelphia, April 21, 2025, https://historyofvaccines.org/blog/papal-patronage-history-vatican-leadership-vaccine-science-and-public-health.

31. Rene F. Najera, Papal Patronage: A History of Vatican Leadership in Vaccine Science and Public Health, April 21, 2025, https://historyofvaccines.org/blog/papal-patronage-hist

ory-vatican-leadership-vaccine-science-and-public-health.

32. Devin Watkins, Pope Francis urges people to get vaccinated against Covid-19, Vatican News, 18 August 2021, https://www.vaticannews.va/en/pope/news/2021-08/pope-francis-appeal-covid-19-vaccines-act-of-love.html.

33. Luis F. Card. Ladaria, S.I., Prefect, S.E. Mons. Giacomo Morandi, Titular Archbishop of Cerveteri, Secretary, Note on the morality of using some anti-Covid-19 vaccines, Congregation for the Doctrine of the Faith, December 21, 2020, https://www.vatican.va/roman_curia/congregations/cfaith/documents/rc_con_cfaith_doc_20201221_nota-vaccini-anticovid_en.html.

34. Herbert Shelton, Vaccines and Serum Evils (c1940's), http://www.whale.to/vaccines/shelton3.html (last visited on August 3, 2023).

35. Id.

36. Steve C. Halbrook, Vaccine Pandemic: Part 2: Opposition to Vaccines by Doctors and Others in History, January 25, 2019, https://www.vaccinesandchristianity.org/2019/01/25/vaccine-pandemic-part-2-opposition-to-vaccines-by-doctors-and-others-in-history/, citing George Starr White, A Lecture Course to Physicians on Natural Methods in Diagnosis and Treatment: Aids to Human Helpers (Los Angeles, CA: George Star White, M.D., 1918), 1032.

37. Steve C. Halbrook, Part 2, supra, quoting Charles Creighton, Jenner and Vaccination: A Strange Chapter

of Medical History (London: Swan Sonnenschein & Co., 1889), 353.

38. Charles Creighton, M.A., M.D., Encyclopedia Britannica, Ninth Edition, 1875-1889, http://www.whale.to/a/creighton4.html.

39. Steve C. Halbrook, Part 2, supra, quoting George Starr White, A Lecture Course to Physicians on Natural Methods in Diagnosis and Treatment: Aids to Human Helpers (Los Angeles, CA: George Star White, M.D., 1918), 1032, 1033.

40. Steve C. Halbrook, Part 2, supra.

41. Steve C. Halbrook, Part 2, supra, quoting John W. Hodge, The Vaccination Superstition: Prophylaxis to be Realized Through the Attainment of Health, Not by the Propagation of Disease; Can Vaccination Produce Syphilis? (Niagara Falls, NY: 1902) (Read before the Western New York Homeopathic Medical Society In Buffalo April 11, 1902), 44.

42. Steve C. Halbrook, Part 2, supra, quoting James Martin Peebles, Vaccination a Curse and a Menace to Personal Liberty: With Statistics Showing Its Dangers and Criminality (Los Angeles, CA: Peebles Publishing Company, 1913), 303.

43. Dr. William Howard Hay, Address to The Medical Freedom Society (June 25, 1937), http://www.whale.to/v/hay1.html.

44. Brett Wilcox, Jabbed, How the Vaccine Industry, Medical Establishment and Government Stick It to You and Your Family, at 224 (2018).

45. Brett Wilcox, supra, chapter 1.

46. Brett Wilcox, Jabbed, supra at chapter 23.

47. Brett Wilcox, Jabbed, supra at chapter 23.

48. Brett Wilcox, Jabbed, supra at chapter 23.

49. Edward Hendrie, Antichrist: The Beast Revealed (2015).

50. Physician Group Practice Demonstration, Influenza Vaccination Strategies, CMS, at 6, https://innovation.cms.gov/files/x/pgp-flu-vaccination.pdf (last visited on April 10, 2023).

51. Readers sound off on coed classrooms, vaccines and 'Sesame Street', New York Daily News, November 7, 2015, https://www.nydailynews.com/opinion/nov-7-coed-classrooms-vaccines-sesame-street-article-1.2426184.

52. AMA Supports Tighter Limitations on Immunization Opt Outs, AMA, June 8, 2015, https://web.archive.org/web/20150614042738/https://www.ama-assn.org/ama/pub/news/news/2015/2015-06-08-tighter-limitations-immunization-opt-outs.page.

53. Rong-Gong Lin II, Rosanna Xia, Vaccines required for daycare workers under new California law. Los Angeles Times, October 13, 2015, https://www.latimes.com/local/lanow/la-me-ln-vaccines-required-for-daycare-workers-under-new-california-law-20151012-story.html.

54. Smallpox, CDC, https://www.cdc.gov/smallpox/index.html#:~:text=Thousands%20of%20years%20ago%2C%20variola,United%20States%20occurred%20in%201949. (last visited on February 11, 2023).

55. Dr. A.R. Campbell, M.D. -- Discoverer of the Cause of Smallpox, https://www.reformation.org/campbell.html (last visited on February 11, 2023).

56. Dr. A.R. Campbell, M.D., supra.

57. Smallpox, CDC, https://www.cdc.gov/smallpox/index.html#:~:text=Thousands%20of%20years%20ago%2C%20variola,United%20States%20occurred%20in%201949. (last visited on February 11, 2023).

58. Tomas S. Cowan and Sally Morell, The Contaigion Myth, at 30 (2020).

59. Vincent Ianelli, M.D., The Hospital Rock Engravings of Farmington, Connecticut, March 18, 2018, https://vaxopedia.org/2018/03/18/the-hospital-rock-engravings-of-farmington-connecticut/.

60. Toby Rogers, Pfizer COVID Vaccine Fails Risk-Benefit Analysis in Children 5 to 11, The Defender, November 5, 2021, https://childrenshealthdefense.org/defender/fda-pfizer-covid-vaccine-risk-benefit-analysis-nntv-children/.

61. Coronavirus disease (COVID-19): Herd immunity, lockdowns and COVID-19, World Health Organization, 31 December 2020, https://www.who.int/news-room/questions-and-answers/item/herd-immunity-lockdowns-and-covid-19.

62. Remarks by President Biden on the COVID-19 Response and the State of Vaccinations, The White House, April 21, 2021,

https://www.whitehouse.gov/briefing-room/speeches-remarks/2021/04/21/remarks-by-president-biden-on-the-covid-19-response-and-the-state-of-vaccinations-2/.

63. Koplan JP. Benefits, risks and costs of immunization programmes. Ciba Found Symp. 1985;110:55-68. doi: 10.1002/9780470720912.ch5. PMID: 3921321.

64. Miller NZ, Goldman GS. Infant mortality rates regressed against number of vaccine doses routinely given: is there a biochemical or synergistic toxicity? Hum Exp Toxicol. 2011 Sep;30(9):1420-8. doi: 10.1177/0960327111407644. Epub 2011 May 4. Erratum in: Hum Exp Toxicol. 2011 Sep;30(9):1429. PMID: 21543527; PMCID: PMC3170075, https://www.ncbi.nlm.nih.gov/pmc/articles/PMC3170075/.

65. Edmund Massey, A Sermon Against the Dangerous and Sinful Practice of Inoculation, at 6 (1722).

66. Edmund Massey, A Sermon Against the Dangerous and Sinful Practice of Inoculation, at 7 (1722).

67. Edmund Massey, A Sermon Against the Dangerous and Sinful Practice of Inoculation, at 13 (1722).

68. Edmund Massey, A Sermon Against the Dangerous and Sinful Practice of Inoculation, at 15 (1722).

69. The Satanic Temple Presents Satancon, https://archive.is/zf48L#selection-1389.0-1389.195 (last visited on February 22, 2023).

70. The Satanic Temple Presents Satancon, https://archive.is/zf48L#selection-1389.0-1389.195 (last visited on February 22, 2023).

71. Edmund Massey, A Sermon Against the Dangerous and Sinful Practice of Inoculation, at 14 (1722).

72. Edmund Massey, supra at p. 15.

73. Paul Offit, Biography, https://www.paul-offit.com/about-paul-offit-md (last visited on January 29, 2023).

74. Are Fetal Cells Used to Make Vaccines?, https://www.chop.edu/centers-programs/vaccine-education-center/video/are-fetal-cells-used-make-vaccines (last visited on January 29, 2023).

75. Patrick Reilly, *Assessing the Catholic Campaign for Human Development, Human Events,* November 20, 1998.

76. *Id.*

77. *Id.*

78. *Id.*

79. *Id.*

80. Katheryn Jean Lopez, *Catholic Campaign for Human Development: Still Entranced by Leftist Activism, Despite Growing Unrest, Human Events,* November 10, 2000.

81. *Id.*

82. *Id.*

83. *Id.*

84. *Id.*

85. KERRI HOUSTON AND PATRICIA FAVA, ALL GORE, AMERICA IN THE BALANCE, p. 59 (2000).

86. Walt Murray, A medical Mort Sahl, Press-Telegram, January 21, 1983, https://thepeoplesdoctor.net/wp-content/uploads/2016/01/ASC17293.pdf.

87. Brett Wilcox, Jabbed, How the Vaccine Industry, Medical Establishment and Government Stick It to You and Your Family (2018), quoting Robert S. Mendelsohn, Confessions of a Medical Heretic (1979).

88. Brett Wilcox, supra, quoting Robert S. Mendelsohn, Confessions of a Medical Heretic (1979).

89. Richard Moskowitz, The Case Against Immunizations, https://sites.google.com/site/doctorrmosk/the-case-against-immunizations (last visited on March 26, 2023).

90. Brett Wilcox, supra, quoting Olivier Clerc, Modern Medicine: The New World Religion: How Beliefs Secretly Influence Medical Dogmas and Practices (2004).

91. Brett Wilcox, quoting Oliver Clerc, supra.

92. Brett Wilcox, Jabbed, How the Vaccine Industry, Medical Establishment and Government Stick It to You and Your Family (2018).

93. Wilcox, supra.

94. Wilcox, supra.

95. Marco Cáceres, The Toxic Logic of Water and Applesauce, The Vaccine Reaction, December 8, 2015, https://thevaccinereaction.org/2015/12/the-toxic-logic-of-water-and-applesauce/.

96. Marco Cáceres, December 8, 2015, supra.

97. Claudia Kalb, Dr. Paul Offit: Debunking the Vaccine-Autism Link, Newsweek, October 24, 2008, https://www.newsweek.com/dr-paul-offit-debunking-vaccine-autism-link-91933.

98. Parents Pack Newsletter, Children's Hospital of Philadelphia, October 2005, archive of September 7, 2006 page, http://web.archive.org/web/20060907100428/http://www.chop.edu/consumer/jsp/division/generic.jsp?id=81553.

99. Andrew Zuckerman, How Panicked Parents Skipping Shots Endanger Us All, Wired, October 19, 2009, https://www.wired.com/2009/10/ff-waronscience/.

100. J.B. Handley, Dr. Paul Offit, The Autism Expert. Doesn't See Patients with Autism?, Age of Autism, October 26, 2009, https://www.ageofautism.com/2009/10/dr-paul-offit-the-autism-expert-doesnt-see-patients-with-autism.html.

101. Brett Wilcox, Jabbed, How the Vaccine Industry, Medical Establishment and Government Stick It to You and Your Family, at 20 (2018).

102. Dan Olmstead, The Age of Polio. Explosion., https://www.ageofautism.com/the-age-of-polio-explosion.html (last visited on February 11, 2023).

103. Dan Olmstead, supra.

104. Tomas S. Cowan and Sally Morell, The Contaigion Myth, at 30 (2020).

105. Jason Bergerhouse, The Germ Theory Is Bogus!, March 27, 2021, https://thrivespinecenter.com/the-germ-theory-is-bogus/, citing Jim West, Thomas S. Cowan, M.D., and Sally Fallon Morell.

106. Suzanne Humphries, M.D., Roman Bystrianyk, Dissolving Illusions, at 242 (2015).

107. Suzanne Humphries, M.D., supra.

108. Jim West, Pesticides and Polio: A Critique of Scientific Literature, August 2, 2003, https://somosbacteriasyvirus.com/pdf/polioyddt.pdf.

109. Jim West, supra.

110. Jim West, supra.

111. Jim West, supra .

112. Suzanne Humphries, M.D., Roman Bystrianyk, Dissolving Illusions, at 222-92 (2015).

113. Suzanne Humphries, M.D., supra.

114. Suzanne Humphries, M.D., supra.

115. Jim West, Pesticides and Polio: A Critique of Scientific Literature, August 2, 2003, https://somosbacteriasyvirus.com/pdf/polioyddt.pdf.

116. Dhiman R, Prakash SC, Sreenivas V, Puliyel J. Correlation between Non-Polio Acute Flaccid Paralysis Rates with Pulse Polio Frequency in India. Int J Environ Res Public Health. 2018 Aug 15;15(8):1755. doi: 10.3390/ijerph15081755. PMID: 30111741; PMCID: PMC6121585. https://pubmed.ncbi.nlm.nih.gov/30111741/.

117. Eleanor McBean, The Poisoned Needle (1957).

118. Jefferey Jaxen, 491,000 Children Paralyzed Over 17 Years, Indian Polio Vaccine Program Study Suggests, GreenMedinfo, September 13th 2018, https://greenmedinfo.com/blog/491000-children-paralyzed-over-17-years-indian-polio-vaccine-program-study-sugges.

119. Helen Branswell, 'The switch' was supposed to be a major step toward eradicating polio. Now it's a quandary, STAT, September 13, 2019, https://www.statnews.com/2019/09/13/the-switch-polio-eradication-quandary/.

120. Brian Shilhavy, Big Pharma and Corporate Media Finally Admit the Oral Polio Vaccine is a Failure – Causes Polio Instead of Preventing It, Health Impact News, Novermber 20, 2019, https://healthimpactnews.com/2019/big-pharma-and-corporate-media-finally-admit-the-oral-polio-vaccine-is-a-failure-causes-polio-instead-of-preventing-it/.

121. More polio cases now caused by vaccine than by wild virus, AP, November 25, 2019, https://apnews.com/article/health-united-nations-ap-top-news-pakistan-international-news-7d8b0e32efd0480fbd12acf27729f6a5.

122. Brian Shilhavy, Big Pharma and Corporate Media Finally Admit the Oral Polio Vaccine is a Failure – Causes Polio Instead of Preventing It, Health Impact News, Novermber 20, 2019, https://healthimpactnews.com/2019/big-pharma-and-corporate-media-finally-admit-the-oral-polio-vaccine-is-a-failure-causes-polio-instead-of-preventing-it/.

123. Polio Vaccination—Still Causing Polio After All These Years, Children's Health Defense, September 24, 2019, https://childrenshealthdefense.org/news/childrens-health/polio-vaccination-still-causing-polio-after-all-these-years/.

124. Measles, Mumps, and Rubella (MMR) Vaccination: What Everyone Should Know, CDC, https://www.cdc.gov/vaccines/vpd/mmr/public/index.html (last visited on February 12, 2023).

125. Measles, Mumps, and Rubella (MMR), supra.

126. Dave Mihalovic, Biologist wins Supreme Court case proving that the measles virus does not exist, SOTT, 27 January 2017, https://www.sott.net/article/340948-Biologist-wins-Supreme-Court-case-proving-that-the-measles-virus-does-not-exist.

127. Dave Mihalovic, SOTT, supra.

128. Dave Mihalovic, SOTT, supra.

129. Germany court orders measles sceptic to pay 100,000 euros, BBC, 12 March 2015, https://www.bbc.com/news/world-europe-31864218.

130. Dave Mihalovic, SOTT, supra.

131. Dave Mihalovic, SOTT, supra.

132. Dave Mihalovic, SOTT, supra.

133. Mike Adams, MMR measles vaccine clinical trial results FAKED by Big Pharma - shocking U.S. court documents reveal all, Janaury 25, 2015, https://graviolateam.blogspot.com/2017/02/mmr-measles-vaccine-clinical-trial.html. Complaint For Violation of the Federal False Claims Act, United States, ex rel., Stephen Kahling and Joan A. Wlochowski v. Merck, U.S. District Court for the District of Eastern Districe of Pennsylvania, Civil Action No. 10 4374, August 27, 2010, https://www.naturalnews.com/gallery/documents/Merck-False-Claims-Act.pdf.

134. Chatom Primary Care v. Merck, Civil Action No. 12 3555, Class Action Complaint, June 12, 2012, https://www.naturalnews.com/gallery/documents/Chatom-Lawsuit-Merck-Mumps.pdf.

135. Mike Adams, January 25, 2015, supra.

136. Joseph Mercola, Two Lawsuits Accuse Merck of Lying about Vaccine Effectiveness, Vaccine Impact, July 10, 2012, https://vaccineimpact.com/2012/two-lawsuits-accuse-merck-of-lying-about-vaccine-effectiveness/.

137. Milton J. Rosenau, M.D., Experiments to Determine Mode of Spread of Influenza, Journal of the American Medical Association, Volume 73, Number 5, August 2, 1919, https://zenodo.org/record/1505669#.X4DQ0y1q3mo.

138. Milton J. Rosenau, supra.

139. Eleanor McBean, The Poisoned Needle (1957).

140. Fredericks L. Gates, M.D., A Report on Antimeningitis Vaccination and Observations on Agglutinins in the Blood of Chronic Meningococcus Carriers, July 20, 2018, https://www.ncbi.nlm.nih.gov/pmc/articles/PMC2126288/pdf/449.pdf.

141. The 1918 "Spanish Flu": Only The Vaccinated Died, May 29, 2020, https://salmartingano.com/the-1918-spanish-flu-only-the-vaccinated-died/.

142. Eleanor McBean, Swine Flu Exposed, 1977, http://www.whale.to/a/mcbean2.html.

143. Eleanor McBean, Swine Flu Exposed, 1977, Chap. 2: Vaccination Condemned, https://www.mnwelldir.org/docs/vaccines/vaccinations_condemned_McBean.htm.

144. E.g., Gabor David Kelen, M.D., Lisa Maragakis, M.D., M.P.H., COVID-19 Vaccine: What You Need to Know, Johns Hopkins, Updated on November 1, 2022, https://www.hopkinsmedicine.org/health/conditions-and-diseases/coronavirus/covid-19-vaccine-what-you-need-to-know#:~:text=Yes%2C%20evidence%20continues%20to%20indicate,had%20COVID%2D19%20or%20not.

145. E.g., Richard Gray, This is how new Covid-19 variants are changing the pandemic, BBC, 27 January 2021, https://www.bbc.com/future/article/20210127-covid-19-variants-how-mutations-are-changing-the-pandemic.

146. Christine Massey, CDC confesses: our DHCPP "experts" have never obtained scientific evidence of any alleged "virus"... including "hantavirus", August 26, 2024, https://christinemasseyfois.substack.com/p/cdc-confesses-our-dhcpp-experts-have.

147. Id.

148. Sally Fallon Morell, Dr. Thomas Cowan, and Dr. Andrew Kaufman, Statement on Virus Isolation (SOVI). "SARS-CoV-2 Has Never Been Isolated or Purified", Global Research, May 17, 2022.

149. Sally Fallon, May 17, 2022, supra.

150. Affidavit of Christine Massey, November 30. 2021, https://drive.google.com/file/d/1axe-YpJIFlV0NRtm47XvYzhQAski_oac/view.

151. Christine Massey, FOIs reveal that health/science institutions around the world (208 and counting!) have no record of SARS-COV-2 isolation/purification, anywhere, ever, https://www.fluoridefreepeel.ca/fois-reveal-that-health-science-institutions-around-the-world-have-no-record-of-sars-cov-2-isolation-purification/ (last visited on September 2, 2022).

152. Pieter Borger, et al., Review report Corman-Drosten et al. Eurosurveillance 2020, November 27, 2020, https://cormandrostenreview.com/report/.

153. Kary B. Mullis, The Nobel Prize, https://www.nobelprize.org/prizes/chemistry/1993/mullis/facts/ (last visited on September 27, 2022).

154. Inventor of COVID test calls Fauci a liar, says it 'doesn't tell you that you're sick'. Narural News, March 17, 2021, https://www.naturalnews.com/2021-03-17-inventor-calls-fauci-a-liar.html#.

155. Id.

156. Apoorva Mandavilli, Your Coronavirus Test Is Positive. Maybe It Shouldn't Be, The New York Times, August 29, 2020, https://www.nytimes.com/2020/08/29/health/coronavirus-testing.html.

157. Amandha Vollmer, PCR Tests Show Positive Because They Respond to Genetic Material Present in All Humans, G. Edward Griffin's Need to Know, August 28, 2020, https://needtoknow.news/2020/08/pcr-tests-show-positive-because-they-respond-to-genetic-material-present-in-all-humans/?utm_source=rss&utm_medium=rss&utm_campaign=pcr-tests-show-positive-because-they-respond-to-genetic-material-present-in-all-humans.

158. Protocol: Real-time RT-PCR assays for the detection of SARS-CoV-2 Institut Pasteur, Parishttps://www.who.int/docs/default-source/coronaviruse/real-time-rt-pcr-assays-for-the-detection-of-sars-cov-2-institut-pasteur-paris.pdf?sfvrsn=3662fcb6_2 (last visited on September 2, 2022).

159. Homo sapiens chromosome 8, GRCh38.p14 Primary Assembly,

https://www.ncbi.nlm.nih.gov/nucleotide/NC_000008.11?report=genbank&log%24=nuclalign&from=63648346&to=63648363 (last visited on September 2, 2022).

160. CDC 2019-Novel Coronavirus (2019-nCoV) Real-Time RT-PCR Diagnostic Panel, Instructions for Use, at page 35, 7/21/2021, https://www.fda.gov/media/134922/download.

161. Edward Hendrie, The PCR Test is Generating False-Positive COVID-19 Results, November 19, 2020, https://greatmountainpublishing.com/2020/11/19/the-pcr-test-is-generating-false-positive-covid-19-results/.

162. Apoorva Mandavilli, *supra*.

163. Apoorva Mandavilli, *supra*.

164. Id.

165. Peter Andrews, *Landmark Legal Ruling Finds That Covid Tests Are Not Fit for Purpose. So What Do the MSM Do? They Ignore It*, RT, 27 November 2020, https://www.rt.com/op-ed/507937-covid-pcr-test-fail/.

166. Id.

167. Potential for False Positive Results with Antigen Tests for Rapid Detection of SARS-CoV-2 - Letter to Clinical Laboratory Staff and Health Care Providers, https://www.fda.gov/medical-devices/letters-health-care-providers/potential-false-positive-results-antigen-tests-rapid-detection-sars-cov-2-letter-clinical-laboratory (last visited on September 2, 2022).

168. Id.

169.*Potential for False Positive Results with Antigen Tests for Rapid Detection of SARS-CoV-2 - Letter to Clinical Laboratory Staff and Health Care Providers*, U.S. Food and Drug Administration, November 3, 2020, https://www.fda.gov/medical-devices/letters-health-care-providers/potential-false-positive-results-antigen-tests-rapid-detection-sars-cov-2-letter-clinical-laboratory.

170.Edward Hendrie, Authoritative Study Shows Zero Transmission of COVID-19 by Asymptomatic Carriers, December 22, 2020, https://greatmountainpublishing.com/2020/12/22/authoritative-study-shows-zero-transmission-of-covid-19-by-asymptomatic-carriers/.

171.Edward Hendrie, Proof that COVID-19 Statistics are Being Padded With Influenza Cases, February 3, 2021, https://greatmountainpublishing.com/2021/02/03/proof-that-covid-19-statistics-are-being-padded-with-influenza-cases/.

172.Edward Hendrie, February 3, 2021, supra.

173.Edward Hendrie, February 3, 2021, supra.

174.Edward Hendrie, World Council For Health Calls for Immediate Recall of All COVID-19 Vaccines, July 30, 2022, https://greatmountainpublishing.com/2022/07/30/world-council-for-health-calls-for-immediate-recall-of-all-covid-19-vaccines/.

175.David Zweig, The Most Important Test You've Never Heard Of, Substack, May 8, 2023, https://davidzweig.substack.com/p/the-most-important-test-youve-never.

176. Allyson M. Pollock, et al., Asymptomatic transmission of covid-19, The BMJ, 21 December 2020, https://www.bmj.com/content/371/bmj.m4851?utm_source=twitter&utm_medium=social&utm_term=hootsuite&utm_content=sme&utm_campaign=usage.

177. Cao, S., Gan, Y., Wang, C. et al. Post-lockdown SARS-CoV-2 nucleic acid screening in nearly ten million residents of Wuhan, China. Nat Commun 11, 5917 (2020). https://doi.org/10.1038/s41467-020-19802-w.

178. David Zweig, May 8, 2023, supra.

179. Catherine A. Hogan, et al., Strand-Specific Reverse Transcription PCR for Detection of Replicating SARS-CoV-2, CDC, Emerging Infectious Diseases, Volume 27, Number 2, February 2021, https://wwwnc.cdc.gov/eid/article/27/2/20-4168_article.

180. David Zweig, May 8, 2023, supra.

181. David Zweig, May 8, 2023, supra.

182. Chuck Callesto, CHD interview of Michael Yeadon, Twitter, May 8, 2023, https://twitter.com/ChuckCallesto/status/1655735185206329345.

183. Leading Report, Twitter, May 11, 2023, https://twitter.com/LeadingReport/status/1656654739659018240.

184. Thomas S. Cowan, M.D., The Contagion Myth, at 68 (2020), https://pattoverascienza.com/wp-content/uploads/2020/08/The_Contagion-MITH_W.pdf.

185. Derek M. Yellon and Sean M. Davidson, Exosomes, Nanoparticles Involved in Cardioprotection?, AHA Journals, 17 January 2014, https://www.ahajournals.org/doi/10.1161/circresaha.113.300636#pane-pcw-references.

186. Stefan Lanka, The Virus Misconception, WISSENSCHAFFTPLUS magazin 01/2020, https://truthseeker.se/wp-content/uploads/The-Virus-Misconception-Part-1-Measles-as-an-example-By-Dr-Stefan-Lanka.pdf.

187. The Contagion Myth, at 69 (2020).

188. The Contagion Myth, at 70 (2020).

189. The Contagion Myth, at 72 (2020).

190. Immunization: The Basics, CDC, https://www.cdc.gov/vaccines/vac-gen/imz-basics.htm (last visited on Janaury 5, 2023).

191. Vaccine Knowledge Project, University of Oxford, https://vk.ovg.ox.ac.uk/vk/vaccine-ingredients#Active%20ingredients (last visited on January 5, 2023).

192. Antigen, Oxford Learner's Dictionaries, https://www.oxfordlearnersdictionaries.com/us/definition/english/antigen (last visited on January 5, 2023).

193. Immunization: The Basics, CDC, https://web.archive.org/web/20210826113846/https://www.cdc.gov/vaccines/vac-gen/imz-basics.htm

(August 26, 2021 archive).

194. Vaccine Knowledge Project, University of Oxford, https://vk.ovg.ox.ac.uk/vk/vaccine-ingredients#Active%20ingredients (last visited on January 5, 2023).

195. Claire Gillespie, Fetal Cell Lines Were Used to Make the Johnson & Johnson COVID Vaccine—Here's What That Means, Health, March 4, 2021, https://www.health.com/condition/vaccines/johnson-and-johnson-fetal-cells-vaccine.

196. Vaccines, Merck, https://www.merck.com/research/vaccines/ (last visited on February 23, 2023).

197. Vaccines, Merck, https://www.merck.com/research/vaccines/ (last visited on February 23, 2023).

198. About our company, Merck, https://www.merck.com/company-overview/ (last viewed on February 23, 2023).

199. Hope Changes Lives, Pfizer, https://www.pfizer.com/ (last visited on February 23, 2023).

200. Pharmaceutical Products, The Janssen Pharmaceutical Companies of Johnson & Johnson, Infectious Diseases & Vaccines, https://www.jnj.com/healthcare-products/prescription. (last visited on February 23, 2023).

201. Moderna Reports Fourth Quarter and Fiscal Year 2022 Financial Results and Provides Business Updates, Moderna, February 23, 2023,

https://investors.modernatx.com/news/news-details/2023/Moderna-Reports-Fourth-Quarter-and-Fiscal-Year-2022-Financial-Results-and-Provides-Business-Updates/default.aspx.

202. Medicine, American Dictionary of the English Language, https://webstersdictionary1828.com/Dictionary/medicine (last visited on February 23, 2023).

203. Medicine, supra.

204. Pharmaceutical, American Dictionary of the English Language, https://webstersdictionary1828.com/Dictionary/Pharmaceutic (last visited on February 23, 2023).

205. Pharmaceutical, Online Etymology Dictionary, https://www.etymonline.com/search?q=pharmaceutical (last visited on February 23, 2023).

206. Pharmacy, Online Etymology Dictionary, https://www.etymonline.com/word/pharmaceutical#etymonline_v_14832 (last visited on February 23, 2023).

207. Vioxx: Revisiting Merck's History of Manipulating Science for Profit, Regardless of Public Health Risk, The New Atlantean, Substack, October 11, 2021, https://newatlantean.substack.com/p/vioxx-revisiting-mercks-history-of.

208. Snigdha Prakash, Timeline: The Rise and Fall of Vioxx, NPR, November 10, 2007, https://www.npr.org/2007/11/10/5470430/timeline-the-rise-and-fall-of-vioxx. Vioxx: Revisiting Merck's History of Manipulating Science for Profit, Regardless

of Public Health Risk, The New Atlantean, Substack, October 11, 2021, https://newatlantean.substack.com/p/vioxx-revisiting-mercks-history-of.

209. Gregory D. Curfman, M.D., Stephen Morrissey, Ph.D., and Jeffrey M. Drazen, M.D., Expression of Concern: Bombardier et al., "Comparison of Upper Gastrointestinal Toxicity of Rofecoxib and Naproxen in Patients with Rheumatoid Arthritis," N Engl J Med 2000;343:1520-8., N Engl J Med 2005; 353:2813-2814, DOI: 10.1056/NEJMe058314, December 29, 2005, https://www.nejm.org/doi/full/10.1056/NEJMe058314.

210. Snigdha Prakash, Timeline: The Rise and Fall of Vioxx, NPR, November 10, 2007, https://www.npr.org/2007/11/10/5470430/timeline-the-rise-and-fall-of-vioxx.

211. U.S. Pharmaceutical Company Merck Sharp & Dohme to Pay Nearly One Billion Dollars Over Promotion of Vioxx®, Merck to Pay $950 Million for Illegal Marketing, Department of Justice Office of Public Affairs, November 22, 2011, https://www.justice.gov/opa/pr/us-pharmaceutical-company-merck-sharp-dohme-pay-nearly-one-billion-dollars-over-promotion.

212. Pfizer's $2.3 Billion Settlement Leaves Victims in the lurch, Alliance for Human Research Protection, https://ahrp.org/pfizers-2-3-billion-settlement-leaves-victims-in-the-lurch/ (last visited on February 24, 2023).

213. Pfizer's $2.3 Billion Settlement, supra.

214. Justice Department Announces Largest Health Care Fraud Settlement in Its History, Pfizer to Pay $2.3 Billion for Fraudulent Marketing, September 2, 2009, https://www.justice.gov/opa/pr/justice-department-announces-largest-health-care-fraud-settlement-its-history.

215. Sammy Almashat, et. al., Twenty-Seven Years of Pharmaceutical Industry Criminal and Civil Penalties: 1991 Through 2017, Public Citizen, March 14, 2018, https://www.citizen.org/wp-content/uploads/2408.pdf.

216. Curis Wayant, Risperdal Lawsuit, Consumer Safety, https://www.consumersafety.org/drug-lawsuits/risperdal/ (last visited on February 24, 2023).

217. Johnson & Johnson to Pay More Than $2.2 Billion to Resolve Criminal and Civil Investigations, U.S. Department of Justice, November 4, 2013, https://www.justice.gov/opa/pr/johnson-johnson-pay-more-22-billion-resolve-criminal-and-civil-investigations.

218. Jack Fortier and Brian Mann, Johnson & Johnson Ordered To Pay Oklahoma $572 Million In Opioid Trial, NPR, August 26, 2019, https://www.npr.org/sections/health-shots/2019/08/26/754481268/judge-in-opioid-trial-rules-johnson-johnson-must-pay-oklahoma-572-million.

219. Jack Fortier and Brian Mann, Johnson & Johnson Ordered To Pay Oklahoma $572 Million In Opioid Trial, NPR, August 26, 2019, https://www.npr.org/sections/health-shots/2019/08/26/754481268/judge-in-opioid-trial-rules-johnson-johnson-must-pay-oklahoma-572-million.

220. Justice Department Announces Global Resolution of Criminal and Civil Investigations with Opioid Manufacturer Purdue Pharma and Civil Settlement with Members of the Sackler Family, Press Release, Ocober 21, 2020, https://www.justice.gov/opa/pr/justice-department-announces-global-resolution-criminal-and-civil-investigations-opioid.

221. Dina Kraft, Sackler Name Is Everywhere at Tel Aviv U., but Not the Opioid Controversy Plaguing the Family, Haaretz, March 4, 2019, https://www.haaretz.com/israel-news/2019-03-04/ty-article/.premium/at-tel-aviv-u-sackler-name-is-everywhere-not-the-opioid-controversy/0000017f-ea91-d0f7-a9ff-eed536350000.

222. Ronny Linder, Tel Aviv University Resists Pressure to Remove Sackler Name Over Opioid Crisis, Haaretz, November 18, 2021, https://www.haaretz.com/israel-news/2021-11-18/ty-article/.premium/tel-aviv-university-resists-pressure-to-remove-sackler-name-over-opioid-crisis/0000017f-e0e2-d7b2-a77f-e3e7fc580000.

223. Harriet Ryan, Lisa Girion and Scott Glover, OxyContin goes global — "We're only just getting started", Los Angeles Times, December 18, 2016, https://www.latimes.com/projects/la-me-oxycontin-part3/.

224. Harriet Ryan, December 18, 2016, supra.

225. Brett Wilcox, Jabbed, How the Vaccine Industry, Medical Establishment and Government Stick It to You and Your Family, at 43-44 (2018).

226. Memo From Alan Bernstein to Larry Hewlett, Regading DTP Vaccine, Wyeth, August 27, 1979, https://www.ageofautism.com/files/wyeth79.pdf.

227. Brett Wilcox, Jabbed, How the Vaccine Industry, Medical Establishment and Government Stick It to You and Your Family, at 43-44 (2018).

228. Brett Wilcox, Jabbed, How the Vaccine Industry, Medical Establishment and Government Stick It to You and Your Family, at 30 (2018), quoting Executive Reorganization and Government Research of the Committee on Government Operations United States Senate, Ninety-Second Congress, Second Session, pages 499-505, April 20-21 and May 3-4, 1972.

229. Brett Wilcox, Jabbed, How the Vaccine Industry, Medical Establishment and Government Stick It to You and Your Family, at 29 (2018), quoting Richard Carter, Breakthrough: The Saga of Jonas Salk, Trident Press, New York, 1965, pp. 318-319.

230. Brett Wilcox, Jabbed, at 28, supra.

231. The Satanic Temple Presents Satancon, https://archive.is/zf48L#selection-1389.0-1389.195 (last visited on February 22, 2023).

232. Brett Wilcox, Jabbed, How the Vaccine Industry, Medical Establishment and Government Stick It to You and Your Family, at 178 (2018)

233. Influenza, CDC, https://www.cdc.gov/nchs/fastats/flu.htm (last visited on April 6, 2023). See also, https://web.archive.org/web/20230406133028/https://

www.cdc.gov/nchs/fastats/flu.htm.

234. Glen Nowak, Planning for the 2004-05 Influenza Vaccination Season: A Communication Situation Analysis, archived September 5, 2004 page, https://web.archive.org/web/20040905095426/https://www.ama-assn.org/ama1/pub/upload/mm/36/2004_flu_nowak.pdf.

235. Laheij RJF, Sturkenboom MCJM, Hassing R, Dieleman J, Stricker BHC, Jansen JBMJ. Risk of Community-Acquired Pneumonia and Use of Gastric Acid–Suppressive Drugs. JAMA. 2004;292(16):1955–1960. doi:10.1001/jama.292.16.1955, https://jamanetwork.com/journals/jama/article-abstract/199672.

236. Jon Rappoport, Bombshell: 18 people died of the flu, not 36,000, September 8, 2012, https://www.naturalnews.com/037129_influenza_death_statistics_CDC.html.

237. Influenza: The Disease, CDC, archived September 27, 2008, page, https://web.archive.org/web/20080927045351/http://www.cdc.gov/flu/about/disease/.

238. Kenneth Stoller, CDC — Influenza Deaths: Request for Correction (RFC), https://aspe.hhs.gov/cdc-influenza-deaths-request-correction-rfc (last visited on April 6, 2023).

239. Seasonal Influenza: The Disease, CDC, archived April 7, 2010, page, https://web.archive.org/web/20100407203929/http://www.cdc.gov/flu/about/disease/.

240. Glen Nowak, Planning for the 2004-05 Influenza Vaccination Season: A Communication Situation Analysis, archived September 5, 2004 page, https://web.archive.org/web/20040905095426/https://www.ama-assn.org/ama1/pub/upload/mm/36/2004_flu_nowak.pdf.

241. Glen Nowak, supra.

242. Glen Nowak, supra.

243. Seasonal Flu Vaccines, CDC, https://www.cdc.gov/flu/prevent/flushot.htm#:~:text=Everyone%206%20months%20and%20older,the%2020 10%2D2011%20flu%20season. (last visited on April 7, 2023).

244. Brett Wilcox, Jabbed, supra at 180, citing Vittorio Demicheli, et al., Vaccines for preventing influenza in healthy adults, February 1, 2018, https://doi.org/10.1002/14651858.CD001269.pub6.

245. Brett Wilcox, Jabbed, supra at 181.

246. Brett Wilcox, Jabbed, supra at 181.

247. Congressional Record, 113th Congress, Vol. 159, No. 59, at E576, April 26, 2013, https://www.govinfo.gov/content/pkg/CREC-2013-04-26/pdf/CREC-2013-04-26.pdf.

248. Dan Burton, "Mercury in Medicine," Congressional Record (May 20, 2003): E1011, E1014, https://www.aapsonline.org/vaccines/mercinmed.pdf.

249. Influenza (Flu) Vaccine and Pregnancy, CDC, https://www.cdc.gov/vaccines/pregnancy/hcp-toolkit/flu-vaccine-pregnancy.html (last visited on April 7,

2023).

250. Brett Wilcox, Jabbed, supra.

251. Daniel Neides, Make 2017 the year to avoid toxins (good luck) and master your domain: Words on Wellness, Cleveland Clinic, January 6, 2017, https://www.cleveland.com/lyndhurst-south-euclid/2017/01/make_2017_the_year_to_avoid_to.html.

252. Statement from Cleveland Clinic, Affirming our support of vaccinations, Cleveland Clinic, January 8, 2017, https://newsroom.clevelandclinic.org/2017/01/08/statement-cleveland-clinic/.

253. Brett Wilcox, Jabbed, supra at 248.

254. Brett Wilcox, Jabbed, How the Vaccine Industry, Medical Establishment and Government
Stick It to You and Your Family, at 249 (2018).

255. Brett Wilcox, Jabbed, supra at 247-48.

256. Brett Wilcox, Jabbed supra at 183.

257. FLUARIX QUADRIVALENT (Influenza Vaccine) injectable suspension, for intramuscular use 2022-2023 Formula Initial U.S. Approval: 2012, at 16, https://www.fda.gov/media/79278/download.

258. FLUARIX QUADRIVALENT (Influenza Vaccine) injectable suspension, for intramuscular use 2022-2023 Formula Initial U.S. Approval: 2012, https://gskpro.com/content/dam/global/hcpportal/en_US/Prescribing_Information/Fluarix_Quadrivalent/pdf/FLUARIX-QUADRIVALENT.PDF.

259. Pfizer-BioNTech COVID-19 Vaccine Frequently Asked Questions, FDA, August 23, 2021, https://web.archive.org/web/20210830124725/https://www.fda.gov/emergency-preparedness-and-response/coronavirus-disease-2019-covid-19/pfizer-biontech-covid-19-vaccine-frequently-asked-questions.

260. Interim Public Health Recommendations for Fully Vaccinated People, CDC, March 8, 2021, https://web.archive.org/web/20210312000532/https://www.cdc.gov/coronavirus/2019-ncov/vaccines/fully-vaccinated-guidance.html.

261. Interim Public Health Recommendations for Fully Vaccinated People, CDC, March 8, 2021, https://web.archive.org/web/20210312000532/https://www.cdc.gov/coronavirus/2019-ncov/vaccines/fully-vaccinated-guidance.html.

262. FDA Takes Key Action in Fight Against COVID-19 By Issuing Emergency Use Authorization for First COVID-19 Vaccine, FDA, December 11, 2020, https://www.fda.gov/news-events/press-announcements/fda-takes-key-action-fight-against-covid-19-issuing-emergency-use-authorization-first-covid-19. See also Pfizer-BioNTech COVID-19 Vaccine Frequently Asked Questions, FDA, August 23, 2021, https://web.archive.org/web/20210830124725/https://www.fda.gov/emergency-preparedness-and-response/coronavirus-disease-2019-covid-19/pfizer-biontech-covid-19-vaccine-frequently-asked-questions.

263. Edward Hendrie, CDC Says Vaccines Are Ineffective in Stopping Infection and Spread of COVID-19, March 13, 2021, https://greatmountainpublishing.com/2021/03/13/cdc-s

ays-vaccines-are-ineffective-in-stopping-infection-and-spread-of-covid-19/.

264. Interim Public Health Recommendations for Fully Vaccinated People, CDC, March 8, 2021, https://web.archive.org/web/20210312000532/https://www.cdc.gov/coronavirus/2019-ncov/vaccines/fully-vaccinated-guidance.html.

265. Id.

266. FDA Takes Key Action in Fight Against COVID-19 By Issuing Emergency Use Authorization for First COVID-19 Vaccine, FDA, December 11, 2020, https://www.fda.gov/news-events/press-announcements/fda-takes-key-action-fight-against-covid-19-issuing-emergency-use-authorization-first-covid-19. See also Pfizer-BioNTech COVID-19 Vaccine Frequently Asked Questions, FDA, August 23, 2021, https://web.archive.org/web/20210830124725/https://www.fda.gov/emergency-preparedness-and-response/coronavirus-disease-2019-covid-19/pfizer-biontech-covid-19-vaccine-frequently-asked-questions.

267. Interim Public Health Recommendations for Fully Vaccinated People, CDC, March 8, 2021, https://web.archive.org/web/20210312000532/https://www.cdc.gov/coronavirus/2019-ncov/vaccines/fully-vaccinated-guidance.html.

268. Id.

269. Id.

270. Id.

271. Id.

272. Id.

273. Statement from CDC Director Rochelle P. Walensky, MD, MPH on Today's MMWR, CDC, July 30, 2021, https://www.cdc.gov/media/releases/2021/s0730-mmwr-covid-19.html.

274. Outbreak of SARS-CoV-2 Infections, Including COVID-19 Vaccine Breakthrough Infections, Associated with Large Public Gatherings — Barnstable County, Massachusetts, July 2021, Morbidity and Mortality Weekly Report, CDC, August 6, 2021, https://www.cdc.gov/mmwr/volumes/70/wr/mm7031e2.htm?s_cid=mm7031e2_w.

275. Rochelle Walensky Statement, July 30, 2021, supra.

276. Dr Birx admits they oversold vaccines- "I knew these vaccines were not going to prevent infection", Natural News, August 1, 2022, https://www.naturalnews.com/2022-08-01-dr-birx-admits-they-oversold-vaccines.html#. See also https://100percentfedup.com/dr-birx-admits-they-oversold-vaccines-i-knew-these-vaccines-were-not-going-to-prevent-infection/, July 22, 2022.

277. Meg Cunningham, Dr. Birx on her relationship with Trump: 'Respectful in public but very clear in private', December 16, 2020, https://abcnews.go.com/Politics/dr-birx-relationship-trump-respectful-public-clear-private/story?id=74760598.

278. Meg Cunningham, Dr. Birx on her relationship with Trump: 'Respectful in public but very clear in

private', December 16, 2020, https://abcnews.go.com/Politics/dr-birx-relationship-trump-respectful-public-clear-private/story?id=74760598.

279. Lawrence Smith, Dr. Deborah Birx applauds Beshear's 'proactive' handling of the coronavirus, WDRB, December 15, 2020, https://www.wdrb.com/news/dr-deborah-birx-applauds-beshears-proactive-handling-of-the-coronavirus/article_72b4f436-3f18-11eb-ac9d-4be187f7f7a6.html.

280. Immunity. (n.d.) Farlex Partner Medical Dictionary. (2012). Retrieved September 9, 2022, from https://medical-dictionary.thefreedictionary.com/immunity.

281. Immunity, Merriam-Webster Dictionary, https://www.merriam-webster.com/dictionary/immunity (last visited on September 9, 2022).

282. Immunity. (n.d.) McGraw-Hill Concise Dictionary of Modern Medicine. (2002). Retrieved September 9, 2022, from https://medical-dictionary.thefreedictionary.com/immunity.

283. Immunity, Merriam-Webster Dictionary, https://www.merriam-webster.com/dictionary/immunity (last visited on September 9, 2022).

284. Remarks by President Biden on the Importance of COVID-?19 Vaccine Requirements, Data Center, Clayco Construction Site Elk Grove Village, Illinois, October 7, 2021, https://www.whitehouse.gov/briefing-room/speeches-remarks/2021/10/07/remarks-by-president-biden-on-the

-importance-of-covid-19-vaccine-requirements/.

285. Special Committee on COVID-19 Pandemic, European Parliament, October 10, 2022, at 15:23:00, https://multimedia.europarl.europa.eu/en/webstreaming/special-committee-on-covid-19-pandemic_20221010-1430-COMMITTEE-COVI.

286. Id.

287. Joseph Choi, Fauci: Vaccinated people become 'dead ends' for the coronavirus, The Hill, May 16, 2021, https://thehill.com/homenews/sunday-talk-shows/553773-fauci-vaccinated-people-become-dead-ends-for-the-coronavirus/.

288. Mark Connors, Barney S. Graham, H. Clifford Lane, et al; SARS-CoV-2 Vaccines: Much Accomplished, Much to Learn. Ann Intern Med.2021;174:687-690. [Epub 19 January 2021]. doi:10.7326. Article posted in May 2021 at: https://www.acpjournals.org/doi/full/10.7326/M21-0111.

289. Joseph Choi, Pfizer chairman: We're not sure if someone can transmit virus after vaccination, The Hill, December 3, 2020, https://thehill.com/news-by-subject/healthcare/528619-pfizer-chairman-were-not-sure-if-someone-can-transmit-virus-after/.

290. Pfizer Inc. Tweet, @Pfizer, January 13, 2020, https://twitter.com/pfizer/status/1349421959222853633?lang=en.

291. Albert Bourla, @AlbertBourla, Twitter, June 8, 2021, from archive dated June 19, 2021, https://web.archive.org/web/20210619045416/https://twitter.com/AlbertBourla.

292. Dr. John Campbell, Simple questions for Pfizer, YouTube, August 5, 2023, https://www.youtube.com/watch?v=hN4o3lJR0yM&t=125s.

293. Sally Fallon Morell, Dr. Thomas Cowan, and Dr. Andrew Kaufman, Statement on Virus Isolation (SOVI). "SARS-CoV-2 Has Never Been Isolated or Purified", Global Research, May 17, 2022.

294. Peter Andrews, *Landmark Legal Ruling Finds That Covid Tests Are Not Fit for Purpose. So What Do the MSM Do? They Ignore It*, RT, 27 November 2020, https://www.rt.com/op-ed/507937-covid-pcr-test-fail/.

295. A Comparison of Official Government Reports Suggests the Fully Vaccinated Are Suffering Antibody Dependent Enhancement, The Expose, January 23, 2022, https://dailyexpose.uk/2022/01/23/world-government-data-shows-covid-vaccinated-suffering-ade/.

296. Edward Hendrie, The COVID-19 Gambit, Edward Hendrie's Newsletter, October 16, 2022, https://hendrie.substack.com/p/the-covid-19-gambit.

297. Vaccines and Related Biological Products Advisory Committee - 10/22/2020, U.S. Food and Drug Administration, at 2:33:40, https://www.youtube.com/watch?v=1XTiL9rUpkg&t=9220s.

298. Id.

299. Denise M. Hinton, Chief Scientist, FDA, Letter to Pfizer Inc., Attention: Ms. Elisa Harkins, August 23, 2021, https://www.fda.gov/media/150386/download.

300. FDA Approves First COVID-19 Vaccine, FDA, August 23, 2021, https://www.fda.gov/news-events/press-announcements/fda-approves-first-covid-19-vaccine.

301. Anjalee Khemlani, Fauci: Early COVID-19 Vaccines Will Only Prevent Symptoms, Not Block the Virus, Yahoo Finance, October 20, 2020, https://www.yahoo.com/now/fauci-vaccines-will-only-prevent-symptoms-not-block-the-virus-195051568.html.

302. Vaccines and Related Biological Products Advisory Committee - 10/22/2020, U.S. Food and Drug Administration, at 2:33:40, https://www.youtube.com/watch?v=1XTiL9rUpkg&t=9220s.

303. AXIOS on HBO: Moderna Chief Medical Officer Tal Zaks (Clip) | HBO, November 23, 2020, https://www.youtube.com/watch?v=po7qt9BZz0s&t=65s.

304. Vaccines and Related Biological Products Advisory Committee Meeting December 17, 2020, FDA Briefing Document, Moderna COVID-19 Vaccine, https://www.fda.gov/media/144434/download.

305. Fact Sheet for Healthcare Providers Administering Vaccine (Vaccination Providers) Emergency Use

Authorization (Eua) of the Pfizer-biontech COVID-19 Vaccine to Prevent Coronavirus, Disease 2019 (Covid-19), 12 August 2021, https://www.fda.gov/media/144413/download.

306. Id.

307. Id.

308. Frequently Asked Questions about COVID-19 Vaccination, FDA, updated November 23, 2021, archive page from December 1, 2021, https://web.archive.org/web/20211201021445/https://www.cdc.gov/coronavirus/2019-ncov/vaccines/faq.html.

309. Id.

310. Frequently Asked Questions about COVID-19 Vaccination, FDA, updated April 19, 2023, https://www.cdc.gov/coronavirus/2019-ncov/vaccines/faq.html.

311. Benefits of Getting A COVID-19 Vaccine, CDC, Updated December 22, 2022, https://www.cdc.gov/coronavirus/2019-ncov/vaccines/vaccine-benefits.html.

312. Andrew Court, Democrat Congressman Stephen Lynch, 65, Tests Positive to COVID-19 after Receiving Both Doses of Pfizer's Vaccine, The Daily Mail, January 30, 2021, https://www.dailymail.co.uk/news/article-9205321/Rep-Stephen-Lynch-65-tests-positive-COVID-19-receiving-doses-Pfizer-vaccine.html?ito=push-notification&ci=73039&si=23070647.

313. Andrew Court, Democrat Congressman Stephen Lynch, 65, Tests Positive to COVID-19 after Receiving Both Doses of Pfizer's Vaccine, The Daily Mail, January 30, 2021, https://www.dailymail.co.uk/news/article-9205321/Rep-Stephen-Lynch-65-tests-positive-COVID-19-receiving-doses-Pfizer-vaccine.html?ito=push-notification&ci=73039&si=23070647.

314. Pfizer-BioNTech COVID-19 Vaccine Frequently Asked Questions, FDA, https://www.fda.gov/emergency-preparedness-and-response/mcm-legal-regulatory-and-policy-framework/pfizer-biontech-covid-19-vaccine-frequently-asked-questions (last visited on August 20, 2021).

315. Id.

316. 60% of People Being Admitted to UK Hospitals Are Unvaccinated - Adviser, Reuters, July 19, 2021, https://www.reuters.com/business/healthcare-pharmaceuticals/60-people-being-admitted-uk-hospitals-had-two-covid-jabs-adviser-2021-07-19/.

317. Pfizer-BioNTech COVID-19 Vaccine Frequently Asked Questions, FDA, https://www.fda.gov/emergency-preparedness-and-response/mcm-legal-regulatory-and-policy-framework/pfizer-biontech-covid-19-vaccine-frequently-asked-questions (last visited on August 20, 2021). See also Pfizer-BioNTech COVID-19 Vaccine Frequently Asked Questions, FDA, August 23, 2021, https://web.archive.org/web/20210830124725/https://www.fda.gov/emergency-preparedness-and-response/coronavirus-disease-2019-covid-19/pfizer-biontech-covid-19-vaccine-frequently-asked-questions.

318. Interim Public Health Recommendations for Fully Vaccinated People, CDC, August 19, 2021, https://www.cdc.gov/coronavirus/2019-ncov/vaccines/fully-vaccinated-guidance.html.

319. Pien Huang, et al., COVID Booster Shots Are Coming. Here's What You Need To Know, NPR, August 19, 2021, https://www.npr.org/sections/health-shots/2021/08/19/1028594715/covid-booster-shots-are-coming-heres-what-you-need-to-know.

320. Emily Kopp, CDC report shows vaccinated people can spread COVID-19, Roll Call, July 30, 2021, https://www.rollcall.com/2021/07/30/cdc-report-shows-vaccinated-people-can-spread-covid-19/.

321. SARS-CoV-2 Variants of Concern and Variants under Investigation in England, Technical Briefing, Public Health England, 18 June 2021, 16https://assets.publishing.service.gov.uk/government/uploads/system/uploads/attachment_data/file/1001359/Variants_of_Concern_VOC_Technical_Briefing_16.pdf.

322. Id. at 12.

323. Suzanne Humphries, Dissolving Illusions, at 74 (2013).

324. Interim Clinical Considerations for Use of COVID-19 Vaccines Currently Approved or Authorized in the United States, CDC, Last Reviewed by the CDC on March 17, 2023, https://www.cdc.gov/vaccines/covid-19/clinical-considerations/interim-considerations-us.html.

325. Helen Millar, COVID-19 vaccine: Does it stop people getting the virus?, Medical News Today, October 27, 2022, https://www.medicalnewstoday.com/articles/mucus-in-chest-that-wont-come-up-covid#is-a-productive-cough-common.

326. Helen Millar, October 27, 2022, supra.

327. Ensuring COVID-19 Vaccine Safety in the US, CDC, Updated Dec. 22, 2022, https://www.cdc.gov/coronavirus/2019-ncov/vaccines/safety.html#print.

328. Dr. John Campbell, Staff increased 20 fold, March 28, 2023, https://www.youtube.com/watch?v=kELiEGA3q4I.

329. Dr. John Campbell, March 28, 2023, supra.

330. Dr. John Campbell, March 28, 2023, supra.

331. Dr. John Campbell, March 28, 2023, supra.

332. Dr. John Campbell, March 28, 2023, supra.

333. Gabor David Kelen, M.D., Lisa Maragakis, M.D., M.P.H., COVID-19 Vaccine: What You Need to Know, Johns Hopkins, March 30, 2021, archived version of article, https://web.archive.org/web/20210330002308/https://www.hopkinsmedicine.org/health/conditions-and-diseases/coronavirus/covid-19-vaccine-what-you-need-to-know.

334. Id.

335. UK Government quietly confirms Triple+ Vaccinated accounted for 92% of COVID Deaths in 2022, The Expose, March 26, 2023, https://expose-news.com/2023/03/26/uk-gov-confirms-vaccinated-accounted-for-92-percent-of-covid-deaths-in-2022/.

336. Gabor David Kelen, M.D., Lisa Maragakis, M.D., M.P.H., COVID-19 Vaccine: What You Need to Know, Johns Hopkins, Updated on November 1, 2022, https://www.hopkinsmedicine.org/health/conditions-and-diseases/coronavirus/covid-19-vaccine-what-you-need-to-know#:~:text=Yes%2C%20evidence%20continues%20to%20indicate,had%20COVID%2D19%20or%20not.

337. Fiona P. Havers, et al., Laboratory-Confirmed COVID-19–Associated Hospitalizations Among Adults During SARS-CoV-2 Omicron BA.2 Variant Predominance — COVID-19–Associated Hospitalization Surveillance Network, 14 States, June 20, 2021–May 31, 2022, CDC, August 26, 2022, https://www.cdc.gov/mmwr/volumes/71/wr/mm7134a3.htm?s_cid=mm7134a3_x.

338. Fiona P. Havers, et al., supra.

339. Edward Hendrie, The CDC Falsely Counts Vaccinated COVID Deaths as Unvaccinated COVID Deaths, December 27, 2021, https://greatmountainpublishing.com/2021/12/27/the-cdc-falsely-counts-vaccinated-covid-deaths-as-unvaccinated-covid-deaths/.

340. Jennifer B. Griffin, Ph.D., et al., SARS-CoV-2 Infections and Hospitalizations Among Persons Aged =16 Years, by Vaccination Status — Los Angeles

County, California, May 1–July 25, 2021, Morbidity and Mortality Weekly Report / August 27, 2021 / Vol. 70 / No. 34, https://www.cdc.gov/mmwr/volumes/70/wr/pdfs/mm7034e5-H.pdf.

341. Monitoring COVID-19 Vaccine Effectiveness, CDC, https://www.cdc.gov/coronavirus/2019-ncov/vaccines/effectiveness/how-they-work.html. The language that had been posted on the CDC website on or before September 3, 2021 at that URL, has been deleted from the CDC website. But See the Washoe County Health District COVID-19 Facts, which quotes from the language since deleted from the CDC website, https://experience.arcgis.com/experience/6b88f7dff38a44d8b174e89a7ce25352/page/page_4/. (last visited on February 3, 2023).

342. Joseph Mercola, Shockingly, CDC Now Lists Vaccinated Deaths as Unvaccinated, Flyby News, September 15, 2021, https://flybynews.wordpress.com/2021/09/15/shockingly-cdc-now-lists-vaccinated-deaths-as-unvaccinated/. Article also found at: https://greatmountainpublishing.com/2021/12/27/the-cdc-falsely-counts-vaccinated-covid-deaths-as-unvaccinated-covid-deaths/.

343. Joseph Mercola, September 15, 2021, supra.

344. Joseph Mercola, September 15, 2021, supra.

345. Edward Hendrie, "Breakthrough" Cases in the Vaccinated Population Are Actually Symptoms of Antibody-Dependent Enhancement Caused by the Covid-19 Vaccines, September 1, 2021,

https://greatmountainpublishing.com/2021/09/01/breakthrough-cases-in-the-vaccinated-population-are-actually-symptoms-of-antibody-dependent-enhancement-caused-by-the-covid-19-vaccines/.

346. Nobel Prize Winner French Virologist Luc Montagnier Explains How COVID-19 Vaccines Are Creating Variants, May 21, 2021, https://greatgameindia.com/covid-19-vaccines-creating-variants/.

347. 80% of the nuns in this Kentucky convent got COVID 2 days after vaccine, Lifesite News, February 25, 2021, https://www.lifesitenews.com/news/several-nuns-die-after-taking-first-shot-of-covid-vaccine/.

348. Washoe County COVID-19 Facts, https://experience.arcgis.com/experience/6b88f7dff38a44d8b174e89a7ce25352/page/page_4/. (last visited on February 3, 2023). See also Agenda Packet, Office of the District Health Officer District Health Officer Staff Report Board Meeting Date: July 22, 2021, Appendix, at page 421, https://www.washoecounty.gov/health/about-us/board-committees/district-board-of-health/2021/files/Agenda-Packet-07-22-2021.pdf.

349. COVID-19 Vaccine Breakthrough Case Investigation and Reporting, CDC, https://www.cdc.gov/vaccines/covid-19/health-departments/breakthrough-cases.html (last visited on August 28, 2021).

350. *CDC 2019-Novel Coronavirus (2019-nCoV) Real-Time RT-PCR Diagnostic Panel*, Catalog # 2019-nCoVEUA-01 1000 reactions, 7, 13, 2020,

https://www.fda.gov/media/134922/download.

351. Vincent Racaniello, *TWiV 641: COVID-19 with Dr. Anthony Fauci,* July 16, 2020, https://www.youtube.com/watch?time_continue=260&v=a_Vy6fgaBPE&feature=emb_logo.

352. COVID-19 Vaccine Breakthrough Case Investigation and Reporting, CDC, https://www.cdc.gov/vaccines/covid-19/health-departments/breakthrough-cases.html (last visited on August 28, 2021).

353. Joseph Mercola, September 15, 2021, supra.

354. Kit Knightly, How the CDC Is Manipulating Data to Prop-up "Vaccine Effectiveness," Off Guardian, May 18, 2021, https://off-guardian.org/2021/05/18/how-the-cdc-is-manipulating-data-to-prop-up-vaccine-effectiveness/.

355. Deaths by Vaccination Status, England, Office for National Statistics, Dataset, https://www.ons.gov.uk/peoplepopulationandcommunity/birthsdeathsandmarriages/deaths/datasets/deathsbyvaccinationstatusengland (last visited on November 22, 2021).

356. Alex Berenson, Vaccinated English Adults under 60 Are Dying at Twice the Rate of Unvaccinated People the Same Age, Novemer 20, 2021, https://alexberenson.substack.com/p/vaccinated-english-adults-under-60.

357. Alex Berenson, November 20, 2021, supra.

358. Alex Berenson, November 20, 2021, supra.

359. Deaths by Vaccination Status, England, UK Office for National Statistics, https://www.ons.gov.uk/peoplepopulationandcommunity/birthsdeathsandmarriages/deaths/datasets/deathsbyvaccinationstatusengland (last visited on November 26, 2021).

360. James Lyons-Weiler, et al., Relative Incidence of Office Visits and Cumulative Rates of Billed Diagnoses Along the Axis of Vaccination, 14 November 2020, https://www.mdpi.com/1660-4601/17/22/8674. On 16 July 2021, the MDPI retracted the article with the following cryptic notice. "The journal retracts the article 'Relative Incidence of Office Visits and Cumulative Rates of Billed Diagnoses along the Axis of Vaccination' cited above. Following publication, concerns were brought to the attention of the editorial office regarding the validity of the conclusions of the published research. Adhering to our complaints procedure, an investigation was conducted that raised several methodological issues and confirmed that the conclusions were not supported by strong scientific data. The article is therefore retracted. This retraction is approved by the Editor in Chief of the journal. The authors did not agree to this retraction." https://www.mdpi.com/1660-4601/18/15/7754/htm. The MDPI did not indicate what were the "methodological issues" or specify how the conclusions "were not supported by strong scientific data." That lack of specificity for such an extraordinary action suggests the retraction of the article by the MDPI was not due to methodological issues or that it was not supported by strong scientific data but was rather due to financial and political pressure put on MDPI.

361. Gunter Kampf, The Epidemiological Relevance of the COVID-19-Vaccinated Population Is Increasing, Tha Lancet, November 19, 2021, https://www.thelancet.com/journals/lanepe/article/PIIS 2666-7762(21)00258-1/fulltext.

362. Gunter Kampf, November 19, 2021, supra.

363. Robert Koch-Institut. Wochentlicher Lagebericht des RKI zur Coronavirus-Krank-heit-2019 (COVID-19). AKTUALISIERTER STAND FUR DEUTSCHLAND 22. Juli 2021. https://www.rki.de/DE/Content/InfAZ/N/Neuartiges_Coronavirus/Situationsberichte/Wochenbericht/Wochenbericht_2021-07-22.pdf?__blob=publicationFile (accessed 28. September 2021).

364. The Robert Koch Institute, Tasks and Aims, https://www.rki.de/EN/Content/Institute/institute_node.html;jsessionid=A6B6D73428CC04A2F8D992C80F881F61.internet061 (last visited on December 31, 2021).

365. Stunning Omicron Data Emerges From Germany Showing Negative COVID-19 Vaccine Efficacy, January 1, 2022, https://lorphicweb.com/stunning-omicron-data-emerges-from-germany-showing-negative-covid-19-vaccine-efficacy/.

366. Id.

367. Ethan Huff, Lancet Science Paper Destroys False Narrative of COVID Vaccines, Reveals Vaccinated Are Perpetuating the Pandemic, NEWSTARGET, December 21, 2021, https://www.newstarget.com/2021-12-21-lancet-paper-destroys-false-narrative-covid-vaccines.html.

368. Coronavirus Disease 2019 (COVID-19) Outbreak, Maryland Department of Health, https://coronavirus.maryland.gov/#Vaccine (last visited on October 24, 2021).

369. Joe Hoft, EXCLUSIVE: Analysis Shows More COVID Deaths in 2021 than 2020 with Large Percent of 2021 Deaths Fully Vaccinated, October 22, 2021, https://www.thegatewaypundit.com/2021/10/exclusive-analysis-shows-covid-deaths-2021-2020-large-percent-2021-deaths-fully-vaccinated/?utm_source=Email&utm_medium=the-gateway-pundit&utm_campaign=daily pm&utm_content=daily.

370. Joe Hoft, EXCLUSIVE: Analysis Shows More COVID Deaths in 2021 than 2020 with Large Percent of 2021 Deaths Fully Vaccinated, October 22, 2021, https://www.thegatewaypundit.com/2021/10/exclusive-analysis-shows-covid-deaths-2021-2020-large-percent-2021-deaths-fully-vaccinated/?utm_source=Email&utm_medium=the-gateway-pundit&utm_campaign=daily pm&utm_content=daily.

371. Jim Hoft, Former CDC Director Robert Redfield Claims More Than 40% COVID-19 Deaths in Maryland Were Fully Vaccinated, The Gateway Pundit, October 27, 2021, https://www.thegatewaypundit.com/2021/10/former-cdc-director-robert-redfield-claims-40-deaths-cases-maryland-fully-vaccinated/.

372. Jim Hoft, October 27, 2021, supra.

373. Coronavirus Disease 2019 (COVID-19) Outbreak, Maryland Department of Health, https://coronavirus.maryland.gov/#Vaccine (last visited on October 24, 2021).

374. Joe Hoft, EXCLUSIVE: Analysis Shows More COVID Deaths in 2021 than 2020 with Large Percent of 2021 Deaths Fully Vaccinated, October 22, 2021, https://www.thegatewaypundit.com/2021/10/exclusive-analysis-shows-covid-deaths-2021-2020-large-percent-2021-deaths-fully-vaccinated/?utm_source=Email&utm_medium=the-gateway-pundit&utm_campaign=dailypm&utm_content=daily.

375. Joe Hoft, October 22, 2021, supra.

376. The United Kingdom Health Security Agency COVID-19 Vaccine Surveillance Report, Publishing Reference: GOV-10158, at 4-6, October 14, 2021, https://assets.publishing.service.gov.uk/government/uploads/system/uploads/attachment_data/file/1025358/Vaccine-surveillance-report-week-41.pdf

377. Alex Berenson, Vaccinated English Adults under 60 Are Dying at Twice the Rate of Unvaccinated People the Same Age, Novemer 20, 2021, https://alexberenson.substack.com/p/vaccinated-english-adults-under-60.

378. Dr. Anthony Fauci: Fully Vaccinated People Carry As Much Virus As Unvaccinated For Delta Variant, MSNBC, July 27, 2021, https://rumble.com/vlt9b1-dr.-anthony-fauci-fully-vaccinated-people-carry-as-much-virus-as-unvaccinat.html.

379. Kyle Becker, Becker News, CDC Director Changes Her Story, Now Admits COVID Vaccines Don't Prevent Virus Transmission, August 7, 2021, https://beckernews.com/cdc-director-changes-her-story-now-admits-covid-vaccines-dont-prevent-virus-transmission-40754/.

380. Yasmeen Abutaleb, et.al., The War Has Changed': Internal CDC Document Urges New Messaging, Warns Delta Infections Likely More Severe, The Washington Post, July 29, 2021, https://www.washingtonpost.com/health/2021/07/29/cdc-mask-guidance/.

381. Boris Johnson Admits That Covid-1984 Jab DOES NOT Protect You From Anything - So What Is The Point?, April 9, 2021, https://www.bitchute.com/video/OQBS0IAIrXEa/.

382. Andrew White, UK's Boris Johnson Admits Vaccines Do Not Prevent Contracting, Spreading COVID-19, National File, October 23, 2021, https://nationalfile.com/uks-boris-johnson-admits-vaccines-do-not-prevent-contracting-spreading-covid-19/.

383. Remarks by President Biden Laying Out the Next Steps in Our Effort to Get More Americans Vaccinated and Combat the Spread of the Delta Variant, July 29, 2021, 4:23 p.m. EDT, https://www.whitehouse.gov/briefing-room/speeches-remarks/2021/07/29/remarks-by-president-biden-laying-out-the-next-steps-in-our-effort-to-get-more-americans-vaccinated-and-combat-the-spread-of-the-delta-variant/.

384. Natalie Rahhal, Pfizer CEO Admits He Is 'Not Certain' Their COVID-19 Shot Will Prevent Vaccinated People from Spreading the Virus - as the Firm Cuts the Number of Doses it Will Ship this Year, Daily Mail, December 4, 2020, https://www.dailymail.co.uk/health/article-9018547/Pfizer-CEO-not-certain-covid-shot-prevents-transmission.html.

385. AXIOS on HBO: Moderna Chief Medical Officer Tal Zaks (Clip) | HBO, November 23, 2020, https://www.youtube.com/watch?v=po7qt9BZz0s&t=65s.

386. 60% of People Being Admitted to UK Hospitals Are Unvaccinated - Adviser, Reuters, July 19, 2021, https://www.reuters.com/business/healthcare-pharmaceuticals/60-people-being-admitted-uk-hospitals-had-two-covid-jabs-adviser-2021-07-19/.

387. Canada: COVID-19 Outbreak at Retirement Home Where 82% of Residents Are "Vaccinated", March 12, 2021, https://thecovidblog.com/2021/03/12/canada-covid-19-outbreak-at-retirement-home-where-82-of-residents-are-vaccinated/.

388. CDC Issues First Set of Guidelines on How Fully Vaccinated People Can Visit Safely with Others, March 8, 2021, https://archive.is/PrcRy#selection-455.0-455.94.

389. Shannon Pettypiece, et al., CDC Recommends the Vaccinated Wear Masks in Areas with Low Vaccination Rates, NBC News, July 27, 2021, https://www.nbcnews.com/politics/white-house/biden-administration-recommend-vaccinated-wear-masks-areas-low-vaccination-rates-n1275012.

390. Emily Kopp, CDC report shows vaccinated people can spread COVID-19, Roll Call, July 30, 2021, https://www.rollcall.com/2021/07/30/cdc-report-shows-vaccinated-people-can-spread-covid-19/.

391. Outbreak of SARS-CoV-2 Infections, Including COVID-19 Vaccine Breakthrough Infections,

Associated with Large Public Gatherings — Barnstable County, Massachusetts, July 2021, CDC, August 6, 2021, https://www.cdc.gov/mmwr/volumes/70/wr/mm7031e2.htm.

392. Nina Pierpont, Covid-19 Vaccine Mandates Are Now Pointless: Covid-19 Vaccines Do Not Keep People from Catching the Prevailing Delta Variant and Passing it to Others, September 9, 2021, https://theexpose.uk/wp-content/uploads/2021/09/Pierpont-Why-mandated-vaccines-are-pointless-final-1.pdf.

393. https://www.instagram.com/tv/CYpnmfioB2K/?utm_medium=copy_link.

394. https://www.instagram.com/tv/CYpnmfioB2K/?utm_medium=copy_link.

395. Jeff Faraudo, Cal Football: Bears Expecting Everyone Back From COVID-19 for the Big Game, Sports Illustrated, November 13, 2021, https://www.si.com/college/cal/news/cal-covid-update-111321.

396. University of California 2021 Football Roster, https://calbears.com/sports/football/roster.

397. Carol Rosenberg and Aishvarya Kavi, a U.S. Navy Combat Ship Is Stranded in Guantánamo Bay with a Virus Outbreak, The New York Times, December 25, 2021, https://www.nytimes.com/2021/12/25/world/navy-ship-covid-guantanamo-bay.html.

398. Darling v. Sacred Heart Health System, 3:21-CV-1787/TKW, (N.D. Fl. 2021), ruling from the bench of

U.S. District Court Judge T. Kent Wetherell, II denying motion for preliminary injunction.

399. COVID-19 Vaccine Breakthrough Infections Reported to CDC — United States, January 1–April 30, 2021, CDC, May 28, 2021, https://www.cdc.gov/mmwr/volumes/70/wr/mm7021e3.htm.

400. Letter from Seanator Edward J. Markey to Dr. Dr. Rochelle P. Walletnsky, Director, CDC, July 22, 2021, https://www.markey.senate.gov/imo/media/doc/cdc_breakthrough_cases_letter.pdf.

401. The Expose, Whilst you were distracted by Boris resigning, the UK Gov. quietly published a report confirming the Vaccinated account for 94% of all COVID-19 Deaths since April, 90% of which were Triple/Quadruple Jabbed, July 11, 2022, https://expose-news.com/2022/07/11/boris-distraction-uk-gov-revealed-triple-vaccinated-94percent-covid-deaths/.

402. The Expose, July 11, 2022, supra.

403. Deaths by vaccination status, England. Office for National Statistics, https://www.ons.gov.uk/peoplepopulationandcommunity/birthsdeathsandmarriages/deaths/datasets/deathsbyvaccinationstatusengland, Release date: 06 July 2022.

404. UK Government quietly confirms Triple+ Vaccinated accounted for 92% of COVID Deaths in 2022, The Expose, March 26, 2023, https://expose-news.com/2023/03/26/uk-gov-confirms-vaccinated-accounted-for-92-percent-of-covid-deaths-in-2022/.

405. Guy Page, 76% of September COVID-19 Deaths Are Vax Breakthroughs, Vermont Daily Chronicle, September 30, 2021, https://vermontdailychronicle.com/2021/09/30/76-of-september-covid-19-deaths-are-vaxxed-breakthroughs/.

406. Protect Yourself & Others, Vermont Department of Public Health, https://www.healthvermont.gov/covid-19/protect-yourself-others (last visited on October 14, 2021).

407. Hall Turner Radio Show, Newsdesk, November 9, 2021, https://halturnerradioshow.com/index.php/en/news-page/world/hospitals-in-antwerp-belgium-75-6-vaxxed-are-now-reporting-100-of-their-covid-cases-are-double-vaccinated.

408. Id.

409. Id.

410. EXCLUSIVE – 89% of COVID-19 Deaths in the past 4 Weeks Were among the Fully Vaccinated According to the Latest Public Health Data, The Expose, November 11, 2021, https://theexpose.uk/2021/11/11/89-percent-of-covid-19-deaths-were-among-the-fully-vaccinated-in-the-past-month/.

411. Public Health Scotland, COVID-19 & Winter Statistical Report, As at 17 January 2022, Publication Date: 19 January 2022, https://publichealthscotland.scot/media/11223/22-01-19-covid19-winter_publication_report.pdf.

412. Id.

413. Id.

414. Id.

415. Public Health Scotland, COVID-19 & Winter Statistical Report, As at 17 January 2022, Publication Date: 19 January 2022, archived from January 19, 2022, https://web.archive.org/web/20220119160752/https://publichealthscotland.scot/media/11223/22-01-19-covid19-winter_publication_report.pdf

416. Public Health Scotland COVID-19 & Winter Statistical Report As at 14 February 2022 Publication date: 16 February 2022, https://publichealthscotland.scot/media/11916/22-02-16-covid19-winter_publication_report.pdf.

417. Ana Da Silva, Health bosses to stop publishing Covid deaths by vaccine status after 'misrepresentation' of figures, The Press and Jounal, February 17, 2022, https://www.pressandjournal.co.uk/fp/politics/scottish-politics/3966759/health-bosses-to-stop-publishing-covid-deaths-by-vaccine-status/.

418. Steve Kirsch, Think vaccines work?, Substack, February 23, 2022, https://stevekirsch.substack.com/p/think-vaccines-work?utm_source=url.

419. Public Health Scotland COVID-19 & Winter Statistical Report As at 10 January 2022 Publication date: 12 January 2022, https://publichealthscotland.scot/media/11076/22-01-12-covid19-winter_publication_report.pdf.

420. Edward Hendrie, COVER-UP: Scotland Health Authorities Will Stop Reporting COVID Deaths by Vaccine Status, February 25, 2022, https://greatmountainpublishing.com/2022/02/25/cover-up-scotland-health-authorities-will-stop-reporting-covid-deaths-by-vaccine-status/.

421. 5.3.6 CUMULATIVE ANALYSIS OF POST-AUTHORIZATION ADVERSE EVENT REPORTS OF PF-07302048 (BNT162B2) RECEIVED THROUGH 28-FEB-2021, https://drtrozzi.org/wp-content/uploads/2022/01/Pfizer-Cumulative-Analysis-of-Post-authorization-Adverse-Event-Reports.pdf.

422. Compare COVID-19 epidemiology update, July 29, 2022, https://health-infobase.canada.ca/covid-19/, with COVID-19 epidemiology update, June 17, 2022, https://web.archive.org/web/20220622061056/https://health-infobase.canada.ca/covid-19/.

423. Trudeau's Government confirms the Quadruple/Triple Vaccinated have accounted for 90% of Covid-19 Deaths across Canada since the beginning of June, The Expose, July 29, 2022, https://expose-news.com/2022/07/29/trudeau-90percent-covid-deaths-vaccinated-canada/?cmid=60835409-a89a-4896-82cd-c51b2d11c704.

424. Id.

425. Id.

426. Cahterine Brown, et al., Outbreak of SARS-CoV-2 Infections, Including COVID-19 Vaccine Breakthrough Infections, Associated with Large Public Gatherings - Barnstable County, Massachusetts, July

2021, August 6, 2021, https://pubmed.ncbi.nlm.nih.gov/34351882/.

427. Nguyen Van Vinh Chau, et al., Transmission of SARS-CoV-2 Delta Variant Among Vaccinated Healthcare Workers, Vietnam, Volume 41, November 2021, 11043, https://doi.org/10.1016/j.eclinm.2021.101143, and also at: https://papers.ssrn.com/sol3/papers.cfm?abstract_id=3897733.

428. Carla Saade, et al., Live virus neutralization testing in convalescent patients and subjects vaccinated against 19A, 20B, 20I/501Y.V1 and 20H/501Y.V2 isolates of SARS-CoV-2, December 2021, https://pubmed.ncbi.nlm.nih.gov/34176436/.

429. Kasen K. Riemersma, et al., Shedding of Infectious SARS-CoV-2 Despite Vaccination, August 24, 2021, https://www.medrxiv.org/content/10.1101/2021.07.31.21261387v4.full.pdf.

430. The United Kingdom Health Security Agency COVID-19 Vaccine Surveillance Report, Publishing Reference: GOV-10227, at 12, October 21, 2021, https://assets.publishing.service.gov.uk/government/uploads/system/uploads/attachment_data/file/1027511/Vaccine-surveillance-report-week-42.pdf.

431. The United Health Kingdom Health Security Agency COVID-19 Vaccine Surveillance Report, Publishing Reference: GOV-10227, at 13, October 21, 2021, https://assets.publishing.service.gov.uk/government/uploads/system/uploads/attachment_data/file/1027511/Va

ccine-surveillance-report-week-42.pdf.

432. Latest UK Health Security Agency report Shows the COVID-19 Vaccines Have NEGATIVE Effectiveness As Low As MINUS 124%, The Expose, October 22, 2021, https://theexpose.uk/2021/10/22/covid-19-vaccines-have-negative-effectiveness-as-low-as-minus-124-percent/.

433. Official Government Reports Suggest the Fully Vaccinated Will Develop Acquired Immunodeficiency Syndrome by Christmas, The Expose, Ocober 27, 2021, https://theexpose.uk/2021/10/27/official-government-reports-suggest-the-fully-vaccinated-will-develop-acquired-immunodeficiency-syndrome-by-christmas/.

434. COVID-19 Vaccine Surveillance Report, Week 42, UK Health Security Agency, Publishing reference: GOV-10227, 21 October 2021, https://assets.publishing.service.gov.uk/government/uploads/system/uploads/attachment_data/file/1027511/Vaccine-surveillance-report-week-42.pdf.

435. Official Government Reports Suggest the Fully Vaccinated Will Develop Acquired Immunodeficiency Syndrome by Christmas, The Expose, Ocober 27, 2021, https://theexpose.uk/2021/10/27/official-government-reports-suggest-the-fully-vaccinated-will-develop-acquired-immunodeficiency-syndrome-by-christmas/.

436. S. V. Subramanian and Akhil Kumar, Increases in COVID-19 Are Unrelated to Levels of Vaccination Across 68 Countries and 2947 Counties in the United States, September 30, 2021,

https://www.ncbi.nlm.nih.gov/pmc/articles/PMC8481107/#CR1.

437. S. V. Subramanian and Akhil Kumar, supra.

438. S. V. Subramanian and Akhil Kumar, supra.

439. Barbara A. Cohn, et al., Breakthrough SARS-CoV-2 infections in 620,000 U.S. Veterans, February 1, 2021 to August 13, 2021, October 14, 2021, https://www.medrxiv.org/content/10.1101/2021.10.13.21264966v1.

440. Joseph A. Ladapo, M.D., Ph.D., State Surgeon General, Guidance for Pediatric COVID-19 Vaccines, March 8, 2022, http://ww11.doh.state.fl.us/comm/_partners/covid19_report_archive/press-release-assets/g2-jtr_QWBT4hJpqr_20220308-1923.pdf.

441. Joseph A. Ladapo, March 8, 2022, supra.

442. Joseph A. Ladapo, March 8, 2022, supra.

443. Joseph A. Ladapo, March 8, 2022, supra.

444. Stay Up to Date with COVID-19 Vaccines Including Boosters, CDC, October 4, 2022, https://www.cdc.gov/coronavirus/2019-ncov/vaccines/stay-up-to-date.html#children.

445. Interim Infection Prevention and Control Recommendations for Healthcare Personnel During the Coronavirus Disease 2019 (COVID-19) Pandemic, September 23, 2022, CDC, COVID-19, https://www.cdc.gov/coronavirus/2019-ncov/hcp/infection-control-recommendations.html#.

446. HHS Winds Down mRNA Vaccine Development Under BARDA, HHS, August 5, 2025, https://www.hhs.gov/press-room/hhs-winds-down-mrna-development-under-barda.html.

447. HHS Winds Down mRNA Vaccine Development Under BARDA, HHS, August 5, 2025, https://www.hhs.gov/press-room/hhs-winds-down-mrna-development-under-barda.html.

448. Secretary Kennedy, HHS, X, August 5, 2025, https://x.com/SecKennedy/status/1952851097019633766.

449. Martin Wucher, et al., COVID-19 mRNA "vaccine" harms research collection, July 1, 2025, https://zenodo.org/records/15787612, Doi: 10.5281/zenodo.15787612.

450. Catherine J Frompovich, An Interview With Research Immunologist Tetyana Obukhanych, PhD, Part 1 of 3, https://studylib.net/doc/7772112/an-interview-with-research-immunologist-tetyana-obukhanyc... (last visited on April 3, 2023).

451. Brett Wilcox, Jabbed, How the Vaccine Industry, Medical Establishment and Government Stick It to You and Your Family, at 97 (2018).

452. Brett Wilcox, Jabbed, supra, at 88.

453. Debra Heine, Dr. McCullough: COVID Vaccines Have Already Killed Up to 50,000 Americans, According to Whistleblowers, American Greatness, June 15, 2021, https://amgreatness.com/2021/06/15/dr-mccullough-co

vid-vaccines-have-already-killed-up-to-50000-americans-according-to-whistleblowers/.

454. Id.

455. Edward Hendrie, The FDA and Pfizer Concealed Evidence That COVID-19 Vaccines Will Cause Myocarditis in Children, November 7, 2021, https://greatmountainpublishing.com/2021/11/07/the-fda-and-pfizer-concealed-evidence-that-covid-19-vaccines-will-cause-myocarditis-in-children/.

456. The COVID Vaccines; Are they Safe and Effective? Presented by Dr. Peter A. McCullough At the United For Healthcare Summit 2022, published July 24, 2022, https://rumble.com/v1dgd7p-dr.-peter-a.-mccullough-united-for-healthcare-summit-2022.html.

457. Covid-19 Vaccine Pharmacovigilance Report, World Council For Health, June 16, 2022, https://worldcouncilforhealth.org/resources/covid-19-vaccine-pharmacovigilance-report.

458. Dr. Katarina Lindley, Independent Pharmacovigilance Report Confirms Evidence for Recall of Covid-19 Vaccines, World Council For Health, July 11, 2022, https://worldcouncilforhealth.org/news/independent-pharmacovigilance-report-recall-of-covid-19-vaccines.

459. Dr. Katarina Lindley, July 11, 2022, supra.

460. Lazarus, Ross, et al., Grant ID: R18 HS 017045, Final Report, Electronic Support for Public Health–Vaccine Adverse Event Reporting System (ESP:VAERS), at 6, 2/01/07 - 09/30/10, Submitted to:

The Agency for Healthcare Research and Quality (AHRQ) U.S. Department of Health and Human Services, https://digital.ahrq.gov/sites/default/files/docs/publication/r18hs017045-lazarus-final-report-2011.pdf.

461. Kimberly Blumenthal, Acute Allergic Reactions to mRNA COVID-19 Vaccines, Journal of the American Medical Association, March 8, 2021, https://jamanetwork.com/journals/jama/fullarticle/2777417.

462. Tom T. Shimabukuro, Reports of Anaphylaxis After Receipt of mRNA COVID-19 Vaccines in the US—December 14, 2020-January 18, 2021, Journal of the American Medical Association, https://jamanetwork.com/journals/jama/fullarticle/2776557.

463. Selected Adverse Events Reported after COVID-19 Vaccination, CDC, March 30, 2021, https://web.archive.org/web/20210405130532/https://www.cdc.gov/coronavirus/2019-ncov/vaccines/safety/adverse-events.html.

464. Kimberly Blumenthal, Acute Allergic Reactions to mRNA COVID-19 Vaccines, Journal of the American Medical Association, March 8, 2021, https://jamanetwork.com/journals/jama/fullarticle/2777417.

465. Letter from Elizabeth A. Brehm to Dr. Rochelle P. Walensky, Director, Centers for Disease Control and Prevention, March 17, 2021, https://www.icandecide.org/wp-content/uploads/2021/03/Letter-to-Dr.-Walensky-re-anaphylaxis.pdf.

466. Id.

467. Id.

468. Megan Redshaw, Latest VAERS Data Show Reports of Blood Clotting Disorders After All Three Emergency Use Authorization Vaccines, The Defender, April 16, 2021, https://childrenshealthdefense.org/defender/vaers-reports-clotting-disorders-all-three-emergency-use-authorization-vaccines/?itm_term=home. See also Tyler Durden, What The CDC's VAERS Database Reveals About "Adverse" Post-Vaccine Reactions, April 18, 2021, https://www.zerohedge.com/covid-19/what-cdcs-vaers-database-reveals-about-adverse-post-vaccine-reactions.

469. Covid-19 Vaccine Pharmacovigilance Report, World Council For Health, June 16, 2022, https://worldcouncilforhealth.org/resources/covid-19-vaccine-pharmacovigilance-report.

470. Covid-19 Vaccine Pharmacovigilance Report, World Council For Health, June 16, 2022, https://worldcouncilforhealth.org/resources/covid-19-vaccine-pharmacovigilance-report.

471. Lazarus, Ross, et al., Grant ID: R18 HS 017045, Final Report, Electronic Support for Public Health–Vaccine Adverse Event Reporting System (ESP:VAERS), at 6, 2/01/07 - 09/30/10, Submitted to: The Agency for Healthcare Research and Quality (AHRQ) U.S. Department of Health and Human Services, https://digital.ahrq.gov/sites/default/files/docs/publication/r18hs017045-lazarus-final-report-2011.pdf.

472. Scott McLachlan, et al., Analysis of COVID-19 vaccine death reports from the Vaccine Adverse Events Reporting System (VAERS) Database Interim: Results and Analysis, ResearchGate, June 2021, https://www.researchgate.net/publication/352837543_Analysis_of_COVID-19_vaccine_death_reports_from_the_Vaccine_Adverse_Events_Reporting_System_VAERS_Database_Interim_Results_and_Analysis.

473. BREAKING – The Covid-19 Vaccines have killed at least 150,000 people in the USA including 574 children according to new Scientific Study, The Expose, September 20, 2021, https://expose-news.com/2021/09/20/covid-19-vaccines-have-killed-at-least-150000-people-in-the-usa/.

474. Ben Armstrong, CDC Data & Scientific Study suggest 1.2 million Americans may already have died due to COVID Vaccination, The Expose, October 4, 2022, https://expose-news.com/2022/10/04/cdc-12-million-americans-dead-covid-vaccination/.

475. Open VEARS, https://www.openvaers.com/ (last visited on July 28, 2022).

476. Megan Redshaw, Latest VAERS Data Show Reports of Blood Clotting Disorders After All Three Emergency Use Authorization Vaccines, The Defender, April 16, 2021, https://childrenshealthdefense.org/defender/vaers-reports-clotting-disorders-all-three-emergency-use-authorization-vaccines/?itm_term=home. See also Tyler Durden, What The CDC's VAERS Database Reveals About "Adverse" Post-Vaccine Reactions, April 18, 2021, https://www.zerohedge.com/covid-19/what-cdcs-vaers-database-reveals-about-adverse-post-vaccine-reactions.

477. Fact Sheet for Recipients and Caregivers Emergency Use Authorization (EUA) of The Janssen COVID-19 Vaccine to Prevent Coronavirus Disease 2019 (COVID-19) in Individuals 18 Years of Age and Older, August 27, 2021, https://www.janssenlabels.com/emergency-use-authorization/Janssen+COVID-19+Vaccine-Recipient-fact-sheet.pdf.

478. See COVID-19 Vaccine Emergency Use Authorization (EUA) Fact Sheets for Recipients and Caregivers, CDC, August 6, 2021, https://www.cdc.gov/vaccines/covid-19/eua/index.html.

479. Vaccines and Related Biological Products Advisory Committee - 10/22/2020, U.S. Food and Drug Administration, at 2:33:40, https://www.youtube.com/watch?v=1XTiL9rUpkg&t=9220s.

480. Shari Roan, Swine Flu 'Debacle' of 1976 Is Recalled, Los Angeles Times, April 27, 2009, https://www.latimes.com/archives/la-xpm-2009-apr-27-sci-swine-history27-story.html#:~:text=Waiting%20in%20long%20lines%20at,receiving%20the%20vaccine%3B%2025%20died.

481. Vaccines and Related Biological Products Advisory Committee - 10/22/2020, U.S. Food and Drug Administration, at 2:33:40, https://www.youtube.com/watch?v=1XTiL9rUpkg&t=9220s.

482. Remarks by President Biden on Fighting the COVID-19 Pandemic, August 18, 2021, https://www.whitehouse.gov/briefing-room/speeches-r

emarks/2021/08/18/remarks-by-president-biden-on-fighting-the-covid-19-pandemic-2/.

483. Remarks by President Biden Laying Out the Next Steps in Our Effort to Get More Americans Vaccinated and Combat the Spread of the Delta Variant, July 29, 2021, 4:23 p.m. EDT, https://www.whitehouse.gov/briefing-room/speeches-remarks/2021/07/29/remarks-by-president-biden-laying-out-the-next-steps-in-our-effort-to-get-more-americans-vaccinated-and-combat-the-spread-of-the-delta-variant/. See also Executive Order 14043 of September 9, 2021, Requiring Coronavirus Disease 2019 Vaccination for Federal Employees, https://www.federalregister.gov/documents/2021/09/14/2021-19927/requiring-coronavirus-disease-2019-vaccination-for-federal-employees.

484. VAERS COVID Vaccine Data, August 13, 2021, https://www.openvaers.com/covid-data.

485. COVID Vaccine Reported Mortality Breakdowns, August 13, 2021, https://www.openvaers.com/covid-data/mortality.

486. American Frontline Doctors v. Xavier Becerra, Secretary of the U.S. Department of Health and Human Services, Petition For Temporary Restraining Order, United States District Court for The Northern District of Alabama, Case 2:21-cv-00702-CLM, May 20, 2021, at 46, https://americasfrontlinedoctors.org/files/tro/. See also CDC: as Many People Have Died from COVID-19 Vaccines as All Vaccines in Last 20 Years Combined, World News Daily, May 8, 2021, https://www.wnd.com/2021/05/cdc-many-people-died-covid-19-vaccines-vaccines-last-20-years-combined/.

487. Id. at 47.

488. Id. at 46.

489. Id.

490. Id.

491. Ethan Huff, Government Caught "Scrubbing" Covid-19 Vaccine Injuries and Deaths, Natural News, May 6, 2021, https://www.naturalnews.com/2021-05-06-government-caught-scrubbing-covid19-vaccine-injuries-deaths.html.

492. Debra Heine, Dr. McCullough: COVID Vaccines Have Already Killed Up to 50,000 Americans, According to Whistleblowers, American Greatness, June 15, 2021, https://amgreatness.com/2021/06/15/dr-mccullough-covid-vaccines-have-already-killed-up-to-50000-americans-according-to-whistleblowers/.

493. Declaration of Jane Doe, Executed on July 13, 2021, Case 2:21-cv-00702-CLM, United States District Court, Northern District of Alabama, Filed 07/19/21.

494. Id.

495. Lazarus, Ross, et al., Grant ID: R18 HS 017045, Final Report, Electronic Support for Public Health–Vaccine Adverse Event Reporting System (ESP:VAERS), at 6, 2/01/07 - 09/30/10, Submitted to: The Agency for Healthcare Research and Quality (AHRQ) U.S. Department of Health and Human Services, https://digital.ahrq.gov/sites/default/files/docs/publication/r18hs017045-lazarus-final-report-2011.pdf.

496. Open VEARS, https://www.openvaers.com/ (last visited on July 28, 2022).

497. The Expose, COVID Vaccines are at least 75x deadlier than all other Vaccines combined according to Medicine Regulators, August 19, 2022, https://expose-news.com/2022/08/19/covid-jabs-75x-deadlier-than-all-vaccines/.

498. Id.

499. AFLDS suit seeks to immediately revoke emergency COVID vaccine use based on disturbing new mortality data, AFLDS Frontline News, November 23, 2021, https://americasfrontlinenews.com/post/aflds-suit-seeks-to-immediately-revoke-emergency-covid-vaccine-use-based-on-disturbing-new-mortality-data. See also Alabama TRO/Complaint/Preliminary Injunction, SFLDS, https://americasfrontlinedoctors.org/2/legal/tro/ (last visited on July 28, 2022).

500. Robert Malone, et al., Cationic Liposome-mediated RNA Transfection, Proc. Nati. Acad. Sci. USA Vol. 86, pp. 6077-6081, August 1989, https://www.pnas.org/content/pnas/86/16/6077.full.pdf. See also Jon A. Wolfe, Robert Malone, et. al., Direct Gene Transfer into Mouse Muscle in Vivo, Science, Vol. 247, Issue 4949, pp. 1465-1468, DOI: 10.1126/science.1690918, 23 March 1990, https://science.sciencemag.org/content/247/4949/1465.abstract.

501. Spike Protein Is Very Dangerous, It's Cytotoxic (Robert Malone, Steve Kirsch, Bret Weinstein), June 13, 2021,

https://www.youtube.com/watch?v=Du2wm5nhTXY.

502. Id.

503. Karen Weintraub, The first 22M Americans have been vaccinated for COVID-19, and initial safety data shows everything is going well, CDC says, USA Today, January 28, 2021, https://www.usatoday.com/story/news/health/2021/01/28/covid-19-vaccines-cdc-safety-data-pfizer-moderna-coronavirus/4281434001/.

504. Karen Weintraub, January 28, 2022, supra.

505. VAERS COVID Vaccine Adverse Event Reports, December 16, 2022, https://web.archive.org/web/20221231001252/https://openvaers.com/covid-data.

506. Karen Weintraub, January 28, 2022, supra.

507. Karen Weintraub, January 28, 2022, supra.

508. Karen Weintraub, January 28, 2022, supra.

509. Karen Weintraub, January 28, 2022, supra.

510. Denis G. Rancourt, et al., Age-stratified COVID-19 vaccine-dose fatality rate for Israel and Australia, Correlation Research in the Public Interest, 9 February 2023, https://correlation-canada.org/report-age-stratified-covid-19-vaccine-dose-fatality-rate-for-israel-and-australia/.

511. Health Alert on mRNA COVID-19 Vaccine Safety, Florida Department of Health, February 15, 2023,

https://www.floridahealth.gov/newsroom/2023/02/20230215-updated-health-alert.pr.html.

512. Florida Surgeon General, Joseph Ladapo, Letter to Robert M. Calif, Commissioner, FDA and Rochelle P. Walensky, Director, (CDC), February 15, 2023, https://www.floridahealth.gov/_documents/newsroom/press-releases/2023/02/20230215-updated-health-alert-letter.pdf?utm_source=floridahealth.gov&utm_medium=referral&utm_campaign=newsroom&utm_content=article&url_trace_7f2r5y6=https%3A%2F%2Fwww.floridahealth.gov%2Fnewsroom%2F2023%2F02%2F20230215-updated-health-alert.pr.html.

513. Id.

514. Fraiman J, Erviti J, Jones M, Greenland S, Whelan P, Kaplan RM, Doshi P. Serious adverse events of special interest following mRNA COVID-19 vaccination in randomized trials in adults. Vaccine. 2022 Sep 22;40(40):5798-5805. doi: 10.1016/j.vaccine.2022.08.036. Epub 2022 Aug 31. PMID: 36055877; PMCID: PMC9428332. https://pubmed.ncbi.nlm.nih.gov/36055877/.

515. Sun CLF, Jaffe E, Levi R. Increased emergency cardiovascular events among under-40 population in Israel during vaccine rollout and third COVID-19 wave. Sci Rep. 2022 Apr 28;12(1):6978. doi: 10.1038/s41598-022-10928-z. PMID: 35484304; PMCID: PMC9048615. https://pubmed.ncbi.nlm.nih.gov/35484304/.

516. Dag Berild J, Bergstad Larsen V, Myrup Thiesson E, et al. Analysis of Thromboembolic and Thrombocytopenic Events After the AZD1222, BNT162b2, and MRNA-1273 COVID-19 Vaccines in

3 Nordic Countries. JAMA Netw Open. 2022;5(6):e2217375. doi:10.1001/jamanetworkopen.2022.17375. https://jamanetwork.com/journals/jamanetworkopen/fullarticle/2793348?utm_source=floridahealth.gov&utm_medium=referral&utm_campaign=newsroom&utm_content=article&url_trace_7f2r5y6=https://www.floridahealth.gov/newsroom/2023/02/20230215-updated-health-alert.pr.html.

517. Cindy Krischer Goodman and Caroline Catherman, CDC Says Florida Surgeon General Draws Wrong Conclusion From COVID Data In His Vaccine Warning, South Florida SunSentinel, February 17, 2023, https://www.sun-sentinel.com/health/fl-ne-ladapo-covid-vaccine-warning-cdc-data-response-20230217-3zufwdbgrbc4fovew3yca2osji-story.html.

518. Dr. Katarina Lindley, Independent Pharmacovigilance Report Confirms Evidence for Recall of Covid-19 Vaccines, World Council For Health, July 11, 2022, https://worldcouncilforhealth.org/news/independent-pharmacovigilance-report-recall-of-covid-19-vaccines.

519. Dr. Katarina Lindley, July 11, 2022, supra.

520. Sam Ogozalek and Kirby Wilson, Florida surgeon general, again questioning COVID vaccines, sends letter to CDC, FDA, Tampa Bay Times, February 17, 2023, https://www.tampabay.com/news/health/2023/02/17/ladapo-surgeon-general-coronavirus-vaccines-mrna-vaers-safety/.

521. Sam Ogozalek and Kirby Wilson, Florida surgeon general, again questioning COVID vaccines, sends letter to CDC, FDA, Tampa Bay Times, February 17, 2023, https://www.tampabay.com/news/health/2023/02/17/ladapo-surgeon-general-coronavirus-vaccines-mrna-vaers-safety/.

522. Arek, Sarkissian, DeSantis calls for grand jury to investigate Covid-19 vaccines, Politico, December 12, 2022, https://www.politico.com/news/2022/12/13/desantis-grand-jury-covid-19-vaccines-00073718.

523. Ron Desantis, Governor of Florida, Petition for Order to Impanel
A Statewide Grand Jury, In Re Statewide Grand Jury, Case No. SC22-____, December 13, 2022, https://www.flgov.com/wp-content/uploads/2022/12/Vaccine-Grand-Jury-Petition.pdf.

524. Sucharit Bhakdi MD, https://www.chelseagreen.com/writer/sucharit-bhakdi-md/ (last visited on February 21, 2023).

525. COVID Shots to "Decimate World Population," Warns Dr. Bhakdi, https://rumble.com/vfpgoh-dr.-bhakdi-interview.html (last visited on February 21, 2023).

526. America's Frontline Doctors et al., v. Xavier Becerra, Secretary of the U.S. Department of Health and Human Services, et al., Civil Action No. 2:21-cv-00702-CLM (N.D. Alabama 2021), https://www.courtlistener.com/docket/59929233/americas-frontline-doctors-etc-v-becerra/.

527. Immunization: The Basics, CDC, September 1, 2021, https://www.cdc.gov/vaccines/vac-gen/imz-basics.htm.

528. Immunization: The Basics, CDC, August 24, 2021 archive date, https://web.archive.org/web/20210824024512/https://www.cdc.gov/vaccines/vac-gen/imz-basics.htm.

529. Immunization: The Basics, CDC, September 1, 2021, https://www.cdc.gov/vaccines/vac-gen/imz-basics.htm.

530. Getting Your COVID-19 Vaccine, CDC, https://www.cdc.gov/coronavirus/2019-ncov/vaccines/expect.html?s_cid=11781:when%20to%20get%20vaccine%20after%20having%20covid:sem.ga:p:RG:GM:gen:PTN:FY22.

531. Nabin K. Shrestha, et al., Necessity of COVID-19 vaccination in previously infected individuals, June 5, 2020, https://www.medrxiv.org/content/10.1101/2021.06.01.21258176v2.

532. Dr. Scot Youngblood at San Diego City Council Meeting, September 20, 2022, https://www.bitchute.com/video/H3onzCie2198/.

533. Id.

534. Megan Loe, Yes, the CDC changed its definition of vaccine to be 'more transparent', News West 9, February 4, 2022, https://www.newswest9.com/article/news/verify/coronavirus-verify/cdc-changed-vaccine-definition-more-transparent/536-03ce7891-2604-4090-b548-b1618d28683

4.

535. Vaccine, Merriam-Webster Dicitonary, January 18, 2021, https://web.archive.org/web/20210118193104/https://www.merriam-webster.com/dictionary/vaccine.

536. Vaccine, Merriam-Webster Dicitonary, https://www.merriam-webster.com/dictionary/vaccine (last visited on February 2, 2023).

537. Biological Weapon, Merriam-Webster Dictionary, https://www.merriam-webster.com/dictionary/biological%20weapon#medicalDictionary (last visited on February 2, 2023).

538. Steve Kirsch, Survey shows over 500,000 killed by the COVID vaccines so far, May 13, 2022, https://stevekirsch.substack.com/p/jackpot-over-500000-killed-by-the#%C2%A7the-bradford-hill-criteria.

539. MacIntyre, C.R., 2021. Using the Bradford-Hill criteria to assess causality in the association between CHADOX1 NCOV-19 vaccine and thrombotic immune thrombocytopenia. Global Biosecurity, 3(1), p.null.DOI: https://doi.org/10.31646/gbio.109.

540. Aarstad, J.; Kvitastein, O.A. Is there a Link between the 2021 COVID-19 Vaccination Uptake in Europe and 2022 Excess All-Cause Mortality?. Preprints 2023, 2023020350. https://doi.org/10.20944/preprints202302.0350.v1.

541. Aarstad, J.; Kvitastein, supra.

542. Mortality and life expectancy statistics, Eurostat, December 14, 2021, http://web.archive.org/web/20211214113409/https://ec

.europa.eu/eurostat/statistics-explained/index.php?title=Mortality_and_life_expectancy_statistics#Number_of_deaths.

543. CDC coding error led to overcount of 72,000 Covid deaths, The Guardian, https://www.theguardian.com/world/2022/mar/24/cdc-coding-error-overcount-covid-deaths (last visited on March 28, 2023).

544. Deaths and Mortality, CDC, https://www.cdc.gov/nchs/fastats/deaths.htm (last visited on March 22, 2023).

545. OECD, https://stats.oecd.org/index.aspx?queryid=104676 (last visited on March 28, 2023).

546. Deaths and Mortality, CDC, https://www.cdc.gov/nchs/fastats/deaths.htm (last visited on March 22, 2023).

547. OECD, https://stats.oecd.org/index.aspx?queryid=104676 (last visited on March 28, 2023).

548. U.S. and World Population Clock, United States Census Bureau, https://www.census.gov/popclock/ (last visited on March 29, 2023).

549. OECD, https://stats.oecd.org/index.aspx?queryid=104676 (last visited on March 28, 2023).

550. U.S. and World Population Clock, United States Census Bureau, https://www.census.gov/popclock/ (last visited on March 29, 2023).

551. OECD, https://stats.oecd.org/index.aspx?queryid=104676 (last visited on March 28, 2023).

552. U.S. and World Population Clock, United States Census Bureau, https://www.census.gov/popclock/ (last visited on March 29, 2023).

553. The Expose calculated the U.S. excess death figure from the beginning of the COVID-19 vaccine rollout on 12/14/2020, until week 38 of 2022 to be 1,106,019. Secret CDC Report confirms over 1.1m Americans have 'Died Suddenly' since the COVID Vaccine Roll-Out; & further Government reports confirm the Vaccines are to blame, The Expose, April 23, 2023, https://expose-news.com/2023/04/23/over-6-million-americans-dead-covid-vaccine/?cmid=4ea57df8-d67e-458f-ad4f-8292f27ad868.

554. Government publishes shocking figures on COVID Vaccine Deaths: 1 in every 73 Vaccinated people died by June 2022 compared to just 1 in every 172 Not-Vaccinated People, The Expose, March 21, 2023, https://expose-news.com/2023/03/21/1-in-73-covid-vaccinated-died-by-june-22/?cmid=91f62e17-7553-4a2c-95c0-f160c94a2e50.

555. The Expose, 1 in every 73, March 21, 2023, supra.

556. The Expose, 1 in every 73, March 21, 2023, supra.

557. Jawad, M., Hone, T., Vamos, E.P. et al. Estimating indirect mortality impacts of armed conflict in civilian populations: panel regression analyses of 193 countries, 1990–2017. BMC Med 18, 266 (2020). https://doi.org/10.1186/s12916-020-01708-5. Also

available at https://bmcmedicine.biomedcentral.com/articles/10.1186/s12916-020-01708-5.

558. European Centre for Disease Prevention and Control, COVID-19 Vaccine Tracker, https://vaccinetracker.ecdc.europa.eu/public/extensions/COVID-19/vaccine-tracker.html#uptake-tab (last visited on March 22, 2023).

559. John Campbell, Vaccination v excess deaths, correlation study, March 21, 2023, https://www.youtube.com/watch?v=iyo2UNQcdpQ&t=3s.

560. Igor Chudov, PROVEN RELATIONSHIP: COVID Boosters and Excess Mortality in 2022, August 30, 2022, https://igorchudov.substack.com/p/proven-relationship-covid-boosters?utm_source=substack&utm_campaign=post_embed&utm_medium=email.

561. Igor Chudov, August 30, 2022, supra.

562. Excess Mortality in England, Office for Health Improvements and Disparities, https://app.powerbi.com/view?r=eyJrIjoiYmUwNmFhMjYtNGZhYS00NDk2LWFlMTAtOTg0OGNhNmFiNGM0IiwidCI6ImVlNGUxNDk5LTRhMzUtNGIyZS1hZDQ3LTVmM2NmOWRlODY2NiIsImMiOjh9 (last visited on March 30, 2023).

563. Igor Chudov, Is UK's Depopulation Caused by Covid Vaccines?, October 15, 2022, https://igorchudov.substack.com/p/is-uks-depopulation-caused-by-covid?utm_source=substack&utm_campaign=post_embed&utm_medium=web.

564. T. Coddington, UK Birth Data- the need to continue following up, October 11, 2022, https://inumero.substack.com/p/uk-birth-data-the-need-to-continue?utm_source=substack&utm_campaign=post_embed&utm_medium=web.

565. Igor Chudov, October 15, 2022, supra.

566. Secret Government Documents confirm COVID-19 Vaccine roll-out caused Excess Deaths in Australia to increase by 5,162%, The Expose, March 23, 2023, https://expose-news.com/2023/03/23/secret-government-documents-confirm-covid-19-vaccine-roll-out-caused-excess-deaths-in-australia-to-increase-by-5162/?cmid=006a759f-21c8-4d4f-837e-e76b83e849a1.

567. Secret Government Documents, The Expose, March 23, 2023, supra.

568. Denis Rancourt, There Was No Pandemic, July 2, 2023, https://denisrancourt.substack.com/p/there-was-no-pandemic.

569. Denis Rancourt, supra.

570. Denis Rancourt, supra.

571. Rancourt, D.G., Baudin, M., Hickey, J., Mercier, J. "COVID-19 vaccine-associated mortality in the Southern Hemisphere". CORRELATION Research in the Public Interest, Report, 17 September 2023. https://correlation-canada.org/covid-19-vaccine-associated-mortality-in-the-Southern-Hemisphere/.

572. Megan Redshaw, Researchers Find COVID Vaccines Causally Linked to Increased Mortality,

Estimate 17 Million Deaths, Epoch Times, September 28, 2023, quoting Rancourt, D.G., supra.

573. Rancourt, supra.

574. Will Jones, Lancet Study on Covid Vaccine Autopsies Finds 74% Were Caused by Vaccine – Study is Removed Within 24 Hours, July 6, 2023, https://dailysceptic.org/2023/07/06/lancet-study-on-covid-vaccine-autopsies-finds-74-were-caused-by-vaccine-journal-removes-study-within-24-hours/.

575. Hulscher, Nicolas and Alexander, Paul E. and Amerling, Richard and Gessling, Heather and Hodkinson, Roger and Makis, William and Risch, Harvey A. and Trozzi, Mark and McCullough, Peter A., A Systematic Review of Autopsy Findings in Deaths after COVID-19 Vaccination. Available at SSRN: https://ssrn.com/abstract=4496137 or http://dx.doi.org/10.2139/ssrn.4496137.

576. Debra Heine, Dr. McCullough: COVID Vaccines Have Already Killed Up to 50,000 Americans, According to Whistleblowers, American Greatness, June 15, 2021, https://amgreatness.com/2021/06/15/dr-mccullough-covid-vaccines-have-already-killed-up-to-50000-americans-according-to-whistleblowers/.

577. Classen JB. COVID-19 RNA Based Vaccines and the Risk of Prion Disease. Microbiol Infect Dis. 2021; 5(1): 1-3, ISSN 2639-9458, February 8, 2021, https://scivisionpub.com/pdfs/covid19-rna-based-vaccines-and-the-risk-of-prion-disease-1503.pdf.

578. Id.

579. Jean-Claude Perez Emergence of a New Creutzfeldt-Jakob Disease: 26 Cases of the Human Version of Mad-Cow Disease, Days After a COVID-19 Injection, January 2023, https://www.researchgate.net/publication/367167725_Emergence_of_a_New_Creutzfeldt-Jakob_Disease_26_Cases_of_the_Human_Version_of_Mad-Cow_Disease_Days_After_a_COVID-19_Injection.

580. Jeff Childers, Prion Shells, Coffee and COVID, DOI:10.5281/zenodo.7540331, January 31, 2023, https://www.coffeeandcovid.com/p/prion-shells-tuesday-january-31-2023?utm_source=post-email-title&publication_id=463409&post_id=100021796&isFreemail=true&utm_medium=email.

581. Classen JB. COVID-19 RNA Based Vaccines and the Risk of Prion Disease. Microbiol Infect Dis. 2021; 5(1): 1-3, ISSN 2639-9458, February 8, 2021, https://scivisionpub.com/pdfs/covid19-rna-based-vaccines-and-the-risk-of-prion-disease-1503.pdf.

582. COVID Shots Could Cause 'Crippling' Neurodegenerative Disease in Young People, MIT Scientist Warns, The Defender, January 14, 2022, https://childrenshealthdefense.org/defender/mit-scientist-stephanie-seneff-neurodegenerative-disease-young-people-covid-shots/.

583. Id.

584. Id.

585. Id.

586. Rose & McCullough, A Report on Myocarditis Adverse Events in the U.S. Vaccine Adverse Events

Reporting System (VAERS) in Association with COVID-19 Injectable Biological Products, October 1, 2021, https://www.ncbi.nlm.nih.gov/pmc/articles/PMC8483988/.

587. Lazarus, Ross, et al., Grant ID: R18 HS 017045, Final Report, Electronic Support for Public Health–Vaccine Adverse Event Reporting System (ESP:VAERS), at 6, 2/01/07 - 09/30/10, Submitted to: The Agency for Healthcare Research and Quality (AHRQ) U.S. Department of Health and Human Services, https://digital.ahrq.gov/sites/default/files/docs/publication/r18hs017045-lazarus-final-report-2011.pdf.

588. Jessica Rose and Peter A. McCullough, A Report on Myocarditis Adverse Events in the U.S. Vaccine Adverse Events Reporting System (VAERS) in Association with COVID-19 Injectable Biological Products, October 1, 2021, https://web.archive.org/web/20211002192421/https://www.ncbi.nlm.nih.gov/pmc/articles/PMC8483988/.

589. Rose & McCullough, A Report on Myocarditis Adverse Events in the U.S. Vaccine Adverse Events Reporting System (VAERS) in Association with COVID-19 Injectable Biological Products, October 1, 2021, https://www.ncbi.nlm.nih.gov/pmc/articles/PMC8483988/.

590. Stay Up to Date with COVID-19 Vaccines Including Boosters, CDC, October 4, 2022, https://www.cdc.gov/coronavirus/2019-ncov/vaccines/stay-up-to-date.html#children.

591. Oster ME, Shay DK, Su JR, et al. Myocarditis Cases Reported After mRNA-Based COVID-19 Vaccination in the US From December 2020 to August 2021. JAMA. 2022;327(4):331–340. doi:10.1001/jama.2021.24110.

592. Heart disease risk skyrockets 13,200% following covid injections, CDC admits, Natural News, June 21, 2023, https://www.naturalnews.com/2023-06-21-heart-disease-risk-13200-percent-covid-vaccination.html.

593. Joseph A. Ladapo, M.D., Ph.D., State Surgeon General, Guidance for mRNA COVID-19 Vaccines, October 7, 2022, https://floridahealthcovid19.gov/wp-content/uploads/2022/10/20221007-guidance-mrna-covid19-vaccines-doc.pdf.

594. Toby Rogers, Ten red flags in the FDA's risk-benefit analysis of Pfizer's EUA application to inject American children 5 to 11 with its mRNA product, October 25, 2021, https://tobyrogers.substack.com/p/ten-red-flags-in-the-fdas-risk-benefit.

595. Toby Rogers, October 25, 2021, supra.

596. Toby Rogers, October 25, 2021, supra.

597. Toby Rogers, October 25, 2021, supra.

598. Jessica Rose and Peter A. McCullough, A Report on Myocarditis Adverse Events in the U.S. Vaccine Adverse Events Reporting System (VAERS) in Association with COVID-19 Injectable Biological Products, October 1, 2021,

https://web.archive.org/web/20211002192421/https://www.ncbi.nlm.nih.gov/pmc/articles/PMC8483988/.

599. Jessica Rose and Peter A. McCullough, supra.

600. Toby Rogers, October 25, 2021, supra.

601. Toby Rogers, October 25, 2021, supra.

602. Aaron Kheriaty, Twitter, November 15, 2021, https://twitter.com/akheriaty/status/1460135683561963520?lang=en.

603. Terrence Fraser, Myocarditis is often mild, contrary to online claims, AP, November 18, 2021, https://apnews.com/article/fact-checking-552859079506.

604. Edward Hendrie, The FDA and Pfizer Concealed Evidence That COVID-19 Vaccines Will Cause Myocarditis in Children, Great Mountain Publishing, November 7, 2021, https://greatmountainpublishing.com/2021/11/07/the-fda-and-pfizer-concealed-evidence-that-covid-19-vaccines-will-cause-myocarditis-in-children/.

605. Doctor Warns How COVID mRNA 'Vaccines' Will Cause Delayed Strokes & Heart Attacks — 'The Worst Is Yet To Come', Christians for Truth, July 14, 2021, https://christiansfortruth.com/doctor-warns-how-covid-mrna-vaccines-will-soon-cause-strokes-heart-attacks-the-worst-is-yet-to-come/.

606. FAQ on Sudden Death and Myocarditis, Myocarditis Foundation, https://www.myocarditisfoundation.org/research-and-grants/faqs/sudden-death-and-myocarditis/ (last visited

on February 2, 2023).

607. Michael Kang, Viral Myocarditis, NIH, September 6, 2022, https://www.ncbi.nlm.nih.gov/books/NBK459259/.

608. Terrence Fraser, Myocarditis is often mild, contrary to online claims, AP, November 18, 2021, https://apnews.com/article/fact-checking-552859079506.

609. Terrence Fraser, November 18, 2021, supra.

610. Michael Kang, Viral Myocarditis, NIH, September 6, 2022, https://www.ncbi.nlm.nih.gov/books/NBK459259/.

611. Terrence Fraser, November 18, 2021, supra.

612. Michael Kang, September 2, 2022, supra.

613. Michael Kang, September 2, 2022, supra.

614. Covid: The Path not Taken - DarkHorse Podcast with Dr. Peter McCullough, December 6, 2021, https://www.youtube.com/watch?v=-zg1j7Zquoc&t=2959s.

615. Tennis world shocked after scores of players drop out of Miami Open, Free West Media, April 2, 2022, https://freewestmedia.com/2022/04/02/tennis-world-shocked-after-scores-of-players-drop-out-of-miami-open/.

616. E.g., Riley Morgan, 'What's going on': Tennis world stunned after Miami Open carnage, Yahoo Sports, 30 March 2022, https://au.sports.yahoo.com/tennis-2022-viewers-shock

ed-bizarre-miami-open-carnage-004007552.html.

617. J.D. Ruccker, March Was Not a Good Month for "Vaccinated" Cyclists, March 31, 2022, https://endmedicaltyranny.substack.com/p/march-was-not-a-good-month-for-vaccinated.

618. J.D. Rucker, Buried Bombshell: Tennis World Rocked as FIFTEEN "Fully Vaccinated" Players Unable to Finish Miami Open, The Liberty Daily, April 2, 2022, https://thelibertydaily.com/buried-bombshell-tennis-world-rocked-as-fifteen-fully-vaccinated-players-unable-to-finish-miami-open/.

619. Jeff Childers, Prion Shells, Coffee and COVID, January 31, 2023, https://www.coffeeandcovid.com/p/prion-shells-tuesday-january-31-2023?utm_source=post-email-title&publication_id=463409&post_id=100021796&isFreemail=true&utm_medium=email.

620. Baruch Fischoff, et al., (editors), FDA, 2011, Communicating Risks and Benefits: An Evidence-Based User's Guide, https://www.fda.gov/media/81597/download.

621. Toby Rogers, Pfizer COVID Vaccine Fails Risk-Benefit Analysis in Children 5 to 11, The Defender, November 5, 2021, https://childrenshealthdefense.org/defender/fda-pfizer-covid-vaccine-risk-benefit-analysis-nntv-children/.

622. Toby Rogers, November 5, 2021, supra.

623. Toby Rogers, November 5, 2021, supra.

624. Edward Dowd, "Cause Unknown," The Epidemic of Sudden Deaths in 2021 and 2022, at 33 (2022).

625. Edward Dowd, "Cause Unknown," The Epidemic of Sudden Deaths in 2021 and 2022, at 33 (2022).

626. E.g., Kevin Airs, Shattered wife relives the horrific moment her fit husband, 35, dropped dead in front of her from a condition linked to Sudden Adult Death Syndrome - and shares the ONE test that could have saved him, Daily Mail, June 18, 2022, https://www.dailymail.co.uk/news/article-10918281/SADS-Sudden-Adult-Death-Syndrome-Moment-young-mums-husband-dropped-dead-her.html.

627. Ethan Huff, Sudden Adult Death Syndrome is the new name for vaccine deaths in the medical establishment's play-pretend reality, Natural News, June 10, 2022, https://www.naturalnews.com/2022-06-10-sads-new-name-vaccine-deaths-medical-establishment.html.

628. Ethan Huff, June 10, 2022, supra.

629. Ethan Huff, June 10, 2022, Supra.

630. Vaccines and Related Biological Products Advisory Committee Meeting, FDA Briefing Document, Moderna COVID-19 Vaccine, December 17, 2020, https://www.fda.gov/media/144434/download.

631. Id.

632. Ronald Brown, Outcome Reporting Bias in COVID-19 mRNA Vaccine Clinical Trials, 26 February 2021, https://www.mdpi.com/1648-9144/57/3/199/htm.

633. Dr. Ron Brown Discusses Outcome Reporting Bias in COVID-19 mRNA Clinical Trials | Interview, TrialSite News, April 10, 2021, https://www.youtube.com/watch?v=Jkwn5I8tLmE.

634. Ronald Brown, February 2021, supra.

635. Presenting Quantitative Efficacy and Risk Information in Direct-to-Consumer Promotional Labeling and Advertisements Guidance for Industry DRAFT GUIDANCE, FDA, Center for Biologics Evaluation and Research (CBER), October 2018, https://www.fda.gov/media/117573/download.

636. Id..

637. Ronald Brown, February 2021, supra.

638. Butterfly of the Week, 22 February '21: Now You See Me, Now You Don't, David Martin World, February 23, 2021, https://www.youtube.com/watch?v=qtPy7Qrd1mg&t=1389s.

639. Vaccines and Related Biological Products Advisory Committee Meeting December 17, 2020, FDA Briefing Document, Moderna COVID-19 Vaccine, https://www.fda.gov/media/144434/download.

640. Id. at 13.

641. Id. at 13.

642. Lindsey R. Baden, et al., Efficacy and Safety of the mRNA-1273 SARS-CoV-2 Vaccine, N Engl J Med 2021; 384:403-416, DOI: 10.1056/NEJMoa2035389, February 4, 2021,

https://www.nejm.org/doi/full/10.1056/NEJMoa2035389.

643. Peter Doshi, Pfizer and Moderna's "95% Effective" Vaccines—we Need More Details and the Raw Data, BMJ, January 4, 2021, https://blogs.bmj.com/bmj/2021/01/04/peter-doshi-pfizer-and-modernas-95-effective-vaccines-we-need-more-details-and-the-raw-data/.

644. Peter Doshi, BMJ, January 4, 2021, supra.

645. Peter Doshi, BMJ, January 4, 2021, supra.

646. Vaccines and Related Biological Products Advisory Committee Meeting, December 10, 2020, FDA Briefing Document Pfizer-BioNTech COVID-19 Vaccine, at 42, https://www.fda.gov/media/144245/download.

647. Id.

648. 80% of the Nuns in this Kentucky Convent Got COVID 2 Days after Vaccine, Life Site News, February 25, 2021, https://www.lifesitenews.com/news/several-nuns-die-after-taking-first-shot-of-covid-vaccine/.

649. The Pfizer Inoculations for COVID-19 More Harm Than Good, https://www.canadiancovidcarealliance.org/wp-content/uploads/2021/12/The-COVID-19-Inoculations-More-Harm-Than-Good-REV-Dec-16-2021.pdf (last visited on February 8, 2023).

650. Id.

651. Id.

652. What Really Happened Inside the COVID-19 Vaccine Trials?, A Midwestern Doctor, March 13, 2023, https://amidwesterndoctor.substack.com/p/what-really-happened-inside-the-covid?utm_source=substack&utm_medium=email.

653. A Midwestern Doctor, March 13, 2023, supra.

654. A Midwestern Doctor, March 13, 2023, supra.

655. Megan Redshaw, U.S. Sen. Johnson Holds News Conference With Families Injured by COVID Vaccines, Ignored by Medical Community, The Defender, June 29, 2021, https://childrenshealthdefense.org/defender/sen-johnson-ken-ruettgers-press-conference-families-injured-covid-vaccines/.

656. The Pfizer Inoculations for COVID-19 More Harm Than Good, https://www.canadiancovidcarealliance.org/wp-content/uploads/2021/12/The-COVID-19-Inoculations-More-Harm-Than-Good-REV-Dec-16-2021.pdf (last visited on February 8, 2023).

657. Megan Redshaw, June 29, 2021, supra.

658. Comment from de Garay, Stephanie Posted by the Food and Drug Administration on Nov 6, 2021, https://www.regulations.gov/comment/FDA-2021-N-1088-12 9763.

659. The Pfizer Inoculations for COVID-19 More Harm Than Good, https://www.canadiancovidcarealliance.org/wp-content

/uploads/2021/12/The-COVID-19-Inoculations-More-Harm-Than-Good-REV-Dec-16-2021.pdf (last visited on February 8, 2023).

660. Jared Hopkins, Pfizer, BioNTech Get $1.95 Billion Covid-19 Vaccine Order From U.S. Government, The Wall Street Jounal, July 22, 2020, https://www.wsj.com/articles/pfizer-biontech-get-1-95-billion-covid-19-vaccine-order-from-u-s-government-11595418221?mod=searchresults&page=1&pos=2.

661. Jared Hopkins, WSJ, July 22, 2020, supra.

662. Jared Hopkins, WSJ, July 22, 2020, supra.

663. Jared Hopkins, WSJ, July 22, 2020, supra.

664. Jared Hopkins, WSJ, July 22, 2020, supra.

665. Jared Hopkins, WSJ, July 22, 2020, supra.

666. Jared Hopkins, WSJ, July 22, 2020, supra.

667. Katie Adams, Pfizer's COVID-19 vaccine becomes highest-selling pharmaceutical in history, Becker's Hospital Review, February 9, 2022, https://www.beckershospitalreview.com/pharmacy/pfizer-s-covid-19-vaccine-becomes-highest-selling-pharmaceutical-in-history.html#:~:text=Pfizer%20on%20Feb.,%2429%20billion%20in%20international%20sales.

668. Matt Grossman, Johnson & Johnson to Begin Human Trials of Covid-19 Vaccine by September, The Wall Street Jounal, March 30, 2020, https://www.wsj.com/articles/johnson-johnson-to-begin-human-trials-on-covid-19-vaccine-by-september-11585569380.

669. Peter Loftus and Matt Grossman, Johnson & Johnson Readies to Start Covid-19 Vaccine Studies, The Wall Street Journal, July 15, 2020, https://www.wsj.com/articles/johnson-johnson-raises-2020-earnings-guidance-11594897686?mod=searchresults&page=1&pos=7.

670. Andrew Court, Democrat Congressman Stephen Lynch, 65, Tests Positive to COVID-19 after Receiving Both Doses of Pfizer's Vaccine, The Daily Mail, January 30, 2021, https://www.dailymail.co.uk/news/article-9205321/Rep-Stephen-Lynch-65-tests-positive-COVID-19-receiving-doses-Pfizer-vaccine.html?ito=push-notification&ci=73039&si=23070647.

671. Carolyn Crist, Early Vaccines Will Prevent Symptoms, Not Virus, WebMD, October 28, 2020, https://www.webmd.com/vaccines/covid-19-vaccine/news/20201027/early-vaccines-wil-prevent-symptoms-not-virus.

672. Sarah Jacoby, Early COVID-19 Vaccines May Prevent Symptoms but Not the Infection, Dr. Fauci Says, Self, October 29, 2021, https://www.self.com/story/early-covid-19-vaccines-prevent-symptoms.

673. See, e.g., Vaccines and Related Biological Products Advisory Committee Meeting December 17, 2020, FDA Briefing Document, Moderna COVID-19 Vaccine, at 13, https://www.fda.gov/media/144434/download.

674. Vinu Arumugham, Evidence that Food Proteins in Vaccines Cause the Development of Food Allergies and Its Implications for Vaccine Policy

(2015) https://www.longdom.org/open-access/evidence-that-food-proteins-in-vaccines-cause-the-development-of-foodallergies-and-its-implications-for-vaccine-policy-2329-6631-1000137.pdf.

675. Id.

676. Id.

677. American College of Allergy, Asthma, and Immunology, Milk Allergy Affects Half of US Food-Allergic Kids under Age 1: Most children with a milk allergy don't carry epinephrine, ScienceDaily, 16 November 2018, www.sciencedaily.com/releases/2018/11/181116083208.htm.

678. Brett Wilcox, Jabbed, How the Vaccine Industry, Medical Establishment and Government Stick It to You and Your Family, at 41-42 (2018), citing Heather Fraser, The Peanut Allergy Epidemic: What's Causing It and How to Stop It (2011).

679. Robyn Charron, How to Cause a Peanut Allergy Epidemic in 4 Easy Steps, The Thinking Moms' Revolution, August 18, 2015, https://thinkingmomsrevolution.com/whats-really-behind-peanut-allergy-epidemic/.

680. Robyn Charron, August 18, 2015, supra.

681. Vaccine Excipient Summary, Appendix B, CDC, https://www.cdc.gov/vaccines/pubs/pinkbook/downloads/appendices/b/excipient-table-2.pdf (last visited on January 28, 2023).

682. Vaccine Excipient Summary, supra.

683. Vaccine Excipient Summary, supra.

684. Medical Management Guidelines for Formaldehyde, CDC, https://wwwn.cdc.gov/TSP/MMG/MMGDetails.aspx?mmgid=216&toxid=39#:~:text=The%20exact%20mechanism%20of%20action,which%20results%20in%20cell%20death (last visited on January 28, 2023).

685. Center for Disease Control, Vaccine Excipient Summary, February 2020, https://www.cdc.gov/vaccines/pubs/pinkbook/downloads/appendices/b/excipient-table-2.pdf?fbclid=IwAR2cxiqnMzWzyV_YCGjFoQ0Qv4kF0V13aO8qe-IH3D8IwHx0dpp6-KTKL_o.

686. Id.

687. Calvin C. Willhite, Nataliya A. Karyakina, Robert A. Yokel, Nagarajkumar Yenugadhati, Thomas M. Wisniewski, Ian M. F. Arnold, Franco Momoli, and Daniel Krewski1, Systematic Review of Potential Health Risks Posed by Pharmaceutical, Occupational and Consumer Exposures to Metallic and Nanoscale Aluminum, Aluminum Oxides, Aluminum Hydroxide and its Soluble Salts, US National Library of Medicine, National Institutes of Health, August 25, 2016, https://www.ncbi.nlm.nih.gov/pmc/articles/PMC4997813/#R40.

688. Howard Frumkin M.D., Dr.P.H., Director, National Center for Environmental Health/Agency for Toxic Substances and Disease Registry, Julie Louise Gerberding, M.D., M.P.H., Administrator, Agency for Toxic Substances and Disease Registry, TOXICOLOGICAL PROFILE FOR ALUMINUM, September 2008,

https://www.atsdr.cdc.gov/toxprofiles/tp22.pdf.

689. Id.

690. Id.

691. Anne Dachel, Dachel Interview: Dr. Paul Thomas, Age of Autism, https://www.ageofautism.com/2017/02/dachel-interview-dr-paul-thomas.html (last visited on April 8, 2023).

692. Thimerosal and Vaccines, CDC, https://www.cdc.gov/vaccinesafety/concerns/thimerosal/index.html (last visited on April 5, 2023).

693. Center for Disease Control, Vaccine Excipient Summary, February 2020, https://www.cdc.gov/vaccines/pubs/pinkbook/downloads/appendices/b/excipient-table-2.pdf?fbclid=IwAR2cxiqnMzWzyV_YCGjFoQ0Qv4kF0V13aO8qe-IH3D8IwHx0dpp6-KTKL_o.

694. Thimerosal and Vaccines, FDA, content current as of February 1, 2018, https://www.fda.gov/vaccines-blood-biologics/safety-availability-biologics/thimerosal-and-vaccines.

695. Thimerosal in Vaccines, FDA, archived page from October 2, 2016, https://web.archive.org/web/20161002220751/http://www.fda.gov/BiologicsBloodVaccines/SafetyAvailability/VaccineSafety/UCM096228 (last visited on April 4, 2023).

696. Geier, David A., Sykes, Lisa K. and Geier, Mark R. (2007) 'A Review of Thimerosal (Merthiolate) and its Ethylmercury Breakdown Product: Specific Historical Considerations Regarding Safety and

Effectiveness', Journal of Toxicology and Environmental Health, Part B, 10:8, 575 - 596, DOI: 10.1080/10937400701389875, https://web.archive.org/web/20170727232138/http://www.progressiveconvergence.com/Review%20of%20Thimerosal%20and%20its%20Ethylmercury%20Breakdown%20Product.pdf. See also M.M. Powell and W.A. Jamieson, Merthiolate as a Germicide, American Jounal of Hygiene, 1931 Vol. 13, pp. 296-310, ref. 3. ISSN: 0096-5294, Record Number: 19312701068, https://www.cabdirect.org/cabdirect/abstract/19312701068. Thmerosal and Autism Timeline, Slide Share, April 11, 2014, https://www.slideshare.net/ashotoftruth/a-shot-of-truth-thimerosal-timeline-33423446. Thimerosal and Autism Timeline, Before It's News, Tuesday, October 21, 2014, https://beforeitsnews.com/terrorism/2014/10/thimerosal-and-autism-timeline-2451042.html.

697. Brett Wilcox, Jabbed, How the Vaccine Industry, Medical Establishment and Government Stick It to You and Your Family, at 125 (2018).

698. Thimerosal and Autism Timeline, supra.

699. Brett Wilcox, Jabbed, supra at 125.

700. Thomas M. Verstraeten, R. Davies, D. Gu, F DeStefano, Increased risk of developmental neurologic impairment after high exposure to thimerosalcontaining vaccine in first month of life, 1999, https://yale62.org/wp-content/uploads/2021/06/Verstraeten-Thomas-M.D.-et-al-CDC-1999.pdf.

701. Hooker B, Kern J, Geier D, Haley B, Sykes L, King P, Geier M. Methodological issues and evidence of malfeasance in research purporting to show thimerosal in vaccines is safe. Biomed Res Int. 2014;2014:247218. doi: 10.1155/2014/247218. Epub 2014 Jun 4. PMID: 24995277; PMCID: PMC4065774, https://www.ncbi.nlm.nih.gov/pmc/articles/PMC4065774/#B20.

702. Fact Sheet for Recipients and Caregivers, Emergency Use Authorization (EUA) of the Moderna COVID-19 Vaccine to Prevent Coronavirus Disease 2019 (COVID-19) in Individuals 18 Years of Age and Older, https://www.fda.gov/media/144638/download. Fact Sheet for Recipients and Caregivers, Emergency Use Authorization (EUA) of the Pfizer-BioNTech COVID-19 Vaccine to Prevent Coronavirus Disease 2019 (COVID-19) in Individuals 18 Years of Age and Older, https://www.fda.gov/media/144414/download.

703. Cosby A. Stone, M.D., M.P.H., et al., Immediate Hypersensitivity to Polyethylene Glycols and Polysorbates: More Common Than We Have Recognized, The Journal of Allergy and Clinical Immunology: In Practice, Volume 7, Issue 5, 2019 May-June, https://www.ncbi.nlm.nih.gov/pmc/articles/PMC6706272/ and https://www.sciencedirect.com/science/article/abs/pii/S2213219818308237?via%3Dihub.

704. These 'Inactive' Ingredients in COVID Vaccines Could Trigger Allergic Reactions, March 12, 2021, https://childrenshealthdefense.org/defender/inactive-ingredients-covid-vaccines-allergic-reactions/.

705. Angel A. Justiz Vaillant, et. al., Immediate Hypersensitivity Reactions, January 2021, https://pubmed.ncbi.nlm.nih.gov/30020687/.

706. These 'Inactive' Ingredients in COVID Vaccines Could Trigger Allergic Reactions, March 12, 2021, https://childrenshealthdefense.org/defender/inactive-ingredients-covid-vaccines-allergic-reactions/.

707. RFK, Jr. Warned FDA Three Months Ago About Ingredient in Pfizer COVID Vaccine That Likely Caused Life-Threatening Reaction in Two UK Healthcare Workers, December 11, 2020, https://childrenshealthdefense.org/defender/pfizer-covid-vaccine-reaction-fda-peg/.

708. Fact Sheet for Recipients and Caregivers, Emergency Use Authorization (EUA) of the Janssen COVID-19 Vaccine to Prevent Coronavirus Disease 2019 (COVID-19) in Individuals 18 Years of Age and Older, https://www.fda.gov/media/146305/download.

709. Vaccine Excipient Summary, Excipients Included in U.S. Vaccines, by Vaccine, 2019-2020 Norther Hemisphere Formulations, CDC, https://www.cdc.gov/vaccines/pubs/pinkbook/downloads/appendices/b/excipient-table-2.pdf?fbclid=IwAR2cxiqnMzWzyV_YCGjFoQ0Qv4kF0V13aO8qe-IH3D8IwHx0dpp6-KTKL_o.

710. Cosby A. Stone, M.D., M.P.H., et al., Immediate Hypersensitivity to Polyethylene Glycols and Polysorbates: More Common Than We Have Recognized, The Journal of Allergy and Clinical Immunology: In Practice, Volume 7, Issue 5, 2019 May-June, https://www.ncbi.nlm.nih.gov/pmc/articles/PMC67062

72/ and https://www.sciencedirect.com/science/article/abs/pii/S2213219818308237?via%3Dihub.

711. These 'Inactive' Ingredients in COVID Vaccines Could Trigger Allergic Reactions, March 12, 2021, https://childrenshealthdefense.org/defender/inactive-ingredients-covid-vaccines-allergic-reactions/.

712. Angel A. Justiz Vaillant, et. al., Immediate Hypersensitivity Reactions, January 2021, https://pubmed.ncbi.nlm.nih.gov/30020687/.

713. Berkely Lovelace, Jr., J&J Says Two Trial Participants Had Severe Allergic Reactions after Getting Covid Vaccine, CNBC, February 26, 2021, https://www.cnbc.com/2021/02/26/jj-says-two-people-had-severe-allergic-reactions-after-getting-covid-vaccine.html.

714. Brett Wilcox, Jabbed, How the Vaccine Industry, Medical Establishment and Government Stick It to You and Your Family, at 41-42 (2018).

715. Eleanor McBean, The Poisoned Needle (1957).

716. Eleanor McBean, The Poisoned Needle (1957).

717. Lioness of Judah Ministry, MIND-BLOWING REVELATION: Why It's IMPOSSIBLE to "Vaccinate" Against Anything and Why "Vaccines" Are the PERFECT POISONS, Ocober 2, 2024, https://lionessofjudah.substack.com/p/mind-blowing-revelation-why-its-impossible?publication_id=581065&utm_campaign=email-post-title&r=2q45gw&utm_medium=email.

718. Id.

719. Id.

720. Id.

721. Arumugham, Vinu, Evidence that Food Proteins in Vaccines Cause the Development of Food Allergies and Its Implications for Vaccine Policy (2015). Journal of Developing Drugs, 2015, DOI: 10.4172/2329-6631.1000137, Available at SSRN: https://ssrn.com/abstract=3571073.

722. Charles Richet Facts, The Nobel Prize in Physiology or Medicine 1913, https://www.nobelprize.org/prizes/medicine/1913/richet/facts/ (last visited on October 7, 2024).

723. Id.

724. Poison, Merriam Webster Dictionary, https://www.merriam-webster.com/dictionary/poison (last visited on December 13, 2024).

725. ICD-10-CM, CDC, June 7, 2024, https://www.cdc.gov/nchs/icd/icd-10-cm/index.html.

726. ICD-9-CM Dignosis Code 978, https://www.icd10data.com/search?s=978&codebook=icd9volume1 (last visited on December 13, 2024).

727. Convert ICD-9-CM Diagnosis 978.4 to ICD-10-CM, https://www.icd10data.com/Convert/978.4 (last visited on December 13, 2024).

728. ICD-9-CM Dignosis Code 978, https://www.icd10data.com/search?s=978&codebook=icd9volume1 (last visited on December 13, 2024).

729. Convert ICD-9-CM Diagnosis 978.5 to ICD-10-CM, https://www.icd10data.com/Convert/978.5 (last visited on December 13, 2024).

730. ICD-9-CM Diagnosis Code 979.4, https://www.icd10data.com/Search?s=979.4&codebook=icd9volume1 (last visited on December 13, 2024).

731. 2025 ICD-10-CM Diagnosis Code T50.B91A, https://www.icd10data.com/ICD10CM/Codes/S00-T88/T36-T50/T50-/T50.B91A (last visited on December 13, 2024).

732. Convert ICD-9-CM Diagnosis 979.5 to ICD-10-CM, https://www.icd10data.com/Convert/979.5 (last visited on December 13, 2024).

733. Vaccine Ingredients – Fetal Cells, Vaccine Education Center, CHOP, https://www.chop.edu/centers-programs/vaccine-education-center/vaccine-ingredients/fetal-tissues (last visited on January 28, 2023).

734. Overview of COVID-19 Vaccines, CDC, November 1, 2022, https://www.cdc.gov/coronavirus/2019-ncov/vaccines/different-vaccines/overview-COVID-19-vaccines.html?CDC_AA_refVal=https%3A%2F%2Fwww.cdc.gov%2Fcoronavirus%2F2019-ncov%2Fvaccines%2Fdifferent-vaccines%2FModerna.html.

735. ImmunizeBC, https://immunizebc.ca/ask-us/questions/are-there-any-animal-products-including-pork-covid-19-vaccines (last visited on January 29, 2023).

736. Claire Gillespie, Fetal Cell Lines Were Used to Make the Johnson & Johnson COVID Vaccine—Here's What That Means, Health, March 4, 2021, https://www.health.com/condition/vaccines/johnson-and-johnson-fetal-cells-vaccine.

737. Danielle Ong, Johnson & Johnson Vaccine Did Use Aborted Fetal Cell Lines: What Does This Mean?, International Business Times, March 4, 2021, https://www.ibtimes.com/johnson-johnson-vaccine-did-use-aborted-fetal-cell-lines-what-does-mean-3156846.

738. Claire Gillespie, March 4, 2021, supra.

739. Kyle Christopher McKenna, Ph.D, Use of Aborted Fetal Tissue in Vaccines and Medical Research Obscures the Value of All Human Life, US National Library of Medicine National Institutes of Health, March 28, 2018, https://www.ncbi.nlm.nih.gov/pmc/articles/PMC6027112/.

740. Id.

741. Id.

742. Vaccines, Abortion, & Fetal Tissue, Right to Life of Michigan, https://rtl.org/educational-materials/vaccines-abortion/, July 9, 2020, quoting Transcript of the Vaccines and Related Biological Products Advisory Committee of the U.S. Food and Drug Administration, hearing date 16 May 2001, 91. See also, https://www.ohiolife.org/vaccines_abortion_fetal_tissue, October 27, 2017.

743. Jack Jenkins, New Novavax Shot Could Appeal to Pro-Life Christian Skeptics, Religious News Service, February 18, 2022, https://www.christianitytoday.com/news/2022/february/novavax-covid-vaccine-cell-lines-pro-life-abortion-christia.html.

744. McKenna KC. Use of Aborted Fetal Tissue in Vaccines and Medical Research Obscures the Value of All Human Life. Linacre Q. 2018 Feb;85(1):13-17. doi: 10.1177/0024363918761715. Epub 2018 Mar 28. PMID: 29970932; PMCID: PMC6027112. Also found at Lyle Christopher McKenna, Use of Aborted Fetal Tissue in Vaccines and Medical Research Obscures the Value of All Human Life, NIH, March 28, 2018, https://www.ncbi.nlm.nih.gov/pmc/articles/PMC6027112/.

745. Sandhya Bangaru, et al., Structural analysis of full-length SARS-CoV-2 spike protein from an advanced vaccine candidate, 20 October 2020, https://www.science.org/doi/10.1126/science.abe1502.

746. Sandhya Bangaru, et al., Structural analysis of full-length SARS-CoV-2 spike protein from an advanced vaccine candidate, 20 October 2020, https://www.science.org/doi/10.1126/science.abe1502.

747. Jack Jenkins, New Novavax Shot Could Appeal to Pro-Life Christian Skeptics, Religious News Service, February 18, 2022, https://www.christianitytoday.com/news/2022/february/novavax-covid-vaccine-cell-lines-pro-life-abortion-christia.html.

748. Sarah Quale, Yes, Novavax Used HEK293, an Aborted Fetal Cell Line, Personhood Alliance,

February 2, 2022, https://personhood.org/yes-novavax-used-hek293-an-aborted-fetal-cell-line-2/.

749. Sara Quale, February 2, 2022, supra.

750. Raymond Obomsawin, Ph.D., Immunity, Infectious Disease, and Vaccination. Video Re-Posted by Edward Hendrie Under Article Heading: The History of Vaccines Proving They Are Ineffective and Dangerous, May 26, 2021, https://greatmountainpublishing.com/2021/05/26/the-history-of-vaccines-proving-they-are-ineffective-and-dangerous/. See also, Ida Honorof and Eleanor McBean, Vaccination, The Silent Killer: A Clear and Present Danger (1977), https://archive.org/details/vaccinationsilen00hono, and Eleanor McBean, The Poisoned Needle (1957), http://www.whale.to/a/mcbean.html.

751. Brett Wilcox, Jabbed, How the Vaccine Industry, Medical Establishment and Government Stick It to You and Your Family (2018), quoting James Howenstine, M.D., A Physicians Guide to Natural Health Products (2002),

752. Edward Hendrie, Study Shows That Vaccinated Children Are Significantly Less Healthy Than Unvaccinated Children, December 20, 2020, https://greatmountainpublishing.com/2020/12/20/study-shows-that-vaccinated-children-are-significantly-less-healthy-than-unvaccinated-children/.

753. Id.

754. James Lyons-Weiler and Paul Thomas, Relative Incidence of Office Visits and Cumulative Rates of

Billed Diagnoses Along the Axis of Vaccination, 22 November 2020, https://www.mdpi.com/1660-4601/17/22/8674/htm.

755. Retraction: Lyons-Weiler, J.; Thomas, P. Relative Incidence of Office Visits and Cumulative Rates of Billed Diagnoses along the Axis of Vaccination. Int. J. Environ. Res. Public Health 2020, 17, 8674, https://www.mdpi.com/1660-4601/18/15/7754/htm.

756. Lyons-Weiler, J., & Russell L, B. (2022). Revisiting Excess Diagnoses of Illnesses and Conditions in Children Whose Parents Provided Informed Permission to Vaccinate Them. International Journal of Vaccine Theory, Practice, and Research, 2(2), 603–618. https://doi.org/10.56098/ijvtpr.v2i2.59. See also https://ijvtpr.com/index.php/IJVTPR/article/view/59/118.

757. Steve Kirsch, The data is clear: the more vaccines you give your child, the more likely it is that they will develop chronic diseases including autism, May 30, 2023, https://stevekirsch.substack.com/p/the-data-is-clear-the-more-vaccines?utm_source=post-email-title&publication_id=548354&post_id=124853131&isFreemail=true&utm_medium=email.

758. Oregon Medical Board, "In the Matter of Paul Norman Thomas, MD, License No. MD15689: Order of Emergency Suspension," State of Oregon, December 3, 2020, https://omb.oregon.gov/Clients/ORMB/OrderDocuments/e579dd35-7e1b-471f-a69a-3a800317ed4c.pdf.

759. James Lyons-Weiler and Paul Thomas, "Relative Incidence of Office Visits and Cumulative Rates of Billed Diagnoses Along the Axis of Vaccination", International Journal of Environmental Research and Public Health, November 22, 2020, https://doi.org/10.3390/ijerph17228674.

760. Retraction: Lyons-Weiler, J.; Thomas, P. Relative Incidence of Office Visits and Cumulative Rates of Billed Diagnoses along the Axis of Vaccination. Int. J. Environ. Res. Public Health 2020, 17, 8674, https://www.mdpi.com/1660-4601/18/15/7754/htm.

761. Jeremy Hammond, March 26, 2021, Oregon Medical Board Suspends Dr. Paul Thomas for Practicing Informed Consent, https://www.jeremyrhammond.com/2021/03/26/oregon-medical-board-suspends-dr-paul-thomas-for-practicing-informed-consent/.

762. Jeremy Hammond, March 26, 2021, supra.

763. IPAK, https://ipaknowledge.org/ (last visited on December 20, 2020).

764. Rhoda Wilson, Big Study Finds Non-Vaccinated are Healthier than Vaccinated, The Expose, April 11, 2022, https://expose-news.com/2022/04/11/study-finds-non-vaccinated-are-healthier-than-vaccinated/.

765. The Control Group, https://www.thecontrolgroup.org/.

766. Garner v. Trump, Verified Petition for Declaratory and Injunctive Relief, December 14, 2020, https://informedconsentdefense.files.wordpress.com/20

20/12/verified-petition-filed.pdf.

767. The Control Group Litigation, Update October 4, 2022, https://informedconsentdefense.org/.

768. Rhoda Wilson, Big Study Finds Non-Vaccinated are Healthier than Vaccinated, The Expose, April 11, 2022, https://expose-news.com/2022/04/11/study-finds-non-vaccinated-are-healthier-than-vaccinated/.

769. Brian S. Hooker, Analysis of health outcomes in vaccinated and unvaccinated children: Developmental delays, asthma, ear infections and gastrointestinal disorders, May 27, 2020, https://journals.sagepub.com/doi/10.1177/2050312120925344.

770. Anthony Mawson, Pilot comparative study on the health of vaccinated and unvaccinated 6- to 12-year-old U.S. children, Journal of Translational Science, 2017, https://childrenshealthdefense.org/wp-content/uploads/Unvaccinated-vaccinated-ASD-ADHD-study-Mawson-2017.pdf.

771. State of health of unvaccinated children, https://www.vaccineinjury.info/survey/results-unvaccinated/results-illnesses.html (last visited on May 31, 2023).

772. Steve Kirsch, The data is clear: the more vaccines you give your child, the more likely it is that they will develop chronic diseases including autism, May 30, 2023, https://stevekirsch.substack.com/p/the-data-is-clear-the-more-vaccines?utm_source=post-email-title&publicati

on_id=548354&post_id=124853131&isFreemail=true&utm_medium=email.

773. Cal-Oregon Unvaccinated Survey, Generation Rescue, June 26, 2007, https://www.lynneshealth.com/resources/Autism/Vacination%20Study.pdf.

774. Robert F. Kennedy Jr., Fully Vaccinated vs. Unvaccinated — Part 1, Children's Health Defense, June 25, 2019, https://childrenshealthdefense.org/child-health-topics/exposing-truth/fully-vaccinated-vs-unvaccinated/.

775. Secret CDC Verstraeten study shows neurological developmental disorders with mercury in vaccines, https://www.vaccineinjury.info/news/978-secret-cdc-verstraeten-study-shows-neurological-developmental-disorders-with-mercury-in-vaccines.html (last visited on September 23, 2024).

776. Id.

777. Robert F. Kennedy Jr., Fully Vaccinated vs. Unvaccinated — Part 1, supra.

778. Secret CDC Verstraeten study, supra.

779. Verstraeten T, Davis RL, DeStefano F, Lieu TA, Rhodes PH, Black SB, Shinefield H, Chen RT; Vaccine Safety Datalink Team. Safety of thimerosal-containing vaccines: a two-phased study of computerized health maintenance organization databases. Pediatrics. 2003 Nov;112(5):1039-48. Erratum in: Pediatrics. 2004 Jan;113(1):184. PMID: 14595043.

780. State of health of unvaccinated children, https://www.vaccineinjury.info/survey/results-unvaccinated/results-illnesses.html (last visited on May 31, 2023).

781. Kreesten Meldgaard Madsen and Anders Hviid, et al., A Population-Based Study of Measles, Mumps, and Rubella Vaccination and Autism, NEJM, November 7, 2002, N Engl J Med 2002; 347:1477-1482, DOI: 10.1056/NEJMoa021134, https://www.nejm.org/doi/full/10.1056/nejmoa021134

782. Steven Kirsch, Proof: author of #1 paper showing no link between vaccines and autism is corrupt, May 29, 2023, https://stevekirsch.substack.com/p/key-paper-showing-no-link-between?utm_source=post-email-title&publication_id=548354&post_id=124221729&isFreemail=true&utm_medium=email.

783. Something Is Rotten in Denmark. October 2003, https://childrenshealthdefense.org/wp-content/uploads/5.15-SOMETHING-IS-ROTTEN-IN-DENMARK.pdf.

784. Paul Thorsen, https://oig.hhs.gov/fraud/fugitives/poul-thorsen/ (last visited on May 31, 2023).

785. Aaby P, Mogensen SW, Rodrigues A, Benn CS. Evidence of Increase in Mortality After the Introduction of Diphtheria-Tetanus-Pertussis Vaccine to Children Aged 6-35 Months in Guinea-Bissau: A Time for Reflection? Front Public Health. 2018 Mar 19;6:79. doi: 10.3389/fpubh.2018.00079. PMID: 29616207; PMCID: PMC5868131, https://www.ncbi.nlm.nih.gov/pmc/articles/PMC5868131/.

786. Aaron Siri Letter Re: Death of Infants in Certain Developing Countries by Systematic Use of a Biologic to Special Rapporteur on Torture and Other Cruel, Inhuman or Degrading Treatment or Punishment, Janauary 28, 2021, https://icandecide.org/wp-content/uploads/2021/06/2021.01.28-Letter-to-Special-Rapporteur-on-Torture.pdf.

787. Aaby P, et al., 2018 March 19, supra.

788. Aaron Siri Letter, January 28, 2021, supra.

789. Koepke R, Eickhoff JC, Ayele RA, Petit AB, Schauer SL, Hopfensperger DJ, Conway JH, Davis JP. Estimating the effectiveness of tetanus-diphtheria-acellular pertussis vaccine (Tdap) for preventing pertussis: evidence of rapidly waning immunity and difference in effectiveness by Tdap brand. J Infect Dis. 2014 Sep 15;210(6):942-53. doi: 10.1093/infdis/jiu322. Epub 2014 Jun 5. PMID: 24903664, https://pubmed.ncbi.nlm.nih.gov/24903664/.

790. Igor Chudov, Are Childhood Vaccines Safe? DTP Vaccine Was Not - and Was Given for Decades!, May 26, 2023, https://igorchudov.substack.com/p/are-childhood-vaccines-safe-dtp-vaccine?utm_source=post-email-title&publication_id=441185&post_id=123856103&isFreemail=true&utm_medium=email.

791. Aaron Siri Letter, January 28, 2021, supra.

792. Aaron Siri Letter, January 28, 2021, supra.

793. What is SIDS?, NIH, https://safetosleep.nichd.nih.gov/about/sids-definition

(last visited on June 23, 2023).

794. What is SIDS?, NIH, supra.

795. A Midwestern Doctor, Healthy Adults are Not the Only Ones Who Have Been Killed by Vaccines, June 16, 2023, https://amidwesterndoctor.substack.com/p/healthy-adults-are-not-the-only-ones?utm_source=profile&utm_medium=reader2.

796. A Midwestern Doctor, The Century of Evidence That Vaccines Cause Infant Deaths, August 24, 2022, https://amidwesterndoctor.substack.com/p/a-century-of-evidence-has-accumulated.

797. Igor Chudov, Florida "Vaccine Hesitancy" REDUCED Infant Mortality in 2021, March 14, 2022, https://igorchudov.substack.com/p/florida-vaccine-hesitancy-reduced.

798. Carina Blackmore, Director, Division of Disease Control and Health Protection, Assessment of County Health Department Immunization Coverage Levels in 2-Year-Old Children (2021), Florida Health Department, June 4, 2021, https://www.floridahealth.gov/programs-and-services/immunization/resources/surveys/_documents/chd-assesment-2021.pdf.

799. Florida Death Statistics in 2021, https://deadorkicking.com/death-statistics/us/florida/2021/ (last visited on May 28, 2023).

800. Carina Blackmore, June 4, 2021, supra.

801. Igor Chudov, March 14, 2021, supra.

802. Edward Hendrie, Most Pediatricians Refuse to Treat Unvaccinated Children Because They Are Paid a Bounty for Every Fully Vaccinated Child in Their Practice above a Certain Threshold, October 16, 2022, https://hendrie.substack.com/p/most-pediatricians-refuse-to-treat.

803. EO 8.7 Routine Universal Immunization of Physicians, Code of Medical Ethics, Immunization, AMA, https://policysearch.ama-assn.org/policyfinder/detail/immunization?uri=%2FAMADoc%2FEthics.xml-E-8.7.xml.

804. Edward Hendrie, The AMA Is Working to Stop Religious Exemptions and Requires Doctors to Encourage Patients to Get Vaccinated, November 19, 2021, https://greatmountainpublishing.com/2021/11/19/the-ama-is-working-to-stop-religious-exemptions-and-requires-doctors-to-encourage-patients-to-get-vaccinated/.

805. AMA Code of Medical Ethics, https://code-medical-ethics.ama-assn.org/faq (last visited on May 28, 2023).

806. Lessons from the Lockdown—Why Are So Many Fewer Children Dying?, Children's Health Defense, June 18, 2020, https://childrenshealthdefense.org/news/lessons-from-the-lockdown-why-are-so-many-fewer-children-dying/.

807. Id.

808. Santoli, Jeanne M et al. Effects of the COVID-19 Pandemic on Routine Pediatric Vaccine Ordering and Administration — United States, 2020. cdc.gov.

https://www.cdc.gov/mmwr/volumes/69/wr/mm6919e2.htm#F1_down.

809. Lessons from the Lockdown, supra.

810. Miller NZ, Goldman GS. Infant mortality rates regressed against number of vaccine doses routinely given: is there a biochemical or synergistic toxicity? Hum Exp Toxicol. 2011 Sep;30(9):1420-8. doi: 10.1177/0960327111407644. Epub 2011 May 4. Erratum in: Hum Exp Toxicol. 2011 Sep;30(9):1429. PMID: 21543527; PMCID: PMC3170075, https://www.ncbi.nlm.nih.gov/pmc/articles/PMC3170075/.

811. Brett Wilcox, Jabbed, How the Vaccine Industry, Medical Establishment and Government
Stick It to You and Your Family (2018), quoting James Howenstine, M.D., A Physicians Guide to Natural Health Products (2002),

812. Id.

813. Steve Zauderer, 69+ Autism Statistics: How Many People Have Autism?, Key Autism Statistics: Rates Of Autism In 2021 and 2022, December 28, 2022, https://www.crossrivertherapy.com/autism-statistics.

814. Child and Adolescent Immunization Schedule by Age, CDC, https://www.cdc.gov/vaccines/schedules/hcp/imz/child-adolescent.html#note-mening (last visited on February 14, 2023).

815. Child and Adolescent Immunization Schedule by Age, CDC, https://www.cdc.gov/vaccines/schedules/hcp/imz/child

-adolescent.html#note-mening (last visited on February 14, 2023).

816. Autism & Aluminum Adjuvants in Vaccines, How Aluminum Adjuvants in Vaccines Can Cause, August 18, 2017, Autismhttp://vaccinepapers.org/wp-content/uploads/Autism-and-aluminum-adjuvants-in-vaccines-1.pdf.

817. Vaccine Aluminum Travels Into The Brain, February 10, 2015, http://vaccinepapers.org/vaccine-aluminum-travels-to-the-brain/.

818. Vaccine Aluminum Travels Into The Brain, supra.

819. Matthew Mold, et al., Aluminium in brain tissue in autism, Journal of Trace Elements in Medicine and Biology, 46 (2018) 76-82, http://vaccinepapers.org/wp-content/uploads/Mold-2018-Aluminium-aluminum-in-brain-tissue-in-autism.pdf.

820. Vaccine Aluminum Travels Into The Brain, February 10, 2015, http://vaccinepapers.org/vaccine-aluminum-travels-to-the-brain/.

821. Gallagher CM, Goodman MS. Hepatitis B vaccination of male neonates and autism diagnosis, NHIS 1997-2002. J Toxicol Environ Health A. 2010;73(24):1665-77. doi: 10.1080/15287394.2010.519317. PMID: 21058170. https://pubmed.ncbi.nlm.nih.gov/21058170/.

822. Mawson AR, Ray BD, Bhuiyan AR, Jacob B (2017) Pilot comparative study on the health of vaccinated and unvaccinated 6- to 12-year-old U.S.

children. J Transl Sci 3: DOI: 10.15761/JTS.1000186, April 24, 2017, https://www.oatext.com/Pilot-comparative-study-on-the-health-of-vaccinated-and-unvaccinated-6-to-12-year-old-U-S-children.php#gsc.tab=0.

823. Edward Hendrie, Vaccines Cause Autism and Allergies, August 5, 2020, https://greatmountainpublishing.com/2020/08/05/vaccines-cause-autism-and-allergies/.

824. Edward Hendrie, August 5, 2020, supra.

825. Andrew Wakefield, et al., Ileal-lymphoid-nodular hyperplasia, non-specific colitis, and pervasive developmental disorder in children, The Lancet, Volume 351, ISSUE 9103, P637-641, February 28, 1998, https://www.thelancet.com/journals/lancet/article/PIIS0140673697110960/fulltext. DOI:https://doi.org/10.1016/S0140-6736(97)11096-0.

826. Anders Hvid, et al., Measles, Mumps, Rubella Vaccination and Autism, 16 April 2019, https://www.acpjournals.org/doi/full/10.7326/M18-2101.

827. Anders Hvid, et al., supra.

828. Anders Hvid, et al., supra.

829. Novo Nordsk Foundation, Who Are We?, https://novonordiskfonden.dk/en/who-we-are/ (last visited on February 13, 2023).

830. Novo Holdings A/S, Annual Report, 2021, https://www.novoholdings.dk/wp-content/uploads/Novo-Holdings-Annual-Report-2021.pdf.

831. Novo Nordisk Foundation, Open Philanthropy, and Bill & Melinda Gates Foundation Launch Initiative to Support New Antiviral Medicines for Future Pandemics, Bill & Melinda Gates Foundation, https://www.gatesfoundation.org/ideas/media-center/press-releases/2022/03/funding-new-antiviral-medicines-and-preventing-future-pandemics (last visited on February 13, 2023).

832. Quats Application, Novo Nordisk A/S/, https://novonordiskpharmatech.com/products/vaccine-production/ (last visited on February 14, 2023). See also What is Cetrimonium bromide (CTAB)?, Novo Nordisk Pharmaceuticals A/S/, https://novonordiskpharmatech.com/products/ctab/ (last visited on February 14, 2023).

833. Quats Application, Novo Nordisk A/S/, https://novonordiskpharmatech.com/products/vaccine-production/ (last visited on February 14, 2023). See also What is Cetrimonium bromide (CTAB)?, Novo Nordisk Pharmaceuticals A/S/, https://novonordiskpharmatech.com/products/ctab/ (last visited on February 14, 2023).

834. Quats Application, supra.

835. Anders Hvid, et al., Measles, Mumps, Rubella Vaccination and Autism, 16 April 2019, https://www.acpjournals.org/doi/full/10.7326/M18-2101.

836. New in Denmark, Health Guidelines for Parents with small Children, Danish Health Authority, 2016, https://www.sst.dk/-/media/Udgivelser/2016/Ny-i-et-fremmed-land/Engelsk_Ny-i-et-fremmed-land.ashx.

837. Rob Stein, A Large Study Provides More Evidence That MMR Vaccines Don't Cause Autism, NPR, March 4, 2019, https://www.npr.org/sections/health-shots/2019/03/04/699997613/a-large-study-provides-more-evidence-that-mmr-vaccines-dont-cause-autism.

838. Rob Stein, March 4, 2019, supra.

839. New in Denmark, Health Guidelines for Parents with small Children, Danish Health Authority, 2016, https://www.sst.dk/-/media/Udgivelser/2016/Ny-i-et-fremmed-land/Engelsk_Ny-i-et-fremmed-land.ashx.

840. Danish Health Authority Guidelines, 2016, supra.

841. Anders Hvid, et al., Measles, Mumps, Rubella Vaccination and Autism, 16 April 2019, https://www.acpjournals.org/doi/full/10.7326/M18-2101.

842. Rob Stein, A Large Study Provides More Evidence That MMR Vaccines Don't Cause Autism, NPR, March 4, 2019, https://www.npr.org/sections/health-shots/2019/03/04/699997613/a-large-study-provides-more-evidence-that-mmr-vaccines-dont-cause-autism.

843. Rob Stein, March 4, 2019 supra.

844. Comment of Pedro Alcantara, Asociacion Espanola de Pediatria, 9 May 2019. Anders Hvid, et al., Measles, Mumps, Rubella Vaccination and Autism, 16 April 2019, https://www.acpjournals.org/doi/full/10.7326/M18-2101.

845. Comment of Anthony R. Mawson, Department of Epidemiology and Biostatistics, School of Public Health, Jackson State University, 28 March 2019. Anders Hvid, et al., Measles, Mumps, Rubella Vaccination and Autism, 16 April 2019, https://www.acpjournals.org/doi/full/10.7326/M18-2101.

846. Brett Wilcox, Jabbed, How the Vaccine Industry, Medical Establishment and Government Stick It to You and Your Family, at 32-33 (2018).

847. Wilcox, Jabbed, supra.

848. Wilcox, Jabbed, supra.

849. Vaccination Recommendations by the AAP, https://www.aap.org/en/patient-care/immunizations/vaccination-recommendations-by-the-aap/ (last visited on June 17, 2023).

850. COVID-19 Vaccines in Infants, Children, and Adolescents, AAP, August 29, 2022, https://doi.org/10.1542/peds.2022-058700.

851. VAERS COVID Vaccine Adverse Event Reports, June 2, 2023, https://openvaers.com/covid-data.

852. Brian Peckford, American Academy of Pediatrics tries hiding Pfizer funding, August 27, 2021, https://peckford42.wordpress.com/2021/08/27/american-academy-of-pediatrics-tries-hiding-pfizer-funding/.

853. Brian Peckford, August 27, 2021, supra.

854. Vaccination Recommendations by the AAP, https://www.aap.org/en/patient-care/immunizations/vaccination-recommendations-by-the-aap/ (last visited on

June 17, 2023).

855. Vaccines—Autism Toolkit, AAP, 2021, https://publications.aap.org/patiented/article-abstract/doi/10.1542/peo_document599/82016/Vaccines-Autism-Toolkit?redirectedFrom=fulltext.

856. Robert E. Weibel, et al., Acute Encephalopathy Followed by Permanent Brain Injury or Death Associated With Further Attenuated Measles Vaccines: A Review of Claims Submitted to the National Vaccine Injury Compensation Program, AAP, March 1998, https://doi.org/10.1542/peds.101.3.383.

857. How Do Vaccines Cause Autism?, https://howdovaccinescauseautism.org/ (last visited on June 17, 2023). See also Ginger Taylor, 214 Research Papers Supporting The Vaccine/Autism Link, April 28, 2014, https://www.scribd.com/doc/220807175/214-Research-Papers-Supporting-the-Vaccine-Autism-Link?utm_source=substack&utm_medium=email#.

858. Steve Kirsch, If vaccines don't cause autism, then how do you explain all this evidence?, June 17, 2023, https://stevekirsch.substack.com/p/if-vaccines-dont-cause-autism-then?utm_source=post-email-title&publication_id=548354&post_id=128881554&isFreemail=true&utm_medium=email.

859. Steve Kirsch, June 17, 2023, supra.

860. Steve Kirsch, June 17, 2023, supra.

861. Steve Kirsch, June 17, 2023, supra.

862. Steve Kirsch, June 17, 2023, supra.

863. Steve Kirsch, June 17, 2023, supra.

864. Pakcage Insert, Gardasil [Quadrivalent Human Papillomavirus (Types 6, 11, 16, 18) Recombinant Vaccine], Merck, http://web.archive.org/web/20060614111131/http://www.merck.com/product/usa/pi_circulars/g/gardasil/gardasil_pi.pdf (last visited on March 15, 2023).

865. Placebo, Merriam-Webster, https://www.merriam-webster.com/dictionary/placebo (last visited on March 16, 2023).

866. Beecher Hk. The Powerful Placebo. JAMA. 1955;159(17):1602–1606. doi:10.1001/jama.1955.02960340022006, https://jamanetwork.com/journals/jama/article-abstract/303530.

867. Doshi P, Bourgeois F, Hong K, et alAdjuvant-containing control arms in pivotal quadrivalent human papillomavirus vaccine trials: restoration of previously unpublished methodologyBMJ Evidence-Based Medicine 2020;25:213-219, https://ebm.bmj.com/content/25/6/213.

868. Package Insert, Gardasil [Human Papillomavirus Quadrivalent (Types 6, 11, 16, and 18) Vaccine, Recombinant], Merck, http://web.archive.org/web/20080916044911/http://www.merck.com/product/usa/pi_circulars/g/gardasil/gardasil_pi.pdf (las visited on March 15, 2023).

869. Doshi P, Bourgeois F, Hong K, et alAdjuvant-containing control arms in pivotal quadrivalent human papillomavirus vaccine trials:

restoration of previously unpublished methodologyBMJ Evidence-Based Medicine 2020;25:213-219, https://ebm.bmj.com/content/25/6/213.

870. Doshi, supra.

871. Doshi, supra.

872. Doshi, supra.

873. Doshi, supra.

874. Anonymous, Turtles All the Way Down, at 52 (2022).

875. Vaccine (Shot) for Hepatitis A, CDC, https://www.cdc.gov/vaccines/parents/diseases/hepa.html (last visited on March 15, 2023).

876. VAQTA® (Hepatitis A Vaccine, Inactivated), Suspension for Intramuscular Injection, Package Insert, Merck & Co.

877. Diphtheria, Tetanus, and Pertussis Vaccines, Vaccine Safety, CDC, https://www.cdc.gov/vaccinesafety/vaccines/dtap-tdap-vaccine.html (last visited on March 15, 2023).

878. Dr. William H. Gaunt, M.D., How to cheat and lie with Vaccine Science, https://nexusnewsfeed.com/article/health-healing/how-to-cheat-and-lie-with-vaccine-science/ (last visited on March 14, 2023).

879. Antonia Geber, M.D., Clinical Review of Biological License Application DAPTACEL (CPDT), Division of Vaccines and Related Products

Applications, Office of Vaccines Research and Review, Center for Biologics Evaluation and Research, Food and Drug Administration, at 54 and 61, 9 April 2002.

880. Antonia Geber, M.D., supra at p. 55.

881. Investigational Drug, NIH, National Cancer Institute, https://www.cancer.gov/publications/dictionaries/cancer-terms/def/investigational-drug (last visited on March 14, 2023).

882. Package Insert, Pneumococcal 7-valent Conjugate Vaccine (Diphtheria CRM197 Protein) Prevnar®, For Pediatric Use Only, For Intramuscular Injection Only.

883. Anonymous, Turtles All the Way Down, at 61 (2022), citing Black S, Shinefield H, Fireman B, Lewis E, Ray P, Hansen JR, Elvin L, Ensor KM, Hackell J, Siber G, Malinoski F, Madore D, Chang I, Kohberger R, Watson W, Austrian R, Edwards K. Efficacy, safety and immunogenicity of heptavalent pneumococcal conjugate vaccine in children. Northern California Kaiser Permanente Vaccine Study Center Group. Pediatr Infect Dis J. 2000 Mar;19(3):187-95. doi: 10.1097/00006454-200003000-00003. PMID: 10749457.

884. Package Insert, Prevnar.

885. PREVNAR-13 Package Insert, PREVNAR 13 (Pneumococcal 13-valent Conjugate Vaccine [Diphtheria CRM197 Protein]) Suspension for intramuscular injection Initial US Approval: 2010.

886. PREVNAR-13 Package Insert, supra.

887. Ransdell Pierson, U.S. advisory panel recommends Prevnar 13 vaccine for elderly, Reuters, August 13, 2014, https://www.reuters.com/article/us-pfizer-prevnar-idUSKBN0GD23I20140813.

888. Jeremy Howick, Coronavirus vaccine: why it's important to know what's in the placebo, The Conversation, September 21, 2020, https://theconversation.com/coronavirus-vaccine-why-its-important-to-know-whats-in-the-placebo-146365.

889. Study # NCT04368728 (v1), Sponsor BioNTech, Study to Describe the Safety, Tolerability, Immunogenicity, and Potential Efficacy of RNA Vaccine Candidates Against COVID-19 in Healthy Adults, April 29, 2020, https://clinicaltrials.gov/ct2/history/NCT04368728?V_1=View#StudyPageTop.

890. Study # NCT04368728 (v1), supra.

891. Letter from Sarah Kotler, Director Division of Freedom of Information, FDA to ICAN, Request Number: 2020-3738, Subject of Request: ingredients of the 'placebo' in the clinical trial NCTR04368728, June 3, 2020, https://icandecide.org/wp-content/uploads/2021/06/Denial-of-Information-Regarding-Placebo-in-Pfizer-COVID-19-Vaccine-Trial.pdf.

892. Virginia Pediatrics Group, https://www.vapg.com/service/vaccines-specialist (last visited on October 19, 2022).

893. Virginia Pediatric Group, https://web.archive.org/web/20200923183720/http://w

ww.vapg.com/docs/VPG%20Vaccination%20Policy%209-2019.pdf (last visited on October 19, 2022).

894. The Real Agenda Behind American Academy of Pediatrics: Weaponizing Children's Mental Health and Vaccines for Profit, The Defender, December 8, 2022, https://childrenshealthdefense.org/defender/profit-american-academy-pediatrics-childrens-mental-health-vaccines/.

895. Ensuring Comprehensive Care and Support for Transgender and Gender-Diverse Children and Adolescents, AAP, October 1, 2008, https://doi.org/10.1542/peds.2018-2162.

896. Sample Vaccine Policy Statement, Immunization Action Coalition, https://www.immunize.org/catg.d/p2067.pdf (last visited on October 19, 2022).

897. Sample Vaccine Policy Statement, supra.

898. The Immunization Action Coalition, https://www.immunize.org/aboutus/ (last visited on Ocober 19, 2022).

899. CDC and WHO Corrupt Financial Entanglements with the Vaccine Industry, Children's Health Defense, https://childrenshealthdefense.org/cdc-who/ (last visited on October 19, 2022).

900. Alex Pietroski, Proof Surfaces Insurance Co Pays Massive Bonuses to Doctors for Vaccinating Babies, Waking Times, August 8, 2017, http://www.wakingtimes.com/proof-surfaces-insurance-co-pays-massive-bonuses-doctors-vaccinating-babies/.

901. Doctors to Texas parents: No vaccination, no office visit, AP, March 13, 2019, https://abc13.com/measles-vaccination-texas-doctors-doctor-refuse-to-see-un-vaccinated-children/5189002/.

902. Vaccine Refusal: AAP Changes Stance on Patient Dismissal, Consulant 360, https://www.consultant360.com/exclusives/vaccine-refusal-aap-changes-stance-patient-dismissal (last visited on October 2, 2022).

903. David Weissman, No vaccination, no service: Some SC pediatricians turning away kids for parents' decisions, Greenville News, May 7, 2019, https://www.greenvilleonline.com/story/news/2019/05/07/some-sc-pediatricians-refuse-service-if-children-dont-get-vaccine-anti-vaxxer-parents/1128830001/.

904. David Weissman, May 7, 2019, supra.

905. Brian Argo, LinkedIn, https://www.linkedin.com/in/brian-argo-2ba882b (last visited on October 2, 2022).

906. 2016 Performance Recognition Program, Provider Incentive Program, Blue Cross Blue Shield, at 15, http://www.whale.to/c/2016-BCN-BCBSM-Incentive-Program-Booklet.pdf (last visited on October 1, 2022).

907. Id.

908. Alison B. Bocian, et al., Size and Age-Sex Distribution of Pediatric Practice: A Study From Pediatric Research in Office Settings, JAMA, January 1999, https://jamanetwork.com/journals/jamapediatrics/fullarticle/344727.

909. WE, How Much Money Do Pediatricians Really Make From Vaccines?, Wellness and Equality, June 20, 2016, https://wellnessandequality.com/2016/06/20/how-much-money-do-pediatricians-really-make-from-vaccines/.

910. WE, How Much Money Do Pediatricians Really Make From Vaccines?, Wellness and Equality, June 20, 2016, https://wellnessandequality.com/2016/06/20/how-much-money-do-pediatricians-really-make-from-vaccines/. No Results Found, 2016 Blue Cross Blue Shield Performance Recognition Program removed from: https://thephysicianalliance.org/wp-content/uploads/2016/03/2016-BCN-BCBSM-Incentive-Program-Booklet.pdf (last visited on February 23, 2023). 2016 Blue Cross Blue Shield Performance Recognition Program available at: https://greatmountainpublishing.com/wp-content/uploads/2021/05/2016-BCN-BCBSM-Incentive-Program-Booklet.pdf (last visited on February 23, 2023). 2016 Blue Cross Blue Shield Performance Recognition Program also available at: http://www.whale.to/c/2016-BCN-BCBSM-Incentive-Program-Booklet.pdf (last visited on February 23, 2023).

911. J.B. Handley, Vaccines Don't Cause Autism, Pediatricians Do., Age of Autism, https://www.ageofautism.com/2010/01/vaccines-dont-cause-autism-pediatricians-do.html (last visited on April 8, 2023).

912. Brett Wilcox, Jabbed, How the Vaccine Industry, Medical Establishment and Government Stick It to You and Your Family, at 250 (2018).

913. Thomas Massey, Your primary care provider was bribed to suggest you should take the COVID vaccine, Twitter, @RepThomasMassie, https://twitter.com/RepThomasMassie/status/1646696738013454336?utm_source=substack&utm_medium=email.

914. Michael Nevradakis, Exclusive: She Made 'The Real Anthony Fauci' Required Reading for Her Students. Here's What Happened Next., The Defender, April 25, 2023, https://childrenshealthdefense.org/defender/lynn-comerford-the-real-anthony-fauci-required-reading-students-csueb/?utm_source=luminate&utm_medium=email&utm_campaign=defender-wk&utm_id=20230430.

915. Michael Nevradakis, The Defender, April 26, 2023, supra.

916. COVID-19 Vaccination Policy, Yale University, February 7, 2023, https://covid19.yale.edu/covid-19-vaccination-policy#:~:text=The%20university%20requires%20all%20students,within%2014%20days%20of%20eligibility.

917. U.S. Department of Health and Human Services Launches Nationwide Network of Trusted Voices to Encourage Vaccination in Next Phase of COVID-19 Public Education Campaign, April 1, 2021, archive copy from April 1, 2021, https://web.archive.org/web/20210401225102/https:/www.hhs.gov/about/news/2021/04/01/hhs-launches-nationwide-network-trusted-voices-encourage-vaccination-next-phase-covid-19-public-education-campaign.html.

918. Maggie Thorp and Jim Thorp, FOIA Reveals Troubling Relationship between HHS/CDC & the

American College of Obstetricians and Gynecologists, America Out Loud, May 7, 2023, https://www.americaoutloud.com/foia-reveals-troubling-relationship-between-hhs-cdc-the-american-college-of-obstetricians-and-gynecologists/?utm_source=substack&utm_medium=email.

919. Maggie Thorp and Jim Thorp, May 7, 2023, supra.

920. Maggie Thorp and Jim Thorp, May 7, 2023, supra.

921. Maggie Thorp and Jim Thorp, May 7, 2023, supra.

922. COVID-19 Vaccines and Pregnancy: Conversation Guide, ACOG, https://www.acog.org/covid-19/covid-19-vaccines-and-pregnancy-conversation-guide-for-clinicians (last visited on May 10, 2023).

923. COVID-19 Vaccines and Pregnancy, supra.

924. Maggie Thorp and Jim Thorp, May 7, 2023, supra.

925. David Bell, M.D., Brownstone Institute, COVID Vaccines Were Never Safe for Pregnant Women, Pfizer's Own Data Show, The Defender, April 28, 2023, https://childrenshealthdefense.org/defender/pfizer-covid-vaccine-pregnancy/.

926. David Bell, supra.

927. Amy Kelly, Report 69: BOMBSHELL – Pfizer and FDA Knew in Early 2021 That Pfizer mRNA COVID "Vaccine" Caused Dire Fetal and Infant Risks, Including Death. They Began an Aggressive Campaign to Vaccinate Pregnant Women Anyway., April 29, 2023,

https://dailyclout.io/bombshell-pfizer-and-the-fda-knew-in-early-2021-that-the-pfizer-mrna-covid-vaccine-caused-dire-fetal-and-infant-risks-they-began-an-aggressive-campaign-to-vaccinate-pregnant-women-anyway/.

928. Amy Kelly, April 29, 2023, supra.

929. Amy Kelly, April 29, 2023, supra.

930. Amy Kelly, April 29, 2023, supra.

931. Supporting CDC and Public Health, CDC Foundation, https://www.cdcfoundation.org/supporting-cdc (last visited on May 11, 2023).

932. Corporations, Foundations & Organizations, CDC Foundation, https://www.cdcfoundation.org/FY2018/organizations (last visited on May 11, 2023).

933. 310 U.S. 296 (1940).

934. 370 U.S. 421 (1962).

935. 597 U.S. 507 (2022).

936. 310 U.S. 296, 303–04 (1940).

937. Id.

938. 197 U.S. 11 (1905).

939. 197 U.S. 11 (1905).

940. 197 U.S. at 30-31 (1905).

941. ___ F.4th ___, No. 22-55908, 2025 WL 2167401 (9th Cir. 2025) (en banc).

942. ___ F.4th ___, No. 22-55908, 2025 WL 2167401 (9th Cir. 2025) (en banc).

943. ___ F.4th ___, No. 22-55908, 2025 WL 2167401 (9th Cir. 2025) (en banc).

944. ___ F.4th ___, No. 22-55908, 2025 WL 2167401 (9th Cir. 2025) (en banc).

945. ___ F.4th ___, No. 22-55908, 2025 WL 2167401 (9th Cir. 2025) (en banc).

946. ___ F.4th ___, No. 22-55908, 2025 WL 2167401 (9th Cir. 2025) (en banc).

947. Cruzan v. Dir., Missouri Dep't of Health, 497 U.S. 261 (1990).

948. Cruzan v. Dir., Missouri Dep't of Health, 497 U.S. 261, 262 (1990).

949. Cruzan v. Dir., Missouri Dep't of Health, 497 U.S. 261, 305 (1990) (quotation marks omitted), quoting Snyder v. Massachusetts, 291 U.S. 97, 105 (1934).

950. Zablocki v. Redhail, 434 U.S. 374, 388 (1978).

951. Washington v. Glucksberg, 521 U.S. 702, 720 (1997) citing Cruzan, 497 U.S. at 278–279.

952. Washington v. Glucksberg, 521 U.S. 702, 721 (1997), quoting Reno v. Flores, 507 U.S. 292, 302 (1993).

953. Washington v. Glucksberg, 521 U.S. 702, 721 (1997), quoting Reno v. Flores, 507 U.S. 292, 302 (1993) (ellipse and quotation marks omitted).

954. Health Freedom Def. Fund, Inc. v. Carvalho, No. 22-55908, 2025 WL 2167401, at *10 (9th Cir. 2025) (en banc).

955. 486 F. Supp. 3d. at 897.

956. 463 F. Supp. 3d 22, (D. Me. 2020).

957. Id.

958. 140 S.Ct. 2603 (2020) (Alito, J., dissenting).

959. Id. at 2604.

960. Id. at 2605.

961. Id. at 2608.

962. Id.

963. 141 S. Ct. 63, 70 (2020) (Gorsuch, J., concurring).

964. 141 S. Ct. 63, 70 (2020) (Gorsuch, J., concurring).

965. Id. at 71.

966. 983 F.3d 620 (2d Cir. 2020).

967. Id. at 635, citing Jacobson v. Massachusetts, 197 U.S. 11, 25 (1905).

968. Kennedy v. Bremerton Sch. Dist., 597 U.S. 507, 532 (2022).

969. 669 F. Supp. 3d 598 (S.D. Miss. 2023).

970. Bosarge v. Edney, 669 F. Supp. 3d 598, 609 (S.D. Miss. 2023), quoting Fulton v. City of Philadelphia, Pennsylvania, 593 U.S. 522, 540 (2021).

971. 494 U.S. 872 (1990).

972. Fulton v. City of Philadelphia, Pennsylvania, 593 U.S. 522, 533 (2021) (quotation marks and citations omitted).

973. Fulton v. City of Philadelphia, Pennsylvania, 593 U.S. 522, 534 (2021).

974. See Dahl v. Bd. of Trs. of W. Michigan Univ., 15 F.4th 728 (6th Cir. 2021).

975. Does 1-11 v. Bd. of Regents of Univ. of Colorado, 100 F.4th 1251, 1277 (10th Cir. 2024), citing Grace United Methodist Church, 451 F.3d at 654 (quoting Lukumi, 508 U.S. at 537–38, 113 S.Ct. 2217) (citing Fraternal Ord. of Police Newark Lodge No. 12, 170 F.3d at 364–66).

976. Does 1-6 v. Mills, 142 S. Ct. 17, 20 (2021) (Gorsuch, J., dissenting).

977. 142 U.S. at 22.

978. Bosarge v. Edney, 669 F. Supp. 3d 598 (S.D. Miss. 2023). ICAN Attorneys Secure Religious Exemption to Vaccination in Mississippi, April 17, 2023, https://icandecide.org/press-release/ican-attorneys-secure-religious-exemption-to-vaccination-in-mississippi/.

979. 669 F. Supp. 3d 598 (S.D. Miss. 2023).

980. Bosarge v. Edney, Verified Complaint for Declaratory and Injunctive Relief, United States

District Court Southern District of Mississippi Southern Division, Civil Action No. 1:22-cv-00233-HSO-BWR, Filed September 1, 2022, https://icandecide.org/wp-content/uploads/2023/04/001-Complaint.pdf. Bosarge v. Edney, 669 F. Supp. 3d 598 (S.D. Miss. 2023).

981. Tandon v. Newsom, 141 S. Ct. 1294, 1296 (2021) (per curiam).

982. 141 S. Ct. 1294, 1297 (2021) (per curiam).

983. 141 S. Ct. 63 (2020).

984. Bosarge v. Edney, 669 F. Supp. 3d 598, 609 (S.D. Miss. 2023).

985. 107 Stat. 1488, 42 U.S.C. § 2000bb et seq.

986. 374 U.S. 398 (1963).

987. 406 U.S. 205 (1972).

988. City of Boerne v. Flores, 521 U.S. 507 (1997).

989. 42 U.S.C.A. § 2000cc-5(7)(A).

990. 42 U.S. Code § 2000bb–1.

991. 42 U.S. Code § 2000bb–1.

992. 573 U.S. 682 (2014).

993. Id. at 701.

994. Id. at 691.

995. Id. at 724.

996. 450 U.S. 707 (1981).

997. Id.

998. Hobby Lobby, 573 U.S. at 725, citing Thomas v. Review Bd. of Indiana Employment Security Div., 450 U.S. 707, 716 (1981).

999. 42 USC § 2000e-2.

1000. 575 U.S. 768, 776 (2015) (Alito, J., concurring).

1001. 42 U.S.C. § 2000e–2.

1002. 575 U.S. 768, 776 (2015) (Alito, J., concurring).

1003. Groff v. DeJoy, 600 U.S. 447 (2023). Mission Hospital Agrees to Pay $89,000 To Settle EEOC Religious Discrimination Lawsuit, Asheville Hospital Fired Employees for Declining Flu Vaccination, Federal Agency Charged, January 12, 2018, https://www.eeoc.gov/newsroom/mission-hospital-agres-pay-89000-settle-eeoc-religious-discrimination-lawsuit.

1004. 61 F.3d 650, 654 (8th Cir. 1995).

1005. Id. at 654.

1006. Id. at 654-55.

1007. Mission Hospital Agrees to Pay $89,000 To Settle EEOC Religious Discrimination Lawsuit, Asheville Hospital Fired Employees for Declining Flu Vaccination, Federal Agency Charged, January 12, 2018, https://www.eeoc.gov/newsroom/mission-hospital-agres-pay-89000-settle-eeoc-religious-discrimination-laws uit.

1008. 600 U.S. 447 (2023), https://www.supremecourt.gov/opinions/22pdf/22-174_k536.pdf.

1009. Saint Vincent Health Center To Pay $300,000 To Settle EEOC Religious Accommodation Lawsuit, Hospital Refused To Grant Employees Religious Belief-Based Exemptions From Flu Vaccination Requirement and Instead Fired Them, Federal Agency Charged, December 23, 2016, https://www.eeoc.gov/newsroom/saint-vincent-health-center-pay-300000-settle-eeoc-religious-accommodation-lawsuit.

1010. See Thomas v. Rev. Bd. of Indiana, 450 U.S. 707, 714 (1981). "[T]he resolution of that question is not to turn upon a judicial perception of the particular belief or practice in question; religious beliefs need not be acceptable, logical, consistent, or comprehensible to others in order to merit First Amendment protection." Id.

1011. Saint Vincent Health Center To Pay $300,000 To Settle EEOC Religious Accommodation Lawsuit, Hospital Refused To Grant Employees Religious Belief-Based Exemptions From Flu Vaccination Requirement and Instead Fired Them, Federal Agency Charged, December 23, 2016, https://www.eeoc.gov/newsroom/saint-vincent-health-center-pay-300000-settle-eeoc-religious-accommodation-lawsuit.

1012. See, e.g., Lowe v. Mills, 68 F.4th 706 (1st Cir.).

1013. 42 U.S.C. § 2000e-7.

1014. Barber v. Colorado Dep't of Revenue, 562 F.3d 1222, 1233 (10th Cir. 2009) (quotation marks omitted), quoting Quinones v. City of Evanston, Ill., 58 F.3d 275, 277 (7th Cir.1995) (citing Williams v. Gen. Foods Corp., 492 F.2d 399, 404 (7th Cir.1974)).

1015. 497 U.S. 261 (1990).

1016. Face Masks, Including Surgical Masks, and Respirators for COVID-19, FDA, https://www.fda.gov/medical-devices/coronavirus-covid-19-and-medical-devices/face-masks-including-surgical-masks-and-respirators-covid-19 (last visited on August 19, 2021).

1017. 497 U.S. at 279.

1018. 497 U.S. at 279.

1019. In Vitro Diagnostics EUAs - Antigen Diagnostic Tests for SARS-CoV-2, FDA, February 17, 2023, https://www.fda.gov/medical-devices/coronavirus-disease-2019-covid-19-emergency-use-authorizations-medical-devices/in-vitro-diagnostics-euas-antigen-diagnostic-tests-sars-cov-2.

1020. Personal Protective Equipment EUAs, FDA, February 9, 2023, https://www.fda.gov/medical-devices/coronavirus-disease-2019-covid-19-emergency-use-authorizations-medical-devices/personal-protective-equipment-euas.

1021. Personal Protective Equipment EUAs, FDA, February 9, 2023, https://www.fda.gov/medical-devices/coronavirus-disease-2019-covid-19-emergency-use-authorizations-medical-devices/personal-protective-equipment-euas.

1022. Interim Infection Prevention and Control Recommendations for Healthcare Personnel During the Coronavirus Disease 2019 (COVID-19) Pandemic, CDC, updated February 2, 2022, https://www.cdc.gov/coronavirus/2019-ncov/hcp/infection-control-recommendations.html#sourcecontrol.

1023. 21 USC § 321(h)(1).

1024. Personal Protective Equipment EUAs, FDA, https://www.fda.gov/medical-devices/coronavirus-disease-2019-covid-19-emergency-use-authorizations-medical-devices/personal-protective-equipment-euas (last visited on September 17, 2022).

1025. Blanket Letter of Authorization for Surgical Masks From FDA to Manufacturers of Surgical Masks, August 15, 2022, https://www.fda.gov/media/140894/download.

1026. Blanket Letter of Authorization for Surgical Masks From FDA to Manufacturers of Surgical Masks, August 15, 2022, https://www.fda.gov/media/140894/download.

1027. See, e.g., Jacobson v. Massachusetts, 197 U.S. 11, 30-31 (1905), and Health Freedom Def. Fund, Inc. v. Carvalho, ___ F.4th ___, No. 22-55908, 2025 WL 2167401 (9th Cir. 2025) (en banc).

1028. Brox v. Woods Hole, 706 F. Supp. 3d 151, 158, n. 15.

1029. See, e.g., Miller v. McDonald, 130 F.4th 258, 267 (2d Cir. 2025).

1030. Brox v. Woods Hole, 706 F. Supp. 3d 151, 158, n. 15.

1031. 706 F. Supp. 3d at 158, n. 15.

1032. Torcaso v. Watkins, 367 U.S. 488, 492-93 (1961). See also Everson v. Bd. of Ed. of Ewing Twp., 330 U.S. 1, 15 (1947).

1033. 367 U.S. at 495.

1034. Kennedy v. Bremerton Sch. Dist., 597 U.S. 507, 537 (2022), quoting Zorach v. Clauson, 343 U.S. 306, 314 (1952).

1035. New Yorkers for Religious Liberty, Inc. v. City of New York, 125 F.4th 319, 330 (2d Cir. 2025), quoting Agostini v. Felton, 521 U.S. 203, 222–23 (1997).

1036. Drummond ex rel. State v. Oklahoma Statewide Virtual Charter Sch. Bd., 558 P.3d 1 (Okla. 2024), judgment aff'd by an equally divided U.S. Supreme Court in 145 S. Ct. 1381 (2025), quoting Everson v. Bd. of Educ. of Ewing Twp., 330 U.S. 1, 15 (1947).

1037. 430 U.S. 705 (1977).

1038. Lee v. Weisman, 505 U.S. 577, 587 (1992).

1039. Lee v. Weisman, 505 U.S. 577 (1992).

1040. Emp. Div., Dep't of Hum. Res. of Oregon v. Smith, 494 U.S. 872, 888–89 (1990).

1041. 15 F.4th 728, 735 (6th Cir. 2021).

1042. Id. at 735.

1043. 16 F.4th 20 (1st Cir. 2021).

1044. 16 F.4th at 26 and 33 (1st Cir. 2021).

1045. Does 1-6 v. Mills, 566 F. Supp. 3d 34, 39 (D. Me.), aff'd, 16 F.4th 20 (1st Cir. 2021).

1046. COVID Dashboard, Maine Center for Disease Control & Prevention, https://www.maine.gov/dhhs/mecdc/data-reports/diseases/infectious-disease/covid-dashboard (last visited on August 7, 2025).

1047. Kristin Held, *COVID-19 Stats Betray the Facts and the American People*, July 20, 2020, https://krisheldmd.wordpress.com/2020/07/20/covid-19-stats-betray-the-facts-and-the-american-people/.

1048. Dr Scott Jensen With Laura Ingraham | The Ridiculous CDC Guidlines, April 9, 2020, https://www.youtube.com/watch?v=_qWmiWf81zI&feature=emb_logo.

1049. COVID Dashboard, Maine Center for Disease Control & Prevention, https://www.maine.gov/dhhs/mecdc/data-reports/diseases/infectious-disease/covid-dashboard (last visited on August 7, 2025).

1050. COVID Dashboard, Maine Center for Disease Control & Prevention, https://www.maine.gov/dhhs/mecdc/data-reports/diseases/infectious-disease/covid-dashboard (last visited on August 7, 2025).

1051. Id. at 33-34.

1052. Id.

1053. Does 1-6 v. Mills, 566 F. Supp. 3d 34, 52 (D. Me. 2021), aff'd, 16 f.4th 20 (1st Cir. 2021).

1054. Jennifer B. Griffin, Ph.D., et al., SARS-CoV-2 Infections and Hospitalizations Among Persons Aged =16 Years, by Vaccination Status — Los Angeles County, California, May 1–July 25, 2021, Morbidity and Mortality Weekly Report / August 27, 2021 / Vol. 70 / No. 34, https://www.cdc.gov/mmwr/volumes/70/wr/pdfs/mm7034e5-H.pdf.

1055. Christine Massey, CDC confesses: our DHCPP "experts" have never obtained scientific evidence of any alleged "virus"... including "hantavirus", August 26, 2024, https://christinemasseyfois.substack.com/p/cdc-confesses-our-dhcpp-experts-have.

1056. Christine Massey, CDC confesses: our DHCPP "experts" have never obtained scientific evidence of any alleged "virus"... including "hantavirus", August 26, 2024, https://christinemasseyfois.substack.com/p/cdc-confesses-our-dhcpp-experts-have.

1057. Edward Hendrie, Proof that COVID-19 Statistics are Being Padded With Influenza Cases, February 3, 2021, https://greatmountainpublishing.com/2021/02/03/proof-that-covid-19-statistics-are-being-padded-with-influenza-cases/.

1058. Edward Hendrie, February 3, 2021, supra.

1059. Edward Hendrie, February 3, 2021, supra.

1060. Friedman v. Clarkstown Cent. Sch. Dist., 75 F. App'x 815, 818–19 (2d Cir. 2003) (unpublished).

1061. 75 F. App'x 815, 818–19 (2d Cir. 2003) (unpublished).

1062. 75 F. App'x 815, 818–19 (2d Cir. 2003) (unpublished).

1063. Philosophy, Webster's American Dictionary of the English Language, https://webstersdictionary1828.com/Dictionary/philosophy (last visited on July 30, 2025).

1064. Philosophy, Webster's American Dictionary of the English Language, https://webstersdictionary1828.com/Dictionary/philosophy (last visited on July 30, 2025).

1065. Philosophy, Webster's American Dictionary of the English Language, https://webstersdictionary1828.com/Dictionary/philosophy (last visited on July 30, 2025).

1066. Theology, Webster's American Dictionary of the English Language, https://webstersdictionary1828.com/Dictionary/theology (last visited on July 30, 2025).

1067. Religion, Webster's American Dictionary of the English Language, https://webstersdictionary1828.com/Dictionary/religion (last visited on July 30, 2025).

1068. The Golden Rule, Understanding Humanism, https://understandinghumanism.org.uk/wp-content/uploads/2021/10/Golden-Rule.pdf (last visited on August 13, 2025).

1069. Definition of Humanism, American Humanist Association, https://americanhumanist.org/what-is-humanism/definition-of-humanism/ (last visited on August 11, 2025).

1070. Definition of Humanism, American Humanist Association, https://americanhumanist.org/what-is-humanism/definition-of-humanism/ (last visited on August 11, 2025).

1071. Definition of Humanism, American Humanist Association, https://americanhumanist.org/what-is-humanism/definition-of-humanism/ (last visited on August 11, 2025).

1072. The Dhamma, Philosophy and Concepts of Buddhism, https://www.hinduwebsite.com/buddhism/buddhist_philosophy.asp (last visited on August 12, 2025).

1073. Id. at 31.

1074. Tandon v. Newsom, 593 U.S. 61, 62 (2021).

1075. Does 1-6 v. Mills, 142 S. Ct. 17, 19–20 (2021) (Alito, J., dissenting) (citation to transcript omitted).

1076. 142 U.S. at 22.

1077. 706 F. Supp. 3d 151 (D. Mass. 2023) (appeal pending).

1078. Id. at 154.

1079. See Brox v. Hole, 83 F.4th 87, 101 (1st Cir. 2023).

1080. Id. at 154, n. 2.

1081. Weekly Updates by Select Demographic and Geographic Characteristics, Comorbidities and other conditions, CDC, https://www.cdc.gov/nchs/nvss/vsrr/covid_weekly/index.htm#Comorbidities, December 21 2012. See also, https://web.archive.org/web/20211221221243/https://www.cdc.gov/nchs/nvss/vsrr/covid_weekly/index.htm#Comorbidities (archived on September 27, 2023).

1082. Danielle Lama, FOX 35 INVESTIGATES: Questions raised after fatal motorcycle crash listed as COVID-19 death, July 18, 2020, https://www.fox35orlando.com/news/fox-35-investigates-questions-raised-after-fatal-motorcycle-crash-listed-as-covid-19-death.

1083. Id. at 154-55.

1084. Id. at 154, n. 2.

1085. HHS Winds Down mRNA Vaccine Development Under BARDA, HHS, August 5, 2025, https://www.hhs.gov/press-room/hhs-winds-down-mrna-development-under-barda.html.

1086. HHS Winds Down mRNA Vaccine Development Under BARDA, HHS, August 5, 2025, https://www.hhs.gov/press-room/hhs-winds-down-mrna-development-under-barda.html.

1087. Secretary Kennedy, HHS, X, August 5, 2025, https://x.com/SecKennedy/status/1952851097019633766.

1088. Martin Wucher, et al., COVID-19 mRNA "vaccine" harms research collection, July 1, 2025, https://zenodo.org/records/15787612, Doi:

10.5281/zenodo.15787612.

1089. Brox v. Woods HOLE., Reply Brief of Appellants, Civil Action No. 22-10242-RGS, 2024 WL 3408022, July 5, 2024.

1090. Brox v. Woods HOLE., Reply Brief of Appellants, Civil Action No. 22-10242-RGS, 2024 WL 3408022, July 5, 2024. (citations omitted)

1091. Brox v. Woods HOLE., Reply Brief of Appellants, Civil Action No. 22-10242-RGS, 2024 WL 3408022, July 5, 2024. (citations omitted) See Brief of Appellants at 33-41 (discussing District Court's substitution of "limit" for "prevent" in appellees' policy document).

1092. COVID-19 Vaccine Breakthrough Infections Reported to CDC — United States, January 1–April 30, 2021, CDC, May 28, 2021, https://www.cdc.gov/mmwr/volumes/70/wr/mm7021e3.htm.

1093. Letter from Seanator Edward J. Markey to Dr. Dr. Rochelle P. Walletnsky, Director, CDC, July 22, 2021, https://www.markey.senate.gov/imo/media/doc/cdc_breakthrough_cases_letter.pdf.

1094. Covid-19 Vaccine Pharmacovigilance Report, World Council For Health, June 16, 2022, https://worldcouncilforhealth.org/resources/covid-19-vaccine-pharmacovigilance-report.

1095. Miles Mogulescu, Meet the Federal Judge Who Could Decide Whether or Not the US Defaults, Common Dreams, May 16, 2023, https://www.commondreams.org/opinion/federal-judge-debt-ceiling-lawsuit.

1096. 706 F. Supp. 3d at 158, n. 15.

1097. 706 F. Supp. 3d at 158, n. 15.

1098. 706 F. Supp. 3d at 158, n. 15.

1099. Brox v. Woods HOLE., Reply Brief of Appellants, Civil Action No. 22-10242-RGS, 2024 WL 3408022, July 5, 2024.

1100. 19 F.4th 1173 (9th Cir. 2021).

1101. Id. at 1181.

1102. Covid Data Tracker, Ctrs. for Disease Control & Prevention, https://covid.cdc.gov/covid-data-tracker/#data-tracker-home (last visited Dec. 1, 2021).

1103. Weekly Updates by Select Demographic and Geographic Characteristics, Comorbidities and other conditions, CDC, https://web.archive.org/web/20211221221243/https://www.cdc.gov/nchs/nvss/vsrr/covid_weekly/index.htm#Comorbidities (archived by internet archive on December 21 2012). See also, https://www.cdc.gov/nchs/nvss/vsrr/covid_weekly/index.htm#Comorbidities (archived by CDC on September 27, 2023).

1104. Weekly Updates by Select Demographic and Geographic Characteristics, Comorbidities and other conditions, CDC, https://web.archive.org/web/20211221221243/https://www.cdc.gov/nchs/nvss/vsrr/covid_weekly/index.htm#

Comorbidities (archived by internet archive on December 21 2012). See also, https://www.cdc.gov/nchs/nvss/vsrr/covid_weekly/index.htm#Comorbidities (archived by CDC on September 27, 2023).

1105. 19 F.4th at 1181.

1106. 19 F.4th at 1181.

1107. Denis G. Rancourt, et al., Age-stratified COVID-19 vaccine-dose fatality rate for Israel and Australia, Correlation Research in the Public Interest, 9 February 2023, https://correlation-canada.org/report-age-stratified-covid-19-vaccine-dose-fatality-rate-for-israel-and-australia/ .

1108. Health Alert on mRNA COVID-19 Vaccine Safety, Florida Department of Health, February 15, 2023, https://www.floridahealth.gov/newsroom/2023/02/20230215-updated-health-alert.pr.html.

1109. Edward Hendrie, The CDC Falsely Counts Vaccinated COVID Deaths as Unvaccinated COVID Deaths, December 27, 2021, https://greatmountainpublishing.com/2021/12/27/the-cdc-falsely-counts-vaccinated-covid-deaths-as-unvaccinated-covid-deaths/.

1110. Doe v. San Diego Unified Sch. Dist., 22 F.4th 1099, 1100–01 (9th Cir. 2022).

1111. Doe v. San Diego Unified Sch. Dist., 19 F.4th 1173, 1178 (9th Cir. 2021).

1112. Doe v. San Diego Unified Sch. Dist., 19 F.4th 1173, 1185 (9th Cir. 2021) (dissent).

1113. Doe v. San Diego Unified Sch. Dist., 19 F.4th 1173, 1185 (9th Cir. 2021) (dissent)

1114. Doe v. San Diego Unified Sch. Dist., 22 F.4th 1099, 1100 (9th Cir. 2022) (paralell citation and block parenthesis omitted).

1115. Doe v. San Diego Unified Sch. Dist., 22 F.4th 1099, 1104–05 (9th Cir. 2022) (dissent from the denial of rehearing en banc).

1116. Doe v. San Diego Unified Sch. Dist., 22 F.4th 1099, 1108–09 (9th Cir. 2022) (dissent from the denial of rehearing en banc).

1117. 130 F.4th 258 (2d Cir. 2025).

1118. Petition for a Writ of Certiorari, July 31, 2025, https://www.supremecourt.gov/DocketPDF/25/25-133/368571/20250731170404791_25-%20Petition.pdf. See Docket Entries, https://www.supremecourt.gov/docket/docketfiles/html/public/25-133.html.

1119. Id. at 263, n.8.

1120. 130 F.4th at 265.

1121. Fulton v. City of Philadelphia, Pennsylvania, 593 U.S. 522, 537 (2021) (quotation marks omitted).

1122. Id. at 269.

1123. 130 F.4th at 269.

1124. Fulton v. City of Philadelphia, Pennsylvania, 593 U.S. 522, 537 (2021) (quotation marks omitted).

1125. Petition for a Writ of Certiorari, July 31, 2025, https://www.supremecourt.gov/DocketPDF/25/25-133/368571/20250731170404791_25-%20Petition.pdf. See Docket Entries, https://www.supremecourt.gov/docket/docketfiles/html/public/25-133.html.

1126. AFLD et al., v. Xavier Becerra, et al., Complaint, United States District Court for the Northern District of Alabama, Case 2:21-cv-00702-CLM, http://www.opensourcetruth.com/wp-content/uploads/2021/06/Doc-10-Original-AFLDs-Complaint.pdf.

1127. Coronavirus Task Force Press Breifing, White House, April 7, 2020, https://www.whitehouse.gov/briefings-statements/remarks-president-trump-vice-president-pence-members-coronavirus-task-force-press-briefing-april-7-2020/.

1128. Coronavirus Task Force Press Breifing, supra.

1129. Illinois Department of Public Health Director Dr. Ngozi Ezike Explains How Covid Deaths Are Classified, Published August 14, 2021, https://www.bitchute.com/video/vsEScGB2ifHx/.

1130. Greg Piper, Lawmakers seek federal grand jury investigation for COVID-19 statistical manipulation, Just the News, October 10, 2021, https://justthenews.com/government/federal-agencies/lawmakers-seek-federal-grand-jury-investigation-covid-19-statistical.

1131. Oregon Senators Kim Thatcher and Dennis Linthicum, Formal Federal Grand Jury Petition Rights To Petition Protected By 18 USC §3332 & Case Law, August 16, 2021, https://standforhealthfreedom.com/wp-content/uploads/2021/09/0-Senate-Letterhead-Grand-Jury-Petition-AUSA.pdf.

1132. Weekly Updates by Select Demographic and Geographic Characteristics, Comorbidities and other conditions, CDC, https://www.cdc.gov/nchs/nvss/vsrr/covid_weekly/index.htm#Comorbidities.

1133. Weekly Updates by Select Demographic and Geographic Characteristics, Comorbidities and other conditions, CDC, https://www.cdc.gov/nchs/nvss/vsrr/covid_weekly/index.htm#Comorbidities (archived by CDC on September 27, 2023).

1134. Tyler Durden, Florida Man Who Died In Motorcycle Wreck Labeled As COVID-19 Death By State, July 19, 2020, https://www.zerohedge.com/political/florida-man-20s-who-died-motorcycle-wreck-labeled-covid-19-death-state.

1135. Danielle Lama, FOX 35 INVESTIGATES: Questions raised after fatal motorcycle crash listed as COVID-19 death, July 18, 2020, https://www.fox35orlando.com/news/fox-35-investigates-questions-raised-after-fatal-motorcycle-crash-listed-as-covid-19-death.

1136. Edward Hendrie, How the Federal Government Has Turned Hospitals into Death Chambers, February

25, 2022, https://greatmountainpublishing.com/2022/02/25/how-the-federal-government-has-turned-hospitals-into-death-chambers/.

1137. Kristin Herd, *COVID-19 Stats Betray the Facts and the American People*, July 20, 2020, https://krisheldmd.wordpress.com/2020/07/20/covid-19-stats-betray-the-facts-and-the-american-people/.

1138. Kristin Herd, July 20, 2020, supra.

1139. Number of new cases of coronavirus (COVID-19) in the United States from January 20, 2020 to January 13, 2021, by day*, Statista, January 14, 2021, http://web.archive.org/web/20210114220926/https://www.statista.com/statistics/1102816/coronavirus-covid19-cases-number-us-americans-by-day/.

1140. Kristin Herd, July 20, 2020, supra.

1141. *Dr Scott Jensen With Laura Ingraham | The Ridiculous CDC Guidlines*, April 9, 2020, https://www.youtube.com/watch?v=_qWmiWf81zI&feature=emb_logo.

1142. Former gubernatorial candidate Dr. Scott Jensen under investigation by Minnesota Board of Medical Practice, NBC, KTTC, January 30, 2023, https://www.kttc.com/2023/01/31/former-gubernatorial-candidate-dr-scott-jensen-under-investigation-by-minnesota-board-medical-practice/.

1143. Id.

1144. *Vital Statistics Reporting Guidance, Guidance for Certifying Deaths Due to Coronavirus Disease*

2019 (COVID–19), U.S. Department of Health and Human Services • Centers for Disease Control and Prevention • National Center for Health Statistics • National Vital Statistics System, Report No. 3, April 2020, https://www.cdc.gov/nchs/data/nvss/vsrg/vsrg03-508.pdf.

1145. Id.

1146. Guidance for Certifying Deaths Due to Coronavirus Disease 2019 (COVID-19), Report No. 3, U.S. Department of Health and Human Services, Centers for Disease Control and Prevention, National Center for Health Statistics, National Vital Statistics System, Released April 2020 – Expanded February 2023, https://www.cdc.gov/nchs/data/nvss/vsrg/vsrg03-508.pdf.

1147. Danielle Waugh, I-Team: Deaths incorrectly attributed to COVID-19 in Palm Beach County, CBS 12 News, July 23, 2020, https://cbs12.com/news/local/i-team-deaths-incorrectly-attributed-to-covid-19-in-palm-beach-county.

1148. *COVID-19 In Virginia*, Dashboard Updated November 5, 2020, Department of Health, https://www.vdh.virginia.gov/coronavirus/covid-19-in-virginia/.

1149. *Coronavirus Disease 2019 (COVID-19) 2020 Interim Case Definition*, Approved August 5, 2020, Centers for Disease Control, https://wwwn.cdc.gov/nndss/conditions/coronavirus-disease-2019-covid-19/case-definition/2020/08/05/.

1150.*Five Things to Remember When Interpreting Epidemiologic Data*, Virginia Department of Health, May 1, 2020, https://www.vdh.virginia.gov/coronavirus/2020/05/01/interpreting-epidemiologic-data/.

1151.Id.

1152.Id.

1153.COVID-19 cases surpass 70,000 in Virginia | Positivity rate increases to 6.6%, NBC12 Newsroom | March 30, 2020 at 9:04 AM EDT - Updated July 12 at 5:39 PM, http://web.archive.org/web/20200713000744/https://www.nbc12.com/2020/07/11/new-covid-cases-up-by-virginia-positivity-rate-increases/.

1154.Michelle Rogers, Fact Check: Hospitals Get Paid More If Patients Listed as COVID-19, on Ventilators, USA TODAY, April 24, 2020, https://www.usatoday.com/story/news/factcheck/2020/04/24/fact-check-medicare-hospitals-paid-more-covid-19-patients-coronavirus/3000638001/.

1155.Michelle Rogers, April 24, 2020, supra.

1156.Michelle Rogers, April 24, 2020, supra.

1157.Michelle Rogers, April 24, 2020, supra.

1158.Andrew Mark Miller, CDC Director Acknowledges Hospitals Have a Monetary Incentive to Overcount Coronavirus Deaths, Washington Examiner, August 1, 2020, https://www.washingtonexaminer.com/news/cdc-director-acknowledges-hospitals-have-a-monetary-incentive-to-overcount-coronavirus-deaths?fbclid=IwAR0v4RCP

BA5WAPyfUoDF1ZbV_MYFStCRKYhs1TBxwAgSb bgr5foBGrrdg3U.

1159. Andrew Mark Miller, August 1, 2020 supra.

1160. Edwin Mora, CDC Chief Agrees There's 'Perverse' Economic 'Incentive' for Hospitals to Inflate Coronavirus Deaths, Breitbart, July 31, 2020, https://www.breitbart.com/politics/2020/07/31/cdc-chief-agrees-theres-perverse-economic-incentive-for-hospitals-to-inflate-coronavirus-deaths/.

1161. Alya Ellison, State-by-state Breakdown of Federal Aid per COVID-19 Case, Becker's Hospitial CFO Report, April 14, 2020, https://www.beckershospitalreview.com/finance/state-by-state-breakdown-of-federal-aid-per-covid-19-case.html.

1162. Id.

1163. AFLD, et. al., v, Xavier Becerra, et al., Motion For Preliminary Injunction, United States District Court for the Northern District of Alabama, Civil Action No. 2:21-cv-00702-CLM, July 19, 2021.

1164. Brian Shilhavy, CENSORED: COVID19 PCR Tests are Scientifically Meaningless – Everything We've Been Told about COVID is a HOAX!, Health Impact News, June 27, 2020, https://healthimpactnews.com/2020/censored-covid19-pcr-tests-are-scientifically-meaningless-everything-weve-been-told-about-covid-is-a-hoax/.

1165. Id.

1166. Lab Alert: Changes to CDC RT-PCR for SARS-CoV-2 Testing, July 21, 2021, https://www.cdc.gov/csels/dls/locs/2021/07-21-2021-lab-alert-Changes_CDC_RT-PCR_SARS-CoV-2_Testing_1.html.

1167.*Data and Surveillance, How is VDH counting COVID-19 deaths?*, Virginia Department of Health, Page Last Updated: October 22, 2020, https://www.vdh.virginia.gov/coronavirus/data-and-surveillance/.

1168.*Weekly Updates by Select Demographic and Geographic Characteristics*, Centers for Disease Control, Page last reviewed: November 4, 2020, https://www.cdc.gov/nchs/nvss/vsrr/covid_weekly/index.htm#Comorbidities.

1169.Chris Vanderveen, Colorado coroner says death listed by state as COVID-19 related has much more to do with alcohol, NBC, 9News, May 14, 2020, https://www.9news.com/article/news/investigations/colorado-coroner-says-death-listed-by-state-as-covid-19-related-has-much-more-to-do-with-alcohol/73-eec4517a-13dd-45bc-bc59-7e50cedf2272.

1170.Chris Vanderveen, May 14, 2020, supra.

1171.Chris Vanderveen, May 14, 2020, supra.

1172.Chris Vanderveen, May 14, 2020, supra.

1173.Kyle Clark and Erin Powell, GOP rep alleges falsified COVID-19 records, calls for indictment of Colorado's top health official, NBC 9News, May 14, 2020, https://www.9news.com/article/news/local/next/gop-rep-alleges-falsified-covid-19-records-calls-for-indictment-of-colorados-top-health-official/73-bf02452f-4615-4 efe-9413-a4826a8105b2.

1174. State-by-State Breakdown: Delivery of Initial $30 Billion of CARES Act Public Health and Social Services Emergency Fund, https://www.hrsa.gov/sites/default/files/hrsa/provider-relief/state-state-breakdown-delivery-initial-30-billion-cares-act.pdf (last visited on May 7, 2023).

1175. COVID-19 CARES Act Funds, Maricopa County, https://www.maricopa.gov/5744/COVID-19-Cares-Act-Funds (last visited on May 7, 2023).

1176. Noah Higgins Dunn, *Fauci Debunks Theories of Low CDC Coronavirus Death Toll: 'There Are 180,000-plus Deaths' in U.S.,* CNBC, September 1, 2020, https://www.msn.com/en-us/health/medical/fauci-debunks-theories-of-low-cdc-coronavirus-death-toll-there-are-180-000-plus-deaths-in-u-s/ar-BB18B8of?ocid=msedgntp.

1177. Id.

1178. *They Finally Admitted It!!!,* July 8, 2020, https://youtu.be/dtpYi1uC_Iw.

1179. Infra.

1180. Infra.

1181. Yanni Gu, A Closer Look at U.S. Deaths Due to COVID-19, Johns Hopkins News-Letter, November 22, 2020, https://web.archive.org/web/20201126223119/https://www.jhunewsletter.com/article/2020/11/a-closer-look-at-u-s-deaths-due-to-covid-19 (retracted).

1182. Infra.

1183. Infra.

1184. Infra.

1185. Yanni Gu, A closer look at U.S. deaths due to COVID-19, Johns Hopkins News-Letter, November 27, 2020, https://www.jhunewsletter.com/article/2020/11/a-closer-look-at-u-s-deaths-due-to-covid-19.

1186. Yoon K Loke and Carl HeneghanWhy no-one can ever recover from COVID-19 in England – a statistical anomaly, The Centre for Evidence-Based Medicine, July 16, 2020, https://www.cebm.net/covid-19/why-no-one-can-ever-recover-from-covid-19-in-england-a-statistical-anomaly/.

1187. Yoon K Loke and Carl Heneghan, supra.

1188. John Johnson, Matt Hancock orders urgent review into 'misleading' PHE coronavirus death statistics, Politics Home, July 17, 2020, https://www.politicshome.com/news/article/matt-hancock-orders-urgent-review-into-misleading-phe-coronavirus-death-statistics.

1189. John Johnson, July 17, 2020, supra.

1190. John Johnson, July 17, 2020, supra.

1191. *Tracking Dr. Anthony Fauci's Comments On Coronavirus*, CNBC, March 26, 2020, comments at 4:55 of video, https://www.youtube.com/watch?v=ShiwHR5OvtM&feature=emb_logo.

1192. *Dr. Fauci and Other CDC & NIH Officials Testify on Coronavirus – March 11*, Rev Transcripts, March 11, 2020, https://www.rev.com/blog/transcripts/dr-fauci-and-other-cdc-nih-officials-testify-on-coronavirus-march-11. *See Also, Coronavirus "10 Times More Lethal than Seasonal Flu": Fauci*, posted March 12, 2020, https://www.youtube.com/watch?v=Ono3BcbTX4Q&feature=youtu.be.

1193. Anthony S. Fauci, M.D., H. Clifford Lane, M.D., and Robert R. Redfield, M.D., *Covid-19 — Navigating the Uncharted*, New England Journal of Medicine, March 26, 2020, https://www.nejm.org/doi/full/10.1056/NEJMe2002387.

1194. Ronald Brown, Public Health Lessons Learned From Biases in Coronavirus Mortality Overestimation, Cambridge University Press, 12 August 2020, https://www.cambridge.org/core/journals/disaster-medicine-and-public-health-preparedness/article/public-health-lessons-learned-from-biases-in-coronavirus-mortality-overestimation/7ACD87D8FD2237285EB667BB28DCC6E9#.

1195. *Tracking Dr. Anthony Fauci's Comments On Coronavirus*, CNBC, March 26, 2020, comments at 4:55 of video, https://www.youtube.com/watch?v=ShiwHR5OvtM&feature=emb_logo.

1196. Anthony S. Fauci, M.D., H. Clifford Lane, M.D., and Robert R. Redfield, M.D., *Covid-19 — Navigating the Uncharted*, New England Journal of Medicine, March 26, 2020, https://www.nejm.org/doi/full/10.1056/NEJMe200238

7.

1197. Caterina Andreano, Dr. Fauci: Wear Goggles or Eye Shields to Prevent Spread of Covid-19; Flu Vaccine a Must, ABC News, July 29, 2020, https://abcnews.go.com/US/dr-fauci-wear-goggles-eye-shields-prevent-spread/story?id=72059055.

1198. Id. Video of interview of Dr. Fauci by ABC News commentator Dr. Jen Ashton imbedded in Caterina Andreano's ABC News article, supra.

1199. Lisa Krieger, *Stanford Researcher Says Coronavirus Isn't as Fatal as We Thought; Critics Say He's Missing the Point*, The Mercury News, May 20, 2020, https://www.mercurynews.com/2020/05/20/stanford-researcher-says-coronavirus-isnt-as-fatal-as-we-thought-critics-say-hes-missing-the-point/.

1200. Trump and coronavirus task force brief from White House | NBC News (Live Stream Recording), Streamed live on Mar 23, 2020, https://www.youtube.com/watch?v=Fx8oJCzRJUk.

1201. Average life expectancy in Europe for those born in 2019, by gender and region, https://www.statista.com/statistics/274514/life-expectancy-in-europe/ (last visited on June 19, 2020).

1202. Tommaso Ebhardt, Chiara Remondini, and Marco Bertacche, 99% of Those Who Died From Virus Had Other Illness, Italy Says, Bloomberg, Bloomberg, March 18, 2020, https://www.bloomberg.com/news/articles/2020-03-18/99-of-those-who-died-from-virus-had-other-illness-italy-says.

1203. See supra.

1204. U.S. Death Rate 1950-2023, Chart and table of the U.S. death rate from 1950 to 2023, https://www.macrotrends.net/countries/USA/united-states/death-rate.

1205. *Weekly Updates by Select Demographic and Geographic Characteristics*, CDC, National Center for Health Statistics, https://www.cdc.gov/nchs/nvss/vsrr/covid_weekly/index.htm#Comorbidities (last visited on November 7, 2020).

1206. Id.

1207. Id.

1208. Patrick Howley, BUSTED: CDC Inflated COVID Numbers, Accused of Violating Federal Law, National File, March 8, 2021, https://nationalfile.com/busted-cdc-inflated-covid-numbers-accused-of-violating-federal-law/.

1209. Id.

1210. Id.

1211. 2003 CDC Medical Examiner's and Coroner's Handbook on Death Registration, https://www.cdc.gov/nchs/data/misc/hb_me.pdf.

1212. Id.

1213. Steven Schaartz, Ph.D., Director - Division of Vital Statistics, National Center for Health Statistics, COVID-19 Alert No. 2, National Vital Statistics System, March 24, 2020, https://www.cdc.gov/nchs/data/nvss/coronavirus/Alert-2-New-ICD-code-introduced-for-COVID-19-deaths.pdf.

1214. Id.

1215. Henry Ealy, et al., COVID-19 Data Collection, Comorbidity & Federal Law: A Historical Retrospective, Public Health Policy Initiative, October 12, 2020, https://jdfor2020.com/wp-content/uploads/2020/11/adf864_165a103206974fdbb14ada6bf8af1541.pdf.

1216. Henry Ealy, et al., COVID-19 Data Collection, Comorbidity & Federal Law: A Historical Retrospective, Public Health Policy Initiative, October 12, 2020, https://jdfor2020.com/wp-content/uploads/2020/11/adf864_165a103206974fdbb14ada6bf8af1541.pdf.

1217. Henry Ealy, et al., October 12, 2020, supra.

1218. COVID-19 Alert No. 2, National Vital Statistics System, March 24, 2020, https://www.cdc.gov/nchs/data/nvss/coronavirus/Alert-2-New-ICD-code-introduced-for-COVID-19-deaths.pdf.

1219. Guidance for Certifying COVID-19 Deaths, March 4, 2020, National Vital Statistics System, https://www.cdc.gov/nchs/data/nvss/coronavirus/alert-1-guidance-for-certifying-covid-19-deaths.pdf.

1220. Guidance for Certifying Deaths Due to Coronavirus Disease 2019 (COVID–19), National Vital Statistics System, April 2020, https://www.cdc.gov/nchs/data/nvss/vsrg/vsrg03-508.p

df.

1221. Guidance for Certifying COVID-19 Deaths, March 4, 2020, National Vital Statistics System, https://www.cdc.gov/nchs/data/nvss/coronavirus/alert-1-guidance-for-certifying-covid-19-deaths.pdf.

1222. Death certificate analysis shows Washington's COVID-19 death count remains inflated, Press Release, December 16, 2020, Freedom Foundation, https://www.freedomfoundation.com/press-release/death-certificate-analysis-shows-washingtons-covid-19-death-count-remains-inflated/.

1223. Maxford Nelson, WA reduces COVID-19 deaths by 200; investigation suggests it's still too high, Freedom Foundation, December 16, 2020, https://www.freedomfoundation.com/covid-19/wa-lowers-covid-19-deaths-by-200-investigation-suggests-its-still-too-high/.

1224. Death cert. analysis, December 16, 2020, supra.

1225. Maxford Nelsen, Washington health officials: Gunshot victims counted as COVID-19 deaths, Liberty Foundation, May 21, 2020, https://www.freedomfoundation.com/washington/washington-health-officials-gunshot-victims-counted-as-covid-19-deaths/.

1226. Maxford Nelsen, May 21, 2020, supra.

1227. Death certificate analysis shows Washington's COVID-19 death count remains inflated, Press Release, December 16, 2020, Freedom Foundation, https://www.freedomfoundation.com/press-release/death-certificate-analysis-shows-washingtons-covid-19-dea th-count-remains-inflated/.

1228. Maxford Nelson, December 16, 2020, supra.

1229. Death cert. analysis December 16, 2020, supra.

1230. @TheOriginalSai, Twitter, January 14, 2023, https://twitter.com/TheOriginalSai/status/1614332319111970816,

1231. IT WAS ALL A LIE: NHS Director confirms Hospitals lied about Cause of Death to create illusion of COVID Pandemic, The Expose, March 20, 2023, https://expose-news.com/2023/03/20/nhs-director-confirms-hospitals-lied-about-covid-deaths/?cmid=6a508dc3-a2e4-47a3-b166-300d2b15cb67.

1232. LIE, The Expose, March 20, 2023, supra.

1233. LIE, The Expose, March 20, 2023, supra.

1234. LIE, The Expose, March 20, 2023, supra.

1235. LIE, The Expose, March 20, 2023, supra.

1236. LIE, The Expose, March 20, 2023, supra.

1237. LIE, The Expose, March 20, 2023, supra.

1238. LIE, The Expose, March 20, 2023, supra.

1239. LIE, The Expose, March 20, 2023, supra.

1240. COVID-19 medical misinformation policy, YouTube, https://support.google.com/youtube/answer/9891785?hl=en (last visited on February 5, 2023).

1241. Arthur Firstenberg, The Invisible Rainbow, A History of Electricity and Life, at 2 (2020).

1242. Verizon launches first U.S. '3G' network, CNN, January 28, 2002, https://www.cnn.com/2002/TECH/ptech/01/28/verizon.3g/.

1243. SARS Basics Fact Sheet, CDC, page last reviewed December 6, 2017, https://www.cdc.gov/sars/about/fs-sars.html.

1244. Lisa Pace, 4G: History, Origin, and More, 4G Release History, December 6, 2022, https://history-computer.com/4g-guide/#:~:text=available%20shortly%20thereafter.-,4G%20reached%20the%20United%20States%20in%202012%2C%20with%20five%20companies,began%20to%20be%20rolled%20out.

1245. 2009 H1N1 Pandemic (H1N1pdm09 virus), last reviewed on June 11, 2019, CDC, https://www.cdc.gov/flu/pandemic-resources/2009-h1n1-pandemic.html.

1246. When was 5G introduced?, Verizon News Center, December 6, 2019, https://www.verizon.com/about/our-company/5g/when-was-5g-introduced.

1247. CDC Museum COVID-19 Timeline, CDC, last reviewed on August 16, 2022, https://www.cdc.gov/museum/timeline/covid19.html.

1248. S. S. SEKER, "Health Effects of 5G and Millimeter Waves," 2019 11th International Conference on Electrical and Electronics Engineering

(ELECO), Bursa, Turkey, 2019, pp. I16-I16, doi: 10.23919/ELECO47770.2019.8990371. https://ieeexplore.ieee.org/abstract/document/8990371.

1249. Lennart Hardell, et al., Comments on the US National Toxicology Program technical reports on toxicology and carcinogenesis study in rats exposed to whole-body radiofrequency radiation at 900 MHz and in mice exposed to whole-body radiofrequency radiation at 1,900 MHz, International Journal of Oncology, October 24, 2018, https://www.spandidos-publications.com/ijo/54/1/111?fbclid=IwAR0NncY5stN1jpPG4w63H7IeYlHbGOy_E5U4o6CaKWfrwrQbSoA13J4Adsk.

1250. Dr. Tom Cowan: 5G Millimetre Waves are a Weapon to make People sick with COVID, https://stop5g.cz/us/dr-tom-cowan-5g-millimetre-waves-are-a-weapon-to-make-people-sick-with-covid/ (last visited on February 15, 2023).

1251. Dr. Tom Cowan, 5G Millimetre Waves, supra.

1252. Dr. Tom Cowan: 5G Millimetre Waves, supra.

1253. Laruen Smiley, 27 Days in Tokyo Bay: What Happened on the Diamond Princess, Wired, April 30, 2020, https://www.wired.com/story/diamond-princess-coronavirus-covid-19-tokyo-bay/.

1254. Princess Gets Access to SES O3b mPOWER Satellite-Based Communications System, Cruise Industry News, February 3, 2020, https://cruiseindustrynews.com/cruise-news/2020/02/princess-gets-access-to-ses-o3b-mpower-satellite-based-communications-system/.

1255. Accelerating 5G roll out via satellite, SES, 22 February 2019, https://www.ses.com/newsroom/accelerating-5g-roll-out-satellite.

1256. Magda Havas, Is there an association between covid-19 cases/deaths and 5G in the United States?, April 22, 2020 (updated May 7, 2020), https://magdahavas.com/5g-and-mm-waves/is-there-an-association-between-covid-19-cases-deaths-and-5g-in-the-united-states/.

1257. Magda Havas, 5G and COVID-19 Deaths, Supra.

1258. Study Shows Direct Correlation between 5G Networks and "Coronavirus" Outbreaks, Radiation Dangers, April 24, 2020, https://radiationdangers.com/2020/04/24/study-shows-direct-correlation-between-5g-networks-and-coronavirus-outbreaks-2/.

1259. Id.

1260. Id.

1261. 5G Radiation - Potential Cause of Covid-19 Pandemic, May 6, 2020, The Legal Pens, http://alchemistcook.blogspot.com/2020/05/the-potential-dangers-of-5g-radiation.html.

1262. China rolls out 'one of the world's largest' 5G networks, BBC News, 1 November 2019, https://www.bbc.com/news/business-50258287.

1263. 5G network coming to Wuhan, Hubei - China, April 16, 2018, http://en.hubei.gov.cn/news/newslist/201804/t20180416_1275769.shtml.

1264. Huawei builds 5G network at Wuhan Huoshenshan Hospital, CGTN, March 13, 2020, https://news.cgtn.com/news/2020-03-13/Huawei-builds-5G-network-at-Wuhan-Huoshenshan-Hospital-OP6qhHRc1G/index.html.

1265. The Contagion Myth and Germ Theory Hoax For Dummies, August 16, 2021, https://truthscrambler.com/2021/08/16/the-contagion-myth-and-germ-theory-hoax-for-dummies/.

1266. John E. Hoover, HEROES: Tribute to Dr Scott Jensen - Part 1, https://www.youtube.com/watch?v=sVmNFoEjv90 (last visited on February 5, 2023). John E. Hoover, HEROES: Tribute to Dr Scott Jensen w/ John Cullen - Part 2, https://www.youtube.com/watch?v=4-JpcPZRU8Y (last visited on February 5, 2023). John E. Hoover, The Final Chapter: Part 3 - HEROES: A Tribute to Dr Scott Jensen, https://www.youtube.com/watch?v=2gJP-L3z6uY&t=1361s (last visited on February 5, 2023).

1267. Edward Hendrie, Proof that COVID-19 Statistics are Being Padded With Influenza Cases, February 3, 2021, Great Mountain Publishing, https://greatmountainpublishing.com/2021/02/03/proof-that-covid-19-statistics-are-being-padded-with-influenza-cases/.

1268. Peter Andrews, Flu Away: Scientists Baffled at Disappearance of Influenza... but Is it Really Gone, or Just Masked by Covid-19?, 26 October 2020, https://www.rt.com/op-ed/504625-covid19-flu-disappeared-replaced/.

1269. Jo MacFarlane, Has Covid killed off the flu? Experts pose the intriguing question as influenza cases nosedive by 98% across the globe, Daily Mail, 24 October 2020, https://www.dailymail.co.uk/health/article-8875201/Has-Covid-killed-flu.html.

1270. Vernon Coleman, https://www.vernoncoleman.com/ (last visited on March 16, 2023).

1271. Rhoda Wilson, Was Covid made in a Lab?, The Expose, March 14, 2023, https://expose-news.com/2023/03/14/was-covid-made-in-a-lab/.

1272. Physician Group Practice Demonstration, Influenza Vaccination Strategies, CMS, at 6, https://innovation.cms.gov/files/x/pgp-flu-vaccination.pdf (last visited on April 10, 2023).

1273. Menu of State Hospital Influenza Vaccination Laws, CDC Office for State, Local and Territorial Support, https://www.cdc.gov/phlp/docs/menu-shfluvacclaws.pdf (last visited on July 16, 2025).

1274. October 26, 2022 CMS Memo to State Survey Agency Directors, Ref: Ref: QSO-23-02-ALL, Subject: Revised Guidance for Staff Vaccination Requirements, from Directors Quality, Safety & Oversight Group (QSOG) and Survey & Operations Group (SOG). See also Medicare and Medicaid Programs; Omnibus COVID-19 Health Care Staff Vaccination, November 5, 2021, https://www.federalregister.gov/documents/2021/11/05/2021-23831/medicare-and-medicaid-programs-omnib us-covid-19-health-care-staff-vaccination#sectno-citation-491.8.

1275. July 25, 2023, CMS Memo to State Survey Agency Directors, Ref: Ref: QSO-23-02-ALL, Subject: EXPIRED: Revised Guidance for Staff Vaccination Requirements, from Director, Quality, Safety & Oversight Group (QSOG), https://www.cms.gov/files/document/qso-23-02-all-expired.pdf.

1276. Media Statement, For Immediate release: Thursday, September 1, 2022, CDC, https://archive.cdc.gov/#/details?url=https://www.cdc.gov/media/releases/2022/s0901-covid-19-booster.html (last visited on July 15, 2025).

1277. United States v. Price, 383 U.S. 787, 794 (1966).

1278. Id. at 794.

1279. Id. at 794, n.7.

1280. 365 U.S. 715 (1961).

1281. Id. at 717.

1282. Id. at 725.

1283. 68 F.4th 706 (1st Cir.).

1284. Id. at 719-20.

1285. 562 F.3d 1222, 1233 (10th Cir. 2009).

1286. Barber v. Colorado Dep't of Revenue, 562 F.3d 1222, 1233 (10th Cir. 2009) (quotation marks omitted), quoting Quinones v. City of Evanston, Ill., 58 F.3d

275, 277 (7th Cir.1995) (citing Williams v. Gen. Foods Corp., 492 F.2d 399, 404 (7th Cir.1974)).

1287. 562 F.3d at 1234 (concurring opinion).

1288. 42 U.S.C. § 2000e-7.

1289. Hernandez v. Commissioner, 490 U.S. 680, 699 (1989).

1290. Emp. Div., Dep't of Hum. Res. of Oregon v. Smith, 494 U.S. 872, 887 (1990), citing Thomas v. Review Bd. of Indiana Employment Security Div., 450 U.S., at 716, 101 S.Ct., at 1431; Presbyterian Church in U.S. v. Mary Elizabeth Blue Hull Memorial Presbyterian Church, 393 U.S., at 450, 89 S.Ct., at 606–07; Jones v. Wolf, 443 U.S. 595, 602–606, 99 S.Ct. 3020, 3024–3027, 61 L.Ed.2d 775 (1979); United States v. Ballard, 322 U.S. 78, 85–87, 64 S.Ct. 882, 885–87, 88 L.Ed. 1148 (1944).

1291. Presbyterian Church in U.S. v. Mary Elizabeth Blue Hull Mem'l Presbyterian Church, 393 U.S. 440, 445–46 (1969), citing Watson v Jones, 80 U.S. 679 (1871).

1292. 450 U.S. 707 (1981).

1293. Id. at 714. See also Thomas v. Rev. Bd. of Indiana, 450 U.S. 707, 714 (1981).

1294. Does 1-11 v. Bd. of Regents of Univ. of Colorado, 100 F.4th 1251, 1257–58 (10th Cir. 2024).

1295. Id.

1296. 100 F.4th 1251 (10th Cir. 2024).

1297. Id. at 1268.

1298. Id. at 1269 (citations omitted).

1299. Church of Lukumi Babalu Aye, Inc. v. City of Hialeah., 508 U.S. 520, 532 (1993).

1300. Masterpiece Cakeshop v. Colorado C.R. Comm'n, 584 U.S. 617, 618–19 (2018).

1301. Larson v. Valente, 456 U.S. 228, 244 (1982).

1302. Colo. Christian Univ., 534 F.3d at 1261.

1303. Id. at 1261, 1267 (quoting Agostini v. Felton, 521 U.S. 203, 232, 117 S.Ct. 1997, 138 L.Ed.2d 391 (1997)).

1304. 100 F.4th at 1271.

1305. Colo. Christian Univ., 534 F.3d at 1263.

1306. Does 1-11 v. Bd. of Regents of Univ. of Colorado, 100 F.4th 1251, 1271–72 (10th Cir. 2024).

1307. See Mitchell v. Helms, 530 U.S. 793, 828 (2000).

1308. Does 1-11 v. Bd. of Regents of Univ. of Colorado, 100 F.4th 1251, 1275 (10th Cir. 2024).

1309. 100 F.4th 1251, 1275 (10th Cir. 2024), quoting Fulton, 141 S. Ct. at 1877.

1310. A Christian Science perspective on vaccination and public health, Christian Science, https://www.christianscience.com/press-room/a-christian-science-perspective-on-vaccination-and-public-health (last visited on July 20, 2025).

1311. Kane v. De Blasio, 19 F.4th 152, 168 (2d Cir. 2021), quoting Hernandez v. Commissioner, 490 U.S. 680, 699 (1989).

1312. 100 F.4th 1251, 1271–72 (10th Cir. 2024).

1313. 100 F.4th at 1271.

1314. Colo. Christian Univ., 534 F.3d at 1263.

1315. Saint Vincent Health Center To Pay $300,000 To Settle EEOC Religious Accommodation Lawsuit, Hospital Refused To Grant Employees Religious Belief-Based Exemptions From Flu Vaccination Requirement and Instead Fired Them, Federal Agency Charged, December 23, 2016, https://www.eeoc.gov/newsroom/saint-vincent-health-center-pay-300000-settle-eeoc-religious-accommodation-lawsuit.

1316. Rene F. Najera, Papal Patronage: A History of Vatican Leadership in Vaccine Science and Public Health, The College of Physicians of Philadelphia, April 21, 2025, https://historyofvaccines.org/blog/papal-patronage-history-vatican-leadership-vaccine-science-and-public-health.

1317. Rene F. Najera, Papal Patronage: A History of Vatican Leadership in Vaccine Science and Public Health, April 21, 2025, https://historyofvaccines.org/blog/papal-patronage-history-vatican-leadership-vaccine-science-and-public-health.

1318. Rene F. Najera, Papal Patronage: A History of Vatican Leadership in Vaccine Science and Public

Health, April 21, 2025, https://historyofvaccines.org/blog/papal-patronage-history-vatican-leadership-vaccine-science-and-public-health.

1319. Devin Watkins, Pope Francis urges people to get vaccinated against Covid-19, Vatican News, 18 August 2021, https://www.vaticannews.va/en/pope/news/2021-08/pope-francis-appeal-covid-19-vaccines-act-of-love.html.

1320. Courtney Mares, Pope Francis: Being 'properly informed' on COVID-19 vaccines is a 'human right', January 28, 2022, https://www.catholicnewsagency.com/news/250244/pope-francis-being-properly-informed-on-covid-19-vaccines-is-a-human-right.

1321. Id.

1322. Luis F. Card. Ladaria, S.I., Prefect, S.E. Mons. Giacomo Morandi, Titular Archbishop of Cerveteri, Secretary, Note on the morality of using some anti-Covid-19 vaccines, Congregation for the Doctrine of the Faith, December 21, 2020, https://www.vatican.va/roman_curia/congregations/cfaith/documents/rc_con_cfaith_doc_20201221_nota-vaccini-anticovid_en.html.

1323. Ethical and Religious Directives for Catholic Health Care Services, 2018, Sixth Edition, UNITED STATES CONFERENCE OF CATHOLIC BISHOPS, https://www.usccb.org/about/doctrine/ethical-and-religious-directives/upload/ethical-religious-directives-catholic-health-service-sixth-edition-2016-06.pdf.

1324. Vaccine Mandates FAQ, Archdiocese of San Francisco, October 7, 2021, https://sfarchdiocese.org/vaccine-mandate-faq/.

1325. Id.

1326. New anti-Covid measures for entry to Vatican and Curia offices, Vatical News, https://web.archive.org/web/20220207131227/https://www.vaticannews.va/en/vatican-city/news/2021-12/covid-19-decree-vatican-cardinal-parolin-measures.html (last visited on July 20, 2025).

1327. Id.

1328. Steven Watson, Report: Vatican Announces Vaccine Mandate For All Employees And Visitors, December 24, 2021, Summit News, https://web.archive.org/web/20220207145226/https://summit.news/2021/12/24/report-vatican-announces-vaccine-mandate-for-all-employees-and-visitors/. Edward Hendrie, The Vatican (Home of the Antichrist) Has Decreed All Workers and Visitors Must Be Vaccinated (Religious Exemptions Will Not Be Allowed) (repost of article by Steve Watson), December 24, 2021, https://greatmountainpublishing.com/2021/12/25/the-vatican-home-of-the-antichrist-has-decreed-all-workers-and-visitors-must-be-vaccinated-religious-exemptions-will-not-be-allowed/.

1329. Catechism of the Catholic Church, § 2032, https://www.vatican.va/archive/ENG0015/__P74.HTM (last visited on July 20, 2025).

1330. Catechism of the Catholic Church, § 2035, https://www.vatican.va/archive/ENG0015/__P74.HTM (last visited on July 20, 2025).

1331. Devin Watkins, Pope Francis urges people to get vaccinated against Covid-19, Vatican News, 18 August 2021, https://www.vaticannews.va/en/pope/news/2021-08/pope-francis-appeal-covid-19-vaccines-act-of-love.html.

1332. Catechism of the Catholic Church, § 2037, https://www.vatican.va/archive/ENG0015/__P74.HTM (last visited on July 20, 2025).

1333. Catechism of the Catholic Church, § 2039, https://www.vatican.va/archive/ENG0015/__P74.HTM (last visited on July 20, 2025).

1334. Edward Hendrie, Solving the Mystery of BABYLON THE GREAT, ISBN: 978-0-9832627-0-1, https://shop.lightningsource.com/b/085?756yVvSlsxEZsCUe5ojV7MAzZpqfER2BTqKRXEFbTZr.

1335. 450 U.S. 707 (1981).

1336. Hobby Lobby, 573 U.S. at 725, citing Thomas v. Review Bd. of Indiana Employment Security Div., 450 U.S. 707, 716 (1981).

1337. 103 F.4th 1241 (6th Cir. 2024).

1338. Id at 1242-43, citing Lucky v. Landmark Med. of Mich., P.C., No. 23-cv-11004, 2023 WL 7095085, at *7 (E.D. Mich. Oct. 26, 2023).

1339. Id. at 1243-44, quoting Hernandez v. Comm'r of Internal Revenue, 490 U.S. 680, 699 (1989).

1340. Id. at 1244 (citation and quotation marks omitted), citing Employment Div. v. Smith, 494 U.S. 872, 887 (1990).

1341. 450 U.S. 707 (1981).

1342. 100 F.4th 1251 (10th Cir. 2024).

1343. Audit of Military Services' Processing of Coronavirus Disease–2019 Vaccination Exemptions and Discharges for Active Duty Service Members, U.S. Department of Defense, Inspector General, U.S. Department of Defense, March 12, 2024, https://media.defense.gov/2024/Mar/14/2003413066/-1/-1/1/DODIG-2024-061_AUDIT_VACCINEEXEMPT_REDACTED_SECURED.PDF.

1344. James M. Inhofe National Defense Authorization Act for Fiscal Year 2023, PL 117-263, December 23, 2022, 136 Stat 2395. Not later than 30 days after the date of the enactment of this Act, the Secretary of Defense shall rescind the mandate that members of the Armed Forces be vaccinated against COVID-19 pursuant to the memorandum dated August 24, 2021, regarding "Mandatory Coronavirus Disease 2019 Vaccination of Department of Defense Service Members".

1345. Id. at 22 and 25.

1346. Id. at 31.

1347. Doster v. Kendall, 54 F.4th 398, 409 (6th Cir. 2022), cert. granted, judgment vacated as moot, 144 S. Ct. 481 (2023), citing 42 U.S.C. § 2000bb-1.

1348. Doster v. Kendall, 54 F.4th 398, 409 (6th Cir. 2022), cert. granted, judgment vacated as moot, 144 S. Ct. 481 (2023), citing 42 U.S.C. § 2000bb-1.

1349. Audit of Military Services' Processing of Coronavirus Disease–2019 Vaccination Exemptions and Discharges for Active Duty Service Members, U.S. Department of Defense, Inspector General, U.S. Department of Defense, March 12, 2024, https://media.defense.gov/2024/Mar/14/2003413066/-1/-1/1/DODIG-2024-061_AUDIT_VACCINEEXEMPT_REDACTED_SECURED.PDF.

1350. U.S. Navy Seals 1-26 v. Biden, 27 F.4th 336 (5th Cir. 2022) (per curiam), rev'd in part, 142 S. Ct. 1301 (2022).

1351. Id.

1352. 27 F.4th 336, 342–43 (5th Cir. 2022).

1353. Austin v. U.S. Navy Seals 1-26, 142 S. Ct. 1301 (2022) (mem.).

1354. 107 Stat. 1488, 42 U.S.C. § 2000bb et seq.

1355. Tandon v. Newsom, 141 S. Ct. 1294, 1296 (2021) (per curiam).

1356. 669 F. Supp. 3d 598 (S.D. Miss. 2023).

1357. Bosarge v. Edney, 669 F. Supp. 3d 598, 609 (S.D. Miss. 2023).

1358. Inspector General Report at 21.

1359. Hobby Lobby, 573 U.S. at 725, citing Thomas v. Review Bd. of Indiana Employment Security Div., 450 U.S. 707, 716 (1981).

1360. Navy Seal 1 v. Austin, 586 F. Supp. 3d 1180 (M.D. Fla. 2022), injunction dissolved and case dismissed as moot, Colonel Fin. Mgmt. Officer v. Austin, No. 8:21-CV-2429-SDM-TGW, 2023 WL

6557806, at *1 (M.D. Fla. May 17, 2023) (unpublished). Contra, Roth v. Austin, 603 F. Supp. 3d 741 (D. Neb. 2022).

1361. Navy Seal 1 v. Austin, 586 F. Supp. 3d 1180 (M.D. Fla. 2022), injunction dissolved and case dismissed as moot, Colonel Fin. Mgmt. Officer v. Austin, No. 8:21-CV-2429-SDM-TGW, 2023 WL 6557806, at *1 (M.D. Fla. May 17, 2023) (unpublished).

1362. Inspector General Report at 11.

1363. Roth v. Austin, 603 F. Supp. 3d 741, 750 (D. Neb. 2022).

1364. 100 F.4th 1251 (10th Cir. 2024).

1365. Id. at 1268.

1366. Id. at 1269 (citations omitted).

1367. 584 U.S. 617, 618–19 (2018).

1368. Masterpiece Cakeshop v. Colorado C.R. Comm'n, 584 U.S. 617, 618–19 (2018).

1369. 450 U.S. 707 (1981).

1370. Does 1-11 v. Bd. of Regents of Univ. of Colorado, 100 F.4th 1251, 1277 (10th Cir. 2024), quoting Mitchell v. Helms, 530 U.S. 793, 828 (2000).

1371. U.S. Navy Seals 1-26 v. Biden, 27 F.4th 336, 343 (5th Cir. 2022) (per curiam), rev's in part, 142 S. Ct. 1301 (2022).

1372. Bosarge v. Edney, 669 F. Supp. 3d 598, 609 (S.D. Miss. 2023).

1373. 54 F.4th 398, 409, 422-23 (6th Cir. 2022), cert. granted, judgment vacated as moot, 144 S. Ct. 481 (2023), citing 42 U.S.C. § 2000bb-1.

1374. 54 F.4th 398, 423 (6th Cir. 2022) (citation to transcript omitted).

1375. 54 F.4th 398, 409, 422-23 (6th Cir. 2022), cert. granted, judgment vacated as moot, 144 S. Ct. 481 (2023), citing 42 U.S.C. § 2000bb-1.

1376. Hobby Lobby, 573 U.S. at 725, citing Thomas v. Review Bd. of Indiana Employment Security Div., 450 U.S. 707, 716 (1981).

1377. Roman Catholic Diocese of Brooklyn v. Cuomo, 141 S. Ct. 63 (2020) (New York regulation that prohibited religious gatherings but permitted similar secular gatherings violated the First Amendment where the secular and religious activities in question presented comparable alleged contagion risks), Tandon v. Newsom, 141 S. Ct. 1294, 1297 (2021) (per curiam) (unconstitutional for the State of California to issue regulations, ostensibly intended to slow the spread of COVID-19, that placed limits on religious gatherings but treated comparable non-religious activities more favorably).

1378. 107 Stat. 1488, 42 U.S.C. § 2000bb et seq.

1379. Church of Lukumi Babalu Aye, Inc. v. City of Hialeah., 508 U.S. 520, 546–47 (1993).

1380. 586 F. Supp. 3d 1180 (M.D. Fla. 2022), injunction dissolved and case dismissed as moot,

Colonel Fin. Mgmt. Officer v. Austin, No. 8:21-CV-2429-SDM-TGW, 2023 WL 6557806, at *1 (M.D. Fla. May 17, 2023) (unpublished).

1381. Id. at 1203.

1382. 586 F. Supp. 3d 1180, 1203, n. 11, citing Coronavirus: DOD Response, U.S. Dept. of Def., https://www.defense.gov/Spotlights/Coronavirus-DOD-Response/ (data as of Nov. 24, 2021, Dec. 22, 2021, and Feb. 9, 2022); see Oren Lieberman, US military has vaccinated more than 97% of service members, CNN Politics, Dec. 16, 2021, https://www.cnn.com/2021/12/16/politics/military-vaccine-numbers/index.html.

1383. 586 F. Supp. 3d 1180 (M.D. Fla. 2022), injunction dissolved and case dismissed as moot, Colonel Fin. Mgmt. Officer v. Austin, No. 8:21-CV-2429-SDM-TGW, 2023 WL 6557806, at *1 (M.D. Fla. May 17, 2023) (unpublished).

1384. Colonel Fin. Mgmt. Officer v. Austin, No. 8:21-CV-2429-SDM-TGW, 2023 WL 6557806, at *1 (M.D. Fla. May 17, 2023) (unpublished).

1385. 603 F. Supp. 3d 741 (D. Neb. 2022).

1386. 603 F. Supp. 3d at 747.

1387. Navy SEAL 1 v. Austin, 600 F. Supp. 3d 1, 16 (D.D.C. 2022), vacated as moot, No. 22-5114, 2023 WL 2482927 (D.C. Cir. Mar. 10, 2023).

1388. 603 F.Supp.3d at 772.

1389. 603 F.Supp.3d at 778.

1390.603 F. Supp. 3d at 750.

1391.Doster v. Kendall, 54 F.4th 398, 409, 422-23 (6th Cir. 2022), cert. granted, judgment vacated as moot, 144 S. Ct. 481 (2023), citing 42 U.S.C. § 2000bb-1, citing Burwell v. Hobby Lobby Stores, Inc., 573 U.S. 682, 726-27(2014) and Gonzales v. O Centro Espirita Beneficente Uniao do Vegetal, 546 U.S. 418 (2006).

1392.Doster v. Kendall, 54 F.4th 398 (6th Cir. 2022), cert. granted, judgment vacated as moot, 144 S. Ct. 481 (2023), citing 42 U.S.C. § 2000bb-1.

1393.Does 1-6 v. Mills, 142 S. Ct. 17, 20 (2021) (Gorsuch, J., dissenting), citing Fulton, 593 U.S., at ——, 141 S.Ct., at 1877; Tandon, 593 U.S., at ——, 141 S.Ct., at 1296-1297; Lukumi, 508 U.S., at 544–545, 113 S.Ct. 2217.

1394.Does 1-6 v. Mills, 142 S. Ct. 17, 20 (2021) (Gorsuch, J., dissenting), citing Yellowbear v. Lampert, 741 F.3d 48, 57 (C.A.10 2014) (quoting J. Clark, Guidelines for the Free Exercise Clause, 83 Harv. L. Rev. 327, 330–331 (1969)) (ellipses and quotation marks deleted).

1395.603 F.Supp.3d at 775.

1396.Id.

1397.603 F.Supp.3d at 767, quoting Air Force Officer v. Austin, No. 5:22-CV-00009-TES, 588 F.Supp.3d 1338, 1353 (M.D. Ga. Feb. 15, 2022) (citing Roman Cath. Diocese of Brooklyn v. Cuomo, —— U.S. ——, 141 S. Ct. 63, 67 (2020)).

1398.AXIOS on HBO: Moderna Chief Medical Officer Tal Zaks (Clip) | HBO, November 23, 2020, https://www.youtube.com/watch?v=po7qt9BZz0s&t=65s.

1399. CDC Issues First Set of Guidelines on How Fully Vaccinated People Can Visit Safely with Others, March 8, 2021, https://archive.is/PrcRy#selection-455.0-455.94.

1400. Interim Public Health Recommendations for Fully Vaccinated People, CDC, March 8, 2021, https://web.archive.org/web/20210312000532/https://www.cdc.gov/coronavirus/2019-ncov/vaccines/fully-vaccinated-guidance.html.

1401. Shannon Pettypiece, et al., CDC Recommends the Vaccinated Wear Masks in Areas with Low Vaccination Rates, NBC News, July 27, 2021, https://www.nbcnews.com/politics/white-house/biden-administration-recommend-vaccinated-wear-masks-areas-low-vaccination-rates-n1275012.

1402. Remarks by President Biden on the Importance of COVID-?19 Vaccine Requirements, Data Center, Clayco Construction Site Elk Grove Village, Illinois, October 7, 2021, https://www.whitehouse.gov/briefing-room/speeches-remarks/2021/10/07/remarks-by-president-biden-on-the-importance-of-covid-19-vaccine-requirements/. See also Executive Order 14043 of September 9, 2021, Requiring Coronavirus Disease 2019 Vaccination for Federal Employees, https://www.federalregister.gov/documents/2021/09/14/2021-19927/requiring-coronavirus-disease-2019-vaccination-for-federal-employees.

1403. Fact Sheet for Recipients and Caregivers Emergency Use Authorization (EUA) of The Moderna

COVID-19 Vaccine to Prevent Coronavirus Disease 2019 (Covid-19) in Individuals 18 Years of Age and Older, https://www.fda.gov/media/144638/download.

1404. 21 U.S. Code § 360bbb–3(e)(1)(A)(i) (emphasis added).

1405. Emergency Use Authorization of Medical Products and Related Authorities, FDA, January 2017, https://www.fda.gov/media/97321/download.

1406. Department of Health and Human Services Centers for Disease Control and Prevention, Advisory Committee on Immunization Practices (ACIP), Summary Report, August 26, 2020, Atlanta, Georgia, https://www.cdc.gov/vaccines/acip/meetings/downloads/min-archive/min-2020-08-508.pdf.

1407. Food and Drug Administration (FDA), Center for Biologics Evaluation and Research (CBER) 161st Vaccines and Related Biological Products Advisory Committee (VRBPAC) Meeting, October 22, 2020, https://www.fda.gov/media/143982/download.

1408. Aaron Siri, Federal Law Prohibits Employers and Others from Requiring Vaccination with a Covid-19 Vaccine Distributed under an EUA, February 23, 2021, See also 21 U.S. Code § 360bbb–3.

1409. Emergency Use Authorization of Medical Products and Related Authorities, January 2017, https://www.fda.gov/regulatory-information/search-fda-guidance-documents/emergency-use-authorization-medical-products-and-related-authorities#footnote46.

1410. Id.

1411. Emergency Use Authorization of Medical Products and Related Authorities, January 2017, https://www.fda.gov/regulatory-information/search-fda-guidance-documents/emergency-use-authorization-medical-products-and-related-authorities#eligible.

1412. Dawn Johnsen, Acting Assistant Attorney General Office of Legal Counsel, Whether Section 564 of the Food, Drug, and Cosmetic Act Prohibits Entities from Requiring the Use of a Vaccine Subject to an Emergency Use, MEMORANDUM OPINION FOR THE DEPUTY COUNSEL TO THE PRESIDENT, July 6, 2021, Authorizationhttps://www.justice.gov/sites/default/files/opinions/attachments/2021/07/26/2021-07-06-mand-vax.pdf

1413. H.R. Rep. No. 108-354, at 782 (2003) (Conf. Rep.) (emphasis added), https://www.congress.gov/congressional-report/108th-congress/house-report/354.

1414. DOD Instruction 6200.02, § E3.4 (Feb. 27, 2008). https://www.esd.whs.mil/Portals/54/Documents/DD/issuances/dodi/620002p.pdf.

1415. Dawn Johnsen, Acting Assistant Attorney General, Office of Legal Counsel, Whether Section 564 of the Food, Drug, and Cosmetic Act Prohibits Entities from Requiring the Use of a Vaccine Subject to an Emergency Use Authorization, Memorandum Opinion for the Deputy Counsel to the President, July 6, 2021, https://www.justice.gov/sites/default/files/opinions/attachments/2021/07/26/2021-07-06-mand-vax.pdf.

1416. Authorization of Emergency Use of Anthrax Vaccine Adsorbed for Prevention of Inhalation Anthrax by Individuals at Heightened Risk of Exposure Due to Attack With Anthrax; Availability, 70 Fed. Reg. 5452, 5455 (Feb. 2, 2005), https://www.federalregister.gov/documents/2005/02/02/05-2028/authorization-of-emergency-use-of-anthrax-vaccine-adsorbed-for-prevention-of-inhalation-anthrax-by.

1417. Authorization of Emergency Use of Anthrax Vaccine Adsorbed for Prevention of Inhalation Anthrax by Individuals at Heightened Risk of Exposure Due to Attack With Anthrax; Extension; Availability, 70 Fed. Reg. 44,657, 44,659–60 (Aug. 3, 2005).

1418. Guidance Emergency Use Authorization of Medical Products, 2007 WL 2319112, at *15.

1419. Opportunity, American Dictionary of the English Language, https://webstersdictionary1828.com/Dictionary/opportunity

1420. Eric S. Dreiband, Assistant Attorney General, The United States' Statement of Interest in Support of Plaintiff's Motion for an Injunction Pending Appeal, Lighthouse Fellowship Church V. Ralph Northam, Case No. 2:20-cv-00204-awa-rjk, United States District Court, Eastern District of Virginia, May 30, 2020, https://www.justice.gov/opa/press-release/file/1273211/download.

1421. Aaron Siri, Attorney for the Informed Consent Action Network, Letter to Dawn Johnsen, Acting

Assistant Attorney General Office of Legal Counsel, August 4, 2021, https://www.icandecide.org/wp-content/uploads/2021/08/Letter-in-Response-to-DOJ-Slip-Opinion-Released-on-July-26-2021.pdf.

1422. Id.

1423. 12VAC5-20-100.

1424. 367 U.S. 568 (1961).

1425. Id. at 602.

1426. Id. at 603.

1427. See United States v. Harrison, 34 F.3d 886, 891 (9th Cir. 1994).

1428. Ky. Rev. Stat. Ann. § 199.011 (West).

1429. Remarks by President Biden Laying Out the Next Steps in Our Effort to Get More Americans Vaccinated and Combat the Spread of the Delta Variant, July 29, 2021, 4:23 p.m. EDT, https://www.whitehouse.gov/briefing-room/speeches-remarks/2021/07/29/remarks-by-president-biden-laying-out-the-next-steps-in-our-effort-to-get-more-americans-vaccinated-and-combat-the-spread-of-the-delta-variant/.

1430. Nightingale, S. L., Prasher, J. M., & Simonson, S. (2007). Emergency Use Authorization (EUA) to Enable Use of Needed Products in Civilian and Military Emergencies, United States. Emerging Infectious Diseases, 13(7), 1046. https://doi.org/10.3201/eid1307.061188, https://wwwnc.cdc.gov/eid/article/13/7/06-1188_article

#r1.

1431. Aaron Siri, Attorney for the Informed Consent Action Network, Letter to Dawn Johnsen, Acting Assistant Attorney General Office of Legal Counsel, August 4, 2021, https://www.icandecide.org/wp-content/uploads/2021/08/Letter-in-Response-to-DOJ-Slip-Opinion-Released-on-July-26-2021.pdf.

1432. Safer Federal Workforce, GSA, https://web.archive.org/web/20210727233714/https://www.saferfederalworkforce.gov/faq/vaccinations/.

1433. Option, Merriam-Webster Dictionary, https://www.merriam-webster.com/dictionary/option.

1434. PL 93–348 (HR 7724), PL 93–348, JULY 12, 1974, 88 Stat 342, https://www.govinfo.gov/content/pkg/STATUTE-88/pdf/STATUTE-88-Pg342.pdf.

1435. Merlin Duval, Director, Center for Disease Control, Memorandum Terminating the Tuskegee Syphilis Study, November 14, 1972, https://catalog.archives.gov/id/650716.

1436. Id.

1437. Id.

1438. The Belmont Report, Office of the Secretary, Ethical Principles and Guidelines for the Protection of Human Subjects of Research, The National Commission for the Protection of Human Subjects of Biomedical and Behavioral Research, April 18, 1979, https://www.hhs.gov/ohrp/regulations-and-policy/belmont-report/read-the-belmont-report/index.html.

1439. Id (emphasis added).

1440. Part 3 – The Belmont Report: Basic Ethical Principles and their Application, U.S. Department of Health and Human Services, June 16, 2021, Publication Date, October 9, 2018, https://www.youtube.com/watch?v=M6AKIlhoFn4.

1441. Padma Nambisan, in An Introduction to Ethical, Safety and Intellectual Property Rights Issues in Biotechnology, 2017, https://www.sciencedirect.com/topics/medicine-and-dentistry/belmont-report (last visited on August 18, 2021).

1442. Id. (emphasis added).

1443. 45 C.F.R. § 46.116, https://www.ecfr.gov/cgi-bin/text-idx?SID=89a8d8aaed03e964d4a9176d34590463&mc=true&node=se45.1.46_1116&rgn=div8 (last visited on August 18, 2021).

1444. See Abdullahi v. Pfizer, 562 F.3d 163, 174-188 (2nd Cir. 2009)..

1445. 290 U.S. 398 (1934).

1446. 486 F. Supp. 3d 883 (W.D. Pa. 2020), complaint and district court judgment vacated as moot, 8 F.4th 226 (3rd Cir. 2021)).

1447. *City of Butler v. Wolf*, 486 F. Supp. 3d 883 (W.D. Pa. 2020), complaint and district court judgment vacated as moot, 8 F.4th 226 (3rd Cir. 2021)).

1448. Id. at 928.

1449. 450 U.S. 707 (1981).

1450. Thomas v. Rev. Bd. of Indiana, 450 U.S. 707, 714 (1981).

1451. Id. at 716.

1452. Id. at 718.

1453. 508 U.S. 520 (1993).

1454. Id. at 531-32.

1455. Id. at 546.

1456. 667 F.3d 727, 740 (6th Cir. 2012).

1457. Id.

1458. Id. at 546-47.

1459. 170 F.3d 359 (3d Cir. 1999).

1460. Requiring Coronavirus Disease 2019 Vaccination for Federal Employees, Exec. Order No. 14043, 86 FR 50989, September 9, 2021.

1461. Feds for Med. Freedom v. Biden, 581 F. Supp. 3d 826 (S.D. Tex.), rev'd on reh'g en banc, 63 F.4th 366 (5th Cir. 2023), cert. granted, judgment vacated, 144 S. Ct. 480 (2023).

1462. 142 S. Ct. 661 (2022).

1463. 142 S. Ct. at 665.

1464. Feds for Med. Freedom v. Biden, 63 F.4th 366 (5th Cir.) (en banc), cert. granted, judgment vacated, 144 S. Ct. 480 (2023).

1465. 144 S. Ct. 480 (2023).

1466. 562 U.S. 223 (2011), https://www.supremecourt.gov/opinions/10pdf/09-152.pdf.

1467. 42 U.S.C. § 300aa–22, https://www.law.cornell.edu/uscode/text/42/300aa-22.

1468. National Vaccine Injury Compensation Program, Children's Health Defense, https://childrenshealthdefense.org/national-vaccine-injury-compensation-program/ (last visited on January 6, 2021).

1469. Mary S. Holland, Liability for Vaccine Injury: The United States, the European Union, and the Developing World, Emory Law Journal, Vol 67, 2018, https://scholarlycommons.law.emory.edu/elj/vol67/iss3/3/.

1470. Mary S. Holland, supra.

1471. National Vaccine Injury Compensation Program, Children's Health Defense, https://childrenshealthdefense.org/national-vaccine-injury-compensation-program/ (last visited on January 6, 2021).

1472. Mary S. Holland, supra.

1473. Mary S. Holland, supra. Quoting Gayle DeLong, Is "Delitigation" Associated with a Change in Product Safety? The Case of Vaccines, Rev. Ind. Org. (June 14, 2017).

1474. 42 U.S.C. § 300aa–22, https://www.law.cornell.edu/uscode/text/42/300aa-22.

1475. 42 U.S.C. § 300aa–27, https://www.law.cornell.edu/uscode/text/42/300aa-27.

1476. 42 U.S.C. § 300aa–27.

1477. 42 U.S.C. § 300aa–27.

1478. 42 U.S.C. § 300aa–27.

1479. RFK, Jr. Proves HHS is in Violation of the "Mandate for Safer Childhood Vaccines" as Stipulated in the Vaccine Injury Compensation Act, Children's Health Defense, September 13, 2018, https://childrenshealthdefense.org/child-health-topics/federal-failures/rfk-jr-proves-hhs-is-in-violation-of-the-mandate-for-safer-childhood-vaccines-as-stipulated-in-the-vaccine-injury-compensation-act/. ICAN v. HHS, Complaint for Declaratory and Injunctive Relief, April 12, 2018, https://childrenshealthdefense.org/wp-content/uploads/rfk-complaint-against-united-states-department-of-health-and-human-services.pdf. See also ICAN & RFK, Jr. Call Out DHHS for Vaccine Safety Violations, Texans for Vaccine Choice, July 18, 2018, https://texansforvaccinechoice.com/ican-rfk-jr-call-out-dhhs-for-vaccine-safety-violations/.

1480. ICAN v. HHS, Stipulation, July 9, 2018, https://childrenshealthdefense.org/wp-content/uploads/rfk-hhs-stipulated-order-july-2018.pdf.

1481. RFK, Jr. Proves HHS is in Violation of the "Mandate for Safer Childhood Vaccines" as Stipulated in the Vaccine Injury Compensation Act, Children's Health Defense, September 13, 2018, https://childrenshealthdefense.org/child-health-topics/federal-failures/rfk-jr-proves-hhs-is-in-violation-of-the-mandate-for-safer-childhood-vaccines-as-stipulated-in-the-vaccine-injury-compensation-act/.

1482. Edward Hendrie, Study Shows That Vaccinated Children Are Significantly Less Healthy Than Unvaccinated Children, December 20, 2020, https://greatmountainpublishing.com/2020/12/20/study-shows-that-vaccinated-children-are-significantly-less-healthy-than-unvaccinated-children/. Edward Hendrie, Vaccines Increase Mortality of Infants, August 17, 2020, https://greatmountainpublishing.com/2020/08/17/vaccines-increase-mortality-of-children/. Edward Hendrie, Vaccines Cause Autism and Allergies, August 5, 2020, https://greatmountainpublishing.com/2020/08/05/vaccines-cause-autism-and-allergies/.

1483. Pfizer to Acquire Arena Pharmaceuticals, December 13, 2021, https://www.pfizer.com/news/press-release/press-release-detail/pfizer-acquire-arena-pharmaceuticals.

1484. Edward Hendrie, Follow the SILENCE: Paper Proving That COVID-19 Vaccines Cause Myocarditis Is Removed From Publication Without Explanation, October 31, 2021, https://greatmountainpublishing.com/2021/10/31/follow-the-silence-paper-proving-that-covid-19-vaccines-cause-myocarditis-is-removed-from-publication-without-explanation/. See also Edward Hendrie, The FDA and Pfizer Concealed Evidence That COVID-19 Vaccines Will Cause Myocarditis in Children, November 7, 2021, https://greatmountainpublishing.com/2021/11/07/the-fda-and-pfizer-concealed-evidence-that-covid-19-vaccines-will-cause-myocarditis-in-children/.

1485. Pfizer buys immuno-inflammatory firm Arena Pharmaceuticals for $6.7b, December 13, 2021, Outsourcing-Pharma, https://www.outsourcing-pharma.com/Article/2021/12/13/Pfizer-buys-immuno-inflammatory-firm-Arena-for-6.7b.

1486. Edward Hendrie, Doctor Finds That His Patients Have Permanent Organ Damage from Blood Clots Caused by COVID-19 Vaccines, Great Mountain Publishing, October 23, 2021, https://greatmountainpublishing.com/2021/10/23/doctor-finds-that-his-patients-have-permanent-organ-damage-from-blood-clots-caused-by-covid-19-vaccines/, quoting CFT Team, Doctor Warns How COVID mRNA 'Vaccines' Will Cause Delayed Strokes & Heart Attacks — 'The Worst Is Yet To Come', July 14, 2021, https://christiansfortruth.com/doctor-warns-how-covid-mrna-vaccines-will-soon-cause-strokes-heart-attacks-the-worst-is-yet-to-come/.

1487. Harvey Eisner, Firehouse Magazine, archived October 7, 1999 page, https://web.archive.org/web/19991007180848/https://www.firehouse.com/magazine/archives/1998/September/progress2.html.

1488. Firefighter Arson, USFA-TR-141/January 2003, Special Report, U.S. Fire Administration, FEMA, archived page from November 9, 2004, ttps://web.archive.org/web/20041109074057/https://www.usfa.fema.gov/downloads/pdf/publications/tr-141.pdf.

1489. Pfizer Completes Acquisition of Global Blood Therapeutics, Pfizer, October 05, 2022, https://www.pfizer.com/news/press-release/press-release-detail/pfizer-completes-acquisition-global-blood-therapeutics.

1490. Top Pathologist confirms Cancer, Infertility & Strange Blood Clots are common side effects of Covid-19 Vaccination, The Expose, April 22, 2023, https://expose-news.com/2023/04/22/cancer-infertility-blood-clots-due-to-covid-vaccination/?cmid=b9c65fea-8808-4668-80f8-1e76ab03f676.

1491. Official Government Reports prove the COVID Vaccines cause Cancer. The Expose, August 21, 2021, https://expose-news.com/2022/08/21/gov-reports-prove-covid-vaccines-cause-cancer/. See also Lynn Redwood, Researchers Show How COVID Damages Immune System, Increasing Cancer Risks — Science Says Vaccines May Do the Same, The Defender, December 20, 2021, https://childrenshealthdefense.org/defender/covid-vaccines-immune-system-cancer-risks/, citing Jiang H, Mei Y-F. SARS–CoV–2 Spike Impairs DNA Damage Repair and Inhibits V(D)J Recombination In Vitro. Viruses. 2021; 13(10):2056. https://doi.org/10.3390/v13102056 (Published: 13 October 2021 / Retracted: 10 May 2022).

1492. Eustace Mullins, Murder by Injection, The Story of the Medical Conspiracy Against America, at 82 (1988).

1493. Eustace Mullins, Murder by Injection, The Story of the Medical Conspiracy Against America, at 82 (1988).

1494. Phil Taylor, The top 10 biopharma M&A deals in 2021, January 18, 2022, Fierce Pharma, https://www.fiercepharma.com/special-report/top-10-bi opharma-m-a-deals-2021.

1495. Pfizer Invests $43 Billion to Battle Cancer, Pfizer, March 13, 2023, https://www.pfizer.com/news/press-release/press-relea se-detail/pfizer-invests-43-billion-battle-cancer.

1496. McKenzie Sigalos, You Can't Sue Pfizer or Moderna If You Have Severe Covid Vaccine Side Effects. The Government Likely Won't Compensate You for Damages Either, CNBC, December 17, 2020, https://www.cnbc.com/2020/12/16/covid-vaccine-side-effects-compensation-lawsuit.html.

1497. Zachary Stieber, Few, If Any, Doses of Spikevax or Comirnaty Available in United States, Despite FDA Approvals, The Epoch Times, February 2, 2022, https://archive.ph/Ry0Xh. See also SpikeVax COVID-19 Vaccine (Moderna), Updated May 28, 2022, https://www.precisionvaccinations.com/vaccines/spike vax-covid-19-vaccine-moderna. "As of July 11, 2022, Moderna's SpikeVax was **available** in Poland, Czech Republic, Caribbean, Denmark, Romania, Hungary, Bulgaria, Slovenia, Slovakia, Croatia, Estonia, Latvia, Lithuania, Serbia, Ukraine, Moldova, Albania, Bosnia-Herzegovina, Kosovo, North Macedonia, Montenegro, Israel, France, the African Union, Australian, Spain, Switzerland, South Korea, the United Kingdom, Switzerland, and was **Approved in the U.S.**" Id.

1498. MacKenzie Sigalos, You Can't Sue Pfizer or Moderna If You Have Severe Covid Vaccine Side Effects. The Government Likely Won't Compensate You for Damages Either, CNBC, December 17, 2020, https://www.cnbc.com/2020/12/16/covid-vaccine-side-effects-compensation-lawsuit.html.

1499. Mary S. Holland, *Liability for Vaccine Injury: The United States, the European Union, and the Developing World*, 67 Emory L. J. 415 (2018). Available at: https://scholarlycommons.law.emory.edu/elj/vol67/iss3/3.

1500. Countermeasures Injury Compensation Program, Request for Benefits Form Instructions, OMB Control No. 0915-0334, Expiration Date: 3/31/2023, https://www.hrsa.gov/sites/default/files/hrsa/cicp/cicp-request-form-instructions.pdf.

1501. Id.

1502. MacKenzie Sigalos, You Can't Sue Pfizer or Moderna If You Have Severe Covid Vaccine Side Effects. The Government Likely Won't Compensate You for Damages Either, CNBC, December 17, 2020, https://www.cnbc.com/2020/12/16/covid-vaccine-side-effects-compensation-lawsuit.html.

1503. A Vaccine Progress Report, The Wall Street Jounal, July 22, 2020, https://www.wsj.com/articles/a-vaccine-progress-report-11595461075?mod=searchresults&page=1&pos=5.

Other books available from Great Mountain Publishing®

YAHWEH Is NOT the LORD JEHOVAH
Edward Hendrie
ISBN: 978-1-943056-19-4

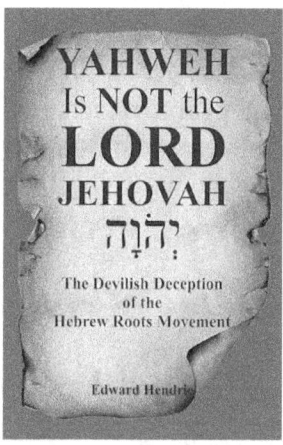

This book is excerpted from Hoax of Biblical Proportions, with some additional material. That book reveals how God's inspired King James Holy Bible exposes Satan's profane Bibles.

Satan knows that God has promised to preserve his words found in the Holy Scriptures, so it would be futile for him to try to destroy them. Thus, Satan's strategy is to obscure God's words by flooding the world with counterfeit Bibles. That way, he can flimflam people into reading his corrupt Bibles instead of God's infallible Scriptures. The devil can then lead men astray from the true gospel.

Hoax of Biblical Proportions proves that the Authorized (King James) Version of the Holy Bible is given by inspiration of God. It will reveal how Satan is using profane Bible versions to divert the world away from God's inspired Holy Scriptures. The changes in the new Bible versions are not merely cosmetic for ease of reading, as claimed by the publishers; they change doctrine. The new Bible versions confuse churches and demoralize the world by proclaiming a different Jesus and a different gospel from what is in God's inspired King James Holy Bible.

Part and parcel of the deception in the new Bible versions is changing the name of God from Jehovah to Yahweh. That change has been popularized by the Hebrew Roots (a.k.a. Sacred Name) movement. Jehovah is the proper English translation of the Hebrew Tetragrammaton (   ) (YHVH). The Hebrew Roots movement invokes Yahweh in place of Jehovah. They falsely claim that Yahweh is the proper pronunciation of the Tetragrammaton. In actuality, invoking Yahweh is a trick to get people to worship a devil in place of God Almighty, Jehovah. God's name is Jehovah; Yahweh is a heathen storm god.

I excerpted the information from Hoax of Biblical Proportions to have a single publication dedicated to helping people understand the devilish deception of the Hebrew Roots movement in its effort to replace the worship of Almighty God, Jehovah, with a heathen god, Yahweh.

Hoax of Biblical Proportions
Edward Hendrie
ISBN: 978-1-943056-18-7

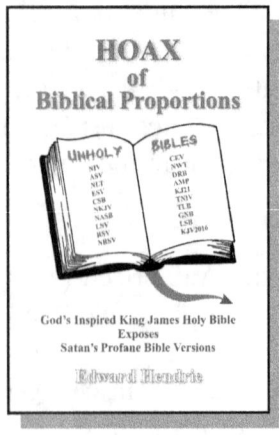

Satan knows that God has promised to preserve his words found in the Holy Scriptures, so it would be futile for him to try to destroy them. Thus, Satan's strategy is to obscure God's words by flooding the world with counterfeit Bibles. That way, he can flimflam people into reading his corrupt Bibles instead of God's infallible Scriptures. The devil can then lead men astray from the true gospel. This book will prove that the Authorized (King James) Version of the Holy Bible is given by inspiration of God. It will reveal how Satan is using profane Bible versions to divert the world away from God's inspired Holy Scriptures. The changes in the new Bible versions are not merely cosmetic for ease of reading, as claimed by the publishers; they change doctrine. The new Bible versions confuse churches and demoralize the world by proclaiming a different Jesus and a different gospel from what is in God's inspired King James Holy Bible.

Vaccine Danger: Quackery and Sin
Edward Hendrie
ISBN: 978-1-943056-17-0

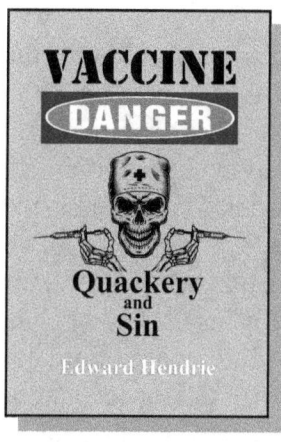

This book reveals the most significant medical fraud in history. The theory that you can prevent illness by injecting poisons into the bodies of healthy people is dangerous quackery and sin. All true science has proven the practice of vaccination to be ineffective and unsafe. But the medical establishment has been lured into the superstitious practice, hook, line, and sinker. It is not merely a matter of ignorance that the debilitating practice flourishes. It is, at its core, being promoted by those who know it is unsafe and ineffective. There is a malevolent spirit behind the practice. It is part of a conspiracy against God and man. While most doctors are unwitting, some are willing minions of that old serpent, called the Devil, and Satan, who are quite happy to kill people for profit. Jesus describes such men: "Ye are of your father the devil, and the lusts of your father ye will do. He was a murderer from the beginning, and abode not in the truth, because there is no truth in him. When he speaketh a lie, he speaketh of his own: for he is a liar, and the father of it." John 8:44.

The Sphere of Influence: The Heliocentric Perversion of the Gospel
Edward Hendrie
ISBN: 978-1-943056-06-4

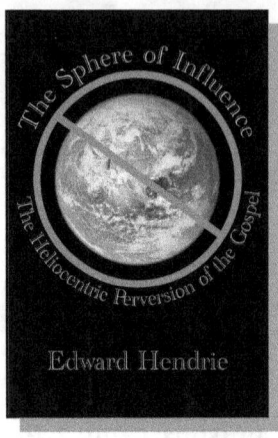

This book is a sequel to *The Greatest Lie on Earth (Expanded Edition): Proof That Our World Is Not a Moving Globe.* It will primarily focus on the infiltration into the church of the superstitious myth of heliocentrism and how that infiltration has served to undermine the gospel. The gospel is the entire Holy Bible, not just some of it. Matthew 4:4. Christian belief is an all or nothing proposition. "All scripture is given by inspiration of God, and is profitable for doctrine, for reproof, for correction, for instruction in righteousness." 2 Timothy 3:16. God's account of his creation is part and parcel of the gospel. A person with genuine faith believes what Jesus said about both heavenly and earthly things. "If I have told you earthly things, and ye believe not, how shall ye believe, if I tell you of heavenly things?" John 3:12. Jesus is God. Jesus created all things in heaven and on earth. See Colossians 1:16-18. God has revealed himself through his creation. "[T]hat which may be known of God is manifest in them; for God hath shewed it unto them. For the invisible things of him from the creation of the world are clearly seen, being understood by the things that are made, even his eternal power and Godhead; so that they are without excuse." Romans 1:19-20. If men have a misunderstanding of God's creation, they will also have a misunderstanding of who God is. If people believe in a creation that does not exist, they consequently also believe in a creator that does not exist. It is essential, therefore, to have an accurate understanding of God's creation. God did not make a movable, spherical earth. If men believe in a heliocentric creation, they will necessarily believe in a heliocentric creator. A heliocentric creation does not exist. So also, a heliocentric creator does not exist. A heliocentric creator is a false god. We have been warned to avoid the preaching of a false gospel, which presents a false Jesus. "For if he that cometh preacheth another Jesus, whom we have not preached, or if ye receive another spirit, which ye have not received, or another gospel, which ye have not accepted, ye might well bear with him." 2 Corinthians 11:4.

The Greatest Lie on Earth
Proof That Our World Is Not a Moving Globe
Edward Hendrie
ISBN-13: 978-1-943056-01-9

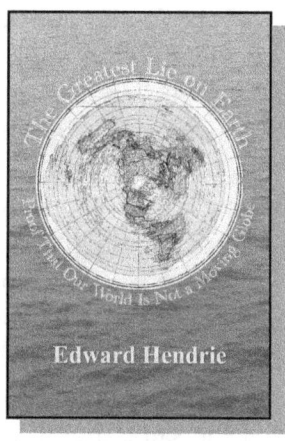

This book reveals the mother of all conspiracies. It sets forth biblical proof and irrefutable evidence that will cause the scales to fall from your eyes and reveal that the world you thought existed is a myth. The most universally accepted scientific belief today is that the earth is a globe, spinning on its axis at a speed of approximately 1,000 miles per hour at the equator, while at the same time it is orbiting the sun at approximately 66,600 miles per hour. All of this is happening as the sun, in turn, is supposed to be hurtling through the Milky Way galaxy at approximately 500,000 miles per hour. The Milky Way galaxy, itself, is alleged to be racing through space at a speed ranging from 300,000 to 1,340,000 miles per hour. What most people are not told is that the purported spinning, orbiting, and speeding through space has never been proven. In fact, every scientific experiment that has ever been performed to determine the motion of the earth has proven that the earth is stationary. Yet, textbooks ignore the scientific proof that contradicts the myth of a spinning and orbiting globe. Christian schools have been hoodwinked into teaching heliocentrism, despite the clear teaching in the Bible that the earth is not a sphere and does not move. This book reveals the evil forces behind the heliocentric deception, and why scientists and the Christian churches have gone along with it.

The Greatest Lie on Earth (Expanded Edition)
Proof That Our World Is Not a Moving Globe
Edward Hendrie
ISBN-13: 978-1943056-03-3

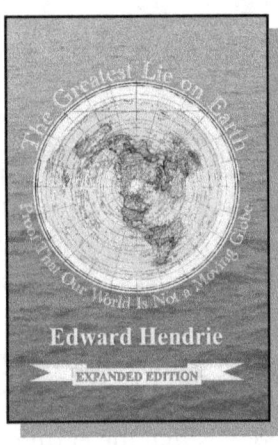

This book is an expanded edition of *The Greatest Lie on Earth*. It contains more than 1,000 pages of authoritative evidence with more than 1,300 endnotes that document proof beyond any doubt that the earth is flat and stationary. The book reveals the mother of all conspiracies. It sets forth biblical proof and irrefutable evidence that will cause the scales to fall from your eyes and reveal that the world you thought existed is a myth. The most universally accepted scientific belief today is that the earth is a globe, spinning on its axis at a speed of approximately 1,000 miles per hour at the equator, while at the same time it is orbiting the sun at approximately 66,600 miles per hour. All of this is happening as the sun, in turn, is supposed to be hurtling through the Milky Way galaxy at approximately 500,000 miles per hour. The Milky Way galaxy, itself, is alleged to be racing through space at a speed ranging from 300,000 to 1,340,000 miles per hour. What most people are not told is that the purported spinning, orbiting, and speeding through space has never been proven. In fact, every scientific experiment that has ever been performed to determine the motion of the earth has proven that the earth is stationary. Yet, textbooks ignore the scientific proof that contradicts the myth of a spinning and orbiting globe. Christian schools have been hoodwinked into teaching heliocentrism, despite the clear teaching in the Bible that the earth is not a sphere and does not move. This book reveals the evil forces behind the heliocentric deception, and why scientists and the Christian churches have gone along with it.

Antichrist: The Beast Revealed
Edward Hendrie
ISBN-13: 978-0-9832627-8-7

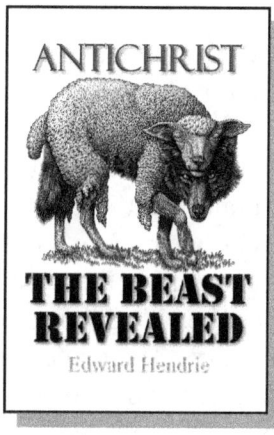

The antichrist is among us, here and now. This book proves it by comparing the biblical prophecies about the antichrist with the evidence that those prophecies have been fulfilled. This book documents the man of sin's esoteric confession that he is the antichrist. You will learn how the antichrist has changed times and laws as prophesied by Daniel, and how he is today sitting in the temple of God, "shewing himself that he is God," in fulfillment of Paul's prophecy in 2 Thessalonians 2:4. The beast of Revelation has come into the world, "after the working of Satan with all power and signs and lying wonders, and with all deceivableness of unrighteousness," as prophesied in 2 Thessalonians 2:10. The antichrist's adeptness as a hypocrite is the reason for his evil success. Indeed, to be the antichrist, his evil character must be concealed beneath a facade of piety. "And no marvel; for Satan himself is transformed into an angel of light. Therefore it is no great thing if his ministers also be transformed as the ministers of righteousness; whose end shall be according to their works." 2 Corinthians 11:14-15. The key to revealing the identity of the antichrist is to uncover his hypocrisy. Because the hypocrisy of the antichrist is so extreme, those who have been hoodwinked by his religious doctrines will be shocked to learn of it. This book exposes the concealed iniquity of the antichrist and juxtaposes it against his publicly proclaimed false persona of righteousness, thus bringing into clear relief that man of sin, the son of perdition, who is truly a ravening wolf in sheep's clothing, speaking lies in hypocrisy. See Matthew 7:15 and 1 Timothy 4:1-3.

9/11-Enemies Foreign and Domestic
Edward Hendrie
ISBN-13: 978-0983262732

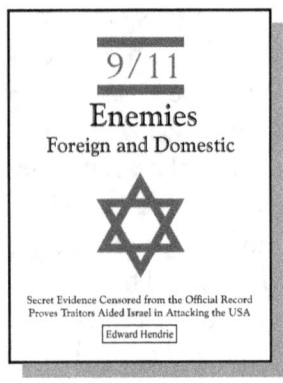

9/11-Enemies Foreign and Domestic proves beyond a reasonable doubt that the U.S. Government's conspiracy theory of the attacks on September 11, 2001, is a preposterous cover story. The evidence in 9/11-Enemies Foreign and Domestic has been suppressed from the official government reports and censored from the mass media. The evidence proves that powerful Zionists ordered the 9/11 attacks, which were perpetrated by Israel's Mossad, aided and abetted by treacherous high officials in the U.S. Government. 9/11-Enemies Foreign and Domestic identifies the traitors by name and details their subversive crimes. There is sufficient evidence in 9/11-Enemies Foreign and Domestic to indict important officials of the U.S. Government for high treason. The reader will understand how the U.S. Government really works and what Sir John Harrington (1561-1612) meant when he said: "Treason doth never prosper: what's the reason? Why if it prosper, none dare call it treason." There are millions of Americans who have taken an oath to defend the U.S. Constitution against all enemies foreign and domestic. The mass media, which is under the control of a disloyal cabal, keeps those patriotic Americans ignorant of the traitors among them. J. Edgar Hoover, former Director of the FBI, explained: "The individual is handicapped by coming face-to-face with a conspiracy so monstrous-he simply cannot believe it exists." 9/11-

Enemies Foreign and Domestic erases any doubt about the existence of the monstrous conspiracy described by Hoover and arms the reader with the knowledge required to save our great nation. "My people are destroyed for lack of knowledge." Hosea 4:6.

Solving the Mystery of BABYLON THE GREAT
Edward Hendrie
ISBN-13: 978-0983262701

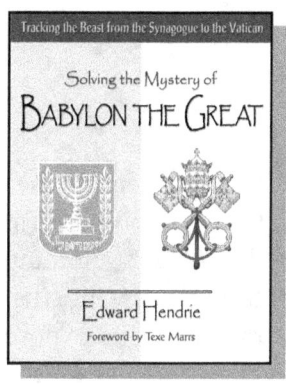

"Attorney and Christian researcher Edward Hendrie investigates and reveals one of the greatest exposés of all time. . . . a book you don't want to miss. Solving the Mystery of Babylon the Great is packed with documentation. Never before have the crypto-Jews who seized the reins of power in Rome been put under such intense scrutiny." Texe Marrs, Power of Prophecy. The evidence presented in this book leads to the ineluctable conclusion that the Roman Catholic Church was established by crypto-Jews as a false "Christian" front for a Judaic/Babylonian religion. That religion is the core of a world conspiracy against man and God. That is not a conspiracy theory based upon speculation, but rather the hard truth based upon authoritative evidence, which is documented in this book. Texe Marrs explains in his foreword to the book: "Who is Mystery Babylon? What is the meaning of the sinister symbols found in these passages? Which city is being described as the 'great city' so full of sin and decadence, and who are its citizens? Why do the woman and beast of Revelation seek the destruction of the holy people, the saints and martyrs of Jesus? What does it all mean for you and me today? Solving the Mystery of Babylon the Great answers these questions and more. Edward Hendrie's discoveries are not based on prejudice but on solid evidence aligned forthrightly with the 'whole counsel of God.' He does not condone nor will he be a part of any project in which Bible verses are taken out of context, or in which scriptures are twisted to mean what they do not say. Again and again you will find that Mr. Hendrie documents his assertions, backing up what he says with historical facts and proofs. Most important is that he buttresses his findings with scriptural understanding. The foundation for his research is sturdy because it is based on the bedrock of God's unshakeable Word."

The Anti-Gospel
Edward Hendrie
ISBN-13: 978-0983262749

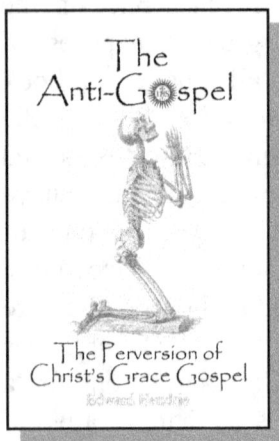

Edward Hendrie uses God's word to strip the sheep's clothing from false Christian ministers and expose them as ravening wolves preaching an anti-gospel. The anti-gospel is based on a myth that all men have a will that is free from the bondage of sin to choose whether to believe in Jesus. The Holy Bible, however, states that all men are spiritually dead and cannot believe in Jesus unless they are born again of the Holy Spirit. Ephesians 2:1-7; John 3:3-8. God has chosen his elect to be saved by his grace through faith in Jesus Christ. Ephesians 1:3-9; 2:8-10. God imbues his elect with the faith needed to believe in Jesus. Hebrews 12:2; John 1:12-13. The devil's false gospel contradicts the word of God and reverses the order of things. Under the anti-gospel, instead of a sovereign God choosing his elect, sovereign man decides whether to choose God. The calling of the Lord Jesus Christ is effectual; all who are chosen for salvation will believe in Jesus. John 6:37-44. The anti-gospel has a false Jesus, who only offers the possibility of salvation, with no assurance. The anti-gospel blasphemously makes God out to be a liar by denying the total depravity of man and the sovereign election of God. All who preach that false gospel are under a curse from God. Galatians 1:6-9.

Bloody Zion
Edward Hendrie
ISBN-13: 978-0983262763

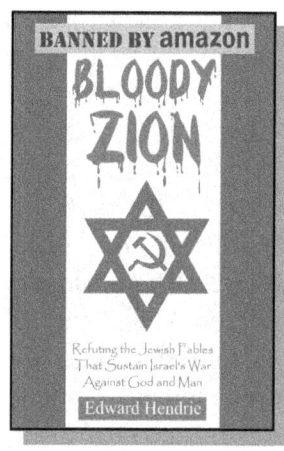

Jesus told Pontius Pilate: "My kingdom is not of this world." John 18:36. God has a spiritual Zion that is in a heavenly Jerusalem. Hebrews 12:22; Revelation 21:10. Jesus Christ is the chief corner stone laid by God in Zion. 1 Peter 2:6. Those who believe in Jesus Christ are living stones in the spiritual house of God. 1 Peter 2:5; Ephesians 2:20-22. Believers are in Jesus and Jesus is in believers. John 14:20; 17:20-23. All who are elected by God to believe in Jesus Christ are part of the heavenly Zion, without regard to whether they are Jews or Gentiles. Romans 10:12. Satan is a great adversary of God, who has created his own mystery religions. During the Babylonian captivity (2 Chronicles 36:20), an occult society of Jews replaced God's commands with Satan's Babylonian dogma. Their new religion became Judaism. Jesus explained the corruption of the Judaic religion: "Howbeit in vain do they worship me, teaching for doctrines the commandments of men." Mark 7:7. Jesus revealed the Satanic origin of Judaism when he stated: "Ye are of your father the devil, and the lusts of your father ye will do." John 8:44. Babylonian Judaism remains the religion of the Jews today. Satan has infected many nominal "Christian" denominations with his Babylonian occultism, which has given rise to "Christian" Zionism. "Christian" Zionism advocates a counterfeit, earthly Zion, within which fleshly

Jews take primacy over the spiritual church of Jesus Christ. This book exposes "Christian" Zionism as a false gospel and subversive political movement that sustains Israel's war against God and man.

Murder, Rape, and Torture in a Catholic Nunnery
Edward Hendrie
ISBN-13: 978-1-943056-00-2

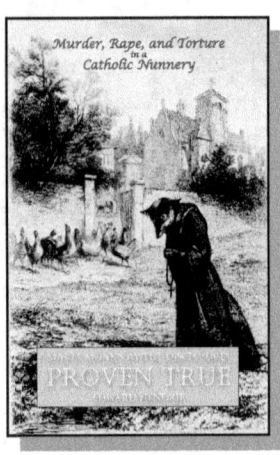

There has probably not been a person more maligned by the powerful forces of the Roman Catholic Church than Maria Monk. In 1836 she published the famous book, *Awful Disclosures of the Hotel Dieu Nunnery of Montreal*. In that book, she told of murder, rape, and torture behind the walls of the cloistered nunnery. Because the evidence was verifiably true, the Catholic hierarchy found it necessary to fabricate evidence and suborn perjury in an attempt to destroy the credibility of Maria Monk. The Catholic Church has kept up the character assassination of Maria Monk now for over 175 years. Even today, there can be found on the internet websites devoted to libeling Maria Monk. Edward Hendrie has examined the evidence and set it forth for the readers to decide for themselves whether Maria Monk was an impostor, as claimed by the Roman Catholic Church, or whether she was a brave victim. An objective view of the evidence leads to the ineluctable conclusion that Maria Monk told the truth about what happened behind the walls of the Hotel Dieu Nunnery of Montreal. The Roman Catholic Church, which is the most powerful religious and political organization in the world, has engaged in an unceasing campaign of vilification against Maria Monk. Their crusade against Maria Monk, however, can only affect the opinion of the uninformed. It cannot change the evidence. The evidence speaks clearly to those who will look at the case objectively. The evidence reveals that the much maligned Maria Monk was a reliable witness who made awful but accurate disclosures about life in a cloistered nunnery.

What Shall I Do to Inherit Eternal Life?
Edward Hendrie
ISBN-13: 978-0983262770

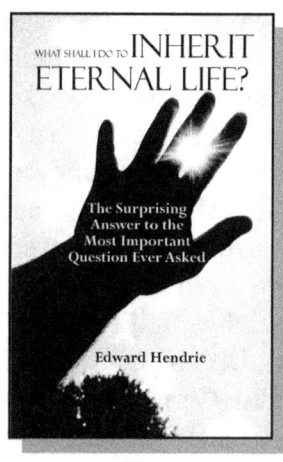

A certain ruler posed to Jesus the most important question ever asked: "Good Master, what shall I do to inherit eternal life?" (Luke 18:18) The man came to the right person. Jesus is God, and therefore his answer to that question is authoritative. This book examines Jesus' surprising answer and definitively explains how one inherits eternal life. This is a book about God's revelation to man. Except for the Holy Bible, this is the most important book you will ever read.

The Damnable Heresy Of Salvation by Dead Faith (Expanded Edition)
Edward Hendrie
ISBN 13: 978-1943056118

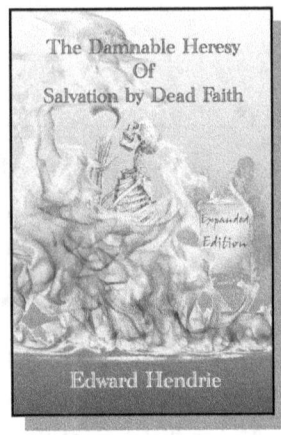

Good works follow salvation; they do not earn salvation. Good works do not save us. The works of faith are those works ordained and performed by God through the believer. They are the result of faith. It is that perfect faith that justifies the believer. "For by grace are ye saved through faith; and that not of yourselves: it is the gift of God: Not of works, lest any man should boast. For we are his workmanship, created in Christ Jesus unto good works, which God hath before ordained that we should walk in them. For we are his workmanship, created in Christ Jesus unto good works, which God hath before ordained that we should walk in them." Ephesians 2:8-10. In Romans, chapters 6 and 8, Paul explains faith without good works cannot save. Paul says that God's elect "walk not after the flesh, but after the Spirit." Romans 8:1. He states that those who do not walk in the Spirit but instead walk in the flesh "shall not inherit the kingdom of God." Galatians 5:15-25. John explains: "If we say that we have fellowship with him, and walk in darkness, we lie, and do not the truth: But if we walk in the light, as he is in the light, we have fellowship one with another, and the blood of Jesus Christ his Son cleanseth us from all sin." 1 John 1:6-7. James asks a rhetorical question: "What doth it profit, my brethren, though a man say he hath faith, and have not works? can faith save him?" James 2:14. James succinctly explains that "faith without works is dead." James 2:20. The pronouncement in James that true faith bears the fruit of good works is a theme found in the gospel. But some perniciously preach that God saves a person by faith that has no good works.

That is one of the "damnable heresies" about which Peter warned. See 2 Peter 2:1-22.

Rome's Responsibility for the Assassination of Abraham Lincoln, With an Appendix Containing Conversations Between Abraham Lincoln and Charles Chiniquy
Thomas M. Harris
ISBN-13: 978-0983262794

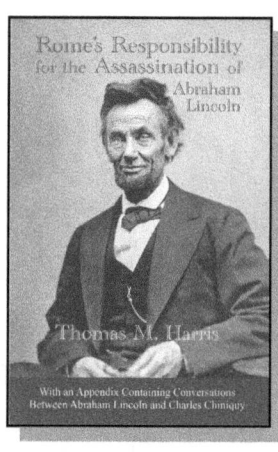

The author of this book, General Thomas Maley Harris, was a medical doctor, who recruited and served as commander of the Tenth West Virginia Volunteers during the Civil War. He rose in rank through meritorious service to become a brigadier general in the Union Army. General Harris established a reputation for faithfulness, industriousness, intelligence, and efficiency. He was noted for his leadership in preparing his troops and leading them in battle. He was brevetted a major general for "gallant conduct in the assault on Petersburg." After the Civil War, General Harris served one term as a representative in the West Virginia legislature, and was West Virginia's Adjutant General from 1869 to 1870. General Harris was a member of the Military Commission that tried and convicted the conspirators who assassinated President Abraham Lincoln. He had first hand knowledge of the sworn testimony of the witnesses in that trial. This book summarizes the salient evidence brought out during the military trial and adds information from other sources to present before the public the ineluctable conclusion that the assassination of Abraham Lincoln was the work of the Roman Catholic Church. The Roman Catholic Church has been largely successful in suppressing the circulation of this book. This book has never been given a place on bookstore shelves, as it exposed too much for the Roman Catholic hierarchy to tolerate. Any display of this book would bring an instant boycott of the bookstore. It is only now, in the age of the internet, where the marketplace of ideas has been opened wide, that this book can be found by those searching for the truth of who was behind the assassination of Abraham Lincoln.

The above books can be ordered from bookstores and from internet sites, including, but not limited to:

https://greatmountainpublishing.com
www.antichristconspiracy.com
www.911enemies.com
www.mysterybabylonthegreat.net
www.antigospel.com
https://play.google.com
www.barnesandnoble.com
www.amazon.com

Edward Hendrie
edwardhendrie@gmail.com

www.ingramcontent.com/pod-product-compliance
Lightning Source LLC
Chambersburg PA
CBHW071202240426
43668CB00032B/1806